Pathophysiology of Vascular Disease

Robert Fitridge • Guilherme Pena
Benjamin Thurston • Prue Cowled
Editors

Pathophysiology of Vascular Disease

A Textbook for Vascular Surgeons

Fourth Edition

Springer

Editors
Robert Fitridge
Vascular Surgery
Adelaide University
Adelaide, SA, Australia

Guilherme Pena
Vascular Surgery Unit
Flinders Medical Centre
Adelaide, SA, Australia

Benjamin Thurston
Vascular and Endovascular Service
Central Adelaide Local Health Network
Adelaide, SA, Australia

Prue Cowled
Discipline of Surgery
Adelaide University
Adelaide, SA, Australia

ISBN 978-3-032-31458-1 ISBN 978-3-032-31459-8 (eBook)
https://doi.org/10.1007/978-3-032-31459-8

This Springer imprint is published by the registered company Springer Nature Switzerland AG
The registered company address is: Gewerbestrasse 11, 6330 Cham, Switzerland

Foreword

It is a pleasure to introduce *Pathophysiology of Vascular Disease*, the companion textbook to Mechanisms of Vascular Disease. These books are enduring references for vascular specialists in Australia and New Zealand, and increasingly, for colleagues around the world. The remarkable uptake of earlier editions—reflected in more than 50,000 chapter downloads of the previous volume—speaks not only to the clinical relevance of the text, but also to its unique ability to bridge fundamental science with contemporary vascular practice.

This new book continues that tradition with substantial renewal. Two entirely new chapters expand the scope of the book into areas of growing clinical and academic importance: "Pathophysiology and Principles of Management of Vascular Malformations" by Iris Baumgartner, and "Multifaceted Applications of Artificial Intelligence in Vascular Surgery" by Fabien Lareyre and colleagues. Together, they reflect both the maturation of vascular anomalies as a subspeciality and the transformative impact that machine learning, computational modelling, and data-driven decision support are beginning to exert on vascular care.

All chapters of the collection have been comprehensively reviewed and updated. The implementation of basic science, including, vascular biology and biomaterial science underpins the fundamentals of pathophysiology of key vascular diseases, providing trainees and practising clinicians with a strong scientific foundation for modern vascular interventions. The addition of key learning points for each chapter further enhances the educational value of the text, ensuring it continues being a core resource for structured vascular training.

This volume exemplifies the collaborative spirit of our speciality: scientists, clinicians, and surgeon-researchers working together to improve understanding, refine treatment, and ultimately advance patient outcomes. I congratulate Robert Fitridge and the Editorial Team, and their contributors for producing a thoroughly modern, rigorously updated edition that will continue to enrich vascular education and practice for years to come.

Professor Emeritus, University of Poitiers
Medical School
Poitiers, France

Jean-Baptiste Ricco

Preface

Pathophysiology of Vascular Disease: A Textbook for Vascular Specialists (Fourth Edition) is a companion textbook to Mechanisms of Vascular Disease: A Textbook for Vascular Specialists. These books comprehensively cover a variety of common and unusual pathologies encountered in vascular surgical practice. They feature detailed information on the latest developments in the pathophysiology and management of conditions including atherosclerosis, aortic aneurysm disease and hereditary aortopathies, multi-organ failure, and vasculitides. Key topics in Pathophysiology of Vascular Disease include radiation biology and radiation safety and vascular malformations. A new chapter provides information on the emerging role of artificial intelligence in vascular practice.

Each chapter contains a set of learning objectives and key references, enabling the reader to quickly identify key points. These books are therefore an ideal resource for both the trainee and practicing clinical vascular surgeon seeking up-to-date information on vascular disease.

Adelaide, SA, Australia — Robert Fitridge
Adelaide, SA, Australia — Guilherme Pena
Adelaide, SA, Australia — Benjamin Thurston
Adelaide, SA, Australia — Prue Cowled

Contents

About the Editors

Robert Fitridge is Professor of Vascular Surgery, Discipline of Surgery, Adelaide University and Consultant Vascular Surgeon, Vascular and Endovascular Service, Central Adelaide Local Health Network, Adelaide, South Australia.

Guilherme Pena is a Consultant Vascular Surgeon, Vascular Unit, Flinders Medical Centre, Bedford Park, South Australia and Affiliate Senior Lecturer, Discipline of Surgery, Adelaide University, Adelaide, South Australia.

Benjamin Thurston is a Consultant Vascular Surgeon, Vascular and Endovascular Service, Central Adelaide Local Health Network, Adelaide, South Australia.

Prue Cowled is an Affiliate Senior Lecturer, Discipline of Surgery, Adelaide University, Adelaide, South Australia.

Abbreviations

α-SMA	Alpha-smooth muscle actin
^{18}F-FDG	^{18}F-fluorodeoxyglucose
^{18}F-NaF	^{18}F-sodium fluoride
3D-IF	3D-image fusion
5-HT2A	5-hydroxytryptamine receptor 2A
AAA	Abdominal aortic aneurysm
AAS	Acute aortic syndromes
AAV	Anti-neutrophil cytoplasmic antibody-associated vasculitis
ABC	Automatic brightness control
ABCA-1	ATP binding cassette subfamily A member 1
ABCG1	ATP binding cassette subfamily G member 1
ABCG5	ATP binding cassette subfamily G member 5
ABCG8	ATP binding cassette subfamily G member 8
ABI	Ankle-brachial index
AC	Abdominal compliance
ACAN	Aggrecan
ACAT-1	Acetyl-CoA acetyltransferase
ACE	Angiotensin converting enzyme
ACR	American College of Rheumatology
ACRL1	Autosomal recessive cutis laxa type 1
ACS	Acute coronary syndrome
ACS	Abdominal compartment syndrome
ACTA2	Alpha-smooth muscle actin
ACVRL1	Activin A receptor type II-like 1(receptor for BMP9)
AD	Aortic dissection
ADA2	Adenosine deaminase-2
ADAMTS13	A disintegrin and metalloprotease with a thrombospondin type 1 motif, member 13
ADAMTS3	A disintegrin and metalloprotease with thrombospondin motifs-3

ADAMTS7	A disintegrin and metalloprotease with thrombospondin type 1 motif 7
ADMA	Asymmetric dimethylarginine
ADP	Adenosine diphosphate
AGEs	Advanced glycation end-products
AHA	American heart association
AI	Artificial intelligence
AIP	Atherogenic index of plasma
AKI	Acute kidney injury
AKT	AKT serine/threonine kinase 1 (protein kinase B)
ALARA	As low as reasonably achievable
ALE	Arbitrary Lagrangian-Eulerian
ALI	Acute limb ischaemia
ALK5	Activine receptor-like kinase 5
ALP	Alkaline phosphatase
AMD	Age-related macular degeneration
AMI	Acute myocardial infarction
AMP	Adenosine monophosphate
ANCA	Anti-neutrophil cytoplasmic antibody
Ang	Angiopoietin
AngII	Angiotensin II
ANGPT2	Angiopoietin 2
ANRIL	Antisense non-coding RNA at the INK4 locus
Anti-GBM	Anti-glomerular basement membrane disease
AP	Antero-posterior
AP-1	Activating protein-1
APC	Activated protein C
APCs	Antigen-presenting cells
APLAS	Antiphospholipid antibody syndrome
APOA1	Apolipoprotein A-I
APOA5	Apolipoprotein A-5
ApoB	Apolipoprotein B
APOC2	Apolipoprotein C-2
APOC3	Apolipoprotein C-3
APOE	Apolipoprotein E
APP	Abdominal perfusion pressure
aPTT	Activated partial thromboplastin time
PTT	Partial thromboplastin time
ARDS	Acute respiratory distress syndrome
ARIH1	Ariadne RBR E3 ubiquitin protein ligase 1
ARVA	Augmented Radiology for Vascular Aneurysm
ASCs	Adipose-derived stem cells
ASCVD	Atherosclerotic cardiovascular disease
ASPH	Aspartate beta-hydroxylase
AST	Aspartate aminotransferase

ASXL1	ASXL transcriptional regulator 1
AT	Antithrombin
ATP	Adenosine triphosphate
ATS	Arterial tortuosity syndrome
AUC	Area under curve
AUROC	Area under the receiver operating characteristic curve
AV	Adenoviral
AVM	Arteriovenous malformations
AVPR1a	Arginine vasopressin receptor 1A
AZA	Azathioprine
B0	B subscript zero (main static magnetic field)
BAPN	3-Aminoproprionitrile
BAV	Bicuspid aortic valve
BC	Boundary conditions
BC	Bacterial cellulose
BCL-2	B cell lymphoma factor 2
BCRL	Breast cancer-related lymphoedema
BD	Behçet's disease
BEIR VII	Biological Effects of Ionising Radiation VII Committee
bFGF	Basic fibroblast growth factor
BGN	Biglycan
BMI	Body mass index
BMP2	Bone morphogenetic protein 2
BMP9/GDF2	Bone morphogenetic protein 9 (gdf2)
BMPR2	Bone morphogenic receptor type 2
BMS	Bare metal stent
BNP	Brain natriuretic peptide
BNP	B-type natriuretic peptide
BRBNS	Blue rubber bleb nevus syndrome
c-MET	Hepatocyte growth factor receptor
C/EBPβ	CCAAT enhancer binding protein beta
C4b	Complement component 4 fragment
CA	Coronary artery
CAA	Coronary artery aneurysms
CAC	Coronary artery calcium
CAD	Coronary artery disease
CAD	Computer-aided design
CADASIL	Cerebral autosomal-dominant arteriopathy with subcortical infarcts and leukoencephalopathy
CAK	Cumulative air kerma
CalDAG-GEFI	Guanine nucleotide exchange factor
CALR	Calreticulin gene
cAMP	Cyclic adenosine monophosphate
CASZ1	Castor zinc finger 1
CBAS	Carmeda bioactive surface

CBCT	Cone-beam CT
CCBE1	Collagen and calcium binding EGF domain-1
CCL2	C-C motif chemokine ligand 2
CCL5	C-C motif chemokine ligand 5
CCLA	Central conducting lymphatic anomalies
CCM	Cerebral cavernous malformations
CCM2	Cerebral cavernous malformation 2
CD31	Endothelial cell surface marker
CDKN2A	Cyclin-dependent kinase inhibitor 2A
CDKN2B	Cyclin-dependent kinase inhibitor 2B
CE	Cholesterol esterase
CE	European conformity marking
CE-MRA	Contrast-enhanced MRA
CEAP	**C**linical signs, a**e**tiology, **A**natomy and **P**athophysiology
CEC	Cholesterol efflux capacity
CETP	Cholesteryl ester transfer protein
CEUS	Contrast enhanced ultrasound
CFD	Computational fluid dynamics
cGMP	Cyclic guanine monophosphate
CHIP	Clonal haematopoiesis of indeterminate potential
CIMLD	Cocaine-induced midline destructive lesions
CIMT	Carotid intima-media thickness
CK	Creatine kinase
CK-MB	Creatine kinase myocardial band
CKD	Chronic kidney disease
Clec-2	C-type lectin domain family 1 member B
CLI	Critical limb ischaemia
CLOVES	Congenital lipomatous overgrowth, vascular malformations, epidermal nevi, and scoliosis
CLTI	Chronic limb-threatening ischaemia
CM	Capillary malformations
CM-AVM	CM-arterio-venous malformation
CNC	Cardiac neural crest
CNN	Convolutional neural network
CNO	Charcot neuroarthropathy
cNOS	Constitutive nitric oxide synthase
CNS	Central nervous system
COL3A1	Collagen type III alpha 1 chain
COMP	Cartilage oligomeric matrix protein
COUP-TFII	N2RF2 (nuclear receptor subfamily 2 group F member 2)
COX	Cyclooxygenase
COX-1	Cyclooxygenase 1
COX-2	Cyclooxygenase-2
CPI	Checkpoint inhibitors
CRC	Colorectal cancer

CRM	Crew resource management
CROW	Charcot restraint orthotic walker
CRP	C-reactive protein
CSF	Cerebral spinal fluid
CT	Computerised tomography
CT angiogram	Computerised tomography angiogram
CTA	Computed tomography angiography
CTGF	Connective tissue growth factor
CV	Cardiovascular
CV	Cryoglobulinaemic vasculitis
CVD	Chronic venous disease
CVI	Chronic venous insufficiency
CVM	Congenital vascular malformations
CVST	Cerebral venous sinus thrombosis
CX3CL1	Fractalkine
CX3CR1	C-X3-C motif chemokine receptor 1
CXC	C-X-C motif chemokine receptor
CXCL10	C-X-C motif chemokine ligand 10
CXCR2	C-X-C motif chemokine receptor 2
CXCR4	C-X-C motif chemokine receptor 4
CyA	Cyclosporine
CYC	Cyclophosphamide
CYP	Cytochrome
CYP27A1	Cytochrome P450 family 27 subfamily A member 1
CYP450	Cytochrome P450
Cys	Cysteine
DAG	Diacylglycerol
DAMP	Danger-associated molecular pattern
DAMPs	Damage-associated molecular patterns
DAP	Dose area product
DAPT	Dual anti-platelet therapy
DASS (LTBP3)	Latent transforming growth factor beta binding protein 3
DCBs	Drug-coated balloons
dECM	Decellularized extracellular matrix
DECT	Dual-energy computed tomography
DES	Drug-eluting stent
DHA	Docosahexanoic acid
DIC	Disseminated intravascular coagulation
DIEP/SIEP	Deep/superficial inferior epigastric perforator flap
DL	Decompression laparotomy
DL	Deep learning
DLL4	Delta-like ligand 4
DLT	Decongestive lymphatic therapy
DM	Diabetes mellitus
DMARDs	Disease modifying antirheumatic drugs

DNMT3A	DNA methyltransferase 3 alpha
DOACs	Direct oral anticoagulants
DOF	Degrees of freedom
DPN	Diabetes-related peripheral neuropathy
DRFCs	Diabetes-related foot complications
DRFIs	Diabetes-related foot infection
DRFO	Diabetes-related foot osteomyelitis
DRFU	Diabetes-related foot ulcer
DRLs	Diagnostic reference levels
DSA	Digital subtraction angiography
dSINE	Distal stent graft-induced new entry
DTS	Dense tubular system
DUS	Duplex ultrasound
DVT	Deep vein thrombosis
EC	Endothelial cells
ECM	Extracellular matrix
ECMO	Extracorporeal membrane oxygenation
ED	Effective dose
EDH	Endothelium-derived hyperpolarisation
EDS	Ehlers-Danlos syndrome
EDTA	Ethylenediamine tetra acetic acid
EDV	End-diastolic velocities
EDV	End diastolic volume
EET	Epoxyeicosatrienoic acid
EFEMP1	Endothelial growth factor-like fibulin extracellular matrix protein 1
EFEMP2	Codes for fibulin-4
eGC	Endothelial glycocalyx
EGDT	Early goal directed therapy
EGFR	Epidermal growth factor receptor
EGPA	Eosinophilic granulomatosis with polyangiitis
EID-CT	Energy-integrating detector computed tomography
EIDs	Energy-integrating detectors
ELAM-1	Endothelial-leukocyte adhesion molecule
ELG	Endoluminal graft
ELISA	Enzyme-linked immunosorbent assay
ELN	Elastin
EMELIN	Elastin microfibril interface-located proteins
EMMPRIN	Extracellular MMP inducer
EMR	Electromagnetic radiation
ENA-78	CXCL5 (C-X-C motif chemokine ligand 5)
EndMT	Endothelial-to-mesenchymal transition
ENG	Endoglin
eNOS	Endothelial nitric oxide synthase
ENPP1	Ectonucleotide pyrophosphatase phosphodiesterase 1

EPA	Eicosapentaenoic acid
EPC	Endothelial progenitor cell
EPCR	Endothelial protein C receptor
EPHB4	Ephrin type-B receptor 4
EPS	Extracellular polymeric substances
ePTFE	Expanded polytetrafluoroethylene
ER	Endoplasmic reticulum
ERK	Extracellular signal-regulated kinases
ESD	Estimated skin dose
ESR	Erythrocyte sedimentation rate
ESVS	European Society for Vascular Surgery
ET	Essential thrombocytosis
ET-1	Endothelin-1
EULAR	European Alliance of Associations for Rheumatology
eV	Electron volts
EVAR	Endovascular abdominal aortic aneurysm repair
EVs	Extracellular vesicles
FAI	Fat attenuation index
FAT4	Codes for a member of the procadherin family
FBLN5	Fibulin 5
FBN1	Fibrillin 1
FBP	Filtered back projection
FCGR	Fc gamma receptor
FCS	Familial chylomicronaemia syndrome
FDB	Familial defective apolipoprotein B-100
FDPs	Fibrin degradation products
FEA	Finite element analysis
FEVAR	Fenestrated endovascular aortic repair
FFT	Fast Fourier transform
FGF	Fibroblast growth factor
FGF-2	Fibroblast growth factor-2
FH	Familial hypercholesterolaemia
FiO2	Fraction of inspired oxygen
FLNA	Codes for Filamin A
FLT4	Fms-like tyrosine kinase 4 (VEGFR3)
FMD	Flow-mediated dilation
FMD	Fibromuscular dysplasia
FOV	Field of view
FOXC2	Forkhead box C2
FOXE3	Codes for Forkhead box E3
FPS	Frames per second
FSI	Fluid-solid interaction
FSPs	Fluorosurfactant polymers
FT	Fluoroscopy time
FTAAD	Familial thoracic aortic aneurysm and dissection

FV	Factor five
FVIII	Factor eight
FVL	Factor five Leiden
FXa	Factor ten a
Gaq	Subunit of G protein complex
GATA2	Codes for a transcription factor
GBM	Glomerular basement membrane
GCA	Giant cell arteritis
GDM	Gestational diabetes mellitus
GDPR	General Data Protection Regulation
GI	Gastrointestinal
GJC2	Gap junction protein, gamma 2, codes for connexin 47
GLA	Generalized lymphatic anomaly
GLP-1R	Glucagon-like peptide-1 receptor
GLP-1RA	Glucagon-like peptide-1receptor agonists
GM-CSF	Granulocyte-macrophage colony-stimulating factor
GNA11	Codes for alpha subunit of G11 (G protein)
GNAQ	G protein subunit alpha q
GP	Glycoprotein
GPA	Granulomatosis with polyangiitis
GPCRs	G-protein coupled receptors
GPELF	Global Programme to Eliminate Lymphatic Filariasis
GPI	Glycosylphosphatidylinositol
GPIHBP1	Glycosylphosphatidylinositol anchored high density lipoprotein binding protein 1
Gq/G11	GTP-binding alpha protein
GSD	Gorham-stout disease
GSV	Great saphenous vein
GWAS	Genome-wide association studies
Gy	Gray
h-FABP	Heart-type fatty acid-binding protein
H_2O_2	Hydrogen peroxide
HARM	Hyperintense acute reperfusion injury marker
HATs	Histone acetyltransferases
HBOT	Hyperbaric oxygen therapy
HBV	Hepatitis B virus
HCN4	Codes for hyperpolarisation activated cyclic nucleotide gated potassium channel 4
HCV	Hepatitis C virus
HDACs	Histone deacetylases
HDL	High-density lipoprotein
HDL-C	High-density lipoprotein cholesterol
HeFH	Heterozygous familial hypercholesterolemia
HES	Hydroxyethyl starch
HFE	Homeostatic iron regulator

Hg	Mercury
HGF	Hepatocyte growth factor
HHT-1 and HHT-2	Hereditary haemorrhagic telangiectasia
HIF	Hypoxia-inducible factors
HIF-1	Hypoxia-inducible factor-1
HIF-1α	Hypoxia-inducible factor-1 alpha
HIFs	Hypoxia-induced factors
HIT	Heparin-induced thrombocytopenia
HIV	Human immunodeficiency virus
HLA	Human leucocyte antigen
HMGB1	High mobility group box 1
HMOX1	Haem oxygenase 1
HMW	High molecular weight
HMWK	High molecular weight kininogen
HOCM	High-osmolar contrast media
HoFH	Homozygous familial hypercholesterolemia
HOTAIR	HOX transcript antisense RNA
HPLC	High-performance liquid chromatography
hsCRP	High-sensitivity C-reactive protein
HSP	Heat shock protein
HTLV1	Human T cell lymphotropic virus type 1
HU	Hounsfield unit
HUV	Hypocomplementaemic urticarial vasculitis
I/R	Ischaemia-reperfusion injury
IA	Intussusceptive angiogenesis
IAH	Intra-abdominal hypertension
IAP	Intra-abdominal pressure
IAV	Intra-abdominal volume
iBTA	In-body tissue architecture
IC	Intermittent claudication
ICA	Internal carotid artery
ICAM	Intercellular cell adhesion molecule
ICAM-1	Intercellular adhesion molecule-1
ICAM-2	Intercellular adhesion molecule-2
ICG	Indocyanine green
ICRP	International Commission on Radiation Protection
ICU	Intensive care unit
ICV	Immune complex vasculitides
IDH1	Isocitrate dehydrogenase 1
IDH2	Isocitrate dehydrogenase 2
IDI	Integrated discrimination improvement
IDL	Intermediate-density lipoprotein
IDSA	Infectious Diseases Society of America
IFN	Interferon
IFN-g	Interferon gamma

IgAV	IgA vasculitis
IgG4-RD	Immunoglobulin G4-related disease
IH	Intimal hyperplasia
II	Image intensifiers
IL	Interleukin
IL-1	Interleukin-1
IL-11	Interleukin-11
IL-17	Interleukin-17
IL-18	Interleukin-18
IL-1a	Interleukin-1alpha
IL-1β	Interleukin 1 beta
IL-4	Interleukin-4
IL-6	Interleukin 6
IL-8	Interleukin-8
IL-10	Interleukin-10
ILT	Intraluminal thrombus
iMAR	Iterative metal artefact reduction
IMH	Intramural hematoma
IMP	Inosine monophosphate
IMT	Intima–media thickness
iNOS	Inducible nitric oxide synthase
IOCM	Iso-osmolar contrast media
IP	Prostaglandin I_2 receptor
IP(3)	1, 4, 5-inositol triphosphate
IP3R	Inositol (1,4,5) trisphosphate receptor
IPH	Intraplaque haemorrhage
IPL	Intense pulsed light laser
IPO8	Importin 8
iPSC	Induced pluripotent stem cell
IR	Iterative reconstruction
irAEs	Immune-related adverse events
IRI	Ischaemia-reperfusion injury
IRP	Interventional reference point
IS	International System of Units
ISR	In situ reconstruction
ISSVA	International Society for the Study of Vascular Anomalies
ITLN1	Intelectin-1
ITPKC	Inositol 1,4,5-triphosphate 3-kinase-C
IVC	Inferior vena cava
IVIg	Intravenous immunoglobulin
IVUS	Intravascular ultrasound
IWGDF	International Working Group on the Diabetic Foot
J	Joule
JAG1	Jagged1 gene
JAK2	Janus kinase 2

JAM-C	Junctional adhesion molecule C
JMJD3	Lysine demethylase 6B
JPS	Juvenile polyposis syndrome
K_{Ca}	Calcium-activated potassium channels
KD	Kawasaki disease
Kerma	*K*inetic *E*nergy *R*eleased in *Matter*
KEV	Kilo-electron-volt
KGD	Lysine-glycine-aspartic acid
KLF	Krüppel-like factor
KLF2	Kruppel-like factor 2
KLF4	Kriippel-like factor-4
KRIT1	Krev/ras interaction trafficking protein 1
KTS	Klippel-trenaunay syndrome
kVp	Kilovoltage peak
L-Arg	L-arginine
LAL	Lysosomal acid lipase
LAO	Left anterior oblique
LCAT	Lecithin–cholesterol acyltransferase
LDH	Lactate dehydrogenase
LDL	Low-density lipoprotein
LDL-C	Low-density lipoprotein cholesterol
LDLR	Low-density lipoprotein receptor
LDS	Loeys-Dietz syndrome
LECs	Lymphatic endothelial cells
LIC	Localised intravascular coagulopathy
LLM	Large language models
LM	Lymphatic malformations
LMF1	Lipase maturation factor 1
LMWH	Low molecular weight heparin
lncRNAs	Long non-coding RNAs
LOCM	Low-osmolar contrast media
LOPS	Loss of protective sensation
LOX	Codes for protein lysine 6 oxidase
LOX-1	Lipoxygenase 1
Lp(a)	Lipoprotein(a)
LPA	Codes for apolipoprotein(a)
LPL	Codes for lipoprotein lipase
LPS	Lipopolysaccharide
LSA	Left subclavian artery
LTA	Light transmittance aggregometry
LTB4	Leukotriene B4
LTBP1,3,4	TGF-β binding protein-isoforms
LUNAR1	Leukaemia-associated non-coding IGF1Rr activator RNA 1
LV	Left ventricular
LVA	Lymphatico-venous anastomosis surgery

LVV	Large vessel vasculitis
LXRa, LXRβ	Liver X receptors
LYVE1	Lymphatic vessel endothelial hyaluronan receptor 1
M-CSF	Macrophage colony-stimulating factor
m^6A	N6-methyladenosine
mA	Milliamperage
MAC	Medial arterial calcification
MAC-1	Macrophage-1 antigen
Mac-2	Galectin 3 (macrophage galactose-specific lectin)
MACE	Major adverse cardiovascular events
MAGP2	Microfibril-associated glycoprotein 2 (same as MFAP5)
MALAT1	Metastasis-associated lung adenocarcinoma transcript 1
MALE	Major adverse limb events
MAP	Mean arterial pressure
MAPK	Mitogen-activated protein kinases (also called ERK)
MAT2A	Codes for methionine adenosyltransferase 2A
MCAP	Megalencephaly-capillary malformation Syndrome
MCP	Monocyte chemoattractant protein
MCP-1	Monocyte chemoattractant protein-1
MCSF	Macrophage colony stimulating factor
MDF	Myocardial depressant factors
MEFV	Mediterranean fever gene
Meg3	Maternally expressed gene 3
MEK1/2	Mitogen-activated protein kinase kinase 1 and 2
MESA	Multi-Ethnic Study of Atherosclerosis
METTL3	Methyltransferase 3
MFAP5	Codes for microfibrillar-associated protein 5
MFS	Marfan syndrome
MGP	Matrix Gla protein
MH1/2	Mad-homology 1 and 2
MHC	Myosin heavy chains
MI	Myocardial infarction
mi-RNAs	Micro-RNAs
MIB1	Codes for MIB E3 ubiquitin protein ligase 1
MIF	Macrophage inhibitory factor
MIP-1α	Macrophage inflammatory protein 1
MIS-C	Multisystem inflammatory syndrome in children
ML	Machine learning
MLC20	20 kDa myosin light chain protein
MLCK	Myosin light chain kinase
MLCp	Myosin light chain phosphorylation
MLCP	Myosin light chain phosphatase
MLD	Manual lymphatic drainage
MLS	Meester-Loeys syndrome
MMF	Mycophenolate mofetil

MMP	Matrix metalloproteinase
MMP2	Matrix metalloproteinase 2
MMP9	Matrix metalloproteinase 9
mmPb LE	Mm of lead equivalence
MMS	Mönckeberg medial sclerosis
MOD	Multi-organ dysfunction
Mpa	Megapascals
MPA	Microscopic polyangiitis
MPL	Thrombopoietin receptor or myeloproliferative leukaemia protein
MPO	Myeloperoxidase
MPXY motif	Methionine-proline-unknown-tyrosine
MR	Magnetic resonance
MRA	Magnetic resonance angiography
MRI	Magnetic resonance imaging
MRI/MRA	Magnetic resonance imaging/angiography
MRL	Magnetic resonance lymphangiography
MrML format	Medical reality modelling language
mRNA	Messenger RNA
MRSA	Methicillin-resistant *Staphylococcus aureus*
MS1	Monocyte state 1
MTHFR	Methylenetetrahydrofolate reductase
mTOR	Mechanistic/mammalian target of rapamycin
MTPJs	Metatarsophalangeal joints
MTX	Methotrexate
MYH11	Myosin heavy chain
MYLK	Codes for smooth muscle myosin light chain kinase
NADPH	Nicotinamide adenine dinucleotide phosphate
NCRP	National Council on Radiation Protection and Measurements
NETs	Neutrophil extracellular traps
NFκB	Nuclear factor kappa B
NGS	Next generation sequencing
NIRL	Near infra-red lymphangiography
NIRS	Near infrared-spectroscopy
NK	Natural killer cells
NLP	Natural language processing
NLRP3	Nucleotide-binding oligomerisation domain-like receptor family pyrin domain containing 3
NMB	Neuromuscular blockade
NO	Nitric oxide
NOS	Nitric oxide synthase
NOTCH	Neurogenic locus notch homolog protein
NOX4	NADPH oxidase 4
NPR3	Codes for natriuretic peptide receptor 3
NPV	Negative prediction value

NPWT	Negative pressure wound therapy
NRI	Net reclassification improvement (OR norepinephrine reuptake inhibitor)
NSAIDs	Non-steroidal anti-inflammatory drugs
NSCLC	Non-small cell lung cancer
O_2^-	Superoxide
OA	Open abdomen
OCI	Operator-controlled imaging
OCP	Oral contraceptive pill
OCT	Optical coherence tomography
OH•	Hydroxyl radical
OM	Osteomyelitis
OPN	Osteopontin
OSLD	Optically stimulated luminescence dosimeters
OSR	Open surgical repair
OxLDL	Oxidised low density lipoprotein
P2Y1	Purinergic receptor P2Y1
P2Y12	Purinergic receptor P2Y12, platelet receptor for adenosine 5'diphosphate (ADP)
$PaCO_2$	Partial pressure of carbon dioxide
PAD	Peripheral artery disease
PAD4	Peptidylarginine deaminase 4
PAF	Platelet activating factor
PAI-1	Plasminogen activator inhibitor-1
PAIs	Plasminogen activator inhibitors
PAMPS	Pathogen-associated molecular patterns
PAN	Polyarteritis nodosa
PAR-1	Protease-activated receptor-1
PAR-4	Protease-activated receptor-4
PARP	Poly (ADP-ribose) polymerase
PARs	Protease-activated receptors
PAU	Penetrating aortic ulcer
PBT	Probe-to-bone test
PC	Protein C
PCCT	Photon-counting computed tomography
PCI	Percutaneous coronary intervention
PCL	Polycaprolactone
PCSK-9	Proprotein convertase subtilisin/kexin type 9
PCT	Procalcitonin
PCU	Polycarbonate polyurethane
PD-1	Programmed cell death protein-1
PD-L1	Programmed cell death ligand-1
PDCD10	Programmed cell death 10 gene
PDE-5	Phosphodiesterase type 5
PDGF	Platelet-derived growth factor

PDGF-β	Platelet-derived growth factor-beta
PDGFR	Platelet-derived growth factor receptor
PDI	Protein disulfide isomerase
PDL	Pulsed dye laser
PECAM-1	Platelet-endothelial cell adhesion molecule-1
PEEP	Positive end-expiratory pressure
PET	Positron emission tomography
PeVD	Pelvic venous disorders
PF4	Platelet factor 4 (CXCL4)
PGA	Polyglycolic acid
PGD_2	Prostaglandin D2
PGE_2	Prostaglandin E2
$PGF_{2\alpha}$	Prostaglandin F2 alpha
PGH_2	Prostaglandin H_2
PGI_2	Prostacyclin (prostaglandin I2)
PGM	Prothrombin gene mutation
PGS	Poly(glycerol sebacate)
PHACE syndrome	Posterior fossa abnormalities, Hemangioma, Arterial anomalies, Cardiac anomalies, and Eye anomalies
PHD	Prolyl hydroxylase domain
$PI(4,5)P_2$	Phosphatidylinositol 4,5-bisphosphate
PI3K	Phosphatidylinositol 3-kinase
PIK3CA	Phosphatidylinositol-4,5-bisphosphate 3-kinase catalytic subunit alpha
PIK3CA/AKT1	Phosphatidylinositol-4,5-bisphosphate 3-kinase catalytic subunit alpha/AKT serine/threonine kinase 1
PKA	Protein kinase A
PKC	Protein kinase C
PKCζ	Protein kinase C zeta
PKG1α	Protein kinase G1α
PLA	Polylactic acid
PLA_2	Phospholipase A_2
PLC	Phospholipase C
PLC	Programmable logic controller
PLCL	Poly(L-lactide-co-caprolactone)
PLGA	Poly(lactic-co-glycolic acid)
PLGF	Placental growth factor
PLOD1	Codes for procollagen-lysine,2-oxoglutarate 5-dioxygenase 1
PM2.5	Fine particulate matter (<2.5 micrometres in size)
PMEPA1	Prostate transmembrane protein, androgen induced 1
PMR	Polymyalgia rheumatica
PNH	Paroxysmal nocturnal haemoglobinuria
POCA	Poly(diol-co-citrate-co-ascorbate)

POCUS	Point-of-care ultrasound
POSS	Polyhedral oligomeric silsesquioxane
PPAR	Peroxisome proliferator-activated receptors
PPIs	Proton pump inhibitors
PPV	Positive prediction value
PR3	Proteinase 3
PRF	Pulse repetition frequency
PRKG1	Codes for type I cGMP-dependent protein kinase
PROS	Pik3ca-related overgrowth spectrum
PROX1	Prospero homeobox 1
PRP	Primary Raynaud's phenomenon
PRRs	Pattern recognition receptors
PRS	Polygenic risk scores
PRTN3	Proteinase 3 gene
PRV	Polycythaemia rubra vera
PS	Protein S
PS	Phosphatidylserine
PSC	Posterior subcapsular cataracts
PSCK9	Proprotein convertase subtilisin/kexin type 9
PSD	Peak skin dose
PSGL-1	P-selectin glycoprotein ligand-1
PSV	Peak systolic velocities
PSVR	Systolic velocity ratio
PT	Prothrombin time
PTA	Percutaneous transluminal angioplasty
PTEN	Phosphatase and tensin homolog
PTFE	Polytetrafluoroethylene
PTPN11	Protein tyrosine phosphatase non-receptor type 11
PTS	Post-thrombotic syndrome
PU	Polyurethane
PVA	Polyvinyl alcohol
PVAT	Perivascular adipose tissue
PVNH	Periventricular nodular heterotopia
PWS	Port-wine stain
PWS	Parkes weber syndrome
QISS	Quiescent-interval -single-shot
qPCR	Quantitative PCR
qRT-PCR	Quantitative reverse transcriptase PCR
r-tPA	Recombinant protein plasminogen activator
r-VCSS	Revised venous clinical severity score
RA	Rheumatoid arthritis
RAAA	Ruptured abdominal aortic aneurysm
Rad	Radiation absorbed dose
RAK	Reference air kerma

RANTES/CCL5	C-C motif chemokine ligand 5 (regulated upon activation, normal T cell expressed and secreted)
RAO	Right anterior oblique
Rap1b	Member of RAS oncogene family
RASA1	RAS p21 protein activator 1
RCC	Renal cell carcinoma
RCT	Randomised controlled trial
Re	Reynolds number
rem	Roentgen Equivalent in Man
RF	Radiofrequency
RGD	Arginine-glycine-aspartic acid
RhoA	Ras homolog family member A
RIAM	Rap1-GTP interacting adapter molecule
RIP-1	Receptor-interacting serine/threonine kinase 1
RLCs	Regulatory light chains
ROBO4	Codes for roundabout guidance receptor 4
ROC	Receiver operating characteristic curve
ROI	Region of interest
ROS	Reactive oxygen species
RP	Raynaud's phenomenon
RPAK	Reference point air kerma
RRT	Renal replacement therapy
RTKs	Receptor tyrosine kinases
RTX	Rituximab
RUNX2	Codes for runt-related transcription factor 2
RV	Right ventricular
SAM	S-adenosylmethionine
SARA	SMAD anchor for receptor activation protein
SASP	Senescence-associated secretory phenotype
SCAD	Spontaneous coronary artery dissection
scRNA-seq	Single-cell RNA sequencing
SCVs	Small colony variants
SDF	Stromal-derived growth factor
SDF-1	Stromal cell-derived factor-1
SDF-1α	Stromal cell-derived factor-1alpha
SECISBP2	Codes for selenocysteine Insertion Sequence Binding Protein 2
SENCR	Smooth muscle and endothelial cell-enriched long-noncoding RNA
SERPINA1	Alpha-1-antitrypsin gene
SF	Silk fibroin
SFA	Superficial femoral artery
sGC	Soluble guanylate cyclase
SGLT-2i	Sodium glucose cotransporter-2 inhibitor
SGLT2	Sodium glucose cotransporter-2

SGS	Shprintzen-Goldberg syndrome
Siah1	Siah E3 ubiquitin protein ligase 1
sICAM-1	Soluble intercellular adhesion molecule-1
SINE	Stent graft induced new entry tear
siRNAs	Small interfering rRNAs
SIRS	Systemic inflammatory response syndrome
SLC2A10	Codes for facilitative glucose transporter GLUT10
SLC40A1	Solute carrier family 40 member 1
SLE	Systemic lupus erythematosus
sLOX-1	Soluble lectin-like oxidised LDL receptor-1
SM	Smooth muscle
SM22a	Transgelin (TAGLN) (also known as smooth muscle protein 22-alpha)
SMA	Smooth muscle actin
SMA	Superior mesenteric artery
SMC	Smooth muscle cell
SMPCs	Smooth muscle progenitor cells
SMuRFs	Standard modifiable risk factors
SNHG12	Small nucleolar RNA host gene
SNP	Single nucleotide polymorphisms
SOFA	Sequential (Sepsis-related) Organ Failure Assessment
SORT1	Sortilin 1
SOS1	Guanine nucleotide exchange factor for RAS proteins,
SOV	Single-organ vasculitis
SOX18	SRY-box transcription factor 18
SP	Substance P
sP-selectin	Soluble P-selectin
SPP	Skin perfusion pressure
SPP1	Secreted phosphoprotein 1
SR-A1	Scavenger receptor-A1
SRB1	Scavenger receptor class B member 1
Src	SRC proto-oncogene, non-receptor tyrosine kinase
SRP	Secondary Raynaud's phenomenon
SSc	Systemic sclerosis
SSC	Surviving sepsis campaign
sST2	Soluble suppression of tumorigenesis-2
SSV	Small saphenous vein
STAT1	Signal transducer and activator of transcription 1
STAT3	Signal transducer and activator of transcription 3
STAT4	Signal transducer and activator of transcription 4
STEMI	ST-segment elevation myocardial infarction
STL format	Stereolithography
STS	Sodium tetradecyl sulphate
Sv	Sievert
sVCAM-1	Soluble vascular cell adhesion molecule-1

SvO2	Mixed venous oxygen saturation
SVP	Symptoms, varices and pathophysiology
SVS	Society for Vascular Surgery
SVV	Small vessel vasculitides
SWS	Sturge-weber syndrome
Syk	Spleen associated tyrosine kinase
TAA	Thoracic aortic aneurysm
TAAA	Thoracoabdominal aortic aneurysm
TAAD	Thoracic aortic aneurysm and dissection
TAB	Temporal artery biopsies
TAC	Temporary abdominal closure
TAFI	Thrombin-activatable fibrinolysis inhibitor
TAK	Takayasu arteritis
TAO	Thromboangiitis obliterans
TBAD	Type B aortic dissection
TBI	Toe-brachial pressure index
TBX20	T-box transcription factor 20
TCC	Total contact cast
TCFA	Thin-cap fibroatheroma
TcPO2	Transcutaneous oxygen tension
TE	Echo time
TEBVs	Tissue-engineered blood vessels
TEE	Transesophageal echocardiograpy
TEK	TEK receptor tyrosine kinase
TET2	Tet methylcytosine dioxygenase 2
TEVAR	Thoracic endovascular aneurysm repair
TEVG	Tissue-engineered vascular grafts
TF	Tissue factor
Tfh	T follicular helper cells
TFPI	Tissue factor pathway inhibitor
TGF	Transforming growth factor
TGF-α	Transforming growth factor alpha
TGF-β	Transforming growth factor-beta
TGF-β/BMP	Transforming growth factor-beta /bone morphogenic protein
TGF-β-R1/TGFb-R2	Type I or II TGF-β receptor unit
TGF-β1	Transforming growth factor beta 1
TGF-β2	Transforming growth factor beta 2
TGF-β3	Transforming growth factor beta 3
TGF-βR1/2	Transforming growth factor beta receptors 1 or 2
THSD4	Thrombospondin type 1 domain containing 4
TI	Inversion time
TIAs	Transient ischaemic attacks
TIE	Tyrosine kinase with immunoglobulin-like and epidermal growth factor-like domain
TIE-2	Tyrosine-protein kinase receptor 2

TIMP	Tissue inhibitors of matrix metalloproteinase
TIMP-3	Tissue inhibitor of matrix metalloproteinases 3
TKIs	Tyrosine kinase inhibitors
TLD	Thermoluminescent
TLR	Toll-like receptors
TLR4	Toll-like receptor 4 gene
TMA	Transmetatarsal amputation
TMAO	Trimethylamine-N-oxide
TNF	Tumour necrosis factor
TNF-α	Tumour necrosis factor alpha
TNFAIP3	Tumour necrosis factor alpha induced protein 3
TNFi	TNF inhibitors
TnI	Troponin I
TnT	Troponin T
TOF	Time-of-flight
TOT	Topical oxygen therapy
TP	Thromboxane
TP	Thromboxane receptor
TP	Toe pressure
tPA	Tissue plasminogen activator
TPa	Thromboxane A(2) receptor alpha
tPA	Tissue-type plasminogen activator
TPβ	Thromboxane A(2) receptor beta
TR	Repetition time
Tregs	Regulatory T cells
TREM-1	Triggering receptor expressed on myeloid cells 1
TREM2	Triggering receptor expressed on myeloid cells 2
TRLs	Triglyceride-rich lipoproteins
TXA_2	Thromboxane A_2
UBA1 gene	Ubiquitin-activating enzyme E1
UBR4	Ubiquitin protein ligase E3 component n-recognin 4,
uPA	Urokinase-type plasminogen activator
USF1	Upstream transcription factor 1
uTBAD	Uncomplicated type B aortic dissection
VACM	Vacuum-assisted wound closure and mesh-mediated fascial traction
vasDCs	Vascular dendritic cells
VC	Vascular calcification
VCAM	Vascular cell adhesion molecule
VCAM-1	Vascular cell adhesion molecule 1
VCAN	Versican
VE	Vascular endothelial
VE-cadherin	Vascular endothelial cadherin
vEDS	Vascular Ehlers-Danlos syndrome
VEGF	Vascular endothelial cell growth factor

VEGFC	Vascular endothelial growth factor C
VEGFD	Vascular endothelial growth factor D
VEGFR	Vascular endothelial growth factor receptor
VEGFR2	Vascular endothelial growth factor receptor 2
VEGFR3	Vascular endothelial growth factor receptor 3 (fms-related receptor tyrosine kinase 4)
VEXAS	Vacuoles, E1 enzyme, X-linked, autoinflammatory, somatic mutation
VITT	Vaccine-induced immune thrombotic thrombocytopenia
VLDL	Very-low-density lipoprotein
VLUs	Venous leg ulcers
VM	Venous malformations
VMCM	Cutaneomucosal venous malformation
VPs	Vulnerable atherosclerotic plaques
VQI	Vascular quality initiative
VRT	Venous refilling time
VSMC	Vascular smooth muscle cell
VTE	Venous thromboembolism
VTE	Vascular tissue engineering
vWF	Von Willebrand Factor
W-P	Weibel-Palade bodies
WBC	White blood cell
WCC	White cell count
WHO	World health organisation
WIfI	Wound, Ischaemia and foot Infection
WSS	Wall shear stress
W	Womersley number

Chapter 1
Pathophysiology and Principles of Management of Vasculitis and Fibromuscular Dysplasia

Maureen Rischmueller and Robert Fitridge

SN Flashcards
Test your learning and check your understanding of this book's contents: use the "Springer Nature Flashcards" app to access questions. To use the app, please follow the instructions below:

1. Go to https://flashcards.springernature.com/login
2. Create a user account by entering your e-mail address and assigning a password.
3. Use the following link to access your SN Flashcards set: ▶ https://sn.pub/wppvze

If the link is missing or does not work, please send an e-mail with the subject "SN Flashcards" and the book title to customerservice@springernature.com

M. Rischmueller (✉)
Rheumatology Department, The Queen Elizabeth Hospital, Woodville South, SA, Australia

Faculty of Health and Medical Sciences, Adelaide University, Adelaide, SA, Australia
e-mail: Maureen.Rischmueller@sa.gov.au

R. Fitridge
Faculty of Health and Medical Sciences, Adelaide University, Adelaide, SA, Australia

Vascular and Endovascular Service, Central Adelaide Local Health Network, Adelaide, SA, Australia
e-mail: Robert.Fitridge@adelaide.edu.au

R. Fitridge et al. (eds.), *Pathophysiology of Vascular Disease*,
https://doi.org/10.1007/978-3-032-31459-8_1

Key Learning Points

- Vasculitis represents a diverse group of inflammatory conditions affecting blood vessels, ranging from localised skin reactions to life-threatening systemic diseases. Early recognition and treatment are crucial to reduce morbidity and mortality. Severity and prognosis depend on the size and distribution of affected vessels.
- Giant cell arteritis (GCA) is a T-cell driven, granulomatous vasculitis primarily affecting large vessels leading to intimal hyperplasia and end-organ ischaemia. It has a biphasic inflammatory process, with Th1/Th17 pathway driving acute inflammation (responsive to corticosteroids) and IL-12/IFNγ-mediated mechanisms promoting chronic vascular inflammation (corticosteroid-resistant). GCA is a medical emergency, requiring prompt diagnosis (which requires imaging or temporal artery biopsy) and treatment to prevent blindness and stroke. Long-term surveillance for aortopathy is important due to the risk of aneurysm formation and dissection.
- Takayasu arteritis (TAK) is a granulomatous vasculitis affecting the aorta and its branches, predominantly in young women. It presents with limb ischaemia, hypertension, and/or renal impairment. Imaging is crucial for diagnosis and monitoring, as CRP and ESR may not be elevated.
- Behçet's disease is a systemic inflammatory disorder with multiorgan involvement including a significant vascular component. Thrombosis (venous and arterial) occurs in unusual locations. Immunosuppressants are the mainstay of treatment for vascular manifestations.
- IgG4-related disease is a systemic fibroinflammatory condition that can mimic vasculitis, particularly in the aorta and its major branches, often presenting as periaortitis or retroperitoneal fibrosis. It may also involve the head and neck, pancreatico-biliary system, or present as Mikulicz syndrome (salivary and lacrimal gland enlargement). While serum IgG4 can be elevated, histopathology is often required for definitive diagnosis. Early recognition and treatment with corticosteroids and/or rituximab are essential to prevent irreversible organ damage and avoid unnecessary surgical intervention.
- Raynaud's phenomenon refers to episodic digital vasospasm triggered by cold or emotion, leading to classic triphasic colour change (white, blue, red). Distinguishing primary Raynaud's (benign, often in younger patients) from secondary Raynaud's, which is associated with connective tissue disorder (especially systemic sclerosis) and has higher risk of complications like digital ulcers, is important. In secondary Raynaud's, impaired endothelium-dependent vasodilation and increased endothelin-1 activity contribute to more severe ischaemia.
- Thromboangiitis obliterans (TAO) (also known as Buerger's disease) is a segmental, occlusive inflammatory disease of small- and medium-sized arteries and veins in the limbs. Strongly associated with tobacco use, it typically affects young male smokers. TAO is histologically distinct from both atherosclerosis and systemic vasculitis, with inflammation primarily affecting the intima and thrombus. The architecture of the vascular walls remains preserved. Angiography often reveals "corkscrew collaterals" (Martorell's sign).

- Cannabis use can induce vessel occlusion and vasospasm, leading to a clinical picture that often mimics TAO, with distal limb ischaemia, digital necrosis, and high risk of amputation. Cannabis cessation is crucial, but often difficult to achieve.
- Fibromuscular dysplasia (FMD) is characterised by abnormal cellular proliferation (fibroblast, smooth muscle cell) in the arterial walls. This leads to a range of vascular abnormalities, including stenosis, aneurysm formation, and dissections. FMD most frequently affects the renal and cerebrovascular arteries. Angiography often reveals a characteristic "string of beads" appearances due to alternating areas of stenosis and dilatation. FMD lesions should be classified according to appearances on imaging as focal or multifocal FMD. FMD primarily affects women and can involve various arteries, including renal, carotid, and coronary arteries. Recent genetic studies have identified the UBR4 gene as a key player in FMD pathogenesis.

1.1 Introduction

Vasculitis covers a broad array of clinicopathological diseases, from transient localised cutaneous reactions to clinical manifestations of systemic diseases, to fulminant life-threatening diseases dominated by widespread inflammation, occlusion, and rupture of blood vessels. There is great diversity in pathophysiology, clinical presentation, diagnosis, and management. Cutaneous lesions such as petechiae, livedo reticularis, purpura, nodules, and ulcers raise the suspicion of vasculitis, which also commonly affects organs and tissues including lungs, kidneys, peripheral nerves, muscles, and the gastrointestinal tract. Patients are often systemically unwell with malaise, fever, weight loss, arthralgia, and normochromic normocytic anaemia and have raised inflammatory markers. History is important and should include the onset and evolution of symptoms, systems review, preceding infections, exposure to drugs and toxins, and relevant family history. Full blood count, electrolytes, renal and hepatic function, C reactive protein (CRP), erythrocyte sedimentation rate (ESR) and, where relevant, viral titres, autoantibodies, and cryoglobulins should be measured. Urinalysis is important to identify renal involvement, typified by red cells, casts, or proteinuria, as prompt treatment may avert irreversible renal failure. Biopsy remains the gold standard for histopathological confirmation of vasculitis, and in addition to formalin fixation, a fresh sample should be provided for immunofluorescent labelling of immune complexes and complement if small vessel vasculitis is suspected. Imaging is paramount when a biopsy is unobtainable and, in large vessel vasculitis, is useful to determine the extent of disease.

Comorbidities are common, including treatment-related toxicities such as corticosteroid-induced obesity, mood disorders, skin fragility, bruising, osteoporotic fractures, peptic ulcer disease, diabetes mellitus, dyslipidaemia, hypertension, accelerated atherosclerosis, cataracts, glaucoma, and immunosuppression predisposing individuals to common and opportunistic infections. Vaccination against influenza, pneumococcus, pertussis, and COVID-19 should be up to date, with consideration of varicella vaccination. Prophylaxis against pneumocystis jiroveci pneumonia should be prescribed for patients taking high doses of corticosteroids and/or rituximab. Patients who screen positive for serum Hepatitis B surface antigen or core antibody should be monitored for viral reactivation and prescribed a nucleoside analogue such as entecavir for at least 18 months following rituximab treatment. All patients commencing treatment with biologic or targeted synthetic immunosuppressive agents should be screened and treated for latent tuberculosis. Additional screening and prophylaxis for latent infections/infestations such as melioidosis, strongyloidiasis, and Human T-cell lymphotropic virus type 1 (HTLV1) should be performed in endemic regions. Vaccination with live vaccines is contraindicated in the setting of immunosuppression because of the risk of disseminated viral disease. Baseline assessment of bone mineral density and treatment to prevent or manage steroid-induced osteoporosis comprise the standard of care. Small and large vessel vasculitis is associated with an increased risk of contemporaneous malignancy, particularly in elderly patients, and clinical examination supplemented by relevant investigations should be undertaken.

The aetiology of most vasculitides is unknown, with management directed towards the prevention and treatment of organ damage, maintenance of a low inflammatory state, titration of therapy according to clinical, serologic and imaging parameters, management of comorbidities, and prevention and management of treatment-related side effects. This chapter will outline the main types of vasculitis encountered in clinical practice, describe known pathogenetic mechanisms, and present management strategies. In addition to vasculitis, Raynaud's phenomenon, thromboangiitis obliterans, cannabis vasculitis, and fibromuscular dysplasia will be discussed.

1.2 Primary Versus Secondary Vasculitis

Vasculitis is caused by immune-mediated inflammation of blood vessels. In most cases, the underlying cause of this reaction is unknown, and the term "primary" is often applied, whereas in a subset of cases the vasculitis is triggered by a known drug or virus or is a manifestation of an underlying systemic disease and is thus termed "secondary". Categorisation into primary versus secondary vasculitis becomes problematic, however, as more aetiologies are discovered. Vasculitis has more recently been divided according to the size and type of blood vessel involved, which has merit given that similar organs and tissues are affected. The discovery of anti-neutrophil cytoplasmic antibodies (ANCAs) associated with a subset of patients with small vessel vasculitis, causative viruses and gene mutations in a subset of patients previously diagnosed with polyarteritis nodosa, and the evolution of modern imaging techniques such as magnetic resonance imaging/angiography (MRI/MRA) and positron emission tomography (PET) have led to further subclassification of vasculitis. Table 1.1 shows the names for vasculitides adopted by the 2012

Table 1.1 Names for vasculitides adopted by the 2012 International Chapel Hill Consensus Conference on the Nomenclature of Vasculitides [1]

Large vessel vasculitis (LVV)
Takayasu arteritis (TAK)
Giant cell arteritis (GCA)
Medium vessel vasculitis (MVV)
Polyarteritis nodosa (PAN)
Kawasaki disease (KD)
Small vessel vasculitis (SVV)
Antineutrophil cytoplasmic antibody (ANCA)-associated vasculitis (AAV)
Microscopic polyangiitis (MPA)
Granulomatosis with polyangiitis (Wegener's) (GPA)
Eosinophilic granulomatosis with polyangiitis (Churg-Strauss) (EGPA)
Immune complex SVV
Anti-glomerular basement membrane (anti-GBM) disease
Cryoglobulinemic vasculitis (CV)
IgA vasculitis (Henoch-Schönlein) (IgAV)
Hypocomplementaemic urticarial vasculitis (HUV) (anti-C1q vasculitis)
Variable vessel vasculitis (VVV)
Behcet's disease (BD)
Cogan's syndrome (CS)
Single-organ vasculitis (SOV)
Cutaneous leukocytoclastic angiitis
Cutaneous arteritis
Primary central nervous system vasculitis
Isolated aortitis
Others
Vasculitis associated with systemic disease
Lupus vasculitis
Rheumatoid vasculitis
Sarcoid vasculitis
Others
Vasculitis associated with probable aetiology
Hepatitis C virus-associated cryoglobulinemic vasculitis
Hepatitis B virus-associated vasculitis
Syphilis-associated aortitis
Drug-associated immune complex vasculitis
Drug-associated ANCA-associated vasculitis
Cancer-associated vasculitis
Others

International Chapel Hill Consensus Conference of the nomenclature of vasculitides [1]. Technology-led advances in our understanding of mechanisms of disease initiation and progression, as well as insights emerging from clinical trials of targeted biologic therapies, will continue to inform this area.

1.3 Large Vessel Vasculitis

1.3.1 Giant Cell Arteritis (Temporal Arteritis)

Giant cell arteritis (GCA) is a granulomatous vasculitis principally involving medium- and large-calibre branches of the aorta and the aorta itself, which if left untreated can lead to permanent blindness and cerebrovascular accidents. It is the commonest form of vasculitis, occurring in patients over the age of 50, and mainly affects people of northern European and Scandinavian descent. There is a female preponderance and worldwide incidence between 1 and 30 per 100,000. The strongest genetic association is with human leucocyte antigen class II gene loci DRB1*04, DQA1*03, and DQB1*03 [2].

GCA is a T cell driven disease characterised by the formation of vessel wall granulomas, intimal hyperplasia, and end-organ ischaemia. T helper cell 1 (Th1) and Th17 pathways and innate immunity appear to be central in its pathogenesis. Activation and maturation of immature vascular dendritic cells (vasDCs) (see Glossary) within the normally immunopriviledged arterial wall leads to recruitment and activation of local innate immune cells such as monocytes and fibroblasts, as well as naive CD4+ T cells. Adventitial *vasa vasora* critically control vessel wall access and drive differentiation of tissue-invasive T cells, which establish tissue residency within autonomous inflammatory lesions [3]. Antigens have been suspected to drive the local activation of vasculogenic CD4 T cells, but data suggest a more generalised defect in their threshold setting. In health, immune checkpoints (see Glossary) provide a physiological brake on T cell activation to curb inflammation-associated tissue destruction. This mechanism has been shown to be disrupted in GCA, as vasDCs fail to express the immunoinhibitory programmed cell death ligand-1 (PD-L1), leaving lesional T cells unchecked. Consequently, programmed cell death protein-1 (PD-1)-positive CD4 T cells can enter the vessel wall, where they produce a broad spectrum of inflammatory cytokines, including interferon-gamma (IFN-γ), interleukin (IL)-17, and IL-21, and have a direct role in driving intimal hyperplasia and intramural neoangiogenesis. The deficiency of the PD-1 immune checkpoint in GCA, promoting unopposed T cell immunity, contrasts with checkpoint hyperactivity in cancer patients in whom excessive PD-L1 expression paralyses the function of antitumour T cells [4].

Diverse macrophage subsets, secreting matrix metalloproteinases which degrade the internal elastic lamina and smooth muscle cells within the media, promote the migration and proliferation of myofibroblasts into and within the intima, ultimately inducing wall capillarisation and intimal hyperplasia, leading to luminal compromise [3]. Macrophages release IL-6 and IL-1β, potent cytokines required for differentiation of Th17 effector cells; levels of circulating IL-6 correlate with the severity of the acute inflammatory response in GCA and fluctuate in line with disease activity. Th1 cells differentiate in the presence of IL-12, thought to be produced by activated vasDCs, and these effector T cells are responsible for the secretion of IFN-γ, a potent activator of macrophages and heavily implicated in promoting mural infiltration, as well as giant cell and granuloma formation. In contrast to IL-6 and IL-17, which appear to wax and wane with disease activity and are highly responsive to corticosteroids, elevated levels of IL-12 and IFN-γ persist within the serum of patients and within temporal artery samples despite months of corticosteroid treatment and higher levels of these cytokines correlate with ischaemic complications.

1.3.1.1 Biphasic Inflammatory Response in GCA

It has been proposed that there is a biphasic inflammatory process, where the Th17 (IL-6/IL-17)-mediated pathway, which is corticosteroid-responsive, drives systemic inflammation in early GCA, while Th1 (IL-12/IFN-γ)-mediated mechanisms promote chronicity and are poorly steroid-responsive. This might explain the disconnect between early control of systemic inflammation and suboptimal numbers of patients achieving long-term remission, with late development of aortic aneurysms [2]. A recent study of patients who had serial temporal artery biopsies (TAB) before and 3–12 months after initiation of therapy revealed that vascular inflammation persisted in most patients, despite normalisation of CRP and ESR [3].

1.3.1.2 Stem-Like CD4+ T Cells Contribute to Aneurysm Formation

Stem-like CD4+ T cells have been shown to survive in perivascular tertiary lymphoid structures in the aortic wall. These cells have high proliferative potential and give rise to effector T cells, promoting chronicity and autonomy of autoimmune tissue inflammation and contributing to aneurysm formation [5]. Imaging studies reveal that clinical remission may be associated with disease activity on ^{18}F-fluorodeoxyglucose (^{18}F-FDG)-PET imaging and MRA, with around 51% of patients in clinical remission having active disease by both MRA and PET [6]. Histopathologic evaluation of the thoracic aorta obtained during surgery revealed active aortitis in most patients with GCA despite being considered in clinical remission several years after GCA diagnosis, and chronic, smouldering aortic inflammation likely contributed to the development of aortic aneurysm and dissection [7]. Transcriptomic profiling of resected ascending aortic aneurysms from patients with GCA, clinically isolated aortitis, and atherosclerotic aneurysms identified differential gene signatures between inflammatory and noninflammatory specimens including immune response genes, allowing identification of potential drug targets through pharmacogenomic network analysis [8].

1.3.1.3 Early Diagnosis Essential to Access Optimal Treatment

GCA may occur de novo, or in patients with known polymyalgia rheumatica (PMR), a related inflammatory condition characterised by pain and stiffness of the shoulder and hip girdles. The most common presenting features of GCA are of occlusive cranial arteritis, such as temporal headache, jaw claudication, facial pain, amaurosis fugax, diplopia, cerebrovascular accident (particularly of the vertebral circulation), and unheralded unilateral or bilateral blindness, which occurs in up to 20% of patients. Limb claudication due to large vessel vasculitis in the absence of cranial arteritis may be the presenting feature of GCA, and some patients present with generalised lethargy, malaise, unexplained weight loss, or pyrexia of unknown origin. Physical signs may be minimal, but include scalp tenderness, nodularity/decreased pulsation of the temporal artery, and in patients with visual symptoms, fundoscopic changes of anterior ischaemic optic neuropathy, retinal arterial occlusions, or choroidal infarction. Presenting features with the highest positive predictive value for GCA include jaw claudication and/or scalp tenderness [2]. Depending on disease duration, normocytic anaemia, thrombocytosis, and/or leukocytosis may be evident, and significant elevation of the ESR and/or CRP is characteristic, although occasionally absent.

In addition to age over 50 years, raised ESR and/or CRP, and positive temporal artery biopsy, current classification criteria for GCA incorporate imaging findings from temporal and axillary arteries using ultrasound, MRI or angiography, and aortic activity on ^{18}F-fluorodeoxyglucose (^{18}F-FDG)-PET [9] (Table 1.2).

GCA is considered a medical emergency because of the high risk of irreversible blindness or stroke if treatment is delayed. In patients sustaining monocular blindness, there is a 50% risk of visual loss in the contralateral eye within 2 weeks.

Histopathology of a temporal artery biopsy (TAB) is the gold standard for diagnosis, but treatment should not be delayed, as pre-TAB corticosteroid exposure does not affect the yield for up to 6 weeks and beyond [10]. Notwithstanding this, early diagnosis of GCA is essential to enable optimal treatment by access to tocilizumab and enable lower initial and total doses of corticosteroids (see below). The sensitivity of TAB for the diagnosis of GCA varies between 39% and 91% because of skip lesions, and the yield can be improved by performing bilateral TAB or achieving a TAB post-fixation length of at least 3 cm [10]. Histologically, the inflammatory infiltrate in GCA is predominantly composed of histiocytes/macrophages and CD4+ lymphocytes, with variable involvement of the three arterial layers, often showing only segmental inflammation in parts of the arterial wall (Fig. 1.1). The lymphocyte population usually includes lesser numbers of CD8+ cytotoxic T cells and CD20+ B cells. Focal fusion of histiocytes and formation of multinucleate giant cells are seen, but these are not required for the diagnosis. The inflammation typically results in breaks, segmental loss, and reduplication of the

Table 1.2 2022 ACR/EULAR classification criteria for giant cell arteritis[a] [9]

Considerations when applying these criteria	
These classification criteria should be applied to classify the patient as having giant cell arteritis when a diagnosis of medium-vessel or large-vessel vasculitis has been made	
Alternative diagnoses mimicking vasculitis should be excluded prior to applying the criteria	
Absolute requirement	
Age ≥ 50 years at time of diagnosis	
Additional clinical criteria	
Morning stiffness in shoulders/neck	+2
Sudden visual loss	+3
Jaw or tongue claudication	+2
New temporal headache	+2
Scalp tenderness	+2
Abnormal examination of the temporal artery	+2
Laboratory, imaging, and biopsy criteria	
Maximum ESR ≥ 50 mm/h or maximum CRP ≥ 10 mg/l	+3
Positive temporal artery biopsy or halo sign on temporal artery ultrasound	+5
Bilateral axillary involvement	+2
FDG-PET activity throughout aorta	+2

[a]Sum the scores for ten items, if present. A score of ≥6 points is needed for the classification of giant cell arteritis

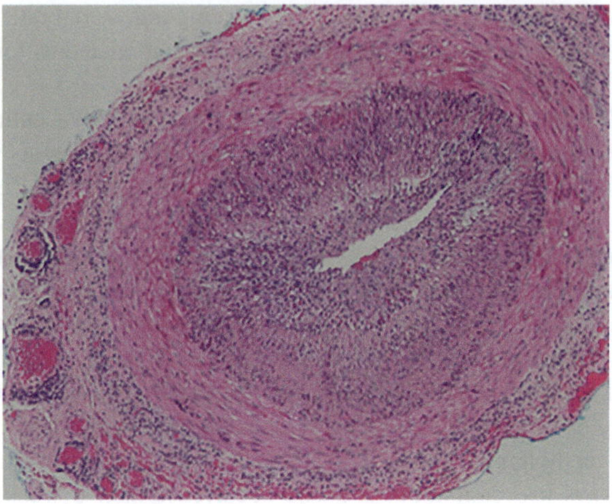

Fig. 1.1 Giant cell arteritis. Histological section taken from temporal artery biopsy shows marked intimal thickening with luminal stenosis associated with dense infiltrate of lymphocytes, histiocytes, and eosinophils, extending to the internal elastic lamina of the media. Only very occasional giant cells are seen

elastic lamina, best seen on elastin stain. This may lead to critical luminal narrowing and aneurysm formation. Following the active phase, inflammatory cell infiltrates may be absent but intimal-medial scarring and injury to the elastic lamina often remain [2].

The European Alliance of Associations for Rheumatology (EULAR) taskforce for imaging in large vessel vasculitis guideline recommends temporal artery ultrasound as the first-line imaging modality for predominantly cranial GCA in centres where experience is at hand, as the test is non-invasive, immediate, and cost effective, and in some centres, is replacing the need for TAB [11]. The temporal artery ultrasound finding of a non-compressible halo sign, caused by oedema of the vessel wall, has a reported sensitivity between 77% and 79% and specificity between 96% and 100% for the diagnosis of GCA. This investigation is dependent on training and expertise of the sonographer, however, and the ability to detect a halo sign declines rapidly after the initiation of corticosteroids, with sensitivity falling to below 50% at 4 days. A diagnostic prediction model for GCA incorporating a probability score and ultrasound findings has been validated and is used in some centres [11]. Confirmation of large vessel GCA not involving cranial vessels requires other imaging techniques, which are also sensitive to corticosteroid therapy. High-resolution MRI has the advantages of the absence of radiation, the contemporaneous detection of structural lesions (such as vessel wall thickening and luminal stenosis/occlusion), and contrast enhancement of the arterial wall presumed (but not proven) to reflect active inflammation [11]. Compared with TAB, ^{18}F-FDG-PET combined with low dose fine cut computed tomography (^{18}F-FDG-PET/CT) performed within 72 h of commencement of corticosteroids had a sensitivity of 92%, specificity of 85%, and negative predictive value of 98% and identified patients with aortitis, who require closer follow-up for late complications such as aneurysm development or aortic regurgitation. Cranial arteritis was evident in temporal, vertebral, maxillary, and occipital arteries, with vasculitis mimics including malignancies found in 20% of patients [12].

The 2021 American College of Rheumatology (ACR)/Vasculitis Foundation guideline for the management of GCA [13] recommends in patients with suspected GCA obtaining a TAB specimen within 2 weeks of starting oral corticosteroids, over waiting longer than 2 weeks for a biopsy, and if TAB is negative, obtaining vascular imaging of the large vessels for diagnosis. All patients with newly diagnosed GCA are recommended to undergo vascular imaging to evaluate large vessel involvement. Performing PET imaging at diagnosis may help to estimate the risk for aortic aneurysm formation [14].

Treatment of GCA consists of high dose corticosteroids, usually 40–60 mg prednisolone daily or 1 mg/kg body weight, augmented by immediate intravenous pulses of high dose methylprednisolone in the presence of ocular involvement. Blindness is almost always irreversible but is a rare occurrence after 2 weeks of high dose corticosteroids. Concomitant treatment with tocilizumab, a monoclonal antibody targeting the interleukin-6 receptor, enables a lower initial and total dose of corticosteroids, reduced relapse rates, and increased quality of life [15], however relapse occurs in over 50% of patients 2 years after discontinuation of a 12 month course of tocilizumab [16]. Access to funded tocilizumab in Australia and elsewhere for GCA relies on documentation of a positive TAB or imaging, in addition to raised inflammatory markers—thus early confirmation enables more rapid access to effective therapy and reduced risk of steroid toxicity.

Therapeutic targets under current investigation include janus kinases, IL-17 [17], and T cell co-stimulatory molecules [18]. Traditional disease-modifying antirheumatic drugs (DMARDs) are not effective in GCA. Treatment with methotrexate (MTX) leads to a significant, though modestly reduced, risk of relapse and lower cumulative corticosteroid doses compared with placebo, but does not reduce the rate of drug-related adverse events. For patients with GCA who have critical or flow-limiting involvement of the vertebral or carotid arteries, addition of low-dose aspirin is recommended [13].

1.3.1.4 Long-Term Surveillance for Aortopathy

CT angiogram (CTA)-defined large vessel vasculitis (LVV) was reported in two-thirds of patients with GCA at the time of diagnosis: aorta 65%, brachiocephalic trunk 47.5%, carotid 35%, subclavian 42.5%, axillary 17.5%, splanchnic 22.5%, renal 7.5%, iliac 15%, femoral arteries 30%; with aortic dilation already present in 15% [19]. Kebed et al. reported the spectrum of aortic involvement in patients with GCA following review of medical records of 4006 patients including those with imaging studies. A total of 1450 patients (36%) had a confirmed diagnosis of GCA. Of these, 974 had aortic imaging. Of the 974 patients with imaging, 435 (45%) had an identified aortopathy. The most common aortopathy was aneurysm/dilation (69%). Overall, an annual aneurysmal growth rate of 1.5 mm/y was calculated. In patients with aneurysm/dilation, aortic dissection occurred in 18 patients (6%), and these patients had a significantly higher aneurysmal growth rate compared with those without dissection (4.5 vs 1.4 mm/y, $p = 0.005$). The median size of the aorta at the time of dissection was 51 mm, with 7 (39%) occurring with a maximal aortic aneurysm/dilation <50 mm [20]. These findings indicate higher aneurysmal growth rate in GCA compared with that reported for degenerative aortic disease, with a significantly higher growth rate in patients who develop dissection. It is recommended that screening for thoracic aortic aneurysm should be undertaken at baseline, and if normal, imaging should be repeated every 2–3 years; the optimal imaging for screening and surveillance and additional clinical risk factors are undetermined. Patients with aortic dilatation should be followed closely, and surgery considered for thoracic aorta diameter > 50 mm.

1.3.2 Takayasu Arteritis

Takayasu arteritis (TAK, previously known as "pulseless disease") is a granulomatous arteritis affecting the aorta and its main branches as well as the pulmonary vasculature, causing aneurysm formation and tissue infarction. Histopathology is similar to GCA with the presence of transmural lymphocytic infiltration and multinucleated giant cells, but involvement of cranial vessels is not a feature, and patients are typically women under 50 years of age. TAK occurs across all races and geographic locations, with a higher incidence in Asians and South Americans [21].

The strongest genetic susceptibility locus for TAK is *HLA-B*52*. Non-HLA susceptibility loci include Fc gamma receptor loci *FCGR2A/FCGR3A*, *IL12B*, and *IL6* [22]. Early vascular lesions consist of T cells, natural killer cells, and macrophages. Granuloma formation and giant cells can subsequently be found in the media of elastic arteries. Late-stage ("burnt out") damage demonstrates extensive fibrosis and intimal hyperplasia, which may lead to aneurysm formation or arterial stenosis (Fig. 1.2). In contrast to GCA, a pathogenic role for B cells has been suggested in TAK by the identification of non-specific polyclonal hypergammaglobulinemia, circulating anti-endothelial antibodies, increased numbers of circulating plasmablasts, B cell infiltration of aortic adventitia, and elevated serum levels of B cell-activating factor in patients with active disease [22].

Patients usually present with symptoms of limb ischaemia, hypertension, and/or renal impairment. Signs on examination include differential brachial blood pressures, inability to palpate peripheral pulses, and subclavian, axillary, abdominal, and femoral bruits. Diagnosis may be confirmed by imaging of the aortic trunk and vessels by MRI, PET, or CT [11]. CRP and ESR are not always elevated. The ACR classification criteria for TAK are shown in Table 1.3 [23].

Corticosteroids are the mainstay of treatment for TAK. Cyclophosphamide (CYC) is usually used initially in conjunction with high dose corticosteroids for severe or organ-threatening disease. Immunosuppressives in addition to corticosteroids are recommended and include MTX, azathioprine (AZA), or tumour necrosis factor (TNF) inhibitors; efficacy of tocilizumab has not been established [13].

TAK is a chronic disease in which inflammatory activity tends to wax and wane, with subclinical radiographic progression seen in more than two thirds of patients [21, 22], thus patients require long-term monitoring and usually immunosuppression. Stenting of arterial stenoses, particularly of renal arteries, is often required, preferably when vessel inflammation has been controlled. Collateral circulation may compensate and improve painful limb claudication over time. Similar to GCA, late complications of aortic root dilatation with aneurysm formation and/or aortic valve regurgitation, or abdominal aortic aneurysm, may require surgical intervention. In patients with large vessel vasculitis (GCA or TAK), MRA, CTA, and/or ultrasound may be used for long-term monitoring of structural damage, particularly to detect stenosis, occlusion, dilatation, and/or aneurysms. The frequency of screening as well as the imaging method applied should be decided on an individual basis [13].

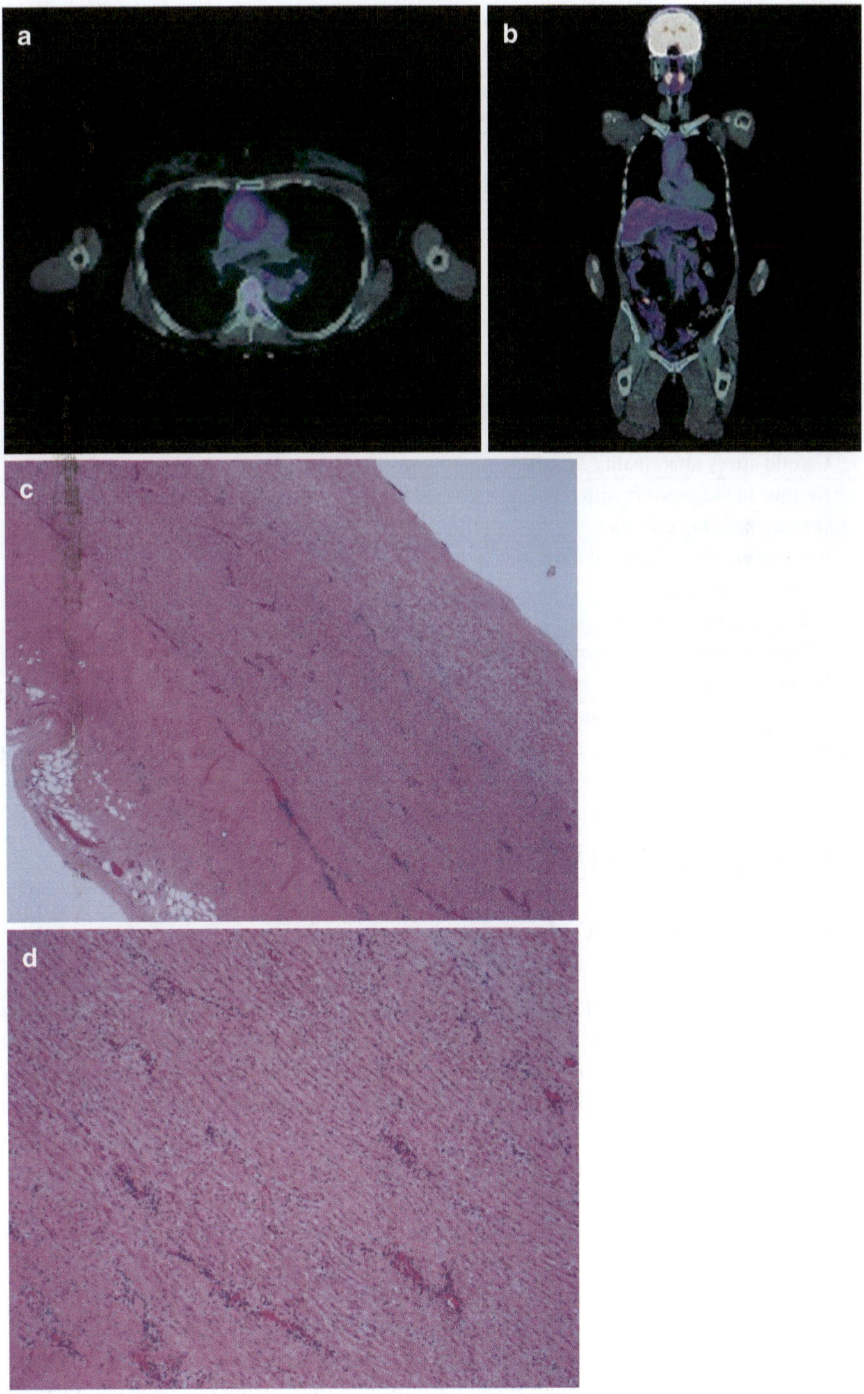

Fig. 1.2 Takayasu arteritis. ^{18}F-FDG-PET/CT showing increased radiotracer avidity associated with the ascending aorta (**a**, **b**). Aortic wall showing patchy lymphocytic inflammatory infiltrate within the media. Elsewhere, there is evidence of dense fibrosis of the aortic wall with extensive disruption of the elastic fibre architecture (**c**, **d**)

Table 1.3 2022 ACR/EULAR classification criteria for Takayasu arteritis[a] [23]

Consideration when applying these criteria	
These classification criteria should be applied to classify the patient as having Takayasu arteritis when a diagnosis of medium-vessel or large-vessel vasculitis has been made	
Alternative diagnoses mimicking vasculitis should be excluded prior to applying the criteria	
Absolute requirements	
Age ≤ 60 years at time of diagnosis	
Evidence of vasculitis on imaging	
Additional clinical criteria	
Female sex	+1
Angina or ischemic cardiac pain	+2
Arm or leg claudication	+2
Vascular bruit	+2
Reduced pulse in upper extremity	+2
Carotid artery abnormality	+2
Systolic blood pressure difference in arms ≥20 mmHg	+1
Additional imaging criteria	
Number of affected arterial territories (select one)	
One arterial territory	+1
Two arterial territories	+2
Three or more arterial territories	+3
Symmetric involvement of paired arteries	+1
Abdominal aorta involvement with renal or mesenteric involvement	+3

[a]Sum the scores for ten items, if present. A score of ≥5 points is needed for the classification of Takayasu arteritis

1.4 Medium Vessel Vasculitis

1.4.1 Polyarteritis Nodosa

Polyarteritis nodosa (PAN) is a rare necrotising vasculitis affecting medium-sized or small muscular arteries. In contrast to microscopic polyangiitis (see below), PAN is not associated with glomerulonephritis or vasculitis of the small vessels (arterioles, capillaries, and venules). PAN occurs most commonly in middle-age with a slight male predominance, with decreasing incidence concomitant with reduced prevalence of hepatitis B virus (HBV) infection.

The aetiopathogenesis of classic PAN is not known, and pathway(s) leading to necrotising inflammation of the blood vessels probably involve both the innate and adaptive immune systems. Loss of function mutations in genes associated with autoinflammatory diseases, such as *CECR1* which codes for adenosine deaminase-2 (ADA2), can lead to a similar phenotype, implicating perturbation of leukocyte growth factors and endothelial instability [24]. HBV infection accounts for 30% of cases previously diagnosed with PAN; vasculitis in this setting has been shown to be caused by viral antigen-containing immune complex deposition on vascular walls with complement fixation and vascular damage. Cutaneous PAN is a designation given to patients presenting with necrotising vasculitis confined to the skin, with occasional musculoskeletal features but no other systemic involvement [24].

The characteristic presentation of PAN is with ischaemia and infarction of numerous organs including the skin causing palpable purpura, livedo reticularis or subcutaneous nodules, nervous system causing stroke or mononeuritis, kidneys causing infarction, hypertension, and renal failure, heart causing myocardial infarction, pericarditis, and congestive cardiac failure, gastrointestinal system causing abdominal pain, infarction, and haemorrhage, and testicles causing painful orchitis. PAN rarely affects the lungs. Systemic symptoms such as fever, weight loss, arthralgia, and myalgia are common.

Diagnosis is established by a combination of clinical features, biopsy (skin, testes, renal), and/or characteristic findings on digital subtraction angiogram, which has a better resolution than CTA. Histopathology reveals segmental transmural inflammation of muscular arteries with evidence of necrosis and disruption of the internal and external elastic lamina. The latter can lead to aneurysmal dilation. Characteristic mesenteric or renal angiographic findings are of multiple aneurysms and irregular constrictions of larger vessels with occlusions of smaller vessels.

Isolated cutaneous PAN often responds to low dose corticosteroids. Higher doses of corticosteroids are the mainstay of treatment for mild classic PAN in combination with MTX, AZA, mycophenolate mofetil (MMF), or leflunomide as steroid-sparing agents. CYC is used in conjunction with corticosteroids in moderate to severe cases. There is emerging evidence for TNF inhibitors (TNFi) for refractory cases and patients with mutations causing ADA2 deficiency and reports of benefit with the B lymphocyte depleting agent rituximab (RTX). The ACR/Vasculitis Foundation Guideline for the management of PAN was published in 2021 [25]. Treated systemic PAN has a 5-year survival rate between 75% and 80%; untreated, it is usually fatal. Treatment for HBV-associated PAN is with anti-viral therapy coupled with short-term corticosteroids, which can lead to total remission of vasculitis with no evidence of recurrence.

1.4.2 Kawasaki Disease

Kawasaki disease (KD) is an acute febrile illness that primarily affects children <5 years old and is the leading cause of acquired heart disease in children in developed countries. Without treatment, approx. 25% of patients develop coronary artery (CA) dilation or CA aneurysms (CAA). The incidence of KD in the USA is 18–25 per 100,000 in children <5 years old; the incidence is 10–30 times higher in northeast Asian countries, including Japan, South Korea, China, and Taiwan. The pathogenesis of KD remains unknown, and the diagnosis is based on established clinical criteria [26].

Current consensus regarding aetiology is that an infectious trigger initiates an abnormal immune response involving innate and adaptive pathways in genetically predisposed children. Several genome-wide association studies and case control studies have identified single nucleotide polymorphisms in genes which code for proteins important in immune activation including *FcgRIIa*, *CD40*, and *BLK*. Other identified pathways of potential importance include vascular endothelial growth factor (VEGF), angiopoietin, transforming growth factor-beta (TGF-β, important in T cell activation and cardiovascular remodelling), and inositol 1,4,5-triphosphate 3-kinase-C (ITPKC, part of a transmembrane signalling pathway). ITPKC influences NLRP3 inflammasome activation through intracellular calcium levels, leading to an increased IL-1β and IL-18 production [27]. Multiple potential infectious triggers have been implicated in KD pathogenesis. In the coronary arteries, immune infiltration of the arterial wall with neutrophils, CD8+ cytotoxic T cells, Ig-A producing plasma cells, and macrophages has been found, accompanied by pro-inflammatory cytokines which vary in proportion and contribution over time [27].

The diagnosis of KD is based on the presence of clinical features of persistent fever in combination with a rash, cervical lymphadenopathy, non-purulent conjunctival injection, changes of the lips and oral cavity (including strawberry tongue, cracked lips, redness of the mucosae), and changes in extremities (swelling and redness of the palms, desquamation in the subacute phase). There is no diagnostic test for KD, and the diagnosis may be delayed or overlooked [27]. Coronary artery lesions are diagnosed by echocardiography in the acute and subacute phases. Close monitoring of CAA is important as ischaemic symptoms or myocardial infarction due to thrombosis or stenosis can occur, most likely in the largest, so-called giant CAA. Apart from the presence of CAA, it is unclear whether KD causes an increased cardiovascular risk due to the vasculitis itself [27].

KD shock syndrome is a rare but severe form of the illness in which patients present with vasodilatory shock, hypotension, and poor perfusion, with or without myocardial dysfunction. Because there is no pathognomonic test for KD, KD and its associated shock syndrome can be difficult to distinguish clinically from other hyperinflammatory disorders. For example, in 2020, with the emergence of SARS-CoV-2 and subsequent recognition of multisystem inflammatory syndrome in children (MIS-C), this new condition became part of the differential diagnosis of KD. MIS-C and KD have clinical similarities, but it has become increasingly clear over the course of the COVID-19 pandemic that they are distinct illnesses. Certain clinical characteristics (e.g. prominent gastrointestinal symptoms [abdominal pain, vomiting, diarrhoea], headache), laboratory findings (e.g. thrombocytopenia, lymphopenia, elevated troponin, or B-type natriuretic peptide (BNP) levels), and cardiac findings (e.g. decreased left ventricular systolic function, pericardial effusion) are more prominent in patients with MIS-C. Rash, conjunctival injection, oral mucosal changes, and CA abnormalities are more common in patients with KD. The incidence of MIS-C has decreased substantially since 2022, potentially because of widespread immunity to SARS-CoV-2 or decreased ability of newer variants of SARS-CoV-2 to cause MIS-C [26].

Treatment consists of high dose intravenous immunoglobulin (IVIg) and is directed at preventing the development of CAA. Unfortunately, 10–20% of patients fail to respond to IVIg and these children need additional treatment with a second dose of IVIg or corticosteroids. Other immunosuppressants used for treatment-resistant, high-risk or refractory disease are inhibitors of IL-1β (anakinra), TNF, calcineurin (cyclosporine [CyA]), and occasionally, CYC. Initial addition of high-dose aspirin is used in many centres, with prospective investigation underway to determine the appropriate dose [26].

1.5 Small Vessel Vasculitis

Small vessel vasculitides (SVV) are a group of relatively uncommon disorders characterised by inflammation of small intraparenchymal arteries, arterioles, capillaries, and venules, which leads to vascular obstruction, tissue ischaemia, and infarction. A complex overlapping set of clinical features involving different organs and systems may occur. According to the 2012 Chapel Hill Consensus Conference, SVV are divided into ANCA-associated vasculitides (AAV) and immune complex vasculitides (ICV) [1]. AAV are necrotising vasculitides frequently associated with proteinase 3 (PR3)-ANCA or myeloperoxidase (MPO)-ANCA; ICV are characterised by wall deposits of immunoglobulin and complement components and include IgA vasculitis (IgAV), cryoglobulinaemic vasculitis (CV), anti-glomerular basement membrane disease (anti-GBM), and hypocomplementaemic urticarial vasculitis (HUV) [1].

1.5.1 Anti-Neutrophil Cytoplasmic Antibody (ANCA)-Associated Vasculitis (AAV)

ANCA are detected by indirect immunofluorescence (IIF) of fixed neutrophils, producing two main patterns: cytoplasmic (C-ANCA), usually caused by antibodies targeting proteinase 3 (PR3), and perinuclear (P-ANCA), the typical pattern of antibodies targeting myeloperoxidase (MPO). A positive C-ANCA or P-ANCA on screening IIF has low specificity and may be seen in other inflammatory conditions and healthy individuals. Confirmation by enzyme-linked immunosorbent assay [28] is required to confirm PR3 or MPO antibody specificity. There are three clinical subgroups of AAV: granulomatosis with polyangiitis (GPA, formerly Wegener's granulomatosis), eosinophilic granulomatosis with polyangiitis (EGPA, formerly Churg-Strauss angiitis), and microscopic polyangiitis (MPA). These are rare and potentially life-threatening multisystem autoimmune diseases.

Environmental factors play a role in pathogenesis, supported by variation in geographical distribution and relationship with exposure to silica, hydrocarbons, and various drugs. Infections such as *Staphylococcus aureus* have often been noted to precede the onset or flares of AAV, with decreased relapse rates reported after use of cotrimoxazole. Genetic associations include *HLA-DRB1*04*, *DPB1*0401*, the proteinase 3 gene (*PRTN3*), and alpha-1-antitrypsin gene (*SERPINA1*) with GPA, *HLA-DRB4* with EGPA, and *HLA-DRB1*0901* with MPA. Toll-like receptor 9 (*TLR 9*) polymorphism is associated with PR3-ANCA but not MPO-ANCA vasculitis. Epigenetic factors include decreased histone demethylation at PR3 and MPO loci [29]. A key role for neutrophils is indicated by amelioration of disease in mouse models in the setting of neutrophil depletion, and abnormal neutrophil extracellular traps containing PR3 and MPO have been demonstrated upon activating neutrophils with ANCA derived from human sera. Macrophages also have a role in propagation of AAV [28]; the predominant effector cells implicated in EGPA are eosinophils [30].

1.5.1.1 Granulomatosis with Polyangiitis (GPA)

The range of clinical presentations is broad and includes granulomatous inflammation of upper and lower airways and vasculitis of small and medium vessels, of which glomerulonephritis is common. Nasal symptoms include nasal obstruction, bloody nasal discharge, epistaxis, chronic sinusitis, and saddle nose deformity. Subglottic stenosis, mastoiditis, otitis media, and orbital pseudotumour are seen less commonly. Systemic features such as fever, arthralgia, and malaise may be absent in the early localised phase. Pulmonary involvement occurs in up to 85% of patients ranging from asymptomatic nodules to massive haemoptysis with respiratory failure. Radiologic features include pulmonary nodular infiltrates, cavities, and bilateral ground glass opacities from pulmonary haemorrhage. Renal involvement in the form of rapidly progressive glomerulonephritis is the presenting manifestation in 20% of patients, increasing to 80% over the disease course. Ocular involvement occurs in 50% in the form of episcleritis, scleritis, and orbital disease. Cutaneous manifestations are usually minor [31].

1.5.1.2 Eosinophilic Granulomatosis with Polyangiitis (EGPA)

This syndrome is characterised by eosinophil-rich granulomatous inflammation of the airways along with small- and medium-vessel vasculitis. Three different disease phases are usually described, namely, prodromal, eosinophilic, and vasculitic. The main clinical feature in the prodromal stage is asthma (which may predate vasculitis by years) and allergic rhinitis with or without polyposis. Upper airway involvement is much milder than in GPA. Peripheral and tissue eosinophilia occurs in the second phase, which may be masked by treatments used for severe asthma, including corticosteroids, IL-5 inhibitors, and IL-4/13 inhibitors [32]. Vasculitic manifestations occur in nerves, heart, lungs, GI tract, and kidneys. Skin involvement is a dominant feature in the form of nodules, urticaria, or ulceration. Neurologic involvement occurs in 60–70% of patients in the form of multiple mononeuropathies or symmetric polyneuropathy; ischaemic optic neuropathy, cranial neuropathies, and stroke are less common. Cardiac involvement is seen in up to 20% of patients in the form of myocarditis, pericarditis, endocarditis, valvulitis, and coronary vasculitis and contributes to half the deaths. Renal involvement in the form of small vessel vasculitis is less common than other AAVs [31].

1.5.1.3 Microscopic Polyangiitis (MPA)

MPA is a necrotising small-vessel AAV. Initially considered a part of PAN, it was recognised as a distinct entity in 1994 [33]. The main manifestations are pauci-immune glomerulonephritis and pulmonary capillaritis. Granulomatous inflammation is absent. Most patients present with rapidly progressive glomerulonephritis and may be oliguric or anuric at the time of presentation, necessitating dialysis. Lung haemorrhage is the most catastrophic manifestation seen in about 10% of patients and is mostly associated with renal involvement. Most patients have constitutional symptoms, with fever, weight loss, arthralgia, and myalgia at the time of presentation. Neurologic involvement is common in the form of mononeuritis multiplex, axonal sensorimotor neuropathy, or cranial nerve involvement. Skin manifestations include purpura, painful ulcers (frequently on the legs), and digital gangrene. Ocular involvement includes scleritis, episcleritis, blepharitis, conjunctivitis, keratitis, uveitis, and retinal vasculitis [31].

Diagnosis of AAV is based on clinical features supported by positive ANCA and biopsy of the involved organ wherever feasible. EGPA is associated with MPO-ANCA in approximately 50% of cases, whereas GPA and MPA are usually associated with PR3-ANCA. The presence of fibrinoid necrosis or crescentic glomerulonephritis is highly suggestive of AAV.

Important mimics of AAV include cocaine-induced midline destructive lesions (CIMDL), lymphoma, infective endocarditis, and VEXAS (see below).

Updated classification criteria for GPA [34] and MPA [35] apply to patients with known vasculitis in whom alternative diagnoses mimicking vasculitis are excluded. Aims of management are to improve patient survival, induce remission, maintain remission, manage treatment-related toxicity, and improve quality of life. Recent guidelines and recommendations informed by clinical trials [36, 37] recommend corticosteroids and RTX for remission induction over CYC. Routine addition of plasma exchange to remission induction therapy is not recommended, even for patients with active glomerulonephritis and/or alveolar haemorrhage, although it may be considered if creatinine is >300 μmol/ml due to active glomerulonephritis—one study reporting improved risk of end stage kidney disease at 12 months albeit with increased risk of serious infections. Another significant change is reduced corticosteroid doses for remission induction, providing non-inferior efficacy, significantly lower adverse effects, and cumulative dose at 6 months <60% of the previous standard dose [38, 39]. Another potentially practice-changing outcome from clinical research in AAV is the finding that avacopan, an oral small-molecule complement C5a receptor blocker which inhibits neutrophil chemoattraction and neutrophil activation, compared with prednisolone for patients with AAV following either CYC or RTX induction, is non-inferior with respect to achievement of remission at week 26 and superior for sustained remission at week 52. Safety and clinical effects of avacopan beyond 52 weeks were not addressed in the trial [40]. Avacopan may be considered as part of a strategy to substantially reduce exposure to corticosteroids in AVV [37]. In patients with non-organ threatening AAV such as sinusitis, lung nodules, purpura, or arthralgia, remission-induction may be undertaken with corticosteroids and MTX, switching to more potent treatments such as corticosteroids + RTX/CYC/AZA/MMF if remission is not achieved, or relapse occurs.

Risk factors for relapse of AAV include the diagnosis of GPA, PR3 positivity, persistently positive ANCA titres, previous relapse, and upper respiratory tract involvement. For remission maintenance, treatment with RTX over MTX or AZA is supported by high-quality randomised controlled trials confirming higher efficacy of RTX [41]. Remission maintenance is recommended with RTX 4–6-monthly for a minimum of 24–48 months; patients who develop hypogammaglobulinaemia associated with recurrent severe infections are recommended to receive immunoglobulin supplementation.

Mepolizumab is a humanised monoclonal antibody which binds free IL-5, an essential cytokine for eosinophil development and proliferation, which is increased in active EGPA. In a phase 3 randomised controlled trial in participants with EGPA, mepolizumab resulted in significantly more weeks in remission and a higher proportion of participants in remission than did placebo, thus allowing for reduced corticosteroid use. Even so, only approximately half the participants treated with mepolizumab had protocol-defined remission [42]. Benralizumab, a monoclonal antibody targeting IL-5 receptors expressed on eosinophils, was non-inferior to mepolizumab for remission induction in patients with relapsing or refractory EGPA. The accrued duration of remission and the time to first relapse were similar in the two groups. Complete withdrawal of oral corticosteroids during weeks 48 through 52 was achieved in 41% of patients who received benralizumab and 26% of those receiving mepolizumab [43]. Emerging therapies for AAV include those targeting B cells.

1.5.2 *Immune Complex Small Vessel Vasculitis*

Immunoglobulin-A vasculitis (IgAV) (previously known as Henoch-Schönlein purpura) predominantly affects capillaries, venules, or arterioles, with IgA1-dominant immune complex deposition. It is the most common childhood vasculitis, affecting 10–20 children per 100,000 annually. More than 90% of patients are under 10 years of age, with a mean age of 6 years; adults tend to have more severe disease. Clinical presentation of IgAV comprises a characteristic tetrad of cutaneous palpable purpura, joint pain, colicky abdominal pain, and renal involvement. Proposed triggers include upper respiratory tract infections, medications, vaccinations, and (in adults) malignancies [44].

The skin rash consists of symmetric erythematous petechiae or papules on the buttocks and lower extremities, which evolve to a typical palpable purpura [45]. Gastrointestinal symptoms occur in about 50% of cases. Abdominal pain is common and may mimic an acute abdomen. The abdominal pain is thought to be due to immune complex deposition in the gut vessel wall. Gastrointestinal complications such as perforation, intussusception, and infarction may occur [45]. Joint involvement includes arthralgias or arthritis often affecting knees and ankles, which often precedes the development of palpable purpura. IgAV kidney involvement is frequent, including haematuria, proteinuria, nephrotic, or nephritic syndrome, with onset usually within a few months of the rash. Severe renal involvement occurs in 7% of cases, most commonly adults, and may lead to end-stage renal disease [45]. Hypertension may develop at the onset or during recovery from IgAV; neurological manifestations are rare [44].

HLA class I and class II *HLA-DRB1* alleles appear to influence predisposition to this disease, and non-HLA gene candidates include those coding for cytokines, chemokines, adhesion molecules, T-cells, aberrant glycosylation of IgA1, nitric oxide production, neoangiogenesis, the renin-angiotensin system, and lipid, pyrin, and homocysteine metabolism [45].

Upper respiratory tract infections precede the majority of cases, with many pathogens implicated. Vascular deposition of IgA1-containing immune complexes plays a pathogenic role, with complement activation, endothelial damage, perivascular leukocytic infiltrates, chemokines, and cytokines being important factors in this process, thus suggesting an IgA-mediated dysregulated immune response to an antigen [44].

Diagnosis is based on clinical criteria and non-mandatory tissue biopsy. Histological features involving the skin are those of a leukocytoclastic vasculitis primarily affecting the small superficial vessels. Vessel walls are infiltrated by neutrophil granulocytes, which partly degenerate and form nuclear dust (leukocytoclasia), located among extravasated erythrocytes (purpura) in the surrounding dermis. The vessel walls are thickened and may be necrotic due to exudation of neutrophils and variable amounts of fibrin. On direct immunofluorescence, IgA and, eventually, complement C3 can be seen deposited in the vessel walls. The process is dynamic, and not all of these features may be seen in a single biopsy [44] (Fig. 1.3).

Treatment is dictated by the severity of organ involvement. Treatment in patients without renal involvement is supportive, including analgesia, rehydration, surgery for intussusception, and wound care. Compression may be used for leg oedema. Nephritis is treated with corticosteroids and/or other immunosuppressive drugs, including MMF, CYC, CyA, RTX, or dapsone. IgAV has been associated with solid tumours, mostly of the gastrointestinal tract, lungs, or urinary tract in men over 60 years of age, and screening for cancer in this subgroup should be considered [44].

Cryoglobulinemic vasculitis (CV) is a small-vessel vasculitis involving mainly the skin, joints, peripheral nervous system, and kidneys, characterised by cryoprecipitable immune complexes which may occur in the settings of chronic infection (mainly hepatitis C virus, HCV), or without infection, particularly in the autoimmune rheumatic disease, primary Sjögren disease and lymphoproliferative disorders [30] (Fig. 1.4). These vasculitides result from the deposition of circulating immune complexes, activation of the classic complement pathway, and recruitment of neutrophils.

Symptoms from HCV-associated CV are mainly cutaneous, rheumatological, and renal. Serological and virological investigations support a pathophysiological role for HCV infection in cryoglobulinaemia with positive anti-HCV testing (80–90% of the patients), circulating HCV-RNA, HCV in lesions, and HCV-RNA in

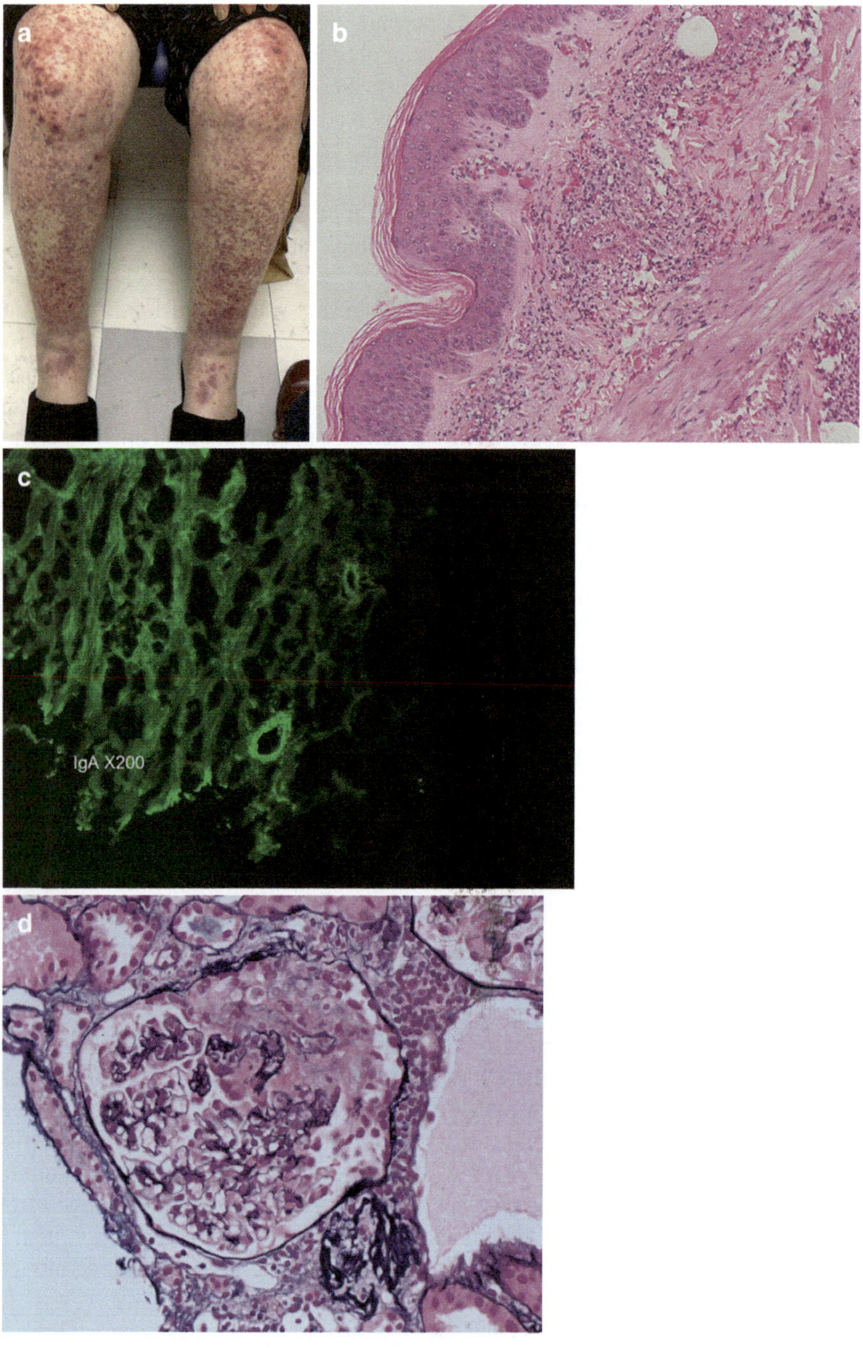

Fig. 1.3 IgA vasculitis. (**a**) Palpable purpura, (**b**) skin biopsy showing leukocytoclastic vasculitis, (**c**) IgA deposition in vessel walls, (**d**) glomerulonephritis with crescent (periodic Schiff-methenamine (PASM) stain)

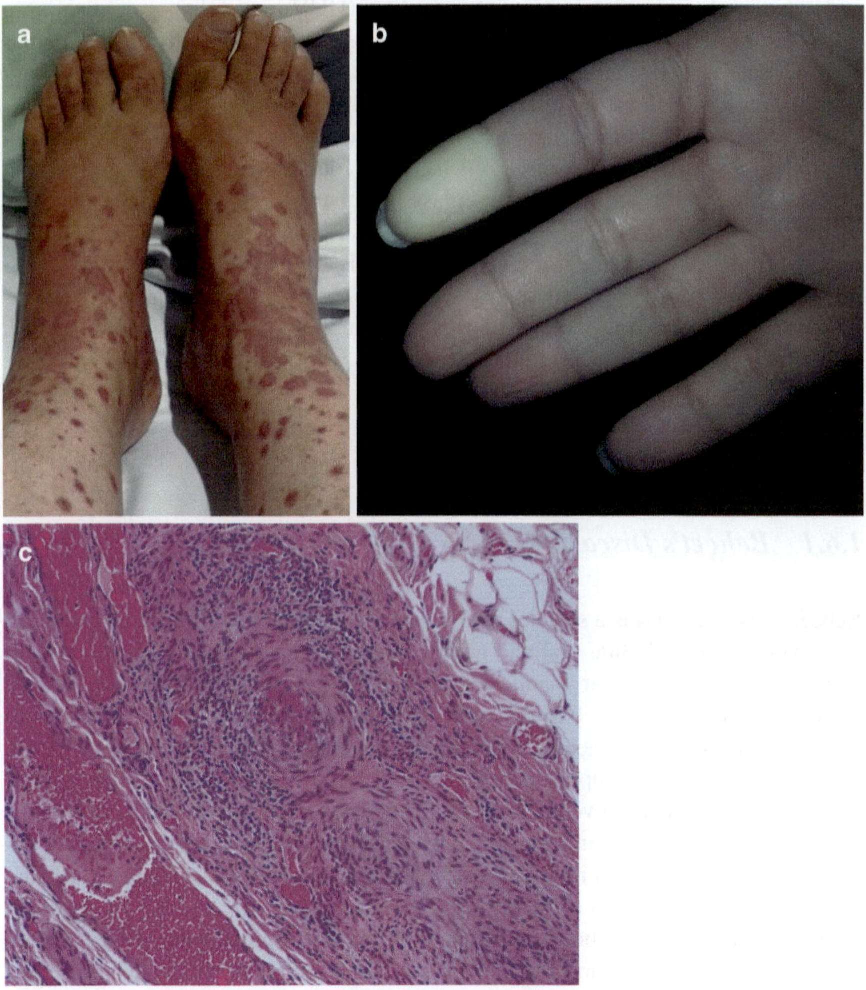

Fig. 1.4 Sjögren disease-related cryoglobulinemic vasculitis. (**a**) Cutaneous palpable purpura, (**b**) Raynaud's phenomenon, (**c**) vasculitis of the gall bladder wall

cryoprecipitate. The 1b HCV genotype is most frequently associated with cryoglobulinaemia, while genotypes 2–3 are associated with cryoglobulinaemia in coinfected HIV–HCV patients. Reported prevalence of cryoglobulins was 45.7% in HCV patients and prevalence of symptoms associated with cryoglobulins was 27%. Cryoglobulinaemia can also be secondary to HBV infection [46]. Eradication of the hepatitis virus leads to resolution of cryoglobulinaemia; short-term corticosteroids and immunosuppressants may be required for symptoms. RTX is in use for mixed cryoglobulinaemia including viral-induced disease in conjunction with antiviral medication [47]. It has a known paradoxical adverse reaction of flare of cryoglobulinaemic vasculitis, particularly in patients with underlying B cell lymphoproliferative disorder [48].

Hypocomplementaemic urticarial vasculitis (HUV, anti-C1q vasculitis) is an uncommon immune complex-mediated entity associated with anti-C1q antibodies and characterised by leukocytoclastic vasculitis, severe angioedema, pulmonary involvement, arthritis/arthralgia, glomerulonephritis, and uveitis. Treatment is symptomatic for mild disease; severe disease is treated with CYC, AZA, or MMF in combination with corticosteroids. CyA has been found useful in patients with progressive airway obstruction. RTX and plasma exchange followed by IVIg has been used in refractory cases [30].

Anti-glomerular basement membrane (anti-GBM) disease is a vasculitis affecting glomerular capillaries, pulmonary capillaries, or both, following GBM deposition of anti-GBM autoantibodies. Lung involvement causes pulmonary haemorrhage, and renal involvement causes glomerulonephritis with necrosis and crescents [1].

1.6 Variable Vessel Vasculitis

1.6.1 Behçet's Disease

Behçet's disease (BD) is a systemic inflammatory disorder characterised by multiorgan involvement including oral and genital ulcers, uveitis, skin lesions, central nervous system, and vascular manifestations [49, 50]. Superficial and deep venous thromboses are the most frequent vascular manifestations, affecting 15–40% of patients. Thrombosis characteristically occurs in unusual sites, including the inferior and superior vena cava, suprahepatic veins with Budd-Chiari syndrome, portal vein, cerebral sinuses, and right ventricle. Arterial involvement, affecting 3–5% of patients, typically presents with aneurysms affecting peripheral, visceral, and pulmonary arteries, the first sign of which may be massive haemorrhage. Vascular events in BD are promoted by inflammation of the vessel wall, with neutrophils playing a key role in the pathogenesis of thrombotic events, and coagulation components such as fibrinogen, thrombin, factor Xa, and factor VIIa amplifying the inflammatory cascade [49].

Pathophysiology of BD involves activation of both innate and adaptive immune pathways triggered by several putative pathogens, with consequent interaction between T lymphocytes (Th1 and Th17 phenotypes) and activated neutrophils. The HLA class I allele *HLA-B*51* is the major genetic risk factor in many populations, especially along the ancient Silk Route which ranged from East Asia to the Middle East and the Mediterranean area. The *HLA-A*26* allele is associated with BD independently of *HLA-B*51*, and polymorphisms in genes encoding IL-10, IL-23 receptor, IL-12 receptor, and STAT4 (signal transducer and activator of transcription 4) have been associated with BD in Turkish, Japanese, and Korean populations. Disease-associated non-synonymous variants in the familial Mediterranean fever gene (*MEFV*), and Toll-like receptor 4 gene (*TLR4*), support the involvement of innate immune responses and bacterial sensing mechanisms in BD pathogenesis [50].

BD typically runs a relapsing and remitting course, and the goal of treatment is to promptly suppress inflammatory exacerbations and recurrences to prevent irreversible organ damage. Ocular, vascular, neurological, and gastrointestinal involvement are associated with a poor prognosis; however, disease manifestations may diminish over time [51]. Control of vascular thrombosis in BD is achieved with immunosuppressant drugs rather than anticoagulants, in particular AZA or CyA in conjunction with low-dose corticosteroids for venous thrombosis, while treatment with CYC or TNFi has been successfully used for arterial involvement [49]. TNFi are also effective for control of mucocutaneous, ocular, neurological, and refractory venous thrombosis. IL-1βi may be useful for refractory disease, especially uveitis, and IL-6Ri for CNS disease [50]. The 2018-updated EULAR recommendations for BD, based on low-level evidence [51], recommend that in addition to TNFi for refractory venous thrombosis, anticoagulants may be added, provided the risk of bleeding in general is low and pulmonary artery aneurysms have been ruled out. For the management of pulmonary artery aneurysms, high dose corticosteroids and CYC are recommended, and also TNFi infliximab for refractory disease. Because of a high mortality rate in surgically treated patients, intervention should be reserved for life-threatening situations, with arterial embolisation the preferred option. For both aortic and peripheral artery aneurysms, medical management should be optimised when possible before surgical intervention, and medical management may be sufficient for small, asymptomatic aneurysms. For both pulmonary and peripheral artery aneurysms, the choice of surgical intervention between graft insertion, ligation, and bypass surgery is dictated by the size and location of the aneurysm and the surgeon's experience. Synthetic grafts are preferable since venous grafts have a higher risk of thrombosis in patients with BD. The first episode of cerebral venous thrombosis should be treated with high-dose corticosteroids followed by tapering. Anticoagulants may be added for a short duration, after screening for vascular disease at other sites [51].

1.6.2 Cogan's Syndrome

Cogan's syndrome is characterised by ocular inflammatory lesions, including interstitial keratitis, uveitis, and episcleritis, and inner ear disease, including sensorineural hearing loss and vestibular dysfunction. Vasculitic manifestations may include arteritis (affecting small, medium, or large arteries), aortitis, aortic aneurysms, and aortic and mitral valvulitis [1].

1.7 Vasculitis Associated with Systemic Disease

1.7.1 Autoimmune Rheumatic Diseases

Small vessel vasculitis may occur in the setting of known autoimmune rheumatic diseases such as rheumatoid arthritis, systemic lupus erythematosus, and Sjögren disease. Biopsy is usually not required, and if performed, will usually show a non-specific leucocytoclastic vasculitis. Vasculitis usually occurs in patients with active systemic disease, to which treatment is directed. In some cases, more aggressive treatment is required for the vasculitis itself. Cryoglobulinaemic vasculitis (discussed above) occurs in 4% of patients with primary Sjögren disease and is a predictor of the development of lymphoma and increased mortality [52].

1.7.2 IgG4-Related Disease (IgG4-RD)

IgG4-RD is a rare systemic sclerosing disorder, initially described in Japan and now increasingly recognised throughout the world. Early recognition and treatment is essential to minimise irreversible organ damage and unnecessary surgical intervention. IgG4-RD occurs most commonly in middle aged to elderly men, with a two to four-fold male preponderance [53]. It is characterised by mass-like sclerosing lesions which can involve almost any anatomic site, and many fibroinflammatory and sclerosing disorders previously considered as distinct entities are now included within the spectrum of IgG4-RD, including sclerosing cholangitis, idiopathic retroperitoneal fibrosis and mesenteritis, some forms of aortitis and periaortitis, and sclerosing sialadenitis of salivary and lacrimal glands including Kuttner tumour and Mikulicz syndrome [53]. Four predominant clinical phenotypes of IgG4-RD have recently been described [54]; (i). pancreato-hepatobiliary disease (31% of patients); (ii). retroperitoneal fibrosis and/or aortitis (24%); (iii). head and neck-limited disease (24%); (iv). classic Mikulicz syndrome with systemic involvement (22%). Aortitis occurred in 10.3% overall, and retroperitoneal fibrosis in 15.8%. In addition to sclerosing abdominal and thoracic aortitis and periaortitis, IgG4-related vasculitis occurs with a predilection for the first and second aortic branches including carotid and coronary arteries [55].

Research into the pathophysiology of IgG4-RD has identified an essential role for oligoclonally expanded CD4+ cytotoxic T lymphocyte populations (CD4+ CTLs), which secrete pro-fibrotic cytokines including IL-1β, TGFβ, and IFN-γ and are capable of perforin- and granzyme B-mediated cytolysis. They accumulate in tissue lesions, representing the dominant T cell population in affected tissues [56]. Patients with IgG4-RD also have elevations of oligoclonally expanded populations of somatically hypermutated plasmablasts, many of which are IgG4+, and because of the profound clinical responses and decline in CD4+ CTLs observed following B-cell depleting therapy, it is considered likely that activated B cells drive the activation of CD4+ CTLs in affected tissues [57]. Upon relapse, distinct plasmablast clones emerge, suggesting de novo recruitment of new plasmablast clones rather than neoplastic oligoclonal proliferations.

T follicular helper (Tfh) and T regulatory (Treg) cells also likely play a critical role in IgG4-RD, particularly with respect to class switching of B cells and induction of aberrant lymphoid follicle formation in tissues. Tfh cytokines IL-21 and IL-4 play a role in germinal centre formation, B-cell differentiation, plasmablast induction, and production of IgG4. IL-10 and TGFβ production by Treg cells also likely contributes to IgG4 class switching and fibrosis, respectively.

The role of plasmablasts and the IgG4 molecule in IgG4-RD remains uncertain. They may act to perpetuate the immune response through reactivity to specific antigens and antigen presentation to CD4+ CTLs. However, given that IgG4 has been shown to be a relatively inactive immunoglobulin subclass, without the ability to fix complement or crosslink antibodies, it has been hypothesised that IgG4 production and the frequent IgG4+ plasma cells may be a secondary or reactive phenomenon to cytokine production, rather than being intrinsically pathogenic. It has also been suggested that IgG4 has anti-inflammatory properties and may be produced in an attempt to mitigate the inflammatory response. It remains uncertain as to which autoantigens may be responsible for the robust immune response in IgG4-RD [53].

Elevation of serum IgG4 level is the most well-known laboratory feature used to support a diagnosis of IgG4-RD; however, up to half of patients with biopsy proven and clinically active IgG4-RD have normal serum IgG4 concentrations [53], and elevated serum IgG4 levels are neither sensitive nor specific for IgG4-RD. Peripheral eosinophilia, polyclonal hypergammaglobulinemia, elevated serum IgE levels, elevated CRP, and hypocomplementemia are relatively common. Histopathology is required for a definitive diagnosis of IgG4-RD and should include two or more characteristic features: (i) a dense lymphoplasmacytic infiltrate, [33] (ii) fibrosis that is typically storiform in pattern (i.e. a matted, irregularly whorled pattern), (iii) obliterative phlebitis, (iv) an increased number of IgG4+ plasma cells per high power field, and (v) an IgG4+/IgG+ plasma cell ratio of >40%. Obliterative phlebitis is the least often identified histologic feature of IgG4-RD, although the most specific [53].

Given the limitations of available biomarkers, a combination of imaging modalities, including CT, MR, and ultrasound, is the cornerstone for evaluating disease burden and activity. ^{18}F-FDG PET/CT has been validated for IgG4-RD assessment and exclusion of concomitant malignancies and provides anatomical and functional information on the extent of organ involvement and disease activity [53].

Due to uncertainty about the molecular mechanisms sustaining IgG4-RD and lack of controlled trial data, treatment is largely based on clinical experience and expert opinion. Prompt intervention is strongly advised in cases affecting vital organs (even sub-clinically) to prevent irreversible organ damage. Given the relapsing-remitting nature of the condition, maintenance therapy should be considered. Immunosuppression is generally advised for cases with prominent lymphoplasmacytic infiltrates on histological examination because they are more likely to respond to pharmacological therapy. Conversely, surgical debulking should be considered for long-standing, end-stage fibrotic lesions since they typically respond poorly to immunosuppression. Temporary stenting is frequently required for bile duct or ureteric strictures.

Corticosteroid therapy leads to swift clinical responses in the majority of patients with IgG4-RD regardless of the clinical presentation and organ involvement, thus representing the first line therapy for inducing remission. IgG4-RD relapses in up to 46% of cases during or after corticosteroid tapering, and conventional steroid-sparing agents such as AZA, MMF, MTX, and CYC have been used as maintenance therapy. In a prospective open-label trial, 97% of patients have responded to RTX at

6 months even in the absence of concomitant corticosteroid treatment, and RTX is indicated as a second-line treatment in IgG4-RD patients with recurrent or refractory disease [53].

1.8 Vasculitis Associated with Probable Aetiology

1.8.1 Infection-Associated Vasculitis

Apart from syphilitic and tuberculous aortitis, a causal relationship between infection and vasculitis has been proven in only few situations, such as HBV with PAN and less commonly SVV and CV, and HCV with CV, discussed above. Relationships between PAN and other infections, particularly streptococcal species, Klebsiella, Pseudomonas, and Yersinia, have been suggested; however, causation has not been strongly established [46]. Cutaneous rashes are associated with COVID-19 infection, including maculopapular, violacious, papular, and erythematous, with histopathologic findings of leucocytoclastic and IgA vasculitis noted [58]. Secondary vasculitis has also been attributed to COVID-19 infection, occurring as early as 2 weeks from the time of infection to later phases, including small vessel, AAV, and large vessel vasculitis typical of GCA, reviewed by Frasier et al. [59].

1.8.2 Drug-Induced Vasculitis

Members of virtually every pharmacological class have been implicated in the development of drug-induced vasculitis, and the mechanisms involved are mainly related to immune complex deposits with antigen excess. Most frequently implicated are sulphonamides, penicillin, allopurinol, and thiazides. Penicillin causes vasculitis by conjugating to serum proteins and mediating immune complex vasculitis. Drug-induced AAV has also been reported, particularly with propylthiouracil, hydralazine, allopurinol, penicillamine, and levamisole in cocaine [60], including a fatal case of methimazole-associated MPO-AAV [61]. Several cross-sectional studies reported a prevalence of propylthiouracil-induced AAV between 20% and 64%. It is essential to withdraw the inciting drug, which usually results in resolution; however, immunosuppressant therapy may be required [62]. A high level of suspicion is required, and a clue that AAV is drug-induced is the co-expression of more than one autoantibody, typically MPO-ANCA, antiphospholipid antibodies, antinuclear antibodies (ANA), and sometimes PR3-ANCA.

1.8.3 Vasculitis Associated with Cancer Immunotherapy

Immunotherapy has revolutionised the treatment of a number of types of metastatic cancer. The family of therapeutic agents known as checkpoint inhibitors (CPIs), which target "exhausted" tumour-specific T lymphocytes to incite them to an active effector phenotype and thence destroy malignant cells, is associated with a new group of immune-related adverse events (irAEs) in almost any organ system. Among these irAEs, rheumatic complications are common and seem to have features that are distinct from irAEs in other organ systems, including a highly variable time of clinical onset and the capacity to persist, possibly indefinitely, after cessation of CPI therapy [63]. Nearly every major category of rheumatic disease, including vasculitis, is mirrored by a category of irAEs resulting from CPIs. GCA with or without polymyalgia rheumatica has been reported after treatment with both anti-cytotoxic T-lymphocyte-associated protein 4 (CTLA4) and anti-PD-1 CPIs. Symptoms mirror the traditional forms of disease, including hip and shoulder girdle stiffness, temporal headache, jaw claudication, and amaurosis fugax. In TAB samples, arteritis, disruption of the elastic lamina, and intimal proliferation have been detected.

Evidence exists that checkpoint dysfunction might contribute directly to GCA pathogenesis and disease activity (discussed above), providing insights into how CPIs might cause autoimmunity. For patients with pre-existing rheumatic diseases who are treated with conventional or biologic DMARDs, as well as for patients with incident rheumatic irAEs who require DMARDs or other immunosuppressive drugs, there is concern that concomitant immunosuppressive therapy may negate the anti-tumour response from CPI therapy. In an analysis of 1959 patients from six international phase 2/3 registration trials across tumour types who received CPI therapy, 834 were treated with immunosuppression for irAEs. Analysis revealed that a higher corticosteroid peak dose for irAEs was associated with worse survival, while cumulative dose was not [64]. Too few patients received second-line immunosuppressants to confirm or reject an association with survival.

1.8.4 Vacuoles, E1 Enzyme, X-Linked, Autoinflammatory, Somatic (VEXAS)

Described in 2020, VEXAS syndrome is an adult-onset autoinflammatory disease primarily affecting males, caused by a somatic mutation of the UBA1 gene in haematopoietic progenitor cells [65]. The name VEXAS is an acronym derived from the core features of disease: V: **V**acuoles are often identified in the bone marrow stem cells of patients presenting with VEXAS. E: The **E**1 ubiquitin conjugating enzyme encoded by the UBA1 gene is mutated in patients. X: The mutated UBA1 gene is recessive and located on the **X**-chromosome and thus the disease is almost exclusively found in individuals with a single X chromosome and thus said to be X-linked. A: Patients with VEXAS present with a wide array of **A**utoinflammatory conditions. S: The mutations which cause VEXAS are **S**omatic: they are acquired throughout life, not inherited, and are not passed on to offspring.

The disease arises in late adulthood (typically after the age of 50) and causes both autoinflammatory and haematologic symptoms. Fever and skin conditions—particularly rashes resembling those seen in Sweet syndrome—are common signs. Other autoinflammatory conditions that can occur in individuals with VEXAS syndrome include periorbital angioedema, uveitis and scleritis, relapsing polychondritis, and polyarteritis nodosa. Inflammation may also affect the lungs.

Haematologic issues include macrocytic anaemia, thrombocytopaenia, and a predisposition towards developing haematologic malignancies, especially myelodysplastic syndrome. On bone marrow examination, abnormal vacuoles are usually present in precursor cells of the myeloid and erythroid lineages.

Vasculitis has been reported in nearly half of all cases with VEXAS syndrome and can affect small, medium, or large arteries. Cutaneous vasculitis subtypes include leukocytoclastic, lymphocytic, eosinophilic, urticarial, and bullous vasculitis; multi-digit gangrene due to mixed cryoglobulinemic vasculitis has also been reported. Systemic vasculitides include AAV, PAN, and GCA [66].

Symptoms are usually responsive to prednisolone but require ongoing doses of 40–60 mg daily. Treatments under investigation which provide limited efficacy include inhibitors of IL-6 (tocilizumab), IL-1 (anakinra), janus kinases (ruxolitinib), and co-stimulatory inhibitors (abatacept). Chemotherapy and stem cell transplant have been used for recalcitrant disease, but prognosis remains poor: VEXAS syndrome becomes more severe over time and carries a high mortality rate.

1.9 Vasculitis Mimics

1.9.1 Raynaud's Phenomenon

Raynaud's phenomenon (RP) is a common disorder manifested by triphasic colour change of the fingers and toes from white (vasoconstriction of pre-capillary arterioles) to blue (cyanosis from deoxygenation of sequestered blood) to red (post-ischaemic hyperaemia), occurring in 5% of the population [67]. RP may be bilateral, may be incited by cold or emotion, and usually presents with normal pulses. It is more prevalent in women than in men, and there may be a genetic predisposition. RP can be divided into primary (PRP) and secondary (SRP), the latter associated with rheumatologic as well as noninflammatory conditions. Those with PRP generally present with symptoms by 30 years of age (whereas those presenting over 40 are almost always affected by SRP) [68]. PRP is painless and is rarely associated with tissue breakdown. The most common disorders associated with SRP are systemic sclerosis (SSc/scleroderma), systemic lupus erythematosus, primary Sjögren's disease, and anti-synthetase syndrome, which are systemic autoimmune diseases associated with significant morbidity and increased mortality. Immediate referral for further evaluation and diagnosis is therefore recommended for patients suspected of having SRP, which may be the first manifestation of one of these conditions. Transition from PRP to SRP may rarely occur, but is unlikely when the original symptoms are minimal, antinuclear antibodies are absent, and nailfold capillaroscopy is normal [67, 69].

Vasomotor tone in the digital circulation results from interaction between endothelium, smooth muscle, autonomic, and sensory nerves. Thus, RP can result from alterations in various pathways. There are physiological differences between PRP and SRP: nutritional capillary blood flow is normally protected from cold-induced sympathetic vasoconstriction; this protection is mildly impaired in patients with PRP and severely interrupted in SSc. This difference probably reflects the presence of endothelial dysfunction in patients with SSc; dysfunctional endothelial cells have reduced reactivity to vasodilators, nitric oxide, and prostacyclin and can express increased thrombotic and inflammatory activity, including the increased release of the vasoconstrictor endothelin-1. The maintenance of nutritional capillary blood flow is normally ensured by the conduction of vasodilatation to upstream vessels which results from flow-mediated activation of the endothelium. Impairment of this protective mechanism, combined with structural limitations of the vascular supply in patients with SSc, probably contributes to compromised nutritional blood flow in patients with this disease, leading to tissue injury and ulceration [67].

The diagnosis of RP is usually made by history or by witnessing an episode or photograph (Fig. 1.4b). Avoidance of cold remains the most effective therapy for RP; systemic and local warming are highly effective at increasing blood flow in the skin. A variety of factors can potentially aggravate the disorder and should be avoided, including smoking and the use of sympathomimetic drugs.

Drug therapy is initiated when nonpharmacologic approaches are ineffective in reducing the severity of vasospastic attacks which are impacting quality of life. Although there is paucity of clinical trials, current evidence supports the use of calcium channel blockers, phosphodiesterase type 5 (PDE-5) inhibitors, and topical nitrates, alone or in combination. There is also some evidence to support the use of selective serotonin reuptake inhibitors such as fluoxetine and angiotensin II–receptor blockers. Prostacyclin inhibits vasoconstriction, thrombosis, inflammation, and pathologic vascular remodelling and stimulates the release of endothelium-derived nitric oxide. A systematic review supported the use of intravenous prostacyclin analogues in patients with severe SRP, with reduced severity of vasospastic attacks, increased healing, and prevention of digital ulcers. Endothelin-1 receptor antagonists failed to reduce the frequency of vasospastic attacks but decreased the development of new digital ulcers in scleroderma [67].

Surgical intervention is only considered in refractory RP, usually in the context of digital ulceration or necrosis in SSc. Cervical sympathectomy is no longer performed due to lack of long-term efficacy and an unacceptable burden of side effects. There are favourable reports for digital (but not cervical) sympathectomy and botulinum toxin injection for RP [70].

1.9.2 Thromboangitis Obliterans (TAO, Buerger's Disease)

TAO is a segmental inflammatory condition affecting small- and medium-sized arteries, veins, and nerves. It typically affects people under the age of 50 years who use tobacco, usually in the form of cigarettes. Atherosclerotic risk factors other than smoking are usually absent. Incidence varies by geographic location, with the highest prevalence of greater than 10 per 100,000 observed in the Middle East, Asia, and South-eastern Europe. Clinical manifestations of TAO include pain in a digit or extremity, digital ischaemia, Raynaud's phenomenon, distal digital ulceration, and extremity claudication. As TAO progresses, it involves more proximal portions of the limb, the most dreaded consequence being extremity gangrene and amputation. Cocaine, amphetamine, and cannabis use can present with features mimicking TAO.

The pathogenesis of TAO is largely unknown. The diagnosis of TAO is clinical, with imaging to exclude other causes of digital ischaemia such as large vessel occlusion and proximal sources of emboli. Commonly more than two extremities are involved, and subclinical disease should be sought. Markers of inflammation and autoantibodies are usually absent, and imaging demonstrates normal inflow arteries. While CTA and MRA may be helpful in excluding atherosclerosis, diagnostic angiography is often needed to demonstrate the distal involvement of arteries. A typical presentation is that of normal proximal arteries, segmental distal arterial occlusion, and corkscrew collaterals (Martorell's sign).

Distinguishing features from atherosclerosis include disease distribution and involvement of both upper and lower extremities, superficial venous thrombosis, and greater severity of pain. Biopsy, usually reserved for atypical cases, demonstrates a highly cellular thrombus and features described below [69].

Several diagnostic criteria approaches have been used to date; however in 2023, an International Consensus has been developed by the Working Group of the VAS-European Independent Foundation in Angiology/Vascular Medicine. This expert group has recommended that for a "definitive" diagnosis of Buerger's disease to be made, the presence of three features (history of current or past smoking, typical features on angiography, and typical histological features) is mandatory. For a diagnosis of "suspected" Buerger's disease, they recommended using a combination of major (history of active smoking) and minor criteria (age at disease onset <45 years, ischaemia of the lower limbs, ischaemia of one or both upper limbs, migratory thrombophlebitis, and red/blue shade of purple discolouration of oedematous fingers or toes). The Working Group recommended that a "suspected" case of Buerger's disease would be confirmed in the presence of the major criterion and four or more minor criteria. When the major criterion (smoking) is absent or <4 minor criteria are present, imaging and laboratory data can facilitate a diagnosis [71].

The evolution of TAO is often categorised into three stages. In the acute phase, inflammation affecting the small-calibre and medium-calibre (1- to 5-mm diameter) arteries and veins is observed. The primary features of TAO during the acute phase include an occlusive, highly cellular arterial thrombus, with inflammatory cell infiltrate in the thrombus and intima. Multinucleate giant cells are seen in thrombi;

however, granulomas are not observed. Although the external elastic lamina of the vessel wall may show some disruption, the internal elastic lamina remains largely intact (in contrast to atherosclerosis).

During the intermediate or subacute phase, there is progressive organisation of the occlusive thrombus, with partial recanalisation and disappearance of the micro-abscesses. A prominent inflammatory infiltrate is still present within the thrombus, but is less prominent in the vessel wall. Immunoglobulin and complement are deposited along the inner aspect of the internal elastic lamina. The chronic phase or end-stage lesion is characterised by thrombus organisation followed by recanalisation, prominent vascularisation of the media, and perivascular fibrosis. Regardless of the pathologic stage, the internal elastic lamina and the architecture of the vascular walls are well preserved in TAO, in contrast to atherosclerosis and other forms of systemic vasculitis. The granulomas seen in other forms of vasculitis (including GCA) are not found in TA and inflammatory cell infiltration is found predominantly in the intimal layer and the thrombus [72]. Immunohistochemistry demonstrates that in the acute phase, most infiltrating cells are $CD3^+$ T-cells and $CD20^+$ B cells are also prominent. Macrophages ($CD68^+$) are seen in the intima and thrombi in the acute and subacute stages. Dendritic cells ($S100^+$) are also present [73].

In the early stages of disease, there is increased expression of vascular cell adhesion molecule 1, intercellular adhesion molecule 1, and E-selectin on endothelial cell membranes. This may lead to activation of the innate immune response and later to a highly cellular intraluminal thrombus. Other purported mechanisms include delayed type hypersensitivity or toxic angiitis induced by smoking, aberrant notch signal activation, endothelial dysfunction, anti-endothelial antibodies, impaired endothelium-dependent vasodilation, abnormalities in endothelin, pro-thrombotic factors, and proinflammatory cytokines [74].

The cornerstone of treatment of TAO is complete abstinence from tobacco. Although high level evidence is lacking, intravenous prostacyclin analogues have been shown to improve ulcer healing and pain, and the endothelin-1 receptor antagonist bosentan can reduce new ischaemic lesions [75]. Distal revascularisation may prevent the need for amputations and improve quality of life; however, revascularisation is often technically not feasible because of diffuse, segmental arterial involvement and the distal nature of the disease. Distal arterial spasm during dissection and poor-quality veins owing to phlebitis are other disease-specific challenges [69, 76]. Recent evidence suggests that endovascular treatment is a valid strategy leading to an acceptable limb salvage rate for TAO patients, and surgical bypass to distal target vessels can play a role in cases of previous failed endovascular treatment or extensive soft tissue loss of the foot [76].

1.9.3 Cannabis Vasculitis

Cannabis consumption is associated with arterial complications including cerebral and myocardial infarction and limb arteritis. In their literature review, Desbois and Cacoub [77] found 80 patients reported in the literature with limb arteritis, of whom

91% were male and with an age range of 18–48 years (mean 28 years), 96% had lower limb involvement, and in 21% upper limbs were affected. Venous thrombosis was present in 22%. Most patients presented with painful distal necrosis of the extremities. Arterial imaging of the lower limbs demonstrated distal occlusions in 97%. Nearly all distal occlusions were indistinguishable from those of Thromboangiitis Obliterans. However, 30% of cases were noted to also have proximal lesions. All patients were heavy chronic cannabis smokers and only one patient was not also smoking tobacco. In this review, 58% underwent limb amputation. Cannabis abstinence is critical for symptom relief but infrequently achieved. Iloprost/epoprostanol is frequently used acutely [78].

Coronary and cerebral angiography in those with cannabis-associated cerebral and infarction often did not demonstrate plaque or haemodynamic lesions, suggesting cannabis induced a reversible vasospasm.

Histology of the arterial wall in cannabis vasculitis has been rarely reported. Disdier noted mild granulocyte and mononuclear cell infiltrate in the arterial media with fragmentation of the internal elastic lamina [79]. Sterne and Ducastaing [80] and also Kaniecki [81] demonstrated arterial thrombosis without acute inflammation in their cases, suggestive of vasospasm causing thrombosis. This is in contrast to the typical inflammatory findings noted in TAO as described above.

1.10 Fibromuscular Dysplasia (FMD)

FMD is a noninflammatory, non-atherosclerotic arterial disease that involves fibroblasts and smooth muscle cells in which there is distorted architecture and abnormal proliferation of the arterial wall of medium- or small-sized arteries.

Over 80% of individuals with FMD are women and the mean age at the time diagnosis is 52 years. The true prevalence of FMD is unknown; however, an incidence of 3–4% was found in a series of potential renal donors who underwent CT Angiography. FMD has traditionally been divided histopathologically into several types according to which arterial layer is affected and to the arteriographic pattern of disease. Medial fibroplasia was the most common type, comprising 80–90% of cases in the renal arteries. However, the recent First International Consensus on the diagnosis and management of fibromuscular dysplasia [82] stated that, in the contemporary endovascular era, where tissue was rarely obtained for histopathological examination, FMD should be classified into two types on the basis of angiographic appearance: (a) focal FMD (approximately 30% of cases) or (b) multifocal FMD (which was characterised by areas of stenosis and dilatation—the "string of beads" appearance). FMD is characterised by intra-arterial fibrotic "webs" that give rise to a "beaded" appearance on imaging studies where the beads are larger than the lumen of the artery.

FMD may affect any major arterial bed, and clinical manifestations depend on its distribution. Hypertension, a result of renal artery involvement, remains the most important clinical consequence of FMD. In some patients, the condition remains asymptomatic and incidentally discovered when imaging is performed for other reasons, while in others it may present with arterial dissection, tortuosity, aneurysm formation, and/or end organ ischaemia. In one series, renal arteries were affected in 75% and the extracranial carotid arteries in 70% of patients with FMD. Intracranial aneurysms have been reported in over 10% of cases in the United States FMD registry. Aneurysms and/or dissection were present in about 40% of patients in the US and European registries [83, 84]. FMD may affect the mesenteric, iliac, femoral, or popliteal arteries and result in visceral aneurysm formation or dissection, intermittent claudication, or (rarely) chronic limb-threatening ischaemia.

Spontaneous coronary artery dissection (SCAD) is the cause of 10–35% of cases of acute myocardial infarction (AMI) in women under 50 years of age and 50% of AMIs occurring in the post-partum period. FMD has been found to be present in 25–86% of cases of SCAD [82, 85].

In view of the association between SCAD and FMD, the International Consensus on the diagnosis and management of fibromuscular dysplasia has recommended "imaging of all vessels from brain to pelvis, at least once" in patients who have had SCAD to assess for FMD and other non-coronary arterial pathologies [82].

In contemporary FMD registries, only 2–7% of patients report an affected relative. There are currently no genetic tests that are specific for FMD. The diagnosis of FMD usually relies on a combination of clinical and imaging findings. CT Angiography (CTA) is the investigation of choice for assessment for renal and carotid/vertebral FMD. MRA can be used if CT is contraindicated. Ultrasound in highly expert hands can be used as a diagnostic test for investigation of renal FMD. However, duplex scanning is of limited value in the diagnosis of cerebrovascular FMD, due to the inability to image high cervical internal carotid lesions, vertebral and intracerebral lesions. Angiography, with pressure gradient measurements across lesion(s), is recommended when intervention for renal artery lesions is indicated.

Recently, a meta-analysis of a genome-wide association study with over 1500 cases found 5 loci independently associated with FMD [86, 87]. Subsequently, a systems genetics approach study was undertaken using blood and fibroblasts obtained by skin biopsy in 83 patients with multi-focal FMD and 71 age and sex-matched healthy controls. Bulk RNA-sequencing of the fibroblasts identified 18 gene regulatory co-expression networks. Four of these networks have acted together as an FMD-associated supernetwork (SN-A) in the arterial wall that is associated with FMD. *UBR4* (ubiquitin protein ligase E3 component n-recognin 4, also known as *P600*) was found to be a major key driver of SN-A. Further studies have demonstrated that *UBR4* plays a major role in a range of FMD-relevant cellular functions including collagen/matrix production and that UBR4 protein is expressed in vascular smooth muscle cells in the arterial wall tunica media, where FMD is known to develop [88].

1.10.1 Management of Fibromuscular Dysplasia

Antiplatelet therapy should be used in cases of FMD when there are no contraindications. Antihypertensive therapy should be consistent with standard guidelines. Good blood pressure control is particularly important in those with intracerebral aneurysms. Statins are not routinely recommended in those with FMD without hyperlipidaemia. Renal angioplasty was only associated with cure of hypertension in 36% of cases in a meta-analysis of 11 series by Trinquart. Younger patients and those with a shorter duration of hypertension were more likely to be cured [89]. Stenting is generally reserved for procedural complications. In the recent ARCADIA-POL study, the initial restenosis rate after renal angioplasty was 51%. Those who were re-treated with angioplasty were found to have a recurrent stenosis rate of 42%. Fifty-eight per cent of those treated with stenting (primarily or secondarily) suffered stent-related complications [90].

In patients with FMD and a renal or visceral artery dissection, short term (3–6 months) of anticoagulation is often prescribed, with ongoing antiplatelet therapy when anticoagulation is ceased. Interventional procedures may be indicated if there is progression of dissection over time, secondary aneurysm development, or progression of end organ malperfusion [82].

There is no data to develop recommendations for thresholds for intervention for renal and visceral artery aneurysms in those with FMD. Generally, the threshold for intervention is lower for splenic, renal, or hepatic aneurysms in women of child-bearing age due to the increased risk of rupture.

Cervical dissection (with or without neurological deficit) due to FMD should be treated in the same fashion as in those without FMD. Carotid pseudoaneurysms resulting from dissection seem to be at low risk of ischaemic events or rupture and can generally be treated conservatively [91].

Percutaneous coronary intervention in SCAD is associated with an elevated risk of complications and thus a conservative (non-interventional) approach is recommended in most cases. Most dissections heal within 30 days [85].

1.11 Summary

Much progress has been made in recent years in understanding pathogenetic mechanisms underlying the broad range of diseases we call vasculitis. The classification of vasculitis continues to evolve as new discoveries are made. The advent of biologic therapy and establishment of clinical trial consortia to enable randomised, double blind, controlled clinical trials in these rare diseases have led to major treatment advances resulting in reduced morbidity and mortality. Basic science research has enabled treatable causes such as viruses and genetic defects to be discovered to enable cures in many cases of diseases which have been once uniformly fatal. New challenges in this area are the ability to identify, treat, and monitor patients with IgG4-related disease more effectively, identify strategies to prevent or safely treat immune-related adverse events caused by cancer immunotherapy without disrupting the anti-tumour effects, increase support for research registries and sample repositories to promote basic research as well as collaborative clinical research for these rare diseases, and improve access to ground-breaking but expensive biologic therapies.

Recognition that, rather than a monophasic illness, giant cell arteritis is a chronic disorder with only a minority of patients achieving long-term remission has thrown down the gauntlet for a deeper understanding of its pathogenesis to discover new therapeutic targets. Finally, given that immune mechanisms are involved in vasculitis mimics with or without an identifiable trigger, such as TAO, further research may identify treatment targets for disease amelioration. Application of big data bioinformatic methodology incorporating genomic, epigenetic, transcriptomic, and metabolomic data holds promise to advance our understanding of the pathogenesis and management of vasculitis.

Acknowledgements We acknowledge the contribution of Sarah Downie-Doyle to the previous edition of this chapter.

Multiple Choice Questions

1. Fibromuscular disease most frequently affects:
    (a) First degree relatives of affected individuals
    (b) Males under 50 years of age
    (c) The renal and cerebrovascular arteries
    (d) Mesenteric arteries
    (e) Is most appropriately classified on the basis of histological appearance

    Answer: (c) The renal and cerebrovascular arteries

2. Thromboangiitis obliterans (Buerger's disease)
    (a) Is associated with elevated markers of inflammation and autoantibodies are usually present
    (b) Tends to involve both upper and lower extremities and superficial venous thrombosis is common
    (c) Initially involves the femoral arteries
    (d) Can frequently be treated with bypass surgery
    (e) Responds well to statin therapy

    Answer: (b) Tends to involve both upper and lower extremities and superficial venous thrombosis is common

References

1. Jennette JC, Falk RJ, Bacon PA, Basu N, Cid MC, Ferrario F, et al. 2012 Revised International Chapel Hill Consensus Conference nomenclature of vasculitides. Arthritis Rheum. 2013;65:1–11. https://doi.org/10.1002/art.37715.
2. Al-Mousawi AZ, Gurney SP, Lorenzi AR, Pohl U, Dayan M, Mollan SP. Reviewing the pathophysiology behind the advances in the management of giant cell arteritis. Ophthalmol Ther. 2019;8:177–93. https://doi.org/10.1007/s40123-019-0171-0.

3. Weyand CM, Watanabe R, Zhang H, Akiyama M, Berry GJ, Goronzy JJ. Cytokines, growth factors and proteases in medium and large vessel vasculitis. Clin Immunol. 2019;206:33–41. https://doi.org/10.1016/j.clim.2019.02.007.
4. Watanabe R, Zhang H, Berry G, Goronzy JJ, Weyand CM. Immune checkpoint dysfunction in medium and large vessel vasculitis. Am J Physiol Heart Circ Physiol. 2017;312:H1052–9. https://doi.org/10.1152/ajpheart.00024.2017.
5. Sato Y, Jain A, Ohtsuki S, Okuyama H, Sturmlechner I, Takashima Y, et al. Stem-like CD4(+) T cells in perivascular tertiary lymphoid structures sustain autoimmune vasculitis. Sci Transl Med. 2023;15:eadh0380. https://doi.org/10.1126/scitranslmed.adh0380.
6. Reichenbach S, Adler S, Bonel H, Cullmann JL, Kuchen S, Bütikofer L, et al. Magnetic resonance angiography in giant cell arteritis: results of a randomized controlled trial of tocilizumab in giant cell arteritis. Rheumatology (Oxford). 2018;57:982–6. https://doi.org/10.1093/rheumatology/key015.
7. Kaymakci MS, Boire NA, Bois MC, Elfishawi MM, Langenfeld HE, Hanson AC, et al. Persistent aortic inflammation in patients with giant cell arteritis. Autoimmun Rev. 2023;22:103411. https://doi.org/10.1016/j.autrev.2023.103411.
8. Hur B, Koster MJ, Jang JS, Weyand CM, Warrington KJ, Sung J. Global transcriptomic profiling identifies differential gene expression signatures between inflammatory and noninflammatory aortic aneurysms. Arthritis Rheumatol. 2022;74:1376–86. https://doi.org/10.1002/art.42138.
9. Ponte C, Grayson PC, Robson JC, Suppiah R, Gribbons KB, Judge A, et al. 2022 American College of Rheumatology/EULAR classification criteria for giant cell arteritis. Ann Rheum Dis. 2022;81:1647–53. https://doi.org/10.1136/ard-2022-223480.
10. Chung SH, Morcos MB, Ng B. Determinants of positive temporal artery biopsies in the Veterans Health Administration National Database Cohort. Arthritis Care Res. 2020;72:699–704. https://doi.org/10.1002/acr.23897.
11. Dejaco C, Ramiro S, Duftner C, Besson FL, Bley TA, Blockmans D, et al. EULAR recommendations for the use of imaging in large vessel vasculitis in clinical practice. Ann Rheum Dis. 2018;77:636–43. https://doi.org/10.1136/annrheumdis-2017-212649.
12. Sammel AM, Hsiao E, Schembri G, Nguyen K, Brewer J, Schrieber L, et al. Diagnostic accuracy of PET/CT scan of the head, neck and chest for giant cell arteritis: the double-blinded giant cell arteritis and PET scan (GAPS) study. Arthritis Rheumatol. 2019;71:1319–28. https://doi.org/10.1002/art.40864.
13. Maz M, Chung SA, Abril A, Langford CA, Gorelik M, Guyatt G, et al. 2021 American College of Rheumatology/Vasculitis Foundation guideline for the management of giant cell arteritis and Takayasu arteritis. Arthritis Rheumatol. 2021;73:1349–65. https://doi.org/10.1002/art.41774.
14. Moreel L, Coudyzer W, Boeckxstaens L, Betrains A, Molenberghs G, Vanderschueren S, et al. Association between vascular (^{18})F-fluorodeoxyglucose uptake at diagnosis and change in aortic dimensions in giant cell arteritis: a cohort study. Ann Intern Med. 2023;176:1321–9. https://doi.org/10.7326/m23-0679.
15. Strand V, Dimonaco S, Tuckwell K, Klearman M, Collinson N, Stone JH. Health-related quality of life in patients with giant cell arteritis treated with tocilizumab in a phase 3 randomised controlled trial. Arthritis Res Ther. 2019;21:64. https://doi.org/10.1186/s13075-019-1837-7.
16. Samec MJ, Rakholiya J, Langenfeld H, Crowson CS, Abril A, Wang B, et al. Relapse risk and safety of long-term tocilizumab use among patients with giant cell arteritis: a single-enterprise cohort study. J Rheumatol. 2023;50:1310–7. https://doi.org/10.3899/jrheum.2022-1214.
17. Venhoff N, Schmidt WA, Bergner R, Rech J, Unger L, Tony HP, et al. Safety and efficacy of secukinumab in patients with giant cell arteritis (TitAIN): a randomised, double-blind, placebo-controlled, phase 2 trial. Lancet Rheumatol. 2023;5:e341–e50. https://doi.org/10.1016/s2665-9913(23)00101-7.
18. Loricera J, Tofade T, Prieto-Peña D, Romero-Yuste S, de Miguel E, Riveros-Frutos A, et al. Effectiveness of janus kinase inhibitors in relapsing giant cell arteritis in real-world clinical

practice and review of the literature. Arthritis Res Ther. 2024;26:116. https://doi.org/10.1186/s13075-024-03314-9.
19. Prieto-González S, Arguis P, García-Martínez A, Espígol-Frigolé G, Tavera-Bahillo I, Butjosa M, et al. Large vessel involvement in biopsy-proven giant cell arteritis: prospective study in 40 newly diagnosed patients using CT angiography. Ann Rheum Dis. 2012;71:1170–6. https://doi.org/10.1136/annrheumdis-2011-200865.
20. Kebed DT, Bois JP, Connolly HM, Scott CG, Bowen JM, Warrington KJ, et al. Spectrum of aortic disease in the giant cell arteritis population. Am J Cardiol. 2018;121:501–8. https://doi.org/10.1016/j.amjcard.2017.11.011.
21. Unizony S, Stone JH, Stone JR. New treatment strategies in large-vessel vasculitis. Curr Opin Rheumatol. 2013;25:3–9. https://doi.org/10.1097/BOR.0b013e32835b133a.
22. Watts RA. Evolving concepts in classification of systemic vasculitis: where are we and what is the way forward? Int J Rheum Dis. 2019;22(Suppl 1):21–7. https://doi.org/10.1111/1756-185X.13304.
23. Grayson PC, Ponte C, Suppiah R, Robson JC, Gribbons KB, Judge A, et al. 2022 American College of Rheumatology/EULAR classification criteria for Takayasu arteritis. Ann Rheum Dis. 2022;81:1654–60. https://doi.org/10.1136/ard-2022-223482.
24. Ozen S. The changing face of polyarteritis nodosa and necrotizing vasculitis. Nat Rev Rheumatol. 2017;13:381–6. https://doi.org/10.1038/nrrheum.2017.68.
25. Chung SA, Gorelik M, Langford CA, Maz M, Abril A, Guyatt G, et al. 2021 American College of Rheumatology/Vasculitis Foundation guideline for the management of polyarteritis nodosa. Arthritis Care Res (Hoboken). 2021;73:1061–70. https://doi.org/10.1002/acr.24633.
26. Jone PN, Tremoulet A, Choueiter N, Dominguez SR, Harahsheh AS, Mitani Y, et al. Update on diagnosis and management of Kawasaki disease: a scientific statement from the American Heart Association. Circulation. 2024;150:e481–500. https://doi.org/10.1161/cir.0000000000001295.
27. Dietz SM, van Stijn D, Burgner D, Levin M, Kuipers IM, Hutten BA, et al. Dissecting Kawasaki disease: a state-of-the-art review. Eur J Pediatr. 2017;176:995–1009. https://doi.org/10.1007/s00431-017-2937-5.
28. Al-Hussain T, Hussein MH, Conca W, Al Mana H, Akhtar M. Pathophysiology of ANCA-associated vasculitis. Adv Anat Pathol. 2017;24:226–34. https://doi.org/10.1097/PAP.0000000000000154.
29. Coit P, Direskeneli H, Sawalha AH. An update on the role of epigenetics in systemic vasculitis. Curr Opin Rheumatol. 2018;30:4–15. https://doi.org/10.1097/BOR.0000000000000451.
30. Lopalco G, Rigante D, Venerito V, Emmi G, Anelli MG, Lapadula G, et al. Management of small vessel vasculitides. Curr Rheumatol Rep. 2016;18:36. https://doi.org/10.1007/s11926-016-0580-1.
31. Sharma A, Dogra S, Sharma K. Granulomatous vasculitis. Dermatol Clin. 2015;33:475–87. https://doi.org/10.1016/j.det.2015.03.012.
32. Ikeda M, Ohshima N, Kawashima M, Shiina M, Kitani M, Suzukawa M. Severe asthma where eosinophilic granulomatosis with polyangiitis became apparent after the discontinuation of dupilumab. Intern Med. 2022;61:755–9. https://doi.org/10.2169/internalmedicine.7990-21.
33. Jennette JC, Falk RJ, Andrassy K, Bacon PA, Churg J, Gross WL, et al. Nomenclature of systemic vasculitides. Arthritis Rheum. 1994;37:187–92. https://doi.org/10.1002/art.1780370206.
34. Robson JC, Grayson PC, Ponte C, Suppiah R, Craven A, Judge A, et al. 2022 American College of Rheumatology/European Alliance of Associations for rheumatology classification criteria for granulomatosis with polyangiitis. Arthritis Rheumatol. 2022;74:393–9. https://doi.org/10.1002/art.41986.
35. Suppiah R, Robson JC, Grayson PC, Ponte C, Craven A, Khalid S, et al. 2022 American College of Rheumatology/European Alliance of Associations for rheumatology classification criteria for microscopic polyangiitis. Arthritis Rheumatol. 2022;74:400–6. https://doi.org/10.1002/art.41983.

36. Chung SA, Langford CA, Maz M, Abril A, Gorelik M, Guyatt G, et al. 2021 American College of Rheumatology/Vasculitis Foundation guideline for the management of antineutrophil cytoplasmic antibody-associated vasculitis. Arthritis Care Res (Hoboken). 2021;73:1088–105. https://doi.org/10.1002/acr.24634.
37. Hellmich B, Sanchez-Alamo B, Schirmer JH, Berti A, Blockmans D, Cid MC, et al. EULAR recommendations for the management of ANCA-associated vasculitis: 2022 update. Ann Rheum Dis. 2024;83:30–47. https://doi.org/10.1136/ard-2022-223764.
38. Walsh M, Merkel PA, Peh CA, Szpirt WM, Puéchal X, Fujimoto S, et al. Plasma exchange and glucocorticoids in severe ANCA-associated vasculitis. N Engl J Med. 2020;382:622–31. https://doi.org/10.1056/NEJMoa1803537.
39. Furuta S, Nakagomi D, Kobayashi Y, Hiraguri M, Sugiyama T, Amano K, et al. Effect of reduced-dose vs high-dose glucocorticoids added to rituximab on remission induction in ANCA-associated vasculitis: a randomized clinical trial. JAMA. 2021;325:2178–87. https://doi.org/10.1001/jama.2021.6615.
40. Jayne DRW, Merkel PA, Schall TJ, Bekker P. Avacopan for the treatment of ANCA-associated vasculitis. N Engl J Med. 2021;384:599–609. https://doi.org/10.1056/NEJMoa2023386.
41. Guillevin L, Pagnoux C, Karras A, Khouatra C, Aumaître O, Cohen P, et al. Rituximab versus azathioprine for maintenance in ANCA-associated vasculitis. N Engl J Med. 2014;371:1771–80. https://doi.org/10.1056/NEJMoa1404231.
42. Wechsler ME, Akuthota P, Jayne D, Khoury P, Klion A, Langford CA, et al. Mepolizumab or placebo for eosinophilic granulomatosis with polyangiitis. N Engl J Med. 2017;376:1921–32. https://doi.org/10.1056/NEJMoa1702079.
43. Wechsler ME, Nair P, Terrier B, Walz B, Bourdin A, Jayne DRW, et al. Benralizumab versus mepolizumab for eosinophilic granulomatosis with polyangiitis. N Engl J Med. 2024;390:911–21. https://doi.org/10.1056/NEJMoa2311155.
44. Hetland LE, Susrud KS, Lindahl KH, Bygum A. Henoch-Schonlein purpura: a literature review. Acta Derm Venereol. 2017;97:1160–6. https://doi.org/10.2340/00015555-2733.
45. Lopez-Mejias R, Castaneda S, Genre F, Remuzgo-Martinez S, Carmona FD, Llorca J, et al. Genetics of immunoglobulin-A vasculitis (Henoch-Schonlein purpura): an updated review. Autoimmun Rev. 2018;17:301–15. https://doi.org/10.1016/j.autrev.2017.11.024.
46. Belizna CC, Hamidou MA, Levesque H, Guillevin L, Shoenfeld Y. Infection and vasculitis. Rheumatology (Oxford). 2009;48:475–82. https://doi.org/10.1093/rheumatology/kep026.
47. Quartuccio L, Bortoluzzi A, Scirè CA, Marangoni A, Del Frate G, Treppo E, et al. Management of mixed cryoglobulinemia with rituximab: evidence and consensus-based recommendations from the Italian Study Group of Cryoglobulinemia (GISC). Clin Rheumatol. 2023;42:359–70. https://doi.org/10.1007/s10067-022-06391-w.
48. Sy-Go JPT, Thongprayoon C, Herrera Hernandez LP, Zoghby Z, Leung N, Manohar S. Rituximab-associated flare of cryoglobulinemic vasculitis. Kidney Int Rep. 2021;6:2840–9. https://doi.org/10.1016/j.ekir.2021.08.024.
49. Emmi G, Bettiol A, Silvestri E, Di Scala G, Becatti M, Fiorillo C, et al. Vascular Behcet's syndrome: an update. Intern Emerg Med. 2018;176:995–1009. https://doi.org/10.1007/s11739-018-1991-y.
50. Emmi G, Silvestri E, Squatrito D, D'Elios MM, Ciucciarelli L, Prisco D, et al. Behçet's syndrome pathophysiology and potential therapeutic targets. Intern Emerg Med. 2014;9:257–65. https://doi.org/10.1007/s11739-013-1036-5.
51. Hatemi G, Christensen R, Bang D, Bodaghi B, Celik AF, Fortune F, et al. 2018 Update of the EULAR recommendations for the management of Behçet's syndrome. Ann Rheum Dis. 2018;77:808–18. https://doi.org/10.1136/annrheumdis-2018-213225.
52. Retamozo S, Gheitasi H, Quartuccio L, Kostov B, Corazza L, Bové A, et al. Cryoglobulinaemic vasculitis at diagnosis predicts mortality in primary Sjögren syndrome: analysis of 515 patients. Rheumatology. 2016;55:1443–51. https://doi.org/10.1093/rheumatology/kew194.
53. Bledsoe JR, Della-Torre E, Rovati L, Deshpande V. IgG4-related disease: review of the histopathologic features, differential diagnosis, and therapeutic approach. APMIS. 2018;126:459–76. https://doi.org/10.1111/apm.12845.

54. Wallace ZS, Zhang Y, Perugino CA, Naden R, Choi HK, Stone JH. Clinical phenotypes of IgG4-related disease: an analysis of two international cross-sectional cohorts. Ann Rheum Dis. 2019;78:406–12. https://doi.org/10.1136/annrheumdis-2018-214603.
55. Katz G, Hedgire SH, Stone JR, Perez-Espina S, Fernandes A, Perugino CA, et al. IgG4-related disease as a variable-vessel vasculitis: a case series of 13 patients with medium-sized coronary artery involvement. Semin Arthritis Rheum. 2023;60:152184. https://doi.org/10.1016/j.semarthrit.2023.152184.
56. Mattoo H, Mahajan VS, Maehara T, Deshpande V, Della-Torre E, Wallace ZS, et al. Clonal expansion of CD4+ cytotoxic T lymphocytes in patients with IgG4-related disease. J Allergy Clin Immunol. 2016;138:825–38. https://doi.org/10.1016/j.jaci.2015.12.1330.
57. Mattoo H, Stone JH, Pillai S. Clonally expanded cytotoxic CD4+ T cells and the pathogenesis of IgG4-related disease. Autoimmunity. 2017;50:19–24. https://doi.org/10.1080/08916934.2017.1280029.
58. Wong K, Farooq Alam Shah MU, Khurshid M, Ullah I, Tahir MJ, Yousaf Z. COVID-19 associated vasculitis: a systematic review of case reports and case series. Ann Med Surg (Lond). 2022;74:103249. https://doi.org/10.1016/j.amsu.2022.103249.
59. Frasier KM, Gallagher-Poehls C, Cochrane M, Roy D. Secondary vasculitis attributable to post-COVID syndrome. Cureus. 2023;15:e44119. https://doi.org/10.7759/cureus.44119.
60. Choi HK, Merkel PA, Walker AM, Niles JL. Drug-associated antineutrophil cytoplasmic antibody–positive vasculitis: prevalence among patients with high titers of antimyeloperoxidase antibodies. Arthritis Rheum. 2000;43:405. https://doi.org/10.1002/1529-0131(200002)43:2<405::aid-anr22>3.0.co;2-5.
61. Hacking S, Uppal NN, Khan N, Ionescu M, Bijol V. Systemic p-ANCA vasculitis with fatal outcome, arising in the setting of methimazole use. Clin Nephrol Case Stud. 2019;7:23–6. https://doi.org/10.5414/CNCS109759.
62. Radic M, Martinovic Kaliterna D, Radic J. Drug-induced vasculitis: a clinical and pathological review. Neth J Med. 2012;70:12–7.
63. Calabrese LH, Calabrese C, Cappelli LC. Rheumatic immune-related adverse events from cancer immunotherapy. Nat Rev Rheumatol. 2018;14:569–79. https://doi.org/10.1038/s41584-018-0074-9.
64. Verheijden RJ, de Groot JS, Fabriek BO, Hew MN, May AM, Suijkerbuijk KPM. Corticosteroids for immune-related adverse events and checkpoint inhibitor efficacy: analysis of six clinical trials. J Clin Oncol. 2024;42:3713–24. https://doi.org/10.1200/jco.24.00191.
65. Beck DB, Ferrada MA, Sikora KA, Ombrello AK, Collins JC, Pei W, et al. Somatic mutations in UBA1 and severe adult-onset autoinflammatory disease. N Engl J Med. 2020;383:2628–38. https://doi.org/10.1056/NEJMoa2026834.
66. Koster MJ, Warrington KJ. VEXAS within the spectrum of rheumatologic disease. Semin Hematol. 2021;58:218–25. https://doi.org/10.1053/j.seminhematol.2021.10.002.
67. Wigley FM, Flavahan NA. Raynaud's phenomenon. N Engl J Med. 2016;375:556–65. https://doi.org/10.1056/NEJMra1507638.
68. Hughes M, Allanore Y, Chung L, Pauling JD, Denton CP, Matucci-Cerinic M. Raynaud phenomenon and digital ulcers in systemic sclerosis. Nat Rev Rheumatol. 2020;16:208–21. https://doi.org/10.1038/s41584-020-0386-4.
69. Weinberg I, Weinberg MD. Non-atherosclerotic arterial disorders of the lower extremities. In: Lanzer P, editor. PanVascular medicine. Berlin, Heidelberg: Springer; 2015. p. 3007–30. https://doi.org/10.1007/978-3-642-37078-6_113.
70. Pauling JD, Hughes M, Pope JE. Raynaud's phenomenon-an update on diagnosis, classification and management. Clin Rheumatol. 2019;38:3317–30. https://doi.org/10.1007/s10067-019-04745-5.
71. Fazeli B, Poredos P, Kozak M, Pecsvarady Z, Catalano M, Al Salman MM, et al. Diagnostic criteria for Buerger's disease: international consensus of VAS – European Independent Foundation in Angiology/Vascular Medicine. Int Angiol. 2023;42:396–401. https://doi.org/10.23736/s0392-9590.23.05098-8.

72. Akar AR, İnan MB, Baran Ç. Thromboangiitis obliterans. Curr Treat Options Rheum. 2016;2:178–95. https://doi.org/10.1007/s40674-016-0047-6.
73. Kobayashi M, Sugimoto M, Komori K. Endarteritis obliterans in the pathogenesis of Buerger's disease from the pathological and immunohistochemical points of view. Circ J. 2014;78:2819–26. https://doi.org/10.1253/circj.cj-14-0656.
74. Dellalibera-Joviliano R, Joviliano EE, Silva JS, Evora PR. Activation of cytokines corroborate with development of inflammation and autoimmunity in thromboangiitis obliterans patients. Clin Exp Immunol. 2012;170:28–35. https://doi.org/10.1111/j.1365-2249.2012.04624.x.
75. Narvaez J, Garcia-Gomez C, Alvarez L, Santo P, Aparicio M, Pascual M, et al. Efficacy of bosentan in patients with refractory thromboangiitis obliterans (Buerger disease): a case series and review of the literature. Medicine (Baltimore). 2016;95:e5511. https://doi.org/10.1097/MD.0000000000005511.
76. Lee CY, Choi K, Kwon H, Ko GY, Han Y, Kwon TW, et al. Outcomes of endovascular treatment versus bypass surgery for critical limb ischemia in patients with thromboangiitis obliterans. PLoS One. 2018;13:e0205305. https://doi.org/10.1371/journal.pone.0205305.
77. Desbois AC, Cacoub P. Cannabis-associated arterial disease. Ann Vasc Surg. 2013;27:996–1005. https://doi.org/10.1016/j.avsg.2013.01.002.
78. Galyfos G, Kerasidis S, Kastrisios G, Giannakakis S, Sachmpazidis I, Anastasiadou C, et al. Conservative treatment of patients with thromboangiitis obliterans or cannabis-associated arteritis presenting with critical lower limb ischaemia. Vasa. 2017;46:471–5. https://doi.org/10.1024/0301-1526/a000649.
79. Disdier P, Granel B, Serratrice J, Constans J, Michon-Pasturel U, Hachulla E, et al. Cannabis arteritis revisited--ten new case reports. Angiology. 2001;52:1–5. https://doi.org/10.1177/000331970105200101.
80. Sterne J, Ducastaing C. Arteritis caused by Cannabis indica. Arch Mal Coeur Vaiss. 1960;53:143–7.
81. Kaniecki T, Huso TH, Haque UJ. Cannabis arteritis revisited: a case report with distinct pathologic features and review of the literature. Rheumatology (Oxford). 2024;63:e190–e2. https://doi.org/10.1093/rheumatology/kead683.
82. Gornik HL, Persu A, Adlam D, Aparicio LS, Azizi M, Boulanger M, et al. First International Consensus on the diagnosis and management of fibromuscular dysplasia. Vasc Med. 2019;24:164–89. https://doi.org/10.1177/1358863x18821816.
83. Kadian-Dodov D, Gornik HL, Gu X, Froehlich J, Bacharach JM, Chi YW, et al. Dissection and aneurysm in patients with fibromuscular dysplasia: findings from the U.S. registry for FMD. J Am Coll Cardiol. 2016;68:176–85. https://doi.org/10.1016/j.jacc.2016.04.044.
84. Plouin PF, Baguet JP, Thony F, Ormezzano O, Azarine A, Silhol F, et al. High prevalence of multiple arterial bed lesions in patients with fibromuscular dysplasia: the ARCADIA registry (assessment of renal and cervical artery dysplasia). Hypertension. 2017;70:652–8. https://doi.org/10.1161/hypertensionaha.117.09539.
85. Le Q, Bhandari A, Fleischer J, Murthy A. Spontaneous coronary artery dissection and fibromuscular dysplasia: a case series and genetic links. Cureus. 2024;16:e54105. https://doi.org/10.7759/cureus.54105.
86. Georges A, Yang ML, Berrandou TE, Bakker MK, Dikilitas O, Kiando SR, et al. Author correction: Genetic investigation of fibromuscular dysplasia identifies risk loci and shared genetics with common cardiovascular diseases. Nat Commun. 2022;13:2251. https://doi.org/10.1038/s41467-022-29921-1.
87. Georges A, Yang ML, Berrandou TE, Bakker MK, Dikilitas O, Kiando SR, et al. Genetic investigation of fibromuscular dysplasia identifies risk loci and shared genetics with common cardiovascular diseases. Nat Commun. 2021;12:6031. https://doi.org/10.1038/s41467-021-26174-2.
88. d'Escamard V, Kadian-Dodov D, Ma L, Lu S, King A, Xu Y, et al. Integrative gene regulatory network analysis discloses key driver genes of fibromuscular dysplasia. Nat Cardiovasc Res. 2024;3:1098–122. https://doi.org/10.1038/s44161-024-00533-w.

89. Trinquart L, Mounier-Vehier C, Sapoval M, Gagnon N, Plouin PF. Efficacy of revascularization for renal artery stenosis caused by fibromuscular dysplasia: a systematic review and meta-analysis. Hypertension. 2010;56:525–32. https://doi.org/10.1161/hypertensionaha.110.152918.
90. Kądziela J, Jóźwik-Plebanek K, Pappaccogli M, van der Niepen P, Prejbisz A, Dobrowolski P, et al. Risks and benefits of renal artery stenting in fibromuscular dysplasia: lessons from the ARCADIA-POL study. Vasc Med. 2024;29:50–7. https://doi.org/10.1177/1358863x231210523.
91. Larsson SC, King A, Madigan J, Levi C, Norris JW, Markus HS. Prognosis of carotid dissecting aneurysms: results from CADISS and a systematic review. Neurology. 2017;88:646–52. https://doi.org/10.1212/wnl.0000000000003617.

Key References

Chung SA, Gorelik M, Langford CA, Maz M, Abril A, Guyatt G, et al. 2021 American College of Rheumatology/Vasculitis Foundation guideline for the management of polyarteritis nodosa. Arthritis Care Res (Hoboken). 2021;73:1061–70. https://doi.org/10.1002/acr.24633.
Gornik HL, Persu A, Adlam D, Aparicio LS, Azizi M, Boulanger M, et al. First International Consensus on the diagnosis and management of fibromuscular dysplasia. Vasc Med. 2019;24:164–89. https://doi.org/10.1177/1358863x18821816.
Hur B, Koster MJ, Jang JS, Weyand CM, Warrington KJ, Sung J. Global transcriptomic profiling identifies differential gene expression signatures between inflammatory and noninflammatory aortic aneurysms. Arthritis Rheumatol. 2022;74:1376–86. https://doi.org/10.1002/art.42138.
Kaymakci MS, Boire NA, Bois MC, Elfishawi MM, Langenfeld HE, Hanson AC, et al. Persistent aortic inflammation in patients with giant cell arteritis. Autoimmun Rev. 2023;22:103411. https://doi.org/10.1016/j.autrev.2023.103411.
Kebed DT, Bois JP, Connolly HM, Scott CG, Bowen JM, Warrington KJ, Makol A, Greason KL, Schaff HV, Anavekar NS. Spectrum of aortic disease in the giant cell arteritis population. Am J Cardiol. 2018;121(4):501–8. https://doi.org/10.1016/j.amjcard.2017.11.011.
Koster MJ, Warrington KJ. VEXAS within the spectrum of rheumatologic disease. Semin Hematol. 2021;58(4):218–25. ISSN 0037-1963. https://doi.org/10.1053/j.seminhematol.2021.10.002.
Maz M, Chung SA, Abril A, Langford CA, Gorelik M, Guyatt G, et al. 2021 American College of Rheumatology/Vasculitis Foundation guideline for the management of giant cell arteritis and Takayasu arteritis. Arthritis Rheumatol. 2021;73:1349–65. https://doi.org/10.1002/art.41774.
Moreel L, Coudyzer W, Boeckxstaens L, Betrains A, Molenberghs G, Vanderschueren S, Claus E, Van Laere K, Blockmans D. Association between vascular ^{18}F-fluorodeoxyglucose uptake at diagnosis and change in aortic dimensions in giant cell arteritis: a cohort study. Ann Intern Med. 2023;176:1321–9. https://doi.org/10.7326/M23-0679.
Sato Y, Jain A, Ohtsuki S, Okuyama H, Sturmlechner I, Takashima Y, et al. Stem-like CD4(+) T cells in perivascular tertiary lymphoid structures sustain autoimmune vasculitis. Sci Transl Med. 2023;15:eadh0380. https://doi.org/10.1126/scitranslmed.adh0380.

Chapter 2
Sepsis and Septic Shock

Benjamin Reddi

SN Flashcards
Test your learning and check your understanding of this book's contents: use the "Springer Nature Flashcards" app to access questions using ▶ https://sn.pub/wppvze. To use the app, please follow the instructions in Chap. 1.

Key Learning Points
- Sepsis is defined as life-threatening organ dysfunction caused by a dysregulated host response to infection.
- The archetypal immune response to infection involves (i) recognising 'non-self' pathogenic material, (ii) recruiting and activating immune effector cells, (iii) localising and neutralising any pathogen, (iv) healing.
- Cytokines such as interleukins and interferon (IFN) attract and activate local and circulating immune cells which amplify the inflammatory cascade and exert direct microbicidal activity.
- Sepsis involves activation of both inflammatory and anti-inflammatory pathways. While anti-inflammatory cytokines and cell types are essential to regulate the immune response, excessive immune suppression in sepsis may impair host defence against infection promoting broad-ranging dysregulation of cardiovascular, coagulation, neuronal, bioenergetic, endocrine, and other systems.
- Early source control plus rational, timely antibiotic selection and evidence-based organ support are crucial to maximise survival. As yet, no specific immunomodulatory therapies have proven beneficial.

B. Reddi (✉)
Intensive Care Unit, Royal Adelaide Hospital, Adelaide, South Australia
e-mail: benjamin.reddi@sa.gov.au

R. Fitridge et al. (eds.), *Pathophysiology of Vascular Disease*,
https://doi.org/10.1007/978-3-032-31459-8_2

- Management of septic circulatory shock is complex; septic shock progresses through three phases—(i) non-progressive phase of effective physiological compensation, (ii) a progressive stage of worsening hypoperfusion and metabolic derangement, and (iii) an irreversible stage at which tissue injury is so severe that restoring circulation cannot prevent death. Fluid, vasopressor, and inotropic therapy should be titrated and responsive to individual patient parameters.

2.1 Introduction and Definitions

Sepsis is the primary cause of death from infection. It has been traditionally conceptualised as an excessive host inflammatory response provoked by uncontrolled infection, and until recently, *sepsis* has been defined as infection causing the development of two or more systemic inflammatory response syndrome (SIRS) criteria (Box 2.1), and *severe sepsis* as sepsis complicated by organ dysfunction [1]. Sepsis, severe sepsis, and *septic shock* 'sepsis-induced hypotension persisting despite adequate fluid resuscitation' were considered increasingly perilous phases of a potentially fatal disease spectrum.

Box 2.1
SIRS (systemic inflammatory response syndrome) is defined as two or more of:

- Temperature >38 °C OR <36 °C
- Heart rate >90/min
- Respiratory rate >20/min or $PaCO_2$ <32 mmHg
- Leucocyte count >12,000/mm^3 or <4000/mm^3 or >10% immature bands

Recently, this paradigm has been challenged. Not only is sepsis now recognised to involve activation of both inflammatory and anti-inflammatory pathways, but also broad-ranging dysregulation of cardiovascular, coagulation, bioenergetic, and other systems. These manifestations are not captured by a simple inflammation-based definition and, not surprisingly, the SIRS-based definition shows limited accuracy in identifying patients at risk of poor outcome [2–4], nor is death limited to those who develop septic shock.

Improved understanding of the pathobiology of sepsis informed the Third International Consensus Definition for Sepsis and Septic Shock (SEPSIS-3): *sepsis is life-threatening organ dysfunction caused by a dysregulated host response to infection* [5]. Organ dysfunction is defined as an increase in the Sequential [Sepsis-related] Organ Failure Assessment (SOFA) score of 2 points or more (Table 2.1) [6] and 'infection' as the invasion of sterile tissue by organisms resulting in infectious pathology. Thus defined, sepsis is associated with >10% in-hospital mortality.

Table 2.1 Sequential [Sepsis-related] Organ Failure Assessment (SOFA) score

	Respiratory	Cardiovascular	Liver	Coagulation	CNS	Renal
Score	PaO_2/FiO_2 mmHg	Mean arterial pressure/ catecholamines	Bilirubin μmol/L	Platelets $\times 10^3/\mu L$	Glasgow coma score	Creatinine μmol/L
0	≥400	MAP ≥70	<20	≥150	15	<110
1	<400	MAP <70	20–32	<150	13–14	110–170
2	<300	Dopamine <5[a] or any dobutamine dose	33–101	<100	10–12	171–299
3	<200[b]	Dopamine 5.1–15[a] or adrenaline ≤0.1[a] or noradrenaline ≤0.1[a]	102–204	<50	6-9	300–440 or Urine output <500 mL/d
4	<100[b]	Dopamine >15[a] or adrenaline >0.1[a] or noradrenaline >0.1[a]	>204	<20	<6	>440 or Urine output <200 mL/d

[a]Catecholamine doses are given as μg/kg/min for at least 1 h
[b]With respiratory support

Non-infectious injuries such as burns, severe trauma, or pancreatitis can elicit a similar process which shares many common features. Patients with sepsis and persisting hypotension requiring vasopressors to maintain mean arterial pressure (MAP) ≥65 mmHg and a serum lactate level >2 mmol/L despite adequate volume resuscitation have *septic shock*, a subtype of sepsis in which underlying circulatory and cellular/metabolic abnormalities are profound enough to substantially increase mortality. Hospital mortality from septic shock exceeds 40% [5]. Although the SEPSIS-3 definition better discriminates those patients with presumed infection at high risk of poor outcome, challenges remain. No unambiguous clinical criteria or investigation results uniquely identify a septic patient and it remains unclear how a clinician identifies a 'dysregulated host response' at the bedside. Furthermore, commonly no causative organism is identified and the diagnosis of infection, and thus sepsis, remains presumptive. Nevertheless, the new definition utilises objective, easily obtained variables, reflects the complex pathobiology of sepsis, and identifies a population of patients with infection at high risk of death. It is widely accepted as the basis for sepsis research and quality assurance.

2.2 Epidemiology

In 2017, an estimated 49 million cases of sepsis were recorded globally. The associated 11 million sepsis-related fatalities represented approximately 20% of all global deaths [7]. Age-standardised sepsis incidence and mortality are decreasing but vary substantially across regions. A systematic review of randomised controlled trials reporting between 2009 and 2019 identified that, on average, 34.7% of patients with septic shock managed in North America, Europe, and Australasia died within 30 days [8]. However, most cases of sepsis occur in the developing world where the age-standardised mortality rate is disproportionately high and the breadth of causative and contributing pathogens—malaria, human immunodeficiency virus, mycobacterium tuberculosis—poses additional challenges. Risk factors for developing sepsis include extremes of age (<2 or >55 years), concurrent chronic and serious illness (such as cancer, diabetes), impaired immunity (including breach of natural barriers, burns, indwelling lines, surgical wounds), and malnutrition.

Healthcare costs are substantial, from critical care requirements during acute illness to ongoing support required for the high proportion of survivors suffering long-term cognitive and functional impairment [9]. A study, including over 12,000 previously employed patients (mean age 43.7 years) admitted with sepsis to a Norwegian hospital between 2010 and 2021, found almost 4 in 10 were out of work 2 years after discharge [10].

2.3 Aetiology

A causative organism is identified in 60–70% of patients with sepsis [11], facilitated by recent improvements in molecular diagnostic testing. A study of consecutive ICU admissions in Japan reported that *Escherichia coli*, *Klebsiella pneumoniae*, *Staphylococcus aureus*, *Streptococcus pneumoniae*, *Streptococcus pyogenes*, and *Enterococcus faecalis* accounted for >50% of cases of sepsis [12], an ecology broadly representative in the developed world.

Likely, organisms vary according to primary site of infection, mode of acquisition, and immune status of the host and local microbiome. For example, in the study above, *Streptococcus*, *S aureus*, *E coli*, *K pneumoniae*, and *P aeruginosa* were dominant causes of respiratory tract infection, while abdominal infections were most often caused by *E coli*, *K pneumoniae*, or *E faecalis*. Hence, a reasoned history guides initial antimicrobial therapy. Fungal infection, while less common than bacterial sepsis, remains an important cause of sepsis-related mortality [13] as are viruses such as *SARS-CoV-2* [14]. A recent study enrolling over 3000 patients with septic shock from Europe, Australasia, and Saudi Arabia identified the most common primary site of infection to be the respiratory tract (34%) followed by abdomen (25%), blood (17%), urinary tract (8%), and skin and soft tissue (7%) [15]. Although less common, CNS and endocardial infections are notable for their high morbidity and mortality. An international point prevalence study of infections in ICU patients found similar proportions although in contrast to the septic shock group, respiratory tract infections accounted for 64% of infections [16]. In the latter study, microbiological culture results were positive in 70% of infected patients; 62% of the positive isolates were gram-negative organisms, 47% were gram-positive, and 19% were fungi. Patients experiencing longer ICU stays had higher rates of infection and more resistant *Staphylococcus*, *Acinetobacter*, *Pseudomonas*, and *Candida* species.

Global and even local antimicrobial resistance patterns vary widely. A 2019 report from the Centre for Disease Control has indicated that more than 2.8 million antibiotic-resistant infections occur annually in the USA, associated with 35,000 deaths [17]. A recent study of US hospitals found that the incidence of methicillin resistance and vancomycin resistance had fallen in *Staphylococcus aureus* and *Enterococcus faecium* isolates, respectively, while third-generation cephalosporin resistance increased from 6·7% in 2007 to 15·3% in 2019 among *Escherichia coli* isolates and carbapenem resistance had increased seven fold in *Enterobacter cloacae* infections [18]. Risk factors include recent antibiotic use, medical instrumentation (e.g. indwelling catheter), and prolonged stay in a healthcare facility [19]. Bacteria and fungi resistant to practically all commonly used antimicrobials have now been described, and empiric antibiotic regimes need to reflect this trend.

2.4 Pathogenesis

Sepsis is a dysregulated immune response to infection leading to organ failure and increased risk of death. The transition to sepsis is unpredictable, contingent upon pathogen load and virulence, host genetics, and immune response profile. For example, certain organisms produce highly toxic substances which spread throughout the circulation to elicit systemic effects (e.g. lipopolysaccharide, streptococcal pyrogenic exotoxin), while polymorphisms of certain host genes coding cytokines, pattern recognition receptors, and other immune/inflammatory proteins are associated with sepsis severity and organ dysfunction. Pathogens drive tissue destruction and organ failure both directly and indirectly, by provoking injurious inflammatory and immunosuppressive responses. Subsequent microvascular and bioenergetic dysregulation contribute to multi-organ failure.

2.4.1 *Direct Host Injury by Pathogens*

Viruses can kill host cells by hijacking the metabolic and synthetic pathways required for cell survival, inducing apoptosis (see Glossary) or by eliciting a cytotoxic immune response. Intracellular bacteria can also elicit a cytotoxic immune response or directly injure and rupture host cells (e.g. *Chlamydia* species). Bacteria also release exotoxins. Some, such as tetanus and botulinum toxins, interrupt signalling pathways, others have an enzymatic function. The anthrax toxin system includes an endoprotease function which promotes immune cell apoptosis. *Staphylococcus aureus* secrete highly destructive proteases that cleave epidermal cells (promoting host invasion), rupture erythrocytes (liberating iron-rich haem for use by the bacterium), and degrade cell membranes. Streptococcal species release pneumolysin, which separates epithelial cell tight junctions, lyses erythrocytes, damages alveolar epithelial cell membranes, and increases permeability of the blood brain barrier to the streptococcus [20]. Diphtheria and pseudomonas cytotoxins inhibit host protein synthesis. *Candida albicans* secrete proteases which promote invasive infection by digesting host extracellular membrane.

2.4.2 Immune Response to Infection

The archetypal immune response involves (i) recognising 'non-self' pathogenic material, (ii) recruiting and activating immune effector cells, (iii) localising and neutralising any pathogen, and (iv) healing.

The innate immune system mediates the initial response to infection. Pattern recognition receptors (PRRs, such as Toll-like receptors (TLRs) and C-type lectin receptors) on the surface of macrophages, neutrophils, dendritic cells, endothelial cells, and natural killer cells recognise structurally conserved molecules (pathogen-associated molecular patterns, PAMPs) shared by pathogens such as lipoteichoic acid, peptidoglycan, lipopolysaccharide (LPS), flagellin, viral RNA, and mannan (a fungal cell wall carbohydrate). Intracellular PRRs (such as NOD-like receptors) recognise cytoplasmic bacterial and viral PAMPs. Besides PAMPs, receptors bind endogenous ligands, termed *damage*-associated molecular patterns (DAMPs), released when host cells undergo non-apoptotic death. These molecules, which include fragments of nuclear and mitochondrial DNA, cytosolic heat shock proteins, and chromatin-associated high mobility group box 1 (HMGB1), instigate the inflammation associated with trauma, burns, and pancreatitis. Interestingly, for example, HMGB1, an ancient, highly conserved protein involved in DNA stabilisation and regulation of transcription, activates inflammatory pathways through receptors (such as TLRs) that also recognise foreign molecules. This ligand-receptor interaction illustrates how both sterile and infectious tissue injury can activate a common inflammatory response [21]. PRR signalling activates transcription factors such as the pivotal NFκB which induce inflammatory cytokine and cell adhesion molecule expression and nitric oxide synthase (NOS) activity and promote immune cell maturation and proliferation [22]. Tumour Necrosis Factor α (TNFα) is thought to be central, being released from macrophages when endotoxin binds to LPS-binding protein. Infusing TNFα can elicit features of sepsis such as fever, tachycardia, upregulation of other inflammatory cytokines, and granulopoiesis. Notably, these inflammatory cytokines activate NFκB in other cells, amplifying the inflammatory cascade [23]. Humoral elements of the immune system such as complement and the contact system of the coagulation cascade (e.g. Factor XII) also recognise conserved elements of the microbial surface and contribute to innate immunity and inflammation [24].

The potentially injurious nature of the inflammatory cytokine storm is illustrated by the observation that suppressing TNFα and complement effector molecules decreases inflammation and improves survival in animal models of sepsis. Cytokines such as TNFα, interleukins, interferon (IFN), and complement fragments C3a and C5a attract and activate local and circulating immune cells which amplify the inflammatory cascade and exert direct microbicidal activity by liberating substances such as lysozyme, platelet activating factor (PAF), and reactive oxygen species (ROS). These effector molecules also activate endothelial cells to express adhesion molecules, facilitating leucocyte recruitment and infiltration. Cells of the innate immune system, for example macrophages and dendritic cells, also act as antigen presenting cells (APCs), displaying antigen through the HLA (human leucocyte antigen) system to T-cells of the adaptive immune system. T-helper (CD4+) cells co-ordinate both innate and antigen-specific T- and B-lymphocyte immune response.

2.4.3 Immunosuppression in Sepsis

Most patients dying with sepsis have unresolved foci of infection at post-mortem. Moreover, patients with sepsis frequently develop secondary nosocomial infections with minimally virulent or opportunistic pathogens such as *Stenotrophomonas*, *Acinetobacter*, *Candida*, or reactivated *Cytomegalovirus*. It is now understood that the initial pro-inflammatory phase of sepsis is soon accompanied by a counter-regulatory anti-inflammatory phase [25]. Consistent with this hypothesis, it has been shown that delayed type hypersensitivity responses (whereby T-cells activated by APCs co-ordinate effector cells) are impaired in animal models of sepsis. A pattern of abundant but hypofunctional neutrophils, lymphopoiesis, and peripheral monocyte suppression has been observed in patients with sepsis and higher disease severity and septic shock. Mechanisms of sepsis-induced immunosuppression include the following:

- Apoptosis of neutrophils, macrophages, dendritic cells, natural killer cells, CD8+ and CD4+ T-lymphocytes, and B-lymphocytes; resistance to apoptosis of anti-inflammatory Treg lymphocytes.
- Immune cell functional exhaustion arising from bioenergetic failure (impaired oxidative phosphorylation and beta-oxidation) (see Glossary).
- Abundant suppressor phenotype monocyte state 1 (MS1) cells [26] and monocyte endotoxin 'tolerance' (diminished HLA expression and cytokine response to infection).
- Pyroptosis (see Glossary) of immune cells driven by PAMP/DAMP activation of cytosolic inflammasomes.
- Shift from pro-inflammatory Th1 to anti-inflammatory Th2 lymphocyte predominance; regulatory T-cell (Treg) expansion.
- Upregulated programmed death ligand 1 (PD-L1) on APCs and programmed death protein (PD-1) expression on T-cells and granulocytes from patients with sepsis, weakening effector immune cell function and inhibiting proliferation [27]. Upregulation of PD-1 correlates with illness severity.
- Downregulation of antigen presentation pathways such as HLA-DR.

These anti-inflammatory immune cell characteristics are associated with an anti-inflammatory cytokine profile (e.g. reduced Interleukin-1 (IL-1) and TNFα, upregulated IL-4 and IL-10) and reduced survival. Splenocytes from patients dying with severe sepsis (median duration 4 days) secrete less TNFα and IL-6 following stimulation with LPS than splenocytes from controls, while both lung and spleen from these septic patients show more inhibitory ligand expression and suppressor cell expansion than tissues from controls [28].

Preliminary data indicate that therapies supporting T-lymphocyte function (such as IL-7 and programmed death ligand-1 antagonism, respectively) may be an effective strategy to treat sepsis [25].

These observations suggest that sepsis arises when the host's response to infection is out of balance, dominated by a maladaptive hyper-inflammatory response to infection or immune suppressed phenotype. What determines the relative intensity of the inflammatory versus anti-inflammatory response remains unknown, but will be key to developing effective sepsis therapies. Unfortunately, host immune dysfunction appears to persist in survivors, associated with poor health outcomes for the subsequent months and years [29].

2.4.4 Microvascular Alterations in Sepsis

TLR and cytokine receptors are also expressed on endothelial cells which are uniquely placed to respond to systemic threats. Endothelial activation by leucocyte and platelet-derived arachidonic acid derivatives, PAF, C3a and C5a, and DAMPs, promotes leucocyte adhesion and trafficking, tissue factor pathway activation, and endothelial permeability. Permeability is also increased by endothelium and glycocalyx injury caused by bacterial toxins, complement, and leucocyte-derived cytotoxic mediators (ROS, lytic enzymes). Localised vascular permeability promotes migration of leucocytes and host defence proteins to areas of tissue injury. In sepsis, however, systemic, uncontrolled vascular permeability leads to hypovolaemia, increased blood viscosity, and generalised oedema. Local oxygen and metabolite diffusion, tissue architecture, capillary blood flow, and lymphatic drainage are compromised contributing to organ dysfunction [30].

Microvascular perfusion is further compromised by a shift to a prothrombotic profile: IL-6, ROS, and bacterial toxins reduce ADAMTS-13 (a disintegrin and metalloproteinase with thrombospondin motifs) activity resulting in highly thrombotic von Willebrand Factor multimers; TNF-α promotes tissue factor expression on macrophages and endothelial cells; tissue factor pathway inhibitor, thrombomodulin, and protein C activity are reduced; plasminogen activator inhibitor is increased. Meanwhile, endothelial cell damage, glycocalyx shedding, and apoptosis expose pro-thrombotic extracellular matrix which, along with thrombin and PAF, activate platelets while disrupting endothelium-dependent platelet inhibition (prostacyclin, CD39). The net consequence is a tendency for thrombosis and microvascular occlusion [31], although reduced platelet function has also been documented [32]. Cross-amplification between coagulation, fibrinolytic, complement, and immune systems, promoted by widespread endothelial activation and damage, propels consumptive coagulopathy throughout the circulation and can precipitate disseminated intravascular coagulation (DIC).

Microvascular occlusion can also arise from the release of neutrophil extracellular traps (NETs), webs of chromatin barbed with antimicrobial proteins which trap and kill microorganisms and bind DAMPs. While beneficial in containing and clearing infection, NETs have been observed to occlude capillaries, exacerbate tissue damage, promote lung injury, and fuel DIC [33].

In addition, regional vasomotor regulation (including metabolic and myogenic regulation) is impaired by glycocalyx damage, endothelial damage, downregulation of endothelial nitric oxide synthase (eNOS), and secretion of local vasoconstrictors such as endothelin and thromboxane A_2.

NETs, clots, reduced erythrocyte deformability, leucocyte aggregates, extrinsic compression from tissue oedema, and vasomotor dysregulation lead to a decrease in the number of functional capillaries and heterogeneity in microvascular perfusion with blood shunted past islands of ischaemic, hypoxic tissue through areas of relatively luxuriant flow. Patchy ischaemia of this nature can be directly visualised in myocardium, renal cortex, gut, and other vascular beds [34].

2.4.5 Metabolic Dysfunction in Sepsis [35]

Fever, tachycardia, and immune activation increase energy expenditure in sepsis. An initial hypermetabolic phase of catabolism driven by inflammatory cytokines such as IL-1, IL-6, and TNFα, associated with insulin resistance and anterior pituitary hormone release, leads to lipolysis, proteolysis, gluconeogenesis, and glycogenolysis liberating substrates for energy production. Conversely, hyperglycaemia can impair neutrophil function, while lipolysis can lead to accumulation of toxic lipid metabolites.

Activated immune cells shift their energy metabolic pathway from oxidative phosphorylation to glycolysis which, although less efficient, produces both rapid energy supply and substrates for immune cell metabolism. The increase in glycolysis is associated with lactate production and arises from reduced pyruvate dehydrogenase activity and suppressed mitochondrial oxidative function.

Mitochondrial dysfunction in sepsis, manifested in reduced oxidative capacity and ATP synthesis, is characterised by any of (i) reduction in mitochondrial number, (ii) ultrastructural mitochondrial damage, and (iii) functional mitochondrial impairment despite normal structure. These heterogeneous appearances are likely underpinned by heterogeneous mechanisms. For example, TNFα and NO inhibit cytochrome c oxidase activity while peroxynitrite (a product of the oxidative burst) inhibits components of the electron transport chain and degrades the mitochondrial membrane and DNA [36]. To what extent suppression of oxidative phosphorylation is a cytokine-mediated adaptive response to limit oxygen consumption, ROS-mediated damage, or to promote aerobic glycolysis, and how much an unwanted consequence of local inflammation is uncertain. Sepsis-induced mitochondrial dysfunction culminates in cytopathic hypoxia, an inability of cells to utilise oxygen even when abundant. Since, in addition to cellular energy delivery, mitochondria also modulate ROS production and apoptosis, mitochondrial injury may be an important contributor to cell injury and death in sepsis.

Microvascular shunting and cytopathic hypoxia underlie the observation that an oxygen extraction deficit and multi-organ dysfunction (MOD) persist despite resolution of systemic haemodynamic variables; hyperlactatemia and tissue hypoxia co-exist with supranormal oxygen delivery and mixed venous oxygen saturation.

2.4.6 Pathological Vasodilation in Septic Shock

Septic shock is characterised by systemic hypotension and tissue hypoperfusion: uncontrolled arterial vasodilation dissipates the head of pressure required to appropriately distribute blood flow, while reduced venomotor tone (coupled with fluid loss through leaky endothelium) reduces stressed circulatory volume (that volume of blood which exerts a distending pressure on the vessel or chamber wall), ventricular preload, and cardiac output.

Pathological vasodilation is a manifestation of reduced baseline vessel tone and calibre and reduced sensitivity to endogenous and administered vasoconstrictors. Inflammatory cytokines promote the production of NO from the amino acid L-arginine by activating inducible NOS (iNOS) in neutrophils and vascular smooth muscle cells. Compared to eNOS, iNOS produces far greater amounts of NO (nanomoles rather than picomoles) and lacks feedback control. iNOS inhibitors improve vascular tone and blood pressure in patients with septic shock but not their outcome [37], perhaps reflecting the complexity of trying to interrupt an endogenous pathway which exerts both useful and toxic effects. Endothelium-derived prostacyclin, the anaphylotoxins C3a and C5a, PAF, adrenomedullin, and other endogenous vasodilators all contribute to pathological vasodilation. Septic shock is associated with initial spikes in plasma corticosteroid and vasopressin levels followed by relative deficiencies in both [38, 39], while ROS oxidise and deactivate circulating noradrenaline. Moreover, even in vitro, sensitivity to α_1-receptor agonists is reduced in arterioles from animals with septic shock potentially as a consequence of receptor downregulation, increased myosin phosphatase activity, and increased ATP sensitive K^+ channel conductance [40, 41].

Immune effector molecules (reactive oxygen species, metalloproteinases, cationic proteins), adaptive immune cytotoxicity (antibodies, natural killer, and CD8+ cells targeting infected cells), immune suppression, oedema, microvascular failure, disordered apoptosis, and metabolic dysregulation contribute to cell injury and death, culminating in MOD.

2.4.7 Sepsis-Induced Organ Dysfunction

Common themes in the MOD syndrome are a causative role for inflammatory cytokines and PAMPs/DAMPs, microvascular and endothelial dysregulation, mitochondrial dysfunction, and often functional impairment rather than necrosis, the latter suggesting that some elements of MOD reflect adaptive changes to reduce cellular stress. Besides apoptosis in immune cells in sepsis, apoptosis has also been observed in parenchymal and epithelial cells; inhibiting apoptosis reduces organ failure in animal models of sepsis. Several lines of enquiry demonstrate that autophagy (see Glossary) is protective in sepsis, mitigating injury in heart, liver, kidney, and brain. Autophagy eliminates cytoplasmic pathogens and damaged host material through a process of lysosome-mediated degradation. Autophagy is critical in resisting pathogens, limiting immune cell damage and apoptosis, and regulating inflammation and tissue injury [42].

2.4.7.1 Heart

In early sepsis, cardiac output may be impaired despite normal contractility because of reduced preload secondary to venodilation, capillary fluid leak, and inadequate diastolic filling time. Sepsis is also associated with elevated pulmonary vascular resistance (hypoxic vasoconstriction, acidosis, adrenergic stimulation, loss of passive recruitment and distension, endothelial injury); elevated right ventricular (RV) afterload compromises RV stroke volume and causes RV dilation (which can compromise left ventricular (LV) filling).

In up to 50% of cases of sepsis, however, intrinsic myocardial systolic and diastolic function are depressed. Notably, despite frequently elevated troponin, cardiomyocyte death is rare in sepsis and does not explain the degree of functional, and importantly reversible, depression observed.

Atrial tachyarrhythmias are common and can compromise cardiac output directly and indirectly by exacerbating ischaemia [43]. Myocardial depression can be induced by PAMPs and cytokines binding to receptors such as TLR-4 on cardiomyocytes (Table 2.2) [44, 45].

Table 2.2 Mechanisms of myocardial dysfunction in sepsis [44, 45]

Pathophysiological mechanism	Causative factors
Downregulated β_1-adrenergic receptors and downstream pathway activity	NO, TNFα, IL-1, other 'myocardial depressant factors' (MDF)
Dysregulated Ca^{2+} transients, Ca^{2+} leak from sarcoplasmic reticulum	NO, ROS, MDF DAMPs, PAMPs binding to TLR Leucocyte binding to cardiomyocyte adhesion molecules [119]
Direct cardiomyocyte injury	Bacterial toxins, ROS, leucocyte degranulation, NETs, microvascular dysfunction, MDF ROS-mediated mitochondrial damage activating apoptosis pathway
Suppressed mitochondrial activity, decreased fatty acid oxidation, reduced oxygen utilisation, and loss of redox homeostasis	DAMPs, PAMPs binding to TLR ROS, NO, cytokines, MDF Peroxisome proliferator-activated receptors (PPAR) downregulation
Mechanically compromised contraction and relaxation	Myocardial oedema

Inflammation and myocardial depression serve as a microcosm of the complex and contradictory pathogenesis of sepsis. Excessive NO promotes endotoxin-mediated myocardial depression, oxidative damage, and cardiomyocyte apoptosis [46]. However, in other contexts, NO appears to attenuate endotoxin-mediated oxidative damage and improves calcium handling, coronary perfusion, and ventricular compliance [45]. Interestingly, survivors tend to have lower ejection fraction and larger LV end diastolic volume (EDV) than non-survivors. This may reflect preserved LV compliance (better diastolic function) and systemic vascular tone in survivors [43].

2.4.7.2 Lung

Neutrophil activation, NET deposition, and endothelial activation lead to pulmonary microvascular dysfunction, breakdown of the alveolocapillary membrane, surfactant failure, and impaired fluid clearance and oedema leading to acute lung injury and Acute Respiratory Distress Syndrome (ARDS).

2.4.7.3 Gut

Direct microbial toxicity and microcirculatory dysfunction in the gut can predispose to translocation of gut bacteria and endotoxin, perpetuating the septic insult. Both sepsis and antimicrobial therapy can alter the gut microbiome, leading to organ dysfunction and immune dysregulation [47].

2.4.7.4 Liver

Liver failure is common in sepsis, manifesting with encephalopathy, hyperbilirubinemia, coagulopathy, and immune and metabolic dysregulation. Hepatocyte apoptosis, pyroptosis, and necrosis are observed; dead and dying immune cells sequestered in the liver architecture expose hepatocytes to oxidative and NET-mediated injury [48].

2.4.7.5 Kidney

Up to 65% of patients with septic shock will develop acute kidney injury (AKI). Once thought to be primarily driven by circulatory insufficiency, it is now recognised that AKI often develops in the context of normal or high renal blood flow. Although microvascular dysfunction and local inflammation can drive tubular injury, the surprisingly bland histopathology and often rapid recovery suggest that some of the tubular dysfunction observed is functional and perhaps adaptive; cytokines, PAMPs, and DAMPs induce cell cycle arrest and downregulate metabolism [49].

2.4.7.6 Brain

Encephalopathy, often manifest as delirium, frequently accompanies sepsis. Mechanisms are poorly understood but include increased blood-brain barrier permeability to leucocytes, toxic mediators and cytokines, mitochondrial and microcirculatory dysfunction, ischaemic lesions, microabscesses, altered cell signalling, and microglial activation [50].

2.5 Clinical Manifestations

A rational history of symptoms, risk factors, and exposures, accompanied by systematic clinical examination, often identifies the presence and source of infection. Patients with sepsis typically present with dysregulated temperature, tachycardia, and tachypnoea with organ dysfunction manifest as altered mental status, respiratory failure, oliguria, ileus, jaundice, or bleeding diathesis. Patients can present with hyperdynamic circulation with bounding pulses and warm peripheries or a low cardiac output state, with cold, mottled skin, lactic acidosis, and narrow pulse pressure, or transition between these states. Hypotension must be considered in the context of pre-morbid blood pressure and the influence of chronic illness and concurrent medication use recognised; for instance, a patient with coronary artery disease will tolerate diastolic hypotension poorly, and beta-blocker therapy may mask tachycardia.

Like other forms of shock, it is proposed that septic shock progresses through three phases—(i) non-progressive phase of effective physiological compensation, (ii) a progressive stage of worsening hypoperfusion and metabolic derangement, and (iii) an irreversible stage at which tissue injury is so severe that resolution of systemic haemodynamic parameters cannot prevent death.

2.6 Investigation

Investigation should focus on identifying a specific anatomic source of infection, the causative organism, and complications of the primary infection [51]. Laboratory signs of sepsis may include leucocytosis or leukopenia, or an increase in peripheral immature granulocyte forms (>10%, usually neutrophils); non-specific inflammatory markers such as C-reactive protein (CRP) and procalcitonin (PCT); derangements localising to the underlying cause of sepsis (e.g. hyperbilirubinemia with cholangitis) or reflecting complications such as tissue ischaemia and organ dysfunction. Common findings are listed in Box 2.2.

Box 2.2
Laboratory findings consistent with the presence of sepsis

- Leukocytosis or leukopenia
- Normal white cell counts with >10% immature forms
- Thrombocytopaenia
- Elevated prothrombin and activated partial thromboplastin time, low fibrinogen, elevated fibrin degradation products
- Hyperglycaemia
- Elevated urea and creatinine
- Arterial hypoxaemia
- Coagulation abnormalities
- Hyperbilirubinaemia, hypoalbuminaemia, deranged liver enzymes
- Elevated troponin
- Adrenal insufficiency (hyponatraemia, hyperkalaemia, normal anion gap acidosis, hypoglycaemia)
- Euthyroid sick syndrome
- Elevated C-reactive protein
- Elevated pro-calcitonin (see text)
- Elevated lactate (tissue hypoperfusion, catecholamine driven aerobic glycolysis, reduced pyruvate dehydrogenase activity, mitochondrial dysfunction)

Both C-reactive protein and procalcitonin have similar sensitivity (0.77vs. 0.78), specificity (0.79), and area under the receiver operating curve (0.85 vs. 0.86) for identifying sepsis [52]. Serum PCT is elevated in response to bacterial infection and falls during recovery, but does not reliably identify sepsis nor differentiate sepsis from other causes of SIRS in critically unwell adult patients, hence PCT is not useful in the decision to initiate antibiotics [51, 53]. A recent network meta-analysis concluded that a PCT-guided antibiotic cessation strategy was associated with shortened antibiotic treatment course and improved survival [54].

Sterilisation of blood cultures can occur within minutes of administering antibiotics and it is recommended that, provided substantial delay to antimicrobial administration is not incurred, blood, cerebrospinal fluid, sputum, urine, or wound cultures be taken before antibiotics are given when sepsis is suspected [51]. Identifying the organism permits de-escalation of antibiotic therapy reducing antibiotic resistance, side effects, costs, and potentially mortality [55]. It is recommended that two or more sets (aerobic and aerobic) of blood cultures be taken. Blood cultures may be drawn together, and yield has not been shown to be improved if timed to temperature spikes [56]. Rapid diagnostic methods such as antigen testing, polymerase chain reaction assays, and microarrays are being translated into clinical practice and will hopefully better inform antibiotic prescribing [57].

Other investigations that may be valuable include plain X-ray, CT or MRI imaging, echocardiographic examination of heart valves, bronchoalveolar lavage, or aspiration of body fluids (e.g. joints).

2.7 Treatment

Sepsis and septic shock are medical emergencies; resuscitation and treatment should take place immediately and concurrently. The concept of 'Early Goal Directed Therapy' (EGDT) was applied to management of septic shock following a seminal study suggesting that protocolised fluid administration, vasopressor therapy, inotrope use, and blood transfusion to achieve target mean arterial pressure, central venous pressure, and central venous oxygen saturation were associated with improved survival [58]. Although the benefits of 'protocolised care' in this single centre study are not replicated in subsequent larger, multi-centre trials, this may reflect in part an improvement in the 'usual care' afforded to patients with sepsis and septic shock [59]. The EGDT concept has served to establish sepsis as a clinical entity demanding timely, multifaceted treatment and triggered an effective research program which has culminated in the development of the evidence-based Surviving Sepsis Campaign (SSC) Guidelines [51, 60] and a progressive reduction in sepsis mortality. Unless otherwise specified, the management approach described in this chapter reflects SSC recommendations.

2.7.1 Initial Resuscitation

As with any acutely unwell patient, the airway should be immediately assessed and secured if necessary. Adequate arterial oxygenation should be achieved using supplementary oxygen or assisted ventilation as appropriate. A trial of nasal high flow oxygen for the management of hypoxic respiratory failure may be preferred over non-invasive ventilation [61]. Severe sepsis is the most common cause of acute ARDS for which evidence-based management guidelines are widely available [62].

'Early, adequate and goal directed' fluid therapy is administered to septic patients with hypotension or impaired perfusion with the goal of restoring intravascular stressed volume, preload, and cardiac output. In patients with septic shock, an initial 30 mL/kg fluid bolus administered within the first 3 h appears safe in most situations (including patients with a history of heart failure or chronic kidney disease) and is recommended [51, 63], albeit on limited evidence.

Below a critical mean arterial pressure (MAP) threshold, autoregulation is exhausted and organ perfusion is limited by MAP. Multiple studies have evaluated the benefits of different MAP targets, ranging from 60 to 85 mmHg, in patients with septic shock treated with vasopressors. Higher pressures have been associated with greater cardiac output, varying effects of tissue perfusion indices, and higher rates of arrhythmia [64–66]. One study which compared a MAP target of 65 mmHg vs 85 mmHg found no mortality difference but a reduction in the need for renal replacement therapy among patients with chronic hypertension in the higher target pressure group [67]. Another study of elderly patients with vasodilatory shock identified no outcome difference between targets of 60 and 65 mmHg, but a reduction in vasopressor exposure in the lower MAP target group [68]. It is generally recommended that an initial blood pressure target of 65 mmHg is reasonable for most patients, while higher targets may be considered in patients with a history of chronic hypertension in whom the effective autoregulation range is elevated. However, blood pressure is not an end in itself; following initial fluid resuscitation, blood pressure, heart rate, tissue perfusion (including brain, kidney, gut, skin), plasma lactate, and mixed venous oxygen saturation (SvO_2) are re-evaluated to identify whether circulatory insufficiency persists. Patients in whom a MAP target has been achieved but lactate clearance and capillary refill time remain impaired benefit from further resuscitation [69].

The decision to administer further fluid therapy or initiate vasopressor can be difficult. The potential benefit of volume expansion, related to an increase in cardiac output and oxygen delivery, must be balanced by the risk of aggravating lung and tissue oedema [70]. Fluid therapy should be carefully titrated; limited volumes administered with regular re-evaluation are preferable to large volumes with infrequent monitoring. A multicentre randomised controlled trial from the US failed to identify a survival difference between a strategy of restrictive fluid therapy and early vasopressor use compared to a liberal fluid strategy for managing refractory sepsis-induced hypotension [71]. Conversely, although contextually different, early fluid bolus administration to sub-Saharan African children with septic shock was shown to increase mortality in a landmark randomised control trial (RCT) [72]. These results may reflect the limitations of RCTs which do not take into account individualised assessment of preload responsiveness.

Using static measures of fluid status such as central venous pressure to guide fluid administration in sepsis has been shown to be physiologically flawed and clinically unreliable [73–75]. Instead, dynamic assessment predicts more accurately which patients are likely to respond to a fluid bolus with an increase in stroke volume (preload responsiveness) [70]; such 'response evaluation'-based fluid management has been shown to improve outcomes [76]. Dynamic assessment of preload responsiveness can be achieved by passive leg raise, assessing cardiopulmonary interactions or directly measuring the change in cardiac output following fluid administration [77, 78].

Crystalloids and colloids appear similarly efficacious [79], although hydroxyethyl starch (HES) is no longer recommended since HES 130/0.42 administration has been associated with poorer outcomes [80]; balanced crystalloid solutions are a rational option and may be associated with better outcomes compared to 0.9% sodium chloride solutions [81]. Although data do not support the routine use of human albumin solutions for initial resuscitation of septic shock [82, 83], where patients have already received substantial volumes of crystalloid, there may be a case for continuing fluid resuscitation with albumin solution [51]. Data suggest that hyperoncotic albumin (see Glossary) solutions may be associated with faster resolution of shock and lower cumulative fluid balance but improvements in patient-centred outcomes are unproven [84].

Later, recognising the association between positive fluid balance and mortality in sepsis [85], a concept of 'de-resuscitation' has gained currency emphasising the need to limit fluid administration and instigate diuresis in patients who are no longer shocked. Fluid overload leads to organ oedema and congestion, and impaired organ function, perfusion, and oxygen flux. Indeed, data suggest that a 'late conservative' may be as important as an 'early adequate' fluid strategy [70]. Resolving shock and absent preload responsiveness, or development of pulmonary oedema or intra-abdominal hypertension, should guide cessation and reversal of fluid loading [86].

Shocked patients with an inadequate or detrimental response to fluid therapy may require vasopressor support. Once euvolaemia is established, noradrenaline ($\alpha_1 > \beta_1$-adrenergic receptor agonist) is recommended as a first line vasopressor augmenting both vasomotor tone and cardiac output (through an increase in cardiac preload and contractility) [87]. Vasopressin mediates vasoconstriction through activation of the arginine vasopressin receptor 1A (AVPR1a) G-protein-coupled receptor and is an effective vasopressor both independently and in combination with noradrenaline. Improved patient outcomes remain uncertain, but vasopressin is an option for cases of refractory vasodilatory shock or to reduce catecholamine toxicity (e.g. cardiac arrhythmia). Use can be complicated by splanchnic, myocardial, and digital ischaemia, but may reduce the risk of tachyarrhythmia [88, 89]. Exogenous angiotensin II has also shown promise as a therapeutic option in vasodilatory shock [90]. Methylene blue inhibits both iNOS and its downstream target-soluble guanylate cyclase, inhibiting cGMP-mediated vasodilation. Methylene blue administration early in septic shock may be associated with reduced time to cessation of vasopressors and time in ICU [91].

Because vasopressor sensitivity is variable throughout the circulation, and some regions are already relatively ischaemic, administering high doses of exogenous vasopressors risks critically impairing vital organ perfusion, especially if hypovolaemia and reduced cardiac output are not addressed.

Although septic shock may be associated with augmented or 'hyperdynamic' circulation because of reduced systemic vascular resistance and tachycardia, some patients have either pre-existing or sepsis-related ventricular systolic and diastolic dysfunction [43]. Echocardiography is an important adjunct to clinical examination. Findings should be interpreted in the context of the prevailing loading conditions, which influence stoke volume and ejection fraction and may be profoundly deranged in sepsis. Systolic dysfunction may respond better to inotropic support and strategies to augment cardiac output [92] rather than further fluid or vasopressor administration. Dobutamine is a rapidly effective, titratable inotrope which improves indices of tissue perfusion, although its use can be complicated by tachyarrhythmia and excessive vasodilation. Dosage should be titrated by monitoring indices of tissue perfusion in response to manipulation of cardiac output. As noted above, normal/high SvO_2 can be misleading in the presence of impaired oxygen extraction and may not reliably identify impaired cardiac output; conversely, low SvO_2 (<65%)

suggests low cardiac output. Levosimendan promotes myocardial contractility and diastolic relaxation and reduces mean pulmonary artery pressure while circumventing the β-receptor and exhibiting a favourable oxygen consumption profile. However, it is costly, difficult to titrate, and associated with arguably worse outcomes than standard care [93].

Preliminary human studies indicate that selective β_1-adrenergic receptor blockade administered to septic patients with tachycardia and preserved cardiac index may improve stroke volume, lactate clearance, microvascular blood flow, and even survival [94]. Putative mechanisms include augmented diastolic filling and improved myocardial efficiency, inhibition of inflammatory and pro-apoptotic pathways, and mitigating myocardial catecholamine toxicity and cytosolic Ca^{2+} overload.

The use of vasoactive and inotropic agents usually requires continuous invasive arterial pressure monitoring and frequently central venous access. Pulse contour analysis devices or echocardiographic monitoring may be helpful. Because of the need for frequent re-evaluation and advanced physiologic monitoring, severe sepsis and septic shock are often managed in an intensive care environment.

2.7.2 Antimicrobial Therapy

The benefits of early initiation of antimicrobial therapy in patients with septic shock are widely recognised; each hour delay in delivery of antibiotic is associated with a mortality cost [95] and administration within 1 h is recommended as a minimum target. Furthermore, indices of organ dysfunction and length of stay are adversely affected by delayed antibiotic therapy [60]. The data relating timing of antibiotics and outcome in patients with more mild sepsis are less clear. Sepsis is often overdiagnosed [96]; according to the Centre for Disease Control, up to 50% of antibiotic prescriptions in the acute setting are inappropriate [97]. Data suggest that overtreatment may increase mortality [98] It is arguable that for a non-shocked patient in whom infection is considered less probable, spending time confirming the diagnosis and obtaining microbiology samples is justifiable [51, 99]. Nevertheless, if sepsis is deemed possible, antibiotics should be administered within 3 h even in the absence of shock. If the likelihood of infection is low, the patient should be monitored and antibiotics deferred to minimise potential harms of antimicrobial therapy (hypersensitivity, kidney injury, Clostridium difficile colitis, thrombocytopaenia, microbiome destruction, antimicrobial resistance) [99].

Initial antibiotic cover should have broad activity against likely causative pathogens while avoiding antibiotic cover of unlikely pathogens. For example, anti-anaerobic antibiotics deplete the healthy microbiome and are often unnecessary. Inappropriate empiric therapy is associated with up to five-fold increase in mortality [100]. The choice will be determined by factors such as the patient's clinical presentation, immune status, recent healthcare facility admission and antibiotic use, and local microbial ecology. Patients vulnerable to infection with multidrug-resistant gram-negative pathogens such as *Pseudomonas*, *Acinetobacter*, or *Klebsiella* should receive a supplementary gram-negative agent, in addition to the empiric regime, to increase the probability that they receive at least one active agent. Similarly, when risk factors for methicillin-resistant *Staphylococcus aureus* (MRSA) exist—such as previous MRSA infection, recent IV antibiotic use, recurrent or chronic skin or wound infection—an anti-MRSA agent should be administered [51]. Broadening cover to ensure potential organisms are covered by one of the administered agents is distinct from 'combination therapy' where antibiotics of different classes are combined to cover the suspected organism with multiple agents; the latter approach is not recommended as undesirable effects are more likely without apparent benefit [101]. Infections associated with high levels of toxin-mediated pathophysiology, such as streptococcal toxic shock syndrome or necrotising soft tissue infections, may benefit from treatment with both a bactericidal and protein synthesis inhibiting antibiotic (e.g. penicillin and clindamycin). Given the time-dependent kill pharmacodynamic characteristics of beta-lactam antibiotics, it is postulated that continuous infusions may be more effective than intermittent administration. RCTs have identified better clinical cure rates with prolonged infusion but no significant mortality benefit [102]. Given the possible benefit and limited risks, prolonged infusion of beta-lactams is conditionally suggested for patients with sepsis [51].

Empiric antifungal cover is considered for patients at risk of fungal infection (Box 2.3), particularly if patients do not defervesce after 3–4 days of antibacterial cover. Empiric antifungals in septic patients without risk factors have not been shown to improve fungal infection-free survival [103].

Box 2.3
Risk factors for fungal infection

- Immunocompromise (neutropenia, malignancy/chemotherapy, transplant, diabetes mellitus, chronic liver, or kidney failure)
- Invasive vascular devices
- Total parenteral nutrition
- Gut perforation, abdominal surgery, pancreatitis
- Prolonged administration of broad-spectrum antibiotics
- Prolonged hospital/ICU admission
- Multisite colonisation
- Intravenous recreational drug use

The role of antivirals is rapidly evolving and guidelines pertaining to specific viral illnesses should be referred to.

Once the causative pathogen and antimicrobial sensitivities are defined, antibiotic therapy should be refined to the narrowest spectrum effective agent. If cultures are negative, monitored de-escalation may be appropriate. Data regarding de-escalation are scant but avoiding unnecessarily prolonged antibiotic exposure is beneficial for both society and patient; unnecessarily prolonged antibiotic therapy promotes *C difficile* colitis, superinfection with multi-drug resistant organisms, and is associated with increased mortality [55].

The optimal duration of antibiotic therapy depends on host, microbe, site, and drug factors; hence, it is not possible to recommend a fixed duration. Nevertheless, of the many studies comparing 'short' (3–8 days) courses guided by clinical resolution vs 'long' (7–15 days) 'fixed duration' courses of antibiotics across a range of infections, shorter courses are generally associated with at least comparable outcomes [51, 104, 105]. Rapid clinical resolution and early effective source control may permit shorter courses, for instance, surgically treated intra-abdominal sepsis and uncomplicated pyelonephritis. There may be benefit in longer courses when source control is challenging (e.g. infected prosthetic material), clinical resolution is slow, immune deficiency exists, or in cases of *S aureus* bacteraemia or fungal infection. Daily assessment for de-escalation of antibiotic therapy is effective and may improve survival. Up to a third of patients diagnosed with sepsis turns out to have a non-infectious condition; the likelihood of the diagnosis should be reviewed regularly and antimicrobials ceased if an alternative diagnosis becomes apparent.

As noted above, PCT measurement can be used to shorten duration of antibiotic therapy in patients with clinically resolving sepsis or support the decision to discontinue antibiotics when ongoing evidence for a presumptive diagnosis of sepsis is weak [51]. The very real threat of antibiotic resistance makes antimicrobial stewardship practices and programmes incumbent on individual practitioners and healthcare institutions [17].

2.7.3 Source Control

When septic shock arises from infection in a site amenable to source control, the time to intervention is a critical determinant of survival [106, 107]. Specifically, abscess drainage, debridement of infected tissue, removal of infected device, or definitive control of an ongoing source of microbial contamination should be undertaken as soon as possible [51]; in some cases, haemodynamic stability cannot be achieved without source control and prolonged efforts at medical stabilisation may be counterproductive.

2.7.4 Corticosteroids

Septic shock appears to be associated with relative adrenal insufficiency arising from dysregulation along the pathway from cortisol production to target cell response [108]. The putative benefits of corticosteroid supplementation are twofold: (i) A generally anti-inflammatory effect—corticosteroids suppress chemokine and cell adhesion molecule expression, antigen presentation and lysosome degranulation, phospholipase A_2-mediated production of arachidonic acid derivatives, and pro-inflammatory cytokine production (e.g. TNFα, IL-1, IL-2, IL-8). Lymphocytic T-cells are shifted from pro-inflammatory Th1 to anti-inflammatory Th2 phenotype. Many anti-inflammatory effects of steroids are mediated through inhibition of the transcription factor NFκB [109]. (ii) Augmenting vasomotor tone—corticosteroids promote α_1-adrenergic receptor sensitivity by increasing inositol trisphosphate (IP_3) release and potentiating downstream sensitivity to protein kinase C. These effects are independent of changes in plasma catecholamine levels, adrenergic receptor expression, or ligand binding affinity. Corticosteroids increase angiotensinogen levels, angiotensin converting enzyme activity and angiotensin density. More generally, corticosteroids promote vasomotor tone by inhibiting inducible nitric oxide release and stimulating endothelin release and modulating vascular smooth muscle cell Na^+ and Ca^{2+} handling [110]. Steroids also promote capillary perfusion independent of global haemodynamic variation [111].

Outcome data regarding corticosteroid therapy in septic shock are conflicting. It has been variably demonstrated that glucocorticoids promote resolution of shock and organ dysfunction, reduce duration of mechanical ventilation, ICU length of stay, blood transfusions, and improve mortality albeit at the potential risk of promoting neuromuscular weakness [15, 112]. Addition of fludrocortisone probably adds benefit. It is suggested that patients requiring ≥0.25 mcg/kg/min of noradrenaline for more than 4 h receive 200 mg hydrocortisone daily [51]. Adrenal function assays in septic shock (e.g. synacthen test, plasma cortisol assay) are difficult to interpret and generally unhelpful.

2.7.5 Adjunctive Therapies

Data supporting specific therapies that target host dysregulation in sepsis and septic shock have proven elusive. Strategies which promote potentially beneficial endogenous pathways (activated protein C [113], thrombomodulin, intravenous immunoglobulins, interferon-γ, granulocyte colony stimulating factor, anti-Enterobacteriaceae monoclonal antibody, vitamin C) or suppress deleterious pathways (TNFα, IL-1, NO, arachidonic acid derivatives, TLR-4 [114]) have been evaluated in patients with septic shock. They have not shown convincing outcome benefit, and none are recommended for use in septic shock.

Blood purification techniques (such as haemofiltration and haemoperfusion) effectively remove inflammatory mediators, but have not translated to improved patient outcomes [115].

Biologically, perhaps the failure of targeting individual mediators (such as TNFα) to improve outcomes is not surprising—inflammatory and immune pathways have built in redundancy and mediators are pleiotropic, promoting both beneficial and maladaptive effects. Targeting one mediator may not significantly redefine the immunological landscape and even if it does, the effects may be unpredictable and dynamic. Administering therapy which neutralises inflammatory mediators may be beneficial during the hyperinflammatory phase of sepsis but fatal if immune-suppression is the dominant feature. For example, while IL-1 antagonism is not beneficial in unselected sepsis, it may be more effective in treating hyperinflammatory, macrophage activation-like syndrome phenotypes of sepsis [116]. Similarly, early data suggest that the efficacy of goal-directed therapy and activated protein C differs by sepsis phenotype.

Higher peak temperature in the first 24 hours after ICU admission has been associated with improved survival in critically ill patients with infection and it remains unclear whether, despite widespread adoption, treatment with antipyretics may increase mortality [117].

Bicarbonate administration may improve outcomes in patients with metabolic acidaemia and acute kidney injury, but can also promote tissue hypoxia and intracellular acidosis. For patients with arterial pH <7.2 and AKI, treatment with sodium bicarbonate may be reasonable [51].

2.7.6 *Red Cell Transfusion*

A restrictive transfusion strategy using a haemoglobin transfusion trigger of 7 g/dL has been shown to be safe and associated with reduced resource utilisation [118]. Nevertheless, transfusion thresholds should be modified according to clinical circumstances (e.g. myocardial ischaemia or evidence of impaired tissue oxygen delivery) [51].

2.8 Conclusion

Sepsis and septic shock are common and often fatal. Our understanding of the pathophysiology is maturing but remains incomplete. We are beginning to appreciate the tensions between adaptive and maladaptive changes, excessive inflammation, and immunoparesis, but have not yet effectively targeted therapies to specific sepsis phenotypes. Patients are best served by a sound application of microbiological principles and physiologically rational approach to supportive therapy.

Multiple Choice Questions

1. Which of the following best defines sepsis?
   (a) Infection with ≥1 SIRS criteria
   (b) Life-threatening organ dysfunction caused by a dysregulated host response to infection.
   (c) Infection causing persistent hypotension despite adequate fluid resuscitation
   (d) Any infection associated with fever and leucocytosis
   (e) Organ dysfunction caused by direct pathogen invasion alone

   Answers: (b) Life-threatening organ dysfunction caused by a dysregulated host response to infection

2. Which of the following correctly describes the immune response in sepsis?
   (a) Sepsis is solely an excessive pro-inflammatory response
   (b) Anti-inflammatory cytokines are suppressed throughout sepsis
   (c) Sepsis activates both inflammatory and anti-inflammatory pathways, and excessive immune suppression may impair host defence
   (d) Interferon and interleukins only modulate metabolic pathways, not immune cell recruitment
   (e) Cytokines play no role in direct microbicidal activity

   Answers: (c) Sepsis activates both inflammatory and anti-inflammatory pathways, and excessive immune suppression may impair host defence
3. Which of the following statements regarding the management of sepsis and septic shock is true?
   (a) Immunomodulatory therapies have consistently shown mortality benefit in sepsis
   (b) Early source control and timely, rational antibiotic therapy are essential to maximise survival
   (c) High-dose corticosteroids are recommended for all patients with sepsis
   (d) Fluid therapy should always follow fixed, non-individualised protocols
   (e) Vasopressors should be avoided in septic shock until all fluid strategies have been exhausted

   Answers: (b) Early source control and timely, rational antibiotic therapy are essential to maximise survival

References

1. Bone RC, Sibbald WJ, Sprung CL. The ACCP-SCCM consensus conference on sepsis and organ failure. Chest. 1992;101:1481–3.
2. Churpek MM, Zadravecz FJ, Winslow C, Howell MD, Edelson DP. Incidence and prognostic value of the systemic inflammatory response syndrome and organ dysfunctions in

ward patients. Am J Respir Crit Care Med. 2015;192:958–64. https://doi.org/10.1164/rccm.201502-0275OC.
3. Kaukonen KM, Bailey M, Pilcher D, Cooper DJ, Bellomo R. Systemic inflammatory response syndrome criteria in defining severe sepsis. N Engl J Med. 2015;372:1629–38. https://doi.org/10.1056/NEJMoa1415236.
4. Serafim R, Gomes JA, Salluh J, Povoa P. A comparison of the quick-SOFA and systemic inflammatory response syndrome criteria for the diagnosis of sepsis and prediction of mortality: a systematic review and meta-analysis. Chest. 2018;153:646–55. https://doi.org/10.1016/j.chest.2017.12.015.
5. Singer M, Deutschman CS, Seymour CW, Shankar-Hari M, Annane D, Bauer M, et al. The third international consensus definitions for sepsis and septic shock (sepsis-3). JAMA. 2016;315:801–10. https://doi.org/10.1001/jama.2016.0287.
6. Vincent JL, Moreno R, Takala J, Willatts S, De Mendonca A, Bruining H, et al. The SOFA (Sepsis-related Organ Failure Assessment) score to describe organ dysfunction/failure. On behalf of the Working Group on Sepsis-Related Problems of the European Society of Intensive Care Medicine. Intensive Care Med. 1996;22:707–10. https://doi.org/10.1007/BF01709751.
7. Rudd KE, Johnson SC, Agesa KM, Shackelford KA, Tsoi D, Kievlan DR, et al. Global, regional, and national sepsis incidence and mortality, 1990–2017: analysis for the Global Burden of Disease Study. Lancet. 2020;395:200–11. https://doi.org/10.1016/S0140-6736(19)32989-7.
8. Bauer M, Gerlach H, Vogelmann T, Preissing F, Stiefel J, Adam D. Mortality in sepsis and septic shock in Europe, North America and Australia between 2009 and 2019-results from a systematic review and meta-analysis. Crit Care. 2020;24:239. https://doi.org/10.1186/s13054-020-02950-2.
9. Iwashyna TJ, Ely EW, Smith DM, Langa KM. Long-term cognitive impairment and functional disability among survivors of severe sepsis. JAMA. 2010;304:1787–94. https://doi.org/10.1001/jama.2010.1553.
10. Skei NV, Moe K, Nilsen TIL, Aasdahl L, Prescott HC, Damas JK, et al. Return to work after hospitalization for sepsis: a nationwide, registry-based cohort study. Crit Care. 2023;27:443. https://doi.org/10.1186/s13054-023-04737-7.
11. Gupta S, Sakhuja A, Kumar G, McGrath E, Nanchal RS, Kashani KB. Culture-negative severe sepsis: nationwide trends and outcomes. Chest. 2016;150:1251–9. https://doi.org/10.1016/j.chest.2016.08.1460.
12. Umemura Y, Ogura H, Takuma K, Fujishima S, Abe T, Kushimoto S, et al. Current spectrum of causative pathogens in sepsis: a prospective nationwide cohort study in Japan. Int J Infect Dis. 2021;103:343–51. https://doi.org/10.1016/j.ijid.2020.11.168.
13. Denning DW. Global incidence and mortality of severe fungal disease. Lancet Infect Dis. 2024;24:e428–e38. https://doi.org/10.1016/S1473-3099(23)00692-8.
14. Gu X, Zhou F, Wang Y, Fan G, Cao B. Respiratory viral sepsis: epidemiology, pathophysiology, diagnosis and treatment. Eur Respir Rev. 2020;29:200038. https://doi.org/10.1183/16000617.0038-2020.
15. Venkatesh B, Finfer S, Cohen J, Rajbhandari D, Arabi Y, Bellomo R, et al. Adjunctive glucocorticoid therapy in patients with septic shock. N Engl J Med. 2018;378:797–808. https://doi.org/10.1056/NEJMoa1705835.
16. Vincent JL, Rello J, Marshall J, Silva E, Anzueto A, Martin CD, et al. International study of the prevalence and outcomes of infection in intensive care units. JAMA. 2009;302:2323–9. https://doi.org/10.1001/jama.2009.1754.
17. Kadri SS. Key takeaways from the U.S. CDC's 2019 antibiotic resistance threats report for frontline providers. Crit Care Med. 2020;48:939–45. https://doi.org/10.1097/CCM.0000000000004371.
18. Pham TM, Zhang Y, Nevers M, Li H, Khader K, Grad YH, et al. Trends in infection incidence and antimicrobial resistance in the US Veterans Affairs Healthcare System: a nationwide

retrospective cohort study (2007–2022). Lancet Infect Dis. 2024;24:1333–46. https://doi.org/10.1016/S1473-3099(24)00416-X.
19. Adler A, Katz DE, Marchaim D. The Continuing Plague of Extended-spectrum beta-lactamase-producing Enterobacteriaceae Infections. Infect Dis Clin N Am. 2016;30:347–75. https://doi.org/10.1016/j.idc.2016.02.003.
20. Hirst RA, Kadioglu A, O'Callaghan C, Andrew PW. The role of pneumolysin in pneumococcal pneumonia and meningitis. Clin Exp Immunol. 2004;138:195–201. https://doi.org/10.1111/j.1365-2249.2004.02611.x.
21. Andersson U, Tracey KJ. HMGB1 is a therapeutic target for sterile inflammation and infection. Annu Rev Immunol. 2011;29:139–62. https://doi.org/10.1146/annurev-immunol-030409-101323.
22. Takeuchi O, Akira S. Pattern recognition receptors and inflammation. Cell. 2010;140:805–20. https://doi.org/10.1016/j.cell.2010.01.022.
23. Guo Q, Jin Y, Chen X, Ye X, Shen X, Lin M, et al. NF-kappaB in biology and targeted therapy: new insights and translational implications. Signal Transduct Target Ther. 2024;9:53. https://doi.org/10.1038/s41392-024-01757-9.
24. Nickel KF, Renne T. Crosstalk of the plasma contact system with bacteria. Thromb Res. 2012;130(Suppl 1):S78–83. https://doi.org/10.1016/j.thromres.2012.08.284.
25. Hotchkiss RS, Monneret G, Payen D. Immunosuppression in sepsis: a novel understanding of the disorder and a new therapeutic approach. Lancet Infect Dis. 2013;13:260–8. https://doi.org/10.1016/S1473-3099(13)70001-X.
26. Leite GGF, de Brabander J, Michels EHA, Butler JM, Cremer OL, Scicluna BP, et al. Monocyte state 1 (MS1) cells in critically ill patients with sepsis or non-infectious conditions: association with disease course and host response. Crit Care. 2024;28:88. https://doi.org/10.1186/s13054-024-04868-5.
27. Liu D, Huang SY, Sun JH, Zhang HC, Cai QL, Gao C, et al. Sepsis-induced immunosuppression: mechanisms, diagnosis and current treatment options. Mil Med Res. 2022;9:56. https://doi.org/10.1186/s40779-022-00422-y.
28. Boomer JS, To K, Chang KC, Takasu O, Osborne DF, Walton AH, et al. Immunosuppression in patients who die of sepsis and multiple organ failure. JAMA. 2011;306:2594–605. https://doi.org/10.1001/jama.2011.1829.
29. Yende S, Kellum JA, Talisa VB, Peck Palmer OM, Chang CH, Filbin MR, et al. Long-term host immune response trajectories among hospitalized patients with sepsis. JAMA Netw Open. 2019;2:e198686. https://doi.org/10.1001/jamanetworkopen.2019.8686.
30. Russell JA, Rush B, Boyd J. Pathophysiology of septic shock. Crit Care Clin. 2018;34:43–61. https://doi.org/10.1016/j.ccc.2017.08.005.
31. Ince C, Mayeux PR, Nguyen T, Gomez H, Kellum JA, Ospina-Tascon GA, et al. The endothelium in sepsis. Shock. 2016;45:259–70. https://doi.org/10.1097/SHK.0000000000000473.
32. Reddi BA, Iannella SM, O'Connor SN, Deane AM, Willoughby SR, Wilson DP. Attenuated platelet aggregation in patients with septic shock is independent from the activity state of myosin light chain phosphorylation or a reduction in Rho kinase-dependent inhibition of myosin light chain phosphatase. Intensive Care Med Exp. 2015;3:37. https://doi.org/10.1186/s40635-014-0037-7.
33. Camicia G, Pozner R, de Larranaga G. Neutrophil extracellular traps in sepsis. Shock. 2014;42:286–94. https://doi.org/10.1097/SHK.0000000000000221.
34. Ince C, Mik EG. Microcirculatory and mitochondrial hypoxia in sepsis, shock, and resuscitation. J Appl Physiol (1985). 2016;120:226–35. https://doi.org/10.1152/japplphysiol.00298.2015.
35. Wasyluk W, Zwolak A. Metabolic alterations in sepsis. J Clin Med. 2021;10:2412. https://doi.org/10.3390/jcm10112412.
36. Harrois A, Huet O, Duranteau J. Alterations of mitochondrial function in sepsis and critical illness. Curr Opin Anaesthesiol. 2009;22:143–9. https://doi.org/10.1097/ACO.0b013e328328d1cc.

37. Bakker J, Grover R, McLuckie A, Holzapfel L, Andersson J, Lodato R, et al. Administration of the nitric oxide synthase inhibitor NG-methyl-L-arginine hydrochloride (546C88) by intravenous infusion for up to 72 hours can promote the resolution of shock in patients with severe sepsis: results of a randomized, double-blind, placebo-controlled multicenter study (study no. 144-002). Crit Care Med. 2004;32:1–12. https://doi.org/10.1097/01.CCM.0000105118.66983.19.
38. Venkatesh B, Prins J, Torpy D, Chapman M, Joyce C, Cooper DJ, et al. Relative adrenal insufficiency in sepsis: match point or deuce? Crit Care Resusc. 2006;8:376–80.
39. Landry DW, Levin HR, Gallant EM, Ashton RC Jr, Seo S, D'Alessandro D, et al. Vasopressin deficiency contributes to the vasodilation of septic shock. Circulation. 1997;95:1122–5. https://doi.org/10.1161/01.cir.95.5.1122.
40. Landry DW, Oliver JA. The ATP-sensitive K+ channel mediates hypotension in endotoxemia and hypoxic lactic acidosis in dog. J Clin Invest. 1992;89:2071–4. https://doi.org/10.1172/JCI115820.
41. Reddi BA, Beltrame JF, Young RL, Wilson DP. Calcium desensitisation in late polymicrobial sepsis is associated with loss of vasopressor sensitivity in a murine model. Intensive Care Med Exp. 2015;3:36. https://doi.org/10.1186/s40635-014-0036-8.
42. Yin X, Xin H, Mao S, Wu G, Guo L. The role of autophagy in sepsis: protection and injury to organs. Front Physiol. 2019;10:1071. https://doi.org/10.3389/fphys.2019.01071.
43. Walley KR. Sepsis-induced myocardial dysfunction. Curr Opin Crit Care. 2018;24:292–9. https://doi.org/10.1097/MCC.0000000000000507.
44. Kakihana Y, Ito T, Nakahara M, Yamaguchi K, Yasuda T. Sepsis-induced myocardial dysfunction: pathophysiology and management. J Intensive Care. 2016;4:22. https://doi.org/10.1186/s40560-016-0148-1.
45. Rudiger A, Singer M. Mechanisms of sepsis-induced cardiac dysfunction. Crit Care Med. 2007;35:1599–608. https://doi.org/10.1097/01.CCM.0000266683.64081.02.
46. Hunter JD, Doddi M. Sepsis and the heart. Br J Anaesth. 2010;104:3–11. https://doi.org/10.1093/bja/aep339.
47. Miller WD, Keskey R, Alverdy JC. Sepsis and the microbiome: a vicious cycle. J Infect Dis. 2021;223:S264–S9. https://doi.org/10.1093/infdis/jiaa682.
48. Beyer D, Hoff J, Sommerfeld O, Zipprich A, Gassler N, Press AT. The liver in sepsis: molecular mechanism of liver failure and their potential for clinical translation. Mol Med. 2022;28:84. https://doi.org/10.1186/s10020-022-00510-8.
49. Zarbock A, Gomez H, Kellum JA. Sepsis-induced acute kidney injury revisited: pathophysiology, prevention and future therapies. Curr Opin Crit Care. 2014;20:588–95. https://doi.org/10.1097/MCC.0000000000000153.
50. Sonneville R, de Montmollin E, Poujade J, Garrouste-Orgeas M, Souweine B, Darmon M, et al. Potentially modifiable factors contributing to sepsis-associated encephalopathy. Intensive Care Med. 2017;43:1075–84. https://doi.org/10.1007/s00134-017-4807-z.
51. Evans L, Rhodes A, Alhazzani W, Antonelli M, Coopersmith CM, French C, et al. Surviving sepsis campaign: international guidelines for management of sepsis and septic shock 2021. Crit Care Med. 2021;49:e1063–e143. https://doi.org/10.1097/CCM.0000000000005337.
52. Wu CC, Lan HM, Han ST, Chaou CH, Yeh CF, Liu SH, et al. Comparison of diagnostic accuracy in sepsis between presepsin, procalcitonin, and C-reactive protein: a systematic review and meta-analysis. Ann Intensive Care. 2017;7:91. https://doi.org/10.1186/s13613-017-0316-z.
53. Tang BM, Eslick GD, Craig JC, McLean AS. Accuracy of procalcitonin for sepsis diagnosis in critically ill patients: systematic review and meta-analysis. Lancet Infect Dis. 2007;7:210–7. https://doi.org/10.1016/S1473-3099(07)70052-X.
54. Kubo K, Sakuraya M, Sugimoto H, Takahashi N, Kano KI, Yoshimura J, et al. Benefits and harms of procalcitonin- or C-reactive protein-guided antimicrobial discontinuation in critically ill adults with sepsis: a systematic review and network meta-analysis. Crit Care Med. 2024;52:e522–e34. https://doi.org/10.1097/CCM.0000000000006366.

55. Garnacho-Montero J, Gutierrez-Pizarraya A, Escoresca-Ortega A, Corcia-Palomo Y, Fernandez-Delgado E, Herrera-Melero I, et al. De-escalation of empirical therapy is associated with lower mortality in patients with severe sepsis and septic shock. Intensive Care Med. 2014;40:32–40. https://doi.org/10.1007/s00134-013-3077-7.
56. Baron EJ, Miller JM, Weinstein MP, Richter SS, Gilligan PH, Thomson RB Jr, et al. A guide to utilization of the microbiology laboratory for diagnosis of infectious diseases: 2013 recommendations by the Infectious Diseases Society of America (IDSA) and the American Society for Microbiology (ASM)(a). Clin Infect Dis. 2013;57:e22–e121. https://doi.org/10.1093/cid/cit278.
57. Burillo A, Bouza E. Use of rapid diagnostic techniques in ICU patients with infections. BMC Infect Dis. 2014;14:593. https://doi.org/10.1186/s12879-014-0593-1.
58. Rivers E, Nguyen B, Havstad S, Ressler J, Muzzin A, Knoblich B, et al. Early goal-directed therapy in the treatment of severe sepsis and septic shock. N Engl J Med. 2001;345:1368–77. https://doi.org/10.1056/NEJMoa010307.
59. Angus DC, Barnato AE, Bell D, Bellomo R, Chong CR, Coats TJ, et al. A systematic review and meta-analysis of early goal-directed therapy for septic shock: the ARISE, ProCESS and ProMISe Investigators. Intensive Care Med. 2015;41:1549–60. https://doi.org/10.1007/s00134-015-3822-1.
60. Rhodes A, Evans LE, Alhazzani W, Levy MM, Antonelli M, Ferrer R, et al. Surviving sepsis campaign: international guidelines for management of sepsis and septic shock: 2016. Crit Care Med. 2017;45:486–552. https://doi.org/10.1097/CCM.0000000000002255.
61. Frat JP, Thille AW, Mercat A, Girault C, Ragot S, Perbet S, et al. High-flow oxygen through nasal cannula in acute hypoxemic respiratory failure. N Engl J Med. 2015;372:2185–96. https://doi.org/10.1056/NEJMoa1503326.
62. Qadir N, Sahetya S, Munshi L, Summers C, Abrams D, Beitler J, et al. An update on management of adult patients with Acute Respiratory Distress Syndrome: an Official American Thoracic Society Clinical Practice Guideline. Am J Respir Crit Care Med. 2024;209:24–36. https://doi.org/10.1164/rccm.202311-2011ST.
63. Liu VX, Morehouse JW, Marelich GP, Soule J, Russell T, Skeath M, et al. Multicenter implementation of a treatment bundle for patients with sepsis and intermediate lactate values. Am J Respir Crit Care Med. 2016;193:1264–70. https://doi.org/10.1164/rccm.201507-1489OC.
64. LeDoux D, Astiz ME, Carpati CM, Rackow EC. Effects of perfusion pressure on tissue perfusion in septic shock. Crit Care Med. 2000;28:2729–32. https://doi.org/10.1097/00003246-200008000-00007.
65. Bourgoin A, Leone M, Delmas A, Garnier F, Albanese J, Martin C. Increasing mean arterial pressure in patients with septic shock: effects on oxygen variables and renal function. Crit Care Med. 2005;33:780–6. https://doi.org/10.1097/01.ccm.0000157788.20591.23.
66. Thooft A, Favory R, Salgado DR, Taccone FS, Donadello K, De Backer D, et al. Effects of changes in arterial pressure on organ perfusion during septic shock. Crit Care. 2011;15:R222. https://doi.org/10.1186/cc10462.
67. Asfar P, Teboul JL, Radermacher P. High versus low blood-pressure target in septic shock. N Engl J Med. 2014;371:283–4. https://doi.org/10.1056/NEJMc1406276.
68. Lamontagne F, Richards-Belle A, Thomas K, Harrison DA, Sadique MZ, Grieve RD, et al. Effect of reduced exposure to vasopressors on 90-day mortality in older critically ill patients with vasodilatory hypotension: a randomized clinical trial. JAMA. 2020;323:938–49. https://doi.org/10.1001/jama.2020.0930.
69. Gu WJ, Zhang Z, Bakker J. Early lactate clearance-guided therapy in patients with sepsis: a meta-analysis with trial sequential analysis of randomized controlled trials. Intensive Care Med. 2015;41:1862–3. https://doi.org/10.1007/s00134-015-3955-2.
70. Malbrain M, Van Regenmortel N, Saugel B, De Tavernier B, Van Gaal PJ, Joannes-Boyau O, et al. Principles of fluid management and stewardship in septic shock: it is time to consider the four D's and the four phases of fluid therapy. Ann Intensive Care. 2018;8:66. https://doi.org/10.1186/s13613-018-0402-x.

71. National Heart L, Blood Institute P, Early Treatment of Acute Lung Injury Clinical Trials N, Shapiro NI, Douglas IS, Brower RG, et al. Early restrictive or liberal fluid management for sepsis-induced hypotension. N Engl J Med. 2023;388:499–510. https://doi.org/10.1056/NEJMoa2212663.
72. Maitland K, Kiguli S, Opoka RO, Engoru C, Olupot-Olupot P, Akech SO, et al. Mortality after fluid bolus in African children with severe infection. N Engl J Med. 2011;364:2483–95. https://doi.org/10.1056/NEJMoa1101549.
73. Reddi BA, Carpenter RH. Venous excess: a new approach to cardiovascular control and its teaching. J Appl Physiol (1985). 2005;98:356–64. https://doi.org/10.1152/japplphysiol.00535.2004.
74. Reddi B, Finnis M, Udy AA, Maiden M, Delaney A, Bellomo R, et al. The relationship between the change in central venous pressure and intravenous fluid volume in patients presenting to the emergency department with septic shock. Intensive Care Med. 2018;44:1591–2. https://doi.org/10.1007/s00134-018-5314-6.
75. Cecconi M, De Backer D, Antonelli M, Beale R, Bakker J, Hofer C, et al. Consensus on circulatory shock and hemodynamic monitoring. Task force of the European Society of Intensive Care Medicine. Intensive Care Med. 2014;40:1795–815. https://doi.org/10.1007/s00134-014-3525-z.
76. Douglas IS, Alapat PM, Corl KA, Exline MC, Forni LG, Holder AL, et al. Fluid response evaluation in sepsis hypotension and shock: a randomized clinical trial. Chest. 2020;158:1431–45. https://doi.org/10.1016/j.chest.2020.04.025.
77. Marik PE, Monnet X, Teboul JL. Hemodynamic parameters to guide fluid therapy. Ann Intensive Care. 2011;1:1. https://doi.org/10.1186/2110-5820-1-1.
78. Monnet X, Marik PE, Teboul JL. Prediction of fluid responsiveness: an update. Ann Intensive Care. 2016;6:111. https://doi.org/10.1186/s13613-016-0216-7.
79. Finfer S, Bellomo R, Boyce N, French J, Myburgh J, Norton R, et al. A comparison of albumin and saline for fluid resuscitation in the intensive care unit. N Engl J Med. 2004;350:2247–56. https://doi.org/10.1056/NEJMoa040232.
80. Perner A, Haase N, Guttormsen AB, Tenhunen J, Klemenzson G, Aneman A, et al. Hydroxyethyl starch 130/0.42 versus Ringer's acetate in severe sepsis. N Engl J Med. 2012;367:124–34. https://doi.org/10.1056/NEJMoa1204242.
81. Brown RM, Wang L, Coston TD, Krishnan NI, Casey JD, Wanderer JP, et al. Balanced crystalloids versus saline in sepsis. A secondary analysis of the SMART clinical trial. Am J Respir Crit Care Med. 2019;200:1487–95. https://doi.org/10.1164/rccm.201903-0557OC.
82. Martin GS, Bassett P. Crystalloids vs. colloids for fluid resuscitation in the Intensive Care Unit: a systematic review and meta-analysis. J Crit Care. 2019;50:144–54. https://doi.org/10.1016/j.jcrc.2018.11.031.
83. Caironi P, Tognoni G, Masson S, Fumagalli R, Pesenti A, Romero M, et al. Albumin replacement in patients with severe sepsis or septic shock. N Engl J Med. 2014;370:1412–21. https://doi.org/10.1056/NEJMoa1305727.
84. Bannard-Smith J, Elrakhawy M, Norman G, Owen R, Felton T, Dark P. The efficacy, safety and effectiveness of hyperoncotic albumin solutions in patients with sepsis: a systematic review and meta-analysis. J Intensive Care Soc. 2024;25:308–18. https://doi.org/10.1177/17511437241259437.
85. Boyd JH, Forbes J, Nakada TA, Walley KR, Russell JA. Fluid resuscitation in septic shock: a positive fluid balance and elevated central venous pressure are associated with increased mortality. Crit Care Med. 2011;39:259–65. https://doi.org/10.1097/CCM.0b013e3181feeb15.
86. Teboul JL, Monnet X. Detecting volume responsiveness and unresponsiveness in intensive care unit patients: two different problems, only one solution. Crit Care. 2009;13:175. https://doi.org/10.1186/cc7979.
87. Hamzaoui O, Georger JF, Monnet X, Ksouri H, Maizel J, Richard C, et al. Early administration of norepinephrine increases cardiac preload and cardiac output in septic patients with life-threatening hypotension. Crit Care. 2010;14:R142. https://doi.org/10.1186/cc9207.

88. Russell JA, Walley KR, Singer J, Gordon AC, Hebert PC, Cooper DJ, et al. Vasopressin versus norepinephrine infusion in patients with septic shock. N Engl J Med. 2008;358:877–87. https://doi.org/10.1056/NEJMoa067373.
89. Gordon AC, Mason AJ, Thirunavukkarasu N, Perkins GD, Cecconi M, Cepkova M, et al. Effect of early vasopressin vs norepinephrine on kidney failure in patients with septic shock: the VANISH randomized clinical trial. JAMA. 2016;316:509–18. https://doi.org/10.1001/jama.2016.10485.
90. Khanna A, English SW, Wang XS, Ham K, Tumlin J, Szerlip H, et al. Angiotensin II for the treatment of vasodilatory shock. N Engl J Med. 2017;377:419–30. https://doi.org/10.1056/NEJMoa1704154.
91. Ibarra-Estrada M, Kattan E, Aguilera-Gonzalez P, Sandoval-Plascencia L, Rico-Jauregui U, Gomez-Partida CA, et al. Early adjunctive methylene blue in patients with septic shock: a randomized controlled trial. Crit Care. 2023;27:110. https://doi.org/10.1186/s13054-023-04397-7.
92. Reddi B, Shanmugan N, Fletcher SN. Heart failure – pathophysiology and inpatient management. BJA Educ. 2017;17:151–60. https://doi.org/10.1093/bjaed/mkw067.
93. Gordon AC, Perkins GD, Singer M, McAuley DF, Orme RM, Santhakumaran S, et al. Levosimendan for the prevention of acute organ dysfunction in sepsis. N Engl J Med. 2016;375:1638–48. https://doi.org/10.1056/NEJMoa1609409.
94. Morelli A, Ertmer C, Westphal M, Rehberg S, Kampmeier T, Ligges S, et al. Effect of heart rate control with esmolol on hemodynamic and clinical outcomes in patients with septic shock: a randomized clinical trial. JAMA. 2013;310:1683–91. https://doi.org/10.1001/jama.2013.278477.
95. Kumar A, Roberts D, Wood KE, Light B, Parrillo JE, Sharma S, et al. Duration of hypotension before initiation of effective antimicrobial therapy is the critical determinant of survival in human septic shock. Crit Care Med. 2006;34:1589–96. https://doi.org/10.1097/01.CCM.0000217961.75225.E9.
96. Klein Klouwenberg PM, Cremer OL, van Vught LA, Ong DS, Frencken JF, Schultz MJ, et al. Likelihood of infection in patients with presumed sepsis at the time of intensive care unit admission: a cohort study. Crit Care. 2015;19:319. https://doi.org/10.1186/s13054-015-1035-1.
97. Dellit TH, Owens RC, McGowan JE Jr, Gerding DN, Weinstein RA, Burke JP, et al. Infectious Diseases Society of America and the Society for Healthcare Epidemiology of America guidelines for developing an institutional program to enhance antimicrobial stewardship. Clin Infect Dis. 2007;44:159–77. https://doi.org/10.1086/510393.
98. Hranjec T, Rosenberger LH, Swenson B, Metzger R, Flohr TR, Politano AD, et al. Aggressive versus conservative initiation of antimicrobial treatment in critically ill surgical patients with suspected intensive-care-unit-acquired infection: a quasi-experimental, before and after observational cohort study. Lancet Infect Dis. 2012;12:774–80. https://doi.org/10.1016/S1473-3099(12)70151-2.
99. Klompas M, Calandra T, Singer M. Antibiotics for sepsis-finding the equilibrium. JAMA. 2018;320:1433–4. https://doi.org/10.1001/jama.2018.12179.
100. Kumar A, Ellis P, Arabi Y, Roberts D, Light B, Parrillo JE, et al. Initiation of inappropriate antimicrobial therapy results in a fivefold reduction of survival in human septic shock. Chest. 2009;136:1237–48. https://doi.org/10.1378/chest.09-0087.
101. Arulkumaran N, Routledge M, Schlebusch S, Lipman J, Conway Morris A. Antimicrobial-associated harm in critical care: a narrative review. Intensive Care Med. 2020;46:225–35. https://doi.org/10.1007/s00134-020-05929-3.
102. Dulhunty JM, Brett SJ, De Waele JJ, Rajbhandari D, Billot L, Cotta MO, et al. Continuous vs intermittent beta-lactam antibiotic infusions in critically ill patients with sepsis: the BLING III randomized clinical trial. JAMA. 2024;332:629–37. https://doi.org/10.1001/jama.2024.9779.
103. Timsit JF, Azoulay E, Schwebel C, Charles PE, Cornet M, Souweine B, et al. Empirical micafungin treatment and survival without invasive fungal infection in adults with ICU-acquired

sepsis, candida colonization, and multiple organ failure: the EMPIRICUS randomized clinical trial. JAMA. 2016;316:1555–64. https://doi.org/10.1001/jama.2016.14655.
104. Mo Y, Booraphun S, Li AY, Domthong P, Kayastha G, Lau YH, et al. Individualised, short-course antibiotic treatment versus usual long-course treatment for ventilator-associated pneumonia (REGARD-VAP): a multicentre, individually randomised, open-label, non-inferiority trial. Lancet Respir Med. 2024;12:399–408. https://doi.org/10.1016/S2213-2600(23)00418-6.
105. Daneman N, Rishu A, Pinto R, Rogers BA, Shehabi Y, Parke R, et al. Antibiotic treatment for 7 versus 14 days in patients with bloodstream infections. N Engl J Med. 2025;392:1065–78. https://doi.org/10.1056/NEJMoa2404991.
106. Azuhata T, Kinoshita K, Kawano D, Komatsu T, Sakurai A, Chiba Y, et al. Time from admission to initiation of surgery for source control is a critical determinant of survival in patients with gastrointestinal perforation with associated septic shock. Crit Care. 2014;18:R87. https://doi.org/10.1186/cc13854.
107. Moss RL, Musemeche CA, Kosloske AM. Necrotizing fasciitis in children: prompt recognition and aggressive therapy improve survival. J Pediatr Surg. 1996;31:1142–6.
108. Annane D. The role of ACTH and corticosteroids for sepsis and septic shock: an update. Front Endocrinol (Lausanne). 2016;7:70. https://doi.org/10.3389/fendo.2016.00070.
109. Liu T, Zhang L, Joo D, Sun SC. NF-kappaB signaling in inflammation. Signal Transduct Target Ther. 2017;2:17023. https://doi.org/10.1038/sigtrans.2017.23.
110. Ullian ME. The role of corticosteriods in the regulation of vascular tone. Cardiovasc Res. 1999;41:55–64.
111. Buchele GL, Silva E, Ospina-Tascon GA, Vincent JL, De Backer D. Effects of hydrocortisone on microcirculatory alterations in patients with septic shock. Crit Care Med. 2009;37:1341–7. https://doi.org/10.1097/ccm.0b013e3181986647.
112. Annane D, Renault A, Brun-Buisson C, Megarbane B, Quenot JP, Siami S, et al. Hydrocortisone plus fludrocortisone for adults with septic shock. N Engl J Med. 2018;378:809–18. https://doi.org/10.1056/NEJMoa1705716.
113. Ranieri VM, Thompson BT, Barie PS, Dhainaut JF, Douglas IS, Finfer S, et al. Drotrecogin alfa (activated) in adults with septic shock. N Engl J Med. 2012;366:2055–64. https://doi.org/10.1056/NEJMoa1202290.
114. Opal SM, Laterre PF, Francois B, LaRosa SP, Angus DC, Mira JP, et al. Effect of eritoran, an antagonist of MD2-TLR4, on mortality in patients with severe sepsis: the ACCESS randomized trial. JAMA. 2013;309:1154–62. https://doi.org/10.1001/jama.2013.2194.
115. Dellinger RP, Bagshaw SM, Antonelli M, Foster DM, Klein DJ, Marshall JC, et al. Effect of targeted polymyxin B hemoperfusion on 28-day mortality in patients with septic shock and elevated endotoxin level: the EUPHRATES randomized clinical trial. JAMA. 2018;320:1455–63. https://doi.org/10.1001/jama.2018.14618.
116. Shakoory B, Carcillo JA, Chatham WW, Amdur RL, Zhao H, Dinarello CA, et al. Interleukin-1 receptor blockade is associated with reduced mortality in sepsis patients with features of macrophage activation syndrome: reanalysis of a prior phase III trial. Crit Care Med. 2016;44:275–81. https://doi.org/10.1097/CCM.0000000000001402.
117. Young PJ, Saxena M, Beasley R, Bellomo R, Bailey M, Pilcher D, et al. Early peak temperature and mortality in critically ill patients with or without infection. Intensive Care Med. 2012;38:437–44. https://doi.org/10.1007/s00134-012-2478-3.
118. Holst LB, Haase N, Wetterslev J, Wernerman J, Guttormsen AB, Karlsson S, et al. Lower versus higher hemoglobin threshold for transfusion in septic shock. N Engl J Med. 2014;371:1381–91. https://doi.org/10.1056/NEJMoa1406617.
119. Davani EY, Dorscheid DR, Lee CH, van Breemen C, Walley KR. Novel regulatory mechanism of cardiomyocyte contractility involving ICAM-1 and the cytoskeleton. Am J Physiol Heart Circ Physiol. 2004;287:H1013–22. https://doi.org/10.1152/ajpheart.01177.2003.

Key References

Evans L, Rhodes A, Alhazzani W, Antonelli M, Coopersmith CM, French C, et al. Surviving sepsis campaign: international guidelines for management of sepsis and septic shock 2021. Crit Care Med. 2021;49:e1063–e143. https://doi.org/10.1097/CCM.0000000000005337.

Umemura Y, Ogura H, Takuma K, Fujishima S, Abe T, Kushimoto S, et al. Current spectrum of causative pathogens in sepsis: a prospective nationwide cohort study in Japan. Int J Infect Dis. 2021;103:343–51. https://doi.org/10.1016/j.ijid.2020.11.168.

Chapter 3
Pathophysiology of Reperfusion Injury

Prue Cowled and Robert Fitridge

SN Flashcards
Test your learning and check your understanding of this book's contents: use the "Springer Nature Flashcards" app to access questions using ▶ https://sn.pub/wppvze. To use the app, please follow the instructions in Chap. 1.

Key Learning Points

- Ischaemia-reperfusion injury (IRI) is the paradoxical local and remote tissue damage which occurs when perfusion is returned to ischaemic tissue.
- Tissue ischaemia occurs when perfusion is less than required to provide tissues with adequate oxygen, glucose and other substances which are required for normal cellular function.
- When oxygen returns to ischaemic tissue, xanthine oxidase catalyses the conversion of hypoxanthine to superoxide anions, which are subsequently converted to reactive oxygen species which cause activation of the endothelium, lipid peroxidation of cellular membranes and the generation of pro-inflammatory eicosanoids.

P. Cowled (✉)
Discipline of Surgery, Adelaide University, The Queen Elizabeth Hospital, Woodville South, SA, Australia
e-mail: prue.cowled@adelaide.edu.au

R. Fitridge
Discipline of Surgery, Adelaide University, The Queen Elizabeth Hospital, Woodville South, SA, Australia

Vascular and Endovascular Service, Royal Adelaide Hospital, Adelaide, SA, Australia
e-mail: robert.fitridge@adelaide.edu.au

R. Fitridge et al. (eds.), *Pathophysiology of Vascular Disease*,
https://doi.org/10.1007/978-3-032-31459-8_3

- Neutrophils are activated during IRI and play a key role in tissue damage by releasing reactive oxygen species and matrix metalloproteinases which subsequently degrade basement membranes, causing fluid and protein leakage.
- Hypoxia and IRI also induce numerous cytokines that play a key role in the development of systemic inflammatory response syndrome and multi-system organ failure associated with IRI.
- The complexity of the pathophysiology of IRI has resulted in the failure of therapeutic interventions to be adopted into clinical practice. Ischaemic preconditioning holds some promise in reducing IRI in vascular surgery, but further larger trials are needed. Ischaemic postconditioning and the effects of volatile anaesthetic agents in ameliorating the severity of IRI also require further investigation.

3.1 Introduction

Ischaemia-reperfusion injury (IRI) is defined as the paradoxical exacerbation of cellular dysfunction and death following restoration of blood flow to previously ischaemic tissues. Re-establishment of blood flow is essential to salvage ischaemic tissues; however, reperfusion itself paradoxically causes further damage, threatening the function and viability of the organ. IRI occurs in a wide range of organs including the heart, lung, kidney, gut, skeletal muscle and brain and may involve not only the ischaemic organ itself but may also induce systemic damage to distant organs, potentially leading to multi-system organ failure. Reperfusion injury is a multi-factorial process which can result in extensive tissue destruction. The aim of this review is to summarise these molecular and cellular mechanisms and thus provide an insight into possible windows for therapeutic intervention.

3.2 Ischaemia

3.2.1 ATP and Mitochondrial Function

Ischaemia occurs when the blood supply is less than the demand required for normal function, resulting in deficiencies in oxygen, glucose and other substances required for metabolism. Derangements in metabolic function begin during this ischaemic phase. Initially, glycogen breakdown by mitochondrial anaerobic glycolysis produces two molecules of adenosine triphosphate (ATP) along with lactic acid, resulting in a decrease in tissue pH, which then acts by negative feedback to inhibit further ATP production (Fig. 3.1). ATP is then sequentially broken down into adenosine diphosphate (ADP), adenosine monophosphate (AMP) and inosine

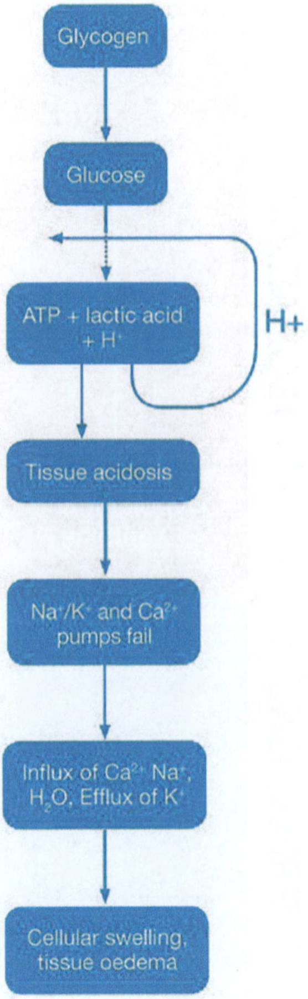

Fig. 3.1 Dysregulation of metabolic pathways during ischaemia. Anaerobic glycolysis during ischaemia results in negative feedback which inhibits ATP production, thereby inducing tissue acidosis, calcium influx and tissue oedema

monophosphate (IMP) and then further into adenosine, inosine, hypoxanthine and xanthine (Fig. 3.2 upper panel).

At the cellular level, a lack of ATP production causes ATP-dependent ionic pumps, including the Na^+/K^+ and Ca^{2+} pumps, to fail, and the transmembrane ionic gradients are lost. Consequently, cytosolic sodium content rises, drawing with it a volume of water to attempt to maintain the osmotic equilibrium and resulting in hydroponic swelling of the cells. To maintain the ionic balance, potassium ions escape from the cell into the interstitial space. Calcium is released from the mitochondria into the cytoplasm and into extracellular spaces, thereby activating mitochondrial calcium-dependent cytosolic proteases including calpain, which then converts the cellular enzyme xanthine dehydrogenase to xanthine oxidase (Fig. 3.2 upper panel). Phospholipases are also activated during ischaemia, degrading membrane lipids and increasing the levels of circulating fatty acids.

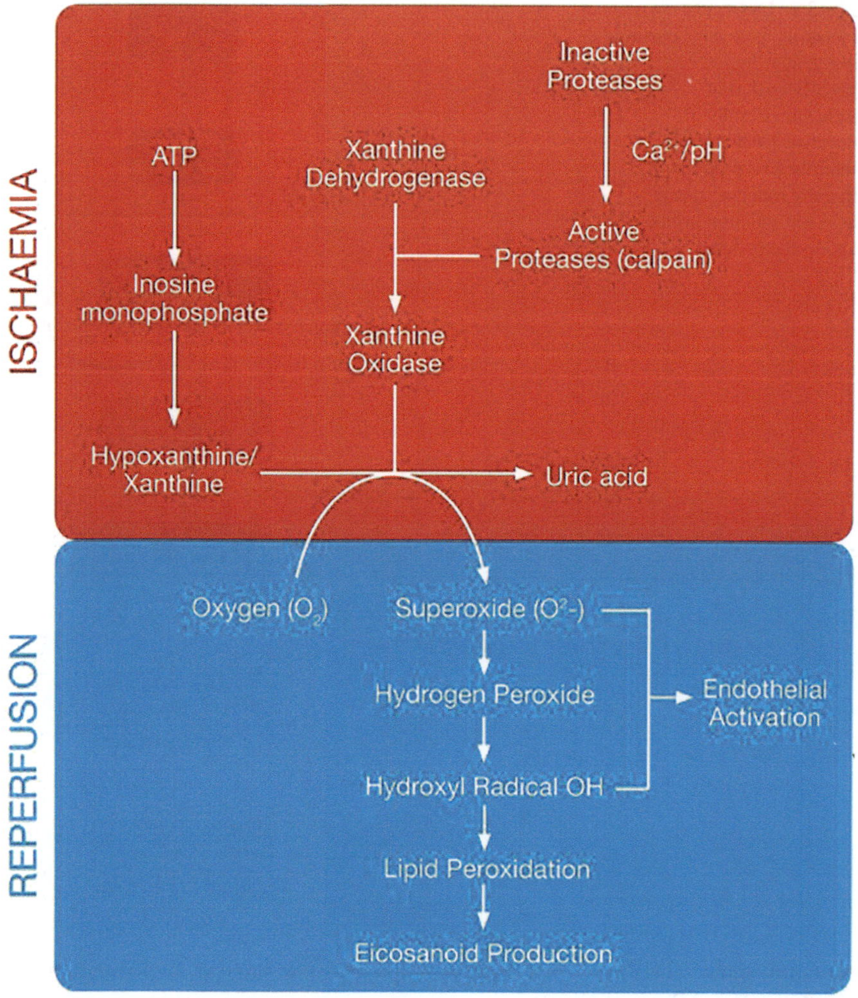

Fig. 3.2 Generation of reactive oxygen species during reperfusion. During ischaemia, ATP is degraded and xanthine dehydrogenase is converted to xanthine oxidase. In the presence of fresh oxygenated blood, xanthine oxidase catalyses the conversion of hypoxanthine to highly reactive and toxic superoxide anions with urea as a by-product. Superoxide then reacts with H^+ to initiate the production of both hydrogen peroxide and the hydroxyl radical, which ultimately mediate lipid peroxidation and tissue damage

3.2.2 Gene Expression During Ischaemia

As well as metabolic derangements, ischaemia induces expression of a large number of genes, which play a major role in the tissue's response to ischaemic damage. An RNA expression micro-array analysis, using mouse soleus muscle rendered ischaemic by femoral artery ligation, found that expression of 962 genes was induced, and 327 genes were repressed [1]. The activated genes were largely clustered into mediators of inflammation, cytokine genes and genes associated with immune cell infiltration. The repressed genes were largely involved in energy production, including mitochondrial respiration and fatty acid oxidation.

Hypoxia itself activates a number of genes, particularly transcription factors, including activating protein-1 (AP-1), hypoxia-inducible factor-1 (HIF-1) and nuclear factor-kappaB (NF-κB). HIF-1 then activates transcription of other genes such as vascular endothelial growth factor (VEGF), erythropoietin and glucose transporter-1, which all play an important role in the cells' adaptive responses to hypoxia (reviewed in [2]). Expression of both HIF-1 and cyclo-oxygenase-2 (COX-2) is also induced in the lungs of rats subjected to haemorrhagic shock. COX-2 promotes the inflammatory response through the rapid and exaggerated production of nitric oxide and prostaglandins, thereby contributing to organ damage [3]. Activation of NF-κB occurs during both the ischaemic and reperfusion phases and will therefore be discussed below.

3.3 Reperfusion

3.3.1 Reactive Oxygen Species

Table 3.1 illustrates the major reactive oxygen species (ROS), which play a role in tissue damage during IRI and the sources of generation of these species. Reactive oxygen species have a destructive role in mediating tissue damage during IRI. During

Table 3.1 Reactive oxygen species involved in IRI

Major ROS
Superoxide anion (O_2^-)
Hydrogen peroxide (H_2O_2)
Hydroxyl radical (OH^λ)
Nitric oxide (NO)
Peroxynitrite ($ONOO^-$)
Minor ROS
Lipid hydroperoxide
Lipid peroxyl radical
Lipid alkoxyl radical
Thiol radical
Sources of ROS during IRI
Xanthine oxidase system
Activated neutrophils
Mitochondrial electron transport chain
Arachidonic acid metabolism
Auto-oxidation of catecholamines

ischaemia, the degradation of ATP produces hypoxanthine (Fig. 3.2, upper panel). Once the ischaemic tissue is re-perfused, an influx of molecular oxygen catalyses xanthine oxidase to degrade hypoxanthine to uric acid and thereby liberating the highly reactive superoxide anion (O_2^-) (Fig. 3.2, lower panel). Superoxide is subsequently converted to hydrogen peroxide (H_2O_2) and the hydroxyl radical ($OH^\bullet$) (Fig. 3.2, lower panel). The major consequence of hydroxyl radical production is peroxidation of the lipid structures of the cell membranes resulting in the production and systemic release of pro-inflammatory eicosanoids, disruption of cell permeability and ultimately cell death. During IRI, ROS also activates endothelial cells, elevating the activity of the transcription factor, NF-κB. Once activated, the endothelial cell produces E-selectin, vascular cell adhesion molecule-1 (VCAM-1), inter-cellular adhesion molecule-1 (ICAM-1), endothelial-leukocyte adhesion molecule (ELAM-1), plasminogen activator inhibitor-1 (PAI-1), tissue factor and interleukin-8 (IL-8). These adhesion molecules contribute to important interactions between the neutrophil and the endothelium and will be discussed in more detail later.

Superoxide anions can be detected within ischaemic muscle and also in the venous effluent of reperfused limbs [4], suggesting an additional role for superoxide damage to distant organs during skeletal muscle reperfusion injury. Xanthine oxidase is located within a spectrum of cell types and tissues to varying degrees, indicating widespread distribution and differing susceptibility to oxidant-mediated IRI. Inhibition of xanthine oxidase activity, by administration of allopurinol prior to ischaemia, reduces the production of superoxide and hence reduces the severity of reperfusion injury in animal models using a range of tissues including skeletal muscle, brain and gut. In an animal model of hindlimb IRI, allopurinol significantly reduced serum tumour necrosis factor-alpha (TNF-α) levels, indicating that systemic inflammation was inhibited [5]. Results in humans are also promising. A systematic review [6] provided evidence that allopurinol was effective in some studies in reducing the severity of post-operative cardiac dysfunction and arrhythmias after coronary artery bypass grafting. In agreement with this hypothesis, a recent randomised clinical trial provided strong evidence that allopurinol pre-treatment of patients with STEMI before a percutaneous coronary intervention procedure led to improved coronary blood flow [7].

3.3.2 *Eicosanoids*

As discussed above, ROS initiate the lipid peroxidation of cellular membranes, releasing arachidonic acid, the main substrate for the production of prostaglandins, thromboxanes and leukotrienes (Fig. 3.2, lower panel). These derivatives of arachidonic acid are collectively known as the eicosanoids, which are signalling molecules that modulate inflammation, immune responses and tissue blood flow and play a major role in the pathophysiology of IRI.

Prostaglandins, synthesised from arachidonic acid via the cyclooxygenase pathway, have a protective vasodilatory effect in IRI. However, since prostaglandins are short-lived molecules, their rapid depletion subsequently leads to uninhibited vasoconstriction, reduced local blood flow and exacerbation of ischaemia. The potential of prostaglandins to ameliorate the degree of metabolic and tissue damage following IRI has been demonstrated in various tissues. In an animal model of myocardial IRI, the prostacyclin analogue, iloprost, demonstrated protective effects against IRI by increasing myocardial contractility [8]. In a placebo-controlled trial of human liver transplantation, administration of prostacyclin was shown to improve post-operative liver graft function [9]. Patients who received prostacyclin also demonstrated better post-operative myocardial oxygen consumption after coronary artery bypass surgery and improved muscle blood flow following skeletal muscle IRI [10].

The ILAILL trial randomised 300 patients treated surgically with acute limb ischaemia to adjuvant iloprost bolus plus iloprost infusion for 4–7 days, versus placebo. At 90-day follow-up, the combined incidence of death and amputation was not significantly different between the groups. However, the overall incidence of fatal or major cardiovascular events was 33% in the placebo cohort and 23% in the iloprost group [11]. In the cohort of patients over 70 years of age, those treated with adjuvant iloprost had a significantly reduced risk of death (6% vs. 15%, $p = 0.03$) and combined death and major amputation (16% vs. 27%, $p = 0.03$) [12]. Similarly, in a randomised clinical trial, 204 patients who underwent open and endovascular procedures for acute limb ischaemia were randomised to receive adjuvant liposomal prostaglandin E1 for 12–14 days or placebo. The combined incidence of perioperative mortality and any major adverse limb events (MALE) at 6 months was significantly lower in the prostaglandin-treated cohort (5.1% vs. 13.2%, $p < 0.05$) [13].

More recent studies have investigated another prostacyclin analogue, treprostinil as a potential therapy for IRI. As well as a number of promising studies of renal IRI models in rats, preliminary results of treprostinil following human liver transplantation demonstrated safety [14]. However, a larger trial is needed to determine if this therapy is effective in reducing IRI Despite these positive studies, adjuvant prostaglandin analogues have not been adopted into routine practice as part of the management of acute limb ischaemia.

Plasma thromboxane A_2, also synthesised from arachidonic acid, increases within minutes following skeletal muscle IRI, thus promoting vasoconstriction and platelet aggregation. These events coincide with a rapid rise in pulmonary artery pressure and a subsequent increase in pulmonary micro-vascular permeability [15], which correlates with sequestration of polymorphonuclear cells in the lungs. In animal models of lower limb IRI, thromboxane synthase inhibitors and synthetic thromboxane A_2 receptor antagonists prevented pulmonary leuko-sequestration, thereby increasing blood flow to re-perfused tissues and preserving tissue viability and function [16]. Together, these studies suggest that administration of thromboxane A_2 antagonists may improve limb salvage rates after surgery for acute ischaemia, but clinical evidence is currently lacking.

Leukotrienes are also synthesised from arachidonic acid through the activation of 5-lipoxygenase and participate in the inflammatory cascade of IRI (reviewed in [17]). Leukotrienes lead to local and systemic injury by their direct proinflammatory action on endothelial and smooth muscle cells and indirectly by their effects on neutrophils. The leukotrienes C_4, D_4 and E_4 modify the endothelial cytoskeleton, leading to increased vascular permeability and enhanced smooth muscle contraction, resulting in vasoconstriction. The lung produces leukotrienes following remote IRI. The direct effects of leukotrienes on pulmonary microvessels lead to increased permeability, transient pulmonary hypertension and the induction of the endothelium to produce thromboxane, resulting in additional vasoconstriction. The leukotriene B_4, released by activated neutrophils, leads to further pulmonary neutrophil accumulation.

The administration of 5-lipoxygenase synthesis inhibitors has been successfully used in animal studies to attenuate IRI. Such agents abolish the elevations in leukotrienes B_4 and C_4 and inhibit neutrophil infiltration normally induced by intestinal IRI, reducing mucosal permeability [18]. In a study of a mouse model of stroke, administration of a lipoxygenase inhibitor 2 h after induction of stroke significantly reduced infarct volume and haemorrhage area [19]. However, there is currently no up-to-date information on their use in a clinical context.

3.3.3 Nitric Oxide

Nitric oxide (NO) is a signalling molecule synthesised from L-arginine by the nitric oxide synthase enzyme (NOS) of which there are three types, constitutive (cNOS), inducible (iNOS) and endothelial (eNOS). An initial surge in NO level in the first 15 min of the ischaemic phase is due to transient eNOS activation. This is followed during early reperfusion by a general decline in endothelial function and loss of functional eNOS, so that NO production falls, along with an increased production of reactive oxygen species. eNOS-derived NO is also necessary for the maintenance of vascular tone. The reduction in eNOS levels that occurs in IRI may therefore predispose to vasoconstriction, a common response seen in IRI. The second surge in NO production is largely due to cytokine-mediated up-regulation of iNOS after about 3 h of reperfusion (reviewed in [20]).

The pathophysiological role of nitric oxide in reperfusion injury is variable, being dependent on the nature of its generation and appears to be tissue specific. In some instances, NO acts as an antioxidant and, in others, combines with the superoxide anion to form the peroxynitrite radical, a potent promoter of lipid peroxidation and hence cellular membrane disruption (reviewed in [20, 21]). Manipulation of nitric oxide production during IRI, using a range of techniques, has recently provided considerable evidence for a principal role for nitric oxide in the aetiology of IRI. Myocardial IRI has been well studied, with paradoxical results, where low doses of NO were found to be protective and high doses harmful. The influence of NO in skeletal muscle IRI has been less well characterised, with some studies suggesting that NO may potentiate cytotoxicity and others suggesting a beneficial role for NO in extremity IRI. In skeletal muscle IRI, NO production may be deleterious and inhibition of NOS activity using a non-specific NOS inhibitor greatly reduced the severity of muscle damage [22].

The assessment of experimental data derived from pharmacological NOS inhibition is difficult due to the non-specificity of NOS inhibitors and administration of these inhibitors at differing times during the injury merely adds to the complexity. In essence, augmentation of NO delivery may be beneficial with respect to protection, particularly in the ischaemic and early reperfusion phase. Inhibition of the iNOS-induced surge in NO production at later times during reperfusion also mediates defence against IRI-induced tissue damage. However, in the clinical setting, systemic distortion of NO kinetics by administering NOS inhibitors would be likely to induce wide-ranging physiological disturbances. Further investigations will be needed to define a role for NOS inhibition in ameliorating the severity of IRI, and local administration of these inhibitors may be required.

However, exogenous administration of NO gas itself may be a useful therapy for IRI. In a mouse model of stroke, administration of NO reduced the levels of inflammatory cytokines, thereby reducing vascular dysfunction [23]. Recent reviews have suggested the possibility of renal protection after transplantation-induced IRI [24]. Similar positive reviews of the role of NO in experimental settings of lung or gastrointestinal IRI have also been published [25, 26]. However, clinical trial evidence for the efficacy of NO for the treatment of IRI is not yet available.

3.3.4 *Endothelin*

Endothelins are potent peptide vasoconstrictors produced by the vascular endothelium. Hypoxia, growth factors, angiotensin II and noradrenaline all stimulate endothelin production, resulting in Ca^{2+}-mediated vasoconstriction. Endothelin-1 is elevated following skeletal muscle IRI during both the ischaemic and reperfusion phases and mediates capillary vasoconstriction, neutrophil aggregation and neutrophil-endothelial interactions. Endothelin-1 inhibitors, including bosentan and tezosentan, inhibit neutrophil infiltration, increase functional capillary density, micro-vascular perfusion and hence tissue viability and function following IRI in a rat model of aortic IRI [27]. In a rat model of spinal cord IRI, bosentan increased expression of VEGF and its receptors, however, a reduction in IRI-induced damage to the spinal cord was not reported [28]. Similarly, in a rat model of intestinal IRI, an endothelin receptor blocker reduced bacterial translocation and inflammation [29]. However, these inhibitors still have not been tested in clinical trials for the treatment of IRI.

3.3.5 *Cytokines*

Hypoxia and IRI both induce the expression of numerous cytokines, TNF-α, interleukins -1 -6 and -8 and platelet-activating factor (PAF), in association with elevations in activity of the transcription factor complex, NF-κB (reviewed in [30]). These cytokines are released systemically and are thus important in the development of systemic inflammatory response syndrome and ultimately multi-system organ failure.

Tumour necrosis factor-alpha (TNF-α) is a 17-kilodalton pro-inflammatory cytokine produced by activated macrophages, monocytes, T-lymphocytes, natural killer cells and fibroblasts. It is a potent chemoattractant and early response cytokine, which subsequently induces expression of IL-1, IL-6, IL-8 and PAF. Elevated serum levels of TNF-α have been detected during cerebral and skeletal muscle IRI and are known to increase neutrophil sequestration and permeability following pulmonary IRI. Serum TNF-α levels increased rapidly in an animal model of aortic clamping, thus inducing up-regulation of iNOS, which increased NO production in the lungs, leading to more severe lung damage [31]. In the same study, inhibition of TNF-α activity prior to limb ischaemia decreased pulmonary NO production and reduced the severity of IRI. TNF-α can also induce the generation of ROS and enhance the susceptibility of the vascular endothelium to neutrophil-mediated injury, by inducing the expression of ICAM-1, which mediates binding of neutrophils to the activated endothelium.

Numerous studies in animal models attest to the potential of TNF-α blockade as a therapeutic modality to reduce the severity of IRI. The introduction of humanised antibodies, including etanercept and infliximab, has provided excellent results in the treatment of other TNF-α-mediated inflammatory diseases, including a number of forms of arthritis and inflammatory bowel disease (reviewed in [32]). However, clinical trials to test the efficacy of TNF-α blockade in human IRI have not yet been reported.

The cytokines interleukin 1-alpha and -beta (IL-1α and IL-1β) are produced during IRI by tissue macrophages, neutrophils and the vascular endothelium. IL-1α is a potent chemotactic agent and stimulates neutrophil infiltration during hepatic IRI. Both IL-1α and TNF-α also increase levels of expression of ICAM-1 on the vascular endothelium. Exposure of endothelial cells in culture to IL-1α and TNF-α induces synthesis of E-selectin, which then interacts with L-selectin on the neutrophil surface, leading to rolling along the endothelial surface. Permanent adhesion of the neutrophil to the endothelium is then mediated by expression of ICAM-1, IL-8 and PAF in the endothelial membrane (Fig. 3.3).

Numerous activating stimuli synthesised during IRI include H_2O_2, thrombin, leukotrienes C_4 and D_4, IL-1β, histamine, bradykinin and ATP; all of which induce the synthesis of PAF by monocytes, macrophages, neutrophils, eosinophils, basophils, platelets and endothelial cells. PAF functions as both an inter- and intra-cellular messenger, having three major effects: vasoconstriction, chemo-attraction and increased micro-vascular permeability. PAF is rapidly produced following skeletal muscle and renal IRI with peak levels after 15 min of reperfusion. PAF enhances the binding of neutrophils to endothelial cells since a PAF-receptor antagonist has been shown to block adhesion of neutrophils to endothelial cells during IRI in a hamster model [33]. Similarly, pre-treatment with the PAF inhibitor lexipafant reduced the severity of intestinal barrier dysfunction and pulmonary and liver permeability in a rat model of intestinal IRI [34]. However, lexipafant is unlikely to be clinically useful as a pharmacotherapy for IRI since, alone, it failed to completely inhibit pulmonary endothelial damage after small bowel IRI in a rat model [35] and there have not been any more recent reports of clinical use of this therapy.

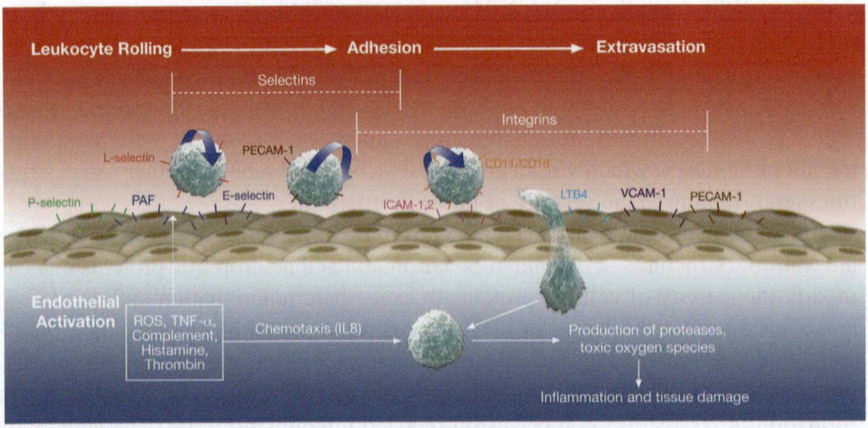

Fig. 3.3 Neutrophil rolling, adhesion to endothelium and extravasation. During reperfusion, activated neutrophils adhere to the activated endothelium and subsequently extravasate into surrounding tissue, resulting in proteolytic degradation of basement membranes. Activated neutrophils also generate toxic reactive oxygen species from molecular oxygen, contributing to tissue degradation during reperfusion

IL-6 is a pro-inflammatory 19–26 kDa protein produced by monocytes, fibroblasts, keratinocytes and endothelial cells in response to IL-1 and TNF-α. IL-6 primes and stimulates the respiratory burst in neutrophils, stimulates endothelial cell expression of ICAM-1 and increases endothelial permeability. IL-6 is produced in hypoperfused skeletal muscle in patients with peripheral arterial disease and is released from the gut into the systemic circulation during reperfusion in aortic aneurysm surgery [36]. In the setting of renal transplantation, IL-6 was released in large amounts from the reperfused transplanted kidney during the first 30 min of reperfusion [37]. A recent randomised clinical trial examined the efficacy of IL-6 inhibition in the setting of STEMI and reported that myocardial salvage was increased in the treatment arm [38].

IL-8 is a potent neutrophil chemotactic and activating factor. It is produced by monocytes, T cells, natural killer (NK) cells, fibroblasts, endothelial cells, eosinophils and neutrophils in response to IL-1, TNF-α, endotoxin, histamine and hypoxia. The chemotactic activity of IL-8 induces diapedesis of activated neutrophils through the endothelium (Fig. 3.3). Elevated levels of serum IL-8 have been detected during early reperfusion following human lung transplantation and predict poor graft function [39]. An anti-IL-8 antibody prevented pulmonary neutrophil infiltration and tissue injury in a rabbit model of lung IRI [40], but there have not yet been any reports testing this modality in human clinical trials.

3.3.6 *Neutrophils and Endothelial Interactions*

Neutrophils play a major role in tissue damage incurred during IRI. Activated neutrophils are a major source of ROS, which are generated through the activity of the membrane-bound nicotinamide adenine dinucleotide phosphate (NADPH) oxidase complex. While oxidising NADPH to NADP+, NADPH oxidase also reduces molecular oxygen to form the superoxide anion. Myeloperoxidase, stored in the azurophilic granules of neutrophils, converts hydrogen peroxide to toxic hypochlorous acid, which, in addition to its direct effects, is also capable of activating proteases. The activated neutrophils also secrete a number of proteases, including matrix metalloproteinases, which will degrade basement membrane and other tissue structures, contributing to the severity of tissue destruction.

Activated neutrophils also secrete neutrophil extracellular traps (NETS), which are web-like structures of decondensed chromatin and neutrophilic proteins that can modify the activity of cellular proteins to exacerbate inflammation and damage of re-perfused tissues (reviewed in [41]). In a porcine model of hindlimb IRI, NETS were produced, raising the possibility of inhibiting NET production as a useful therapy for IRI [42]. Similarly, a mouse model of hindlimb IRI demonstrated robust formation of NETS during reperfusion-induced inflammation [43]. The generation of NETS during IRI can trigger the development of NETosis, a mechanism of programmed cell death (reviewed in [44]).

Neutrophil infiltration is observed at sites of tissue damage in animal models of IRI [45, 46], and depletion of neutrophils before IRI reduces the severity of organ damage in a mouse model of liver IRI [47]. Depletion of neutrophils during cardiac surgery has been extensively investigated as a modality to reduce the severity of post-operative cardiac dysfunction with inconsistent results. Some studies have shown a reduction in markers of cardiac damage and systemic inflammation while others have been less successful in demonstrating a clinically relevant effect [48].

Selectins are a family of transmembrane molecules, expressed on the surface of leucocytes, activated endothelial cells and in platelets (reviewed in [49, 50]). Selectins mediate the initial phase of neutrophil–endothelial cell interactions, often termed rolling (Fig. 3.3), which is essential for their subsequent adhesion and extravasation. L-selectin is expressed constitutively on the surface of neutrophils and initiates the reversible attachment of neutrophils to endothelial cells and platelets. Antibody-mediated blocking of L-selectin, in a rat model of lung IRI, impairs the ability of neutrophils to roll on endothelial cells and reduces neutrophil infiltration following skeletal muscle and pulmonary IRI [51].

P-selectin is stored in the α-granules of platelets and the Weibel-Palade bodies of endothelial cells and is rapidly translocated to the cell surface along with PAF in response to thrombin, histamine, reactive oxygen species, complement and TNF-α. Typically, peak levels of endothelial P-selectin are detected 6 h after reperfusion. Endothelial P-selectin plays a vital role in the rolling of neutrophils along the activated endothelium. Activation of the endothelium by proinflammatory mediators also results in de novo transcription and synthesis of E-selectin. Expression of endothelial E-selectin is induced during both renal and cerebral IRI. The focal expression of E-selectin at sites of endothelial activation promotes neutrophil adhesion and infiltration into adjacent tissues. In support of a vital role for E-selectin in mediating tissue damage during IRI, a study showed that antibodies against E-selectin reduced infarct size following cerebral IRI in mice [52].

Blocking the activity of selectins shows promise in ameliorating the severity of tissue damage in a number of animal models of IRI [53]. In support of their use in a clinical setting, a clinical trial (SELECT-ACS) tested the efficacy of administration of the P-Selectin antibody, inclacumab, administered before percutaneous coronary intervention, in reducing the severity of post-procedure myocardial damage. Blocking P-selectin with inclacumab significantly reduced the severity of myocardial damage and was most effective when given less than 3 h before the procedure [54]. However, no more recent clinical trials testing this therapy have been reported.

The integrin and immunoglobulin supergene families of adhesion molecules mediate the strong adhesion of activated neutrophils to the endothelium and hence allow their subsequent extravasation during IRI. The integrins form a large family of cell surface adhesion molecules that mediate inter-cellular recognition and cellular binding to the extracellular matrix. The neutrophil β_2-integrin adhesion glycoprotein complex consists of a common polypeptide chain, CD18, which is non-covalently linked to three different α-polypeptide chains (CD11a, CD11b, CD11c). CD11a/CD18 is expressed on all leucocytes and mediates the attachment of stimulated neutrophils to the vascular endothelium through a specific interaction with ICAM-1 and ICAM-2. Chemotactic cytokines (IL-1, TNF-α) and ROS all induce neutrophil adherence to the endothelium by CD11/CD18-dependent mechanisms. The CD11b/18 complex on activated neutrophils interacts with ICAM-1 on the surface of the endothelial cell to mediate firm adhesion of neutrophils prior to their extravasation (reviewed in [55]). All these molecules are required for the development of lung injury following skeletal muscle IRI. Using an anti-CD18 monoclonal antibody, inhibition of CD18-mediated leucocyte adhesion prevented vasoconstriction and increased micro-vascular permeability and vascular resistance in animal models of skeletal muscle IRI. However, despite encouraging animal studies, the clinical efficacy of blocking CD11/CD18-mediated interactions in IRI remains doubtful (reviewed in [56]). Clinical trials in humans failed to demonstrate any effect of CD11/CD18 in reducing infarct size following primary coronary angioplasty in the setting of acute myocardial infarction. A review published in 2005 [57] summarised the results from a number of clinical trials using antibodies to CD11/CD18, including for myocardial infarct and stroke, all of which failed to show any significant benefit to the patient. There have been no significant developments in the field since that date, and this approach seems unlikely to be clinically useful.

The immunoglobulin supergene family (ligands for integrins) contains a large number of molecules with multiple Immunoglobulin-G-like domains. Several members of this family are involved in leukocyte-endothelial cell interactions including ICAM-1, VCAM-1 and platelet-endothelial cell adhesion molecule (PECAM-1). Levels of expression of ICAM-1 on endothelial cells are enhanced by exposure to circulating TNF-α that is generated in response to IRI. VCAM-1 was elevated during renal IRI in a mouse model but, unlike ICAM-1, was independent of TNF-α, since renal IRI in TNF-α knockout mice also up-regulated VCAM-1. PECAM-1 is expressed constitutively on platelets, leucocytes and endothelial cells. IRI induces elevated PECAM-1 levels, thereby enhancing activation of neutrophil-endothelial interactions mediated by β-integrins and exacerbating neutrophil extravasation and tissue damage. In a mouse model of stroke, leucocytes infiltration into the damaged brain was inhibited by a monoclonal PECAM antibody [58, 59].

The therapeutic potential of blocking the activity of adhesion molecules has been tested in animal models with encouraging results. Using monoclonal antibodies, inhibition of ICAM-1 activity attenuated neutrophil adhesion in the liver, reduced pulmonary sequestration and oedema following skeletal muscle IRI and also reduced intestinal dysfunction following IRI [34]. Antisense oligonucleotides to ICAM-1 ameliorated renal IRI and prevented delayed graft dysfunction in a rat model of renal transplantation [60]. However, results obtained in clinical trials have not been as positive. A clinical trial which tested anti-ICAM-1 antibody therapy in ischaemic stroke (enlimomab acute stroke trial) concluded that this therapy was not an effective treatment and may significantly worsen stroke outcome, raising significant doubts regarding the efficacy of this therapeutic modality, and there have been no further investigations since then [61].

3.3.7 Complement Activation

Complement activation and deposition also contributes significantly to the pathogenesis of IRI. Using an isolated canine gracilis model, Rubin and colleagues have demonstrated that reperfusion of skeletal muscle is associated with systemic depletion of the complement protein, factor B, indicative of activation of the alternative complement pathway [62]. The complex C5b-9 is also deposited into the endothelial cell membrane after IRI, leading to osmotic lysis [63]. Unequivocal evidence for the importance of complement activation during skeletal muscle IRI has been provided from experiments where limb ischaemia was induced in C5-deficient mice. These mice had approximately 50% less tissue damage than the wild-type animals [34].

Inhibition of the complement cascade has been demonstrated to improve outcomes following IRI in a number of different animal models. Complement depletion of circulating plasma improved the initial blood flow and decreased muscle necrosis and injury after ischaemia and prolonged reperfusion in dogs. Complement blockade also prevented leucocytes adhesion, leading to better capillary perfusion and muscle cell viability and attenuated the increase in permeability index in tissues [62]. Pulmonary damage following bilateral hind limb ischaemia was significantly reduced when the soluble complement receptor was administered to rats, thus inhibiting complement activity [64]. In a rat model of ruptured aneurysm followed by cross-clamping and reperfusion, administration of a C5 complement inhibitor reduced shock and acute lung injury [65].

An additive role of both complement and neutrophils in mediating skeletal muscle IRI has also been observed, with a greater reduction in histological damage in neutropenic C5-deficient animals than in neutropenic or C5-deficient mice alone [34]. These data continue to demonstrate the multi-factorial nature of tissue damage induced during IRI since complement blockade alone failed to completely ameliorate tissue damage. However, clinical efficacy remains uncertain as a clinical trial in renal transplantation failed to show that administration of anti-C5 monoclonal antibody eculizumab had any effect on delayed graft function [66].

3.3.8 Toll-Like Receptors and the Innate Immune System

Toll-like receptors (TLRs) are a class of proteins that play a key role in the innate immune system, and TLR signalling is an important mediator of the inflammatory response during IRI. In particular, TLR-4 has been increasingly recognised as playing a critical role in the pathogenesis of IRI [67]. TLR-4 recognises danger-associated molecular patterns (DAMPs), protein complexes released from damaged and dying cells following IRI. DAMPS released from damaged cells include heat shock proteins (HSPs), some of which can enhance tissue damage during IRI while other HSPs may be protective [68]. Activation of TLR-4 by DAMPs also promotes the release of many of the pro-inflammatory cytokines described above, including IL-1β, IL-6 and TNF-α. TLR-4 also facilitates leucocytes migration and infiltration and also activates the innate and adaptive immune system (reviewed in [69]).

3.4 Tissue Destruction

3.4.1 Proteases and Metalloproteinases

The matrix metalloproteinases (MMPs) are a family of zinc-dependent enzymes that have the ability to degrade components of the extracellular matrix. Together with their inhibitors, the tissue inhibitors of metalloproteinases (TIMPs), they are the major physiological regulators of the extracellular matrix. MMPs are intimately involved in all processes that necessitate degradation or synthesis of the extracellular matrix, and important roles for these enzymes have been identified in wound healing, periodontal disease, cancer metastasis and, of particular relevance, vascular disease including the development of aneurysms, atherosclerotic plaques and reperfusion injury.

Elevations of MMP-2 and MMP-9 have been detected following pulmonary, hepatic and cardiac IRI [70]. MMPs are also elevated following cerebral IRI, corresponding with opening of the blood-brain barrier, degradation of the basal lamina, increased capillary permeability and cerebral oedema [71]. Definitive roles for MMP-9 in the pathophysiology of cerebral IRI have been demonstrated by using both selective MMP-9 inhibitors and MMP-9 knockout mice, which both significantly reduced cerebral infarct size [64]. MMP-2 may have a late role in renal IRI with an elevation detected as late as 8 weeks after IRI [65]. However, the MMP inhibitor, batimastat, did not alter the severity of renal dysfunction in a rat model of renal IRI [72]. In contrast, the MMP inhibitor doxycycline preserved renal function in a rat model of renal IRI [73].

Barr and co-workers [74] examined brain MRI scans from acute ischaemic stroke patients and correlated systemic plasma MMP-9 levels with a hyperintense acute reperfusion injury marker (HARM), measured by MRI 24 h later. Plasma MMP-9 was a significant predictor of elevated HARM measures, supporting the hypothesis that elevated MMP-9 is associated with disruption of the blood-brain barrier after ischaemic stroke. These results raise the possibility that inhibition of MMP-9 may be a useful modality to reduce the severity of cerebral damage, but to date, no clinical trials have tested this possibility.

Studies in our laboratory have demonstrated both a local and systemic role for MMP-2 and MMP-9 in the degradation of type IV collagen in pulmonary tissues and in skeletal muscle following lower limb IRI [46]. Permanent ischaemia alone, without reperfusion, also resulted in elevation of MMP-2 and MMP-9, correlating with destruction of the basement membrane components, type IV collagen and laminin.

3.4.2 Cell Death Mechanisms in IRI

The mechanisms of tissue destruction during IRI are complex and multi-factorial (reviewed in [75]). Tissue destruction resulting from IRI can be due to either necrosis or a range of programmed cell death mechanisms including apoptosis, ferroptosis and necroptosis (reviewed in [76]).

Necrosis is an uncontrolled form of cell death, often caused by traumatic injury and is frequently detected during IRI. It can be easily identified by morphologic damage, cell swelling and plasma membrane rupture. Cellular contents are then released into the surrounding tissues, frequently leading to inflammation.

Autophagy (see Glossary) has a dual role in IRI. As a cellular self-degradation and clearance mechanism, autophagy can confer protection during the initial phases of cellular injury, yet potentially exacerbate damage in the later stages, by facilitating the apoptotic cascade and exacerbating cellular injury. In mild or moderate IRI, it reduces oxidative stress by facilitating the degradation and recycling of damaged organelles and proteins via the lysosomal pathway. This process is essential for maintaining cellular energy balance, homeostasis and adapting to diverse stress conditions. However, excess autophagy can be triggered by the generation of high levels of reactive oxygen species from the mitochondria of damaged cells during IRI [77, 78].

3.4.3 Apoptotic Cell Death During Ischaemia-Reperfusion Injury

Apoptosis is a form of programmed cell death, which is an active process characterised by a series of gene-directed events leading to a characteristic cell morphology, development of apoptotic bodies, controlled DNA fragmentation and eventually death of the cell. The role of apoptosis in IRI-induced tissue damage has been widely investigated. Oxidative stress and the production of ROS will induce apoptosis, the characteristics of which can readily be recognised following cerebral IRI. Similarly, renal [79] and cardiac IRI all result in detectable levels of apoptosis in the damaged tissue. Apoptosis therefore appears to play a fundamental role in cellular damage occurring during IRI in a number of tissues.

However, the role of apoptosis in skeletal muscle IRI remains controversial. Studies conducted in our laboratory, [45] in agreement with Knight and co-workers, [80] have failed to detect any evidence of apoptosis in rat skeletal myocytes following IRI. This implicates a tissue-specific mechanism of cell death following IRI. Blocking the apoptotic cascade, using specific inhibitors directed against pro-apoptotic caspase enzymes, has been partially effective in animal models, reducing the severity and infarct size following hepatic and cardiac IRI [81]. However, clinical trials to test this therapy have not yet been reported.

3.4.4 Necroptosis and Ferroptosis

Necroptosis represents a recently identified form of programmed cell death that combines the features of both apoptosis and necrosis. Necroptotic cells display the morphological features of necrosis but not of apoptosis. When compared to apoptosis, where cellular components from the damaged cell are isolated in apoptotic bodies, necroptosis involves the leakage of cellular contents into the surrounding tissues, generating an inflammatory response (reviewed in [76]). The mechanism of necroptosis is highly regulated by intra-cellular protein signals generated during IRI, including TNF-α [82], ubiquitination and activation of the kinase domain of receptor-interacting protein1 (RIP1), ultimately leading to expression of damage-associated molecular patterns (DAMPs) (reviewed in [83]). It has been suggested that necroptosis inhibitors may be useful to reduce the severity of IRI, but more research is needed [84].

Ferroptosis is an iron-dependent, superoxide-driven, non-apoptotic form of regulated cell death characterised by lipid peroxidation and iron overload which also forms an integral mechanism of tissue destruction during reperfusion [85, 86]. In cardiac reperfusion, damage to mitochondria forms an integral part of cellular damage resulting from ferroptosis, and this mechanism may also be a target for therapeutic intervention, but further study is needed.

3.4.5 *No Reflow Phenomenon*

No reflow is the failure of microvascular perfusion, following restoration of flow to previously ischaemic tissue. The cause of this phenomenon has not been fully elucidated (reviewed in [87, 88]) but is certainly multi-factorial. Cytokines and activated neutrophils act synergistically to produce micro-vascular barrier dysfunction. The resultant increase in permeability leads to the exudation of fluids and proteins, increasing the interstitial pressure and decreasing the intravascular pressure. In addition, CD18-dependent leucocytes plugging produces partial occlusion of post-capillary venules, further contributing to no-reflow. Neutrophil depletion virtually abolishes the phenomenon in the brain, confirming a vital role for neutrophils in no-reflow [89].

3.5 Therapeutic Approaches to Ischaemia-Reperfusion Injury

3.5.1 *Ischaemic Preconditioning*

Ischaemic preconditioning consists of brief and repetitive episodes of IRI before the induction of sustained organ ischaemia and can be effective in reducing the severity of tissue damage. The preconditioning effect can be delivered remotely instead of to the target organ. This treatment could be useful in a number of operative settings including transplantation, coronary bypass grafting and elective major vascular surgical procedures, where the onset of ischaemia can be tightly controlled. In these settings, brief extremity IRI (10 min) administered by tourniquet before surgery, has been widely investigated and shows promise as a therapy to reduce the severity of IRI.

Animal models of IRI have been used to investigate mechanisms of ischaemic preconditioning but the basic molecular mechanisms remain unclear, probably due to the multiple signal transduction pathways involved in this phenomenon. However, it is generally recognised that brief ischaemic preconditioning induces a cascade of intra-cellular kinases, which subsequently modify mitochondrial function. A study in a rat model of lower limb IRI illustrated clearly that two brief 10-min episodes of IRI before a full 60 min of ischaemia followed by reperfusion was effective in reducing proinflammatory neutrophil-endothelium interactions. This effect was noted in both the lower limb itself and in remote tissues, illustrating the systemic nature of this phenomenon [90].

A number of clinical trials have also been reported which have investigated the efficacy of ischaemic preconditioning with varying degrees of success (reviewed in [91, 92]). Remote preconditioning significantly protected against post-operative myocardial injury, myocardial infarction, and renal impairment [93]. An excellent "proof of concept" study of ischaemic preconditioning was reported in the setting of evolving ST-elevation acute myocardial infarction. Subjects were randomised while in the ambulance and received intermittent arm ischaemia during transport to hospital (four cycles of 5-min inflation and 5-min deflation of a blood-pressure cuff). The primary endpoint was the myocardial salvage index 30 days after primary percutaneous coronary intervention, measured by myocardial perfusion imaging. The data showed convincingly that remote ischaemic conditioning before hospital admission increased myocardial salvage [94].

A small randomised clinical trial aimed to determine if remote lower limb ischaemic preconditioning before endovascular aneurysm repair (EVAR) could reduce the severity of renal and cardiac damage [95]. A significant reduction in urinary biomarkers of renal injury was detected in the preconditioning cohort but this small pilot trial was unable to detect any effect on clinical endpoints. However, in the setting of open AAA repair where operative ischaemia is profound, promising results were obtained. In the context of vascular surgical procedures, a pilot randomised controlled trial reported on composite clinical endpoints for 200 patients undergoing open AAA repair, EVAR, carotid endarterectomy or lower limb revascularisation. Patients were randomised to receive four cycles of 5 min of forearm ischaemia before surgery. The results, however, did not show any significant differences between outcomes in the groups, and the authors suggest a larger trial is required [96]. A non-significant result was also recently reported in a similar patient cohort where no change in arterial stiffness could be detected as a result of preconditioning [97]. A recent systematic review and meta-analysis came to similar conclusions, stating that there was insufficient evidence that preconditioning improved outcomes after open AAA repair or EVAR, but the studies were underpowered and that there was considerable methodological heterogeneity [98]. A more recent randomised clinical trial tested remote preconditioning in the settings of open abdominal aortic aneurysm repair, surgical lower limb revascularisation surgery or carotid endarterectomy. Remote ischaemic preconditioning reduced the leakage of high-sensitivity troponin T and pro-b-type natriuretic peptide. Therefore, it may offer cardioprotection in patients undergoing non-cardiac vascular surgery, but further studies are required [99].

3.5.2 *Ischaemic Postconditioning*

Ischaemic postconditioning is defined as rapid sequential intermittent interruption of blood flow applied during the early moments of reperfusion. This interruption can be either local (to the ischaemic organ) or remote, typically where a limb is occluded for a short time. This technique is particularly relevant where the initial ischaemic insult could not have been predicted, thus a preconditioning approach to limiting tissue damage could not have been applied. Experimental animal models have been used to successfully show attenuation of organ injury, including the heart, spinal cord, brain, kidney, liver, muscle, lung and intestines (reviewed in [100]). The mechanisms of postconditioning are not yet entirely clear but appear to involve multiple signalling pathways and molecules, including protein kinases, ROS, proinflammatory cytokines and NO, as well as alterations in mitochondrial function (reviewed in [101, 102]).

Animal models of relevance to vascular surgical procedures have been tested widely and results show promise as an effective therapy to reduce the severity of IRI. In a rat model of lower limb ischaemia induced by aortic clamping, rats underwent 180 min of ischaemia followed by postconditioning consisting of six cycles of 10 s aortic occlusion followed by 10 s unclamping at the beginning of reperfusion. Postconditioning caused a significant reduction in both the severity of systemic inflammatory responses and the degree of remote pulmonary and renal damage [103]. In a similar study in the rat [104], 60 min infrarenal aortic cross-clamping followed by intermittent four times 15 s reperfusion-15 s ischaemic episodes before reperfusion, was effective in reducing production of ROS, leucocytes-endothelial activation and cytokine production. A more recent study in a rat model of myocardial IRI demonstrated that remote postconditioning reduced the severity of myocardial apoptosis. Multiple signal transduction pathways were up-regulated by remote postconditioning, including cytokine activity, Toll-like receptors and TNF-α [102].

Based on the experimental models, ischaemic postconditioning thus appears to show promise as an effective therapy in vascular surgery to reduce reperfusion injuries after aortic surgery and revascularisation procedures (reviewed in [105]). Some clinical studies have verified these findings. Controlled limb reperfusion following revascularisation for acute limb ischaemia resulted in lower levels of systemically circulating products resulting from muscle breakdown, including lactate and potassium levels [106]. This study did not determine if clinical outcomes were improved in these patients. However, after an acute ischaemic stroke, remote ischaemic postconditioning failed to show any improved quality of life [107]. In the future, the duration of the occlusion and reperfusion periods will be critical to the degree of protection and useful algorithms are needed to plan therapeutic strategies after a significant ischaemic insult.

3.5.3 Conditioning Effects of Volatile Anaesthetics

Anaesthetics have been widely demonstrated to reduce the severity of IRI-induced damage in the setting of myocardial ischaemia and reperfusion during cardiac surgery (reviewed in [108]). However, there is conflicting evidence regarding the relative contributions of preconditioning, conditioning during ischaemia and postconditioning to the significant cardioprotection provided by anaesthetics. The molecular mechanisms and signal transduction pathways involved in protection are an area of active investigation. A proteomic study demonstrated that volatile anaesthetics (isofluorane, sevofluorane or desfluorane) induced long-lasting changes in the expression of 106 proteins in the rat myocardium [109] and also in the hippocampus [110]. Mitochondrial protein expression after myocardial IRI was also significantly altered by sevofluorane preconditioning [111].

Anaesthetic-induced postconditioning mechanisms are also multi-factorial. Volatile anaesthetics are known to inhibit neutrophil adhesion in the coronary arteries during the reperfusion phase, thereby inhibiting the inflammatory action of activated neutrophils in post-ischaemic tissues (Fig. 3.3). Evidence also suggests that inhibition by anaesthetics of the opening of the mitochondrial permeability pore may be a key mechanism of anaesthetic-induced preconditioning [112].

There is conflicting clinical evidence for the cardioprotective effects of volatile anaesthetics during cardiac surgery. A meta-analysis examined randomised trials comparing volatile with non-volatile anaesthesia in coronary bypass surgery. There was no significant difference in myocardial ischaemia, myocardial infarct, intensive care unit length of stay or in-hospital mortality. However, patients receiving volatile anaesthetics had significantly higher cardiac function indices, lower troponin I serum concentrations and a lower requirement for inotropic support [113]. A large multi-centre study also provided excellent evidence that volatile anaesthesia significantly reduced mortality after coronary bypass grafting [114]. However, more recent studies have not all been so promising. Sevoflurane anaesthesia did not protect the myocardium against IRI associated with cardiac surgery as assessed by troponin release [115]. In contrast, patients given sevofluorane anaesthesia during renal transplantation had significantly better early graft survival when compared to those given isofluorane [116].

3.5.4 Pharmacological Treatments

As discussed in many of the sections above, a wide range of pharmacological therapies have been tested in both animal models and in clinical practice. Although many of the animal interventions show considerable promise in reducing the severity of IRI, results from clinical trials have uniformly been disappointing. A Cochrane Review reported on treatments to reduce IRI during liver resection under vascular control [117]. They identified 15 randomised trials, which examined 11 pharmacological interventions (methylprednisolone, multi-vitamin antioxidant infusion, vitamin E infusion, amrinone, prostaglandin E1, pentoxifylline, mannitol, trimetazidine, dextrose, allopurinol and a thromboxane A2 synthetase inhibitor). Although some therapies improved liver enzyme levels, there were no significant differences between the groups for mortality, liver failure, or perioperative morbidity. A second Cochrane review from the same authors [118] examined the effects of prostaglandin E1, pentoxifylline, dopexamine, dopamine, ulinastatin, gantaile, sevoflurane, and propofol during liver IRI and reached the same conclusion that there were no significant differences.

Statin therapies have been widely accepted into clinical practice and there is also considerable evidence, both experimental and clinical, that statins will reduce the severity of IRI in a range of settings. Statins inhibit a range of cellular responses to IRI-induced inflammation, including inhibition of NF-κB activity, which leads to decreased transcription of MMPs, adhesion molecule and cytokine genes. The binding of adhesion molecules on activated neutrophils to endothelial cell surface receptors is also blocked. Secretion of MMPs from activated neutrophils is also inhibited by statins. In the endothelium, levels of expression of eNOS mRNA are increased and the eNOS protein is activated, while expression of endothelin-1 is inhibited. All of these effects will ameliorate the severity of tissue damage during IRI (reviewed in [119]).

Trials of lower limb IRI in the rat were carried out in our laboratory and illustrated that pre-treatment for a week with simvastatin before IRI markedly protected both skeletal muscle and remote organs including the lungs and kidneys [22, 120]. A review [121] discussed the efficacy of statins to ameliorate IRI in patients undergoing a range of vascular surgical procedures. In the setting of infrainguinal bypass for peripheral arterial disease, the indications that statins may protect against IRI during surgery are not definitive with some conflicting results, although 1-year mortality was improved. Evidence for any effect of statin treatment on the severity of post-operative complications after AAA repair is lacking, although a retrospective observational study showed that all-cause mortality was reduced in those on long-term statin therapy [122]. However, since all vascular patients should be receiving statin treatment for secondary prevention of cardiovascular disease, prospective randomised trials to obtain definitive results can no longer ethically be performed.

Other pharmacological mediators have been tested as potential therapies to reduce IRI with varying results. N-acetyl cysteine, an antioxidant, was tested in a randomised controlled trial as an early intervention in STEMI patients who were about to undergo percutaneous coronary intervention. A significant reduction in infarct size was detected, supporting a potential therapeutic role of n-acetyl cysteine in reducing the severity of IRI [123]. Other drug therapies, including metoprolol [124] and cyclosporine [125], have been tested in clinical trials addressing myocardial IRI with conflicting results and further research is needed.

3.6 Summary

In summary, IRI is a highly complex series of interwoven pro-inflammatory and pathological events. The production, release and activation of cytokines, ROS, proteases and complement if left unchecked lead to both local and systemic injury with potentially fatal consequences. The failure of therapeutic interventions to translate into routine clinical practice is a reflection of this complexity and redundancy within the system. New therapeutic agents directed towards multiple areas within this cascade may be required to overcome this difficult clinical challenge.

Multiple Choice Questions

1. What are the major mechanisms of cell death in reperfusion injury?

   (a) Activation and proteolytic activity of matrix metalloproteinases
   (b) Necrosis
   (c) Programmed cell death, including apoptosis, necroptosis and ferroptosis
   (d) Cytokine-mediated activation of neutrophils
   (e) No-reflow phenomenon

   Answers: (c) Programmed cell death, including apoptosis, necroptosis and ferroptosis

2. Which therapeutic intervention shows most promise as an effective treatment for reperfusion injury?

   (a) Ischaemic preconditioning
   (b) Inhibition of matrix metalloproteinase activity
   (c) Administration of pharmacological agents
   (d) Inhibition of release of reactive oxygen species in early reperfusion
   (e) Inhibition of nitric oxide generation

   Answers: (a) Ischaemic preconditioning

References

1. Paoni NF, Peale F, Wang F, Errett-Baroncini C, Steinmetz H, Toy K, et al. Time course of skeletal muscle repair and gene expression following acute hind limb ischemia in mice. Physiol Genomics. 2002;11:263–72. https://doi.org/10.1152/physiolgenomics.00110.2002.
2. Safronova O, Morita I. Transcriptome remodeling in hypoxic inflammation. J Dent Res. 2010;89:430–44. https://doi.org/10.1177/0022034510366813.
3. Hierholzer C, Harbrecht BG, Billiar TR, Tweardy DJ. Hypoxia-inducible factor-1 activation and cyclo-oxygenase-2 induction are early reperfusion-independent inflammatory events in hemorrhagic shock. Arch Orthop Trauma Surg. 2001;121:219–22. https://doi.org/10.1007/s004020000211.
4. Yokoyama K, Kimura M, Nakamura K, Itoman M. Time course of post-ischemic superoxide generation in venous effluent from reperfused rabbit hindlimbs. J Reconstr Microsurg. 1999;15:215–21. https://doi.org/10.1055/s-2007-1000094.
5. Gomes RZ, Romanek GM, Przybycien M, Amaral DC, Akahane HG. Evaluation of the effect of allopurinol as a protective factor in post ischemia and reperfusion inflammation in Wistar rats. Acta Cir Bras. 2016;31:126–32. https://doi.org/10.1590/s0102-865020160020000007.
6. Pacher P, Nivorozhkin A, Szabo C. Therapeutic effects of xanthine oxidase inhibitors: renaissance half a century after the discovery of allopurinol. Pharmacol Rev. 2006;58:87–114. https://doi.org/10.1124/pr.58.1.6.
7. Kermani-Alghoraishi M, Sanei H, Heshmat-Ghahdarijani K, Ghahramani R, Honarvar M, Sadeghi M. Impact of allopurinol pretreatment on coronary blood flow and revascularization outcomes after percutaneous coronary intervention in acute STEMI patients: a random-

ized double blind clinical trial. ARYA Atheroscler. 2023;19:1–9. https://doi.org/10.48305/arya.2023.11577.2121.
8. Tumer NB, Erol G, Tekeli Kunt A, Doganci S. Effect of iloprost, a prostacyclin analogue, on myocardial ischemia-reperfusion injury. Heart Surg Forum. 2019;22:E027–e31. https://doi.org/10.1532/hsf.2076.
9. Neumann UP, Kaisers U, Langrehr JM, Glanemann M, Muller AR, Lang M, et al. Administration of prostacyclin after liver transplantation: a placebo controlled randomized trial. Clin Transpl. 2000;14:70–4. https://doi.org/10.1034/j.1399-0012.2000.140113.x.
10. Rowlands TE, Gough MJ, Homer-Vanniasinkam S. Do prostaglandins have a salutary role in skeletal muscle ischaemia-reperfusion injury? Eur J Vasc Endovasc Surg. 1999;18:439–44. https://doi.org/10.1053/ejvs.1999.0929.
11. de Donato G, Gussoni G, de Donato G, Andreozzi GM, Bonizzoni E, Mazzone A, et al. The ILAILL study: iloprost as adjuvant to surgery for acute ischemia of lower limbs: a randomized, placebo-controlled, double-blind study by the Italian Society for Vascular and Endovascular Surgery. Ann Surg. 2006;244:185–93. https://doi.org/10.1097/01.sla.0000217555.49001.ca.
12. de Donato G, Gussoni G, de Donato G, Cao P, Setacci C, Pratesi C, et al. Acute limb ischemia in elderly patients: can iloprost be useful as an adjuvant to surgery? Results from the ILAILL study. Eur J Vasc Endovasc Surg. 2007;34:194–8. https://doi.org/10.1016/j.ejvs.2007.02.002.
13. Li J, Wang B, Wang Y, Wu F, Li P, Li Y, et al. Therapeutic effect of liposomal prostaglandin E1 in acute lower limb ischemia as an adjuvant to hybrid procedures. Exp Ther Med. 2013;5:1760–4. https://doi.org/10.3892/etm.2013.1061.
14. Almazroo OA, Miah MK, Pillai VC, Shaik IH, Xu R, Dharmayan S, et al. An evaluation of the safety and preliminary efficacy of peri- and post-operative treprostinil in preventing ischemia and reperfusion injury in adult orthotopic liver transplant recipients. Clin Transpl. 2021;35:e14298. https://doi.org/10.1111/ctr.14298.
15. Slupski M, Szadujkis-Szadurska K, Szadujkis-Szadurski R, Szadujkis-Szadurski L, Wlodarczyk Z, Andruszkiewicz J, et al. Nitric oxide and thromboxane A2 modulate pulmonary pressure after ischemia and intestinal reperfusion. Transplant Proc. 2006;38:334–7. https://doi.org/10.1016/j.transproceed.2005.12.085.
16. Mazolewski PJ, Roth AC, Suchy H, Stephenson LL, Zamboni WA. Role of the thromboxane A2 receptor in the vasoactive response to ischemia-reperfusion injury. Plast Reconstr Surg. 1999;104:1393–6. https://doi.org/10.1097/00006534-199910000-00023.
17. He Z, Wang DW. The roles of eicosanoids in myocardial diseases. Adv Pharmacol. 2023;97:167–200. https://doi.org/10.1016/bs.apha.2022.11.001.
18. Mangino MJ, Murphy MK, Anderson CB. Effects of the arachidonate 5-lipoxygenase synthesis inhibitor A-64077 in intestinal ischemia-reperfusion injury. J Pharmacol Exp Ther. 1994;269:75–81.
19. Karatas H, Eun Jung J, Lo EH, van Leyen K. Inhibiting 12/15-lipoxygenase to treat acute stroke in permanent and tPA induced thrombolysis models. Brain Res. 2018;1678:123–8. https://doi.org/10.1016/j.brainres.2017.10.024.
20. Khanna A, Cowled PA, Fitridge RA. Nitric oxide and skeletal muscle reperfusion injury: current controversies (research review). J Surg Res. 2005;128:98–107. https://doi.org/10.1016/j.jss.2005.04.020.
21. Lee HM, Choi JW, Choi MS. Role of nitric oxide and protein S-nitrosylation in ischemia-reperfusion injury. Antioxidants (Basel). 2021;11:57. https://doi.org/10.3390/antiox11010057.
22. Cowled PA, Khanna A, Laws PE, Field JB, Varelias A, Fitridge RA. Statins inhibit neutrophil infiltration in skeletal muscle reperfusion injury. J Surg Res. 2007;141:267–76. https://doi.org/10.1016/j.jss.2006.11.021.
23. Sienel RI, Mamrak U, Biller J, Roth S, Zellner A, Parakaw T, et al. Inhaled nitric oxide suppresses neuroinflammation in experimental ischemic stroke. J Neuroinflammation. 2023;20:301. https://doi.org/10.1186/s12974-023-02988-3.

24. Dugbartey GJ. Nitric oxide in kidney transplantation. Biomed Pharmacother. 2023;167:115530. https://doi.org/10.1016/j.biopha.2023.115530.
25. Dugbartey GJ. Therapeutic benefits of nitric oxide in lung transplantation. Biomed Pharmacother. 2023;167:115549. https://doi.org/10.1016/j.biopha.2023.115549.
26. Dugbartey GJ, Nanteer D, Osae I. Nitric oxide protects intestinal mucosal barrier function and prevents acute graft rejection after intestinal transplantation: a mini-review. Nitric Oxide. 2024;149:1–6. https://doi.org/10.1016/j.niox.2024.05.001.
27. Kiris I, Narin C, Gulmen S, Yilmaz N, Sutcu R, Kapucuoglu N. Endothelin receptor antagonism by tezosentan attenuates lung injury induced by aortic ischemia-reperfusion. Ann Vasc Surg. 2009;23:382–91. https://doi.org/10.1016/j.avsg.2008.10.003.
28. Gong S, Seng Z, Wang W, Lv J, Dong Q, Yan B, et al. Bosentan protects the spinal cord from ischemia reperfusion injury in rats through vascular endothelial growth factor receptors. Spinal Cord. 2015;53:19–23. https://doi.org/10.1038/sc.2014.147.
29. Ucar BI, Erikci A, Kosemehmetoglu K, Ozkul C, Iskit AB, Ucar G, et al. Effects of endothelin receptor blockade and COX inhibition on intestinal I/R injury in a rat model: experimental research. Int J Surg. 2020;83:89–97. https://doi.org/10.1016/j.ijsu.2020.08.061.
30. Lutz J, Thurmel K, Heemann U. Anti-inflammatory treatment strategies for ischemia/reperfusion injury in transplantation. J Inflamm (Lond). 2010;7:27. https://doi.org/10.1186/1476-9255-7-27.
31. Tassiopoulos AK, Carlin RE, Gao Y, Pedoto A, Finck CM, Landas SK, et al. Role of nitric oxide and tumor necrosis factor on lung injury caused by ischemia/reperfusion of the lower extremities. J Vasc Surg. 1997;26:647–56. https://doi.org/10.1016/s0741-5214(97)70065-x.
32. Evangelatos G, Bamias G, Kitas GD, Kollias G, Sfikakis PP. The second decade of anti-TNF-α therapy in clinical practice: new lessons and future directions in the COVID-19 era. Rheumatol Int. 2022;42:1493–511. https://doi.org/10.1007/s00296-022-05136-x.
33. Duran WN, Milazzo VJ, Sabido F, Hobson RW 2nd. Platelet-activating factor modulates leukocyte adhesion to endothelium in ischemia-reperfusion. Microvasc Res. 1996;51:108–15. https://doi.org/10.1006/mvre.1996.0011.
34. Sun Z, Wang X, Lasson A, Bojesson A, Annborn M, Andersson R. Effects of inhibition of PAF, ICAM-1 and PECAM-1 on gut barrier failure caused by intestinal ischemia and reperfusion. Scand J Gastroenterol. 2001;36:55–65. https://doi.org/10.1080/00365520150218066.
35. Borjesson A, Wang X, Sun Z, Inghammar M, Truedsson L, Andersson R. Early treatment with lexipafant, a platelet-activating factor-receptor antagonist, is not sufficient to prevent pulmonary endothelial damage after intestinal ischaemia and reperfusion in rats. Dig Liver Dis. 2002;34:190–6. https://doi.org/10.1016/s1590-8658(02)80192-x.
36. Norwood MG, Bown MJ, Sutton AJ, Nicholson ML, Sayers RD. Interleukin 6 production during abdominal aortic aneurysm repair arises from the gastrointestinal tract and not the legs. Br J Surg. 2004;91:1153–6. https://doi.org/10.1002/bjs.4691.
37. de Vries DK, Lindeman JH, Tsikas D, de Heer E, Roos A, de Fijter JW, et al. Early renal ischemia-reperfusion injury in humans is dominated by IL-6 release from the allograft. Am J Transplant. 2009;9:1574–84. https://doi.org/10.1111/j.1600-6143.2009.02675.x.
38. Broch K, Anstensrud AK, Woxholt S, Sharma K, Tøllefsen IM, Bendz B, et al. Randomized trial of interleukin-6 receptor inhibition in patients with acute ST-segment elevation myocardial infarction. J Am Coll Cardiol. 2021;77:1845–55. https://doi.org/10.1016/j.jacc.2021.02.049.
39. De Perrot M, Sekine Y, Fischer S, Waddell TK, McRae K, Liu M, et al. Interleukin-8 release during early reperfusion predicts graft function in human lung transplantation. Am J Respir Crit Care Med. 2002;165:211–5. https://doi.org/10.1164/ajrccm.165.2.2011151.
40. Sekido N, Mukaida N, Harada A, Nakanishi I, Watanabe Y, Matsushima K. Prevention of lung reperfusion injury in rabbits by a monoclonal antibody against interleukin-8. Nature. 1993;365:654–7. https://doi.org/10.1038/365654a0.

41. Li X, Ma Y, Wang D. The role of P-selectin/PSGL-1 in regulating NETs as a novel mechanism in cerebral ischemic injury. Front Neurol. 2024;15:1442613. https://doi.org/10.3389/fneur.2024.1442613.
42. Zollet V, Arenas Hoyos I, Hirsiger S, Brahim BB, Petrucci MF, Casoni D, et al. Neutrophil extracellular traps and citrullinated fibrinogen contribute to injury in a porcine model of limb ischemia and reperfusion. Front Immunol. 2024;15:1436926. https://doi.org/10.3389/fimmu.2024.1436926.
43. Edwards NJ, Hwang C, Marini S, Pagani CA, Spreadborough PJ, Rowe CJ, et al. The role of neutrophil extracellular traps and TLR signaling in skeletal muscle ischemia reperfusion injury. FASEB J. 2020;34:15753–70. https://doi.org/10.1096/fj.202000994RR.
44. Huang J, Hong W, Wan M, Zheng L. Molecular mechanisms and therapeutic target of NETosis in diseases. MedComm (2020). 2022;3:e162. https://doi.org/10.1002/mco2.162.
45. Cowled PA, Leonardos L, Millard SH, Fitridge RA. Apoptotic cell death makes a minor contribution to reperfusion injury in skeletal muscle in the rat. Eur J Vasc Endovasc Surg. 2001;21:28–34. https://doi.org/10.1053/ejvs.2000.1209.
46. Roach DM, Fitridge RA, Laws PE, Millard SH, Varelias A, Cowled PA. Up-regulation of MMP-2 and MMP-9 leads to degradation of type IV collagen during skeletal muscle reperfusion injury; protection by the MMP inhibitor, doxycycline. Eur J Vasc Endovasc Surg. 2002;23:260–9. https://doi.org/10.1053/ejvs.2002.1598.
47. Martinez-Mier G, Toledo-Pereyra LH, McDuffie JE, Warner RL, Ward PA. Neutrophil depletion and chemokine response after liver ischemia and reperfusion. J Investig Surg. 2001;14:99–107. https://doi.org/10.1080/08941930152024228.
48. Khan AI, Patidar GK, Lakshmy R, Makhija N, Talwar S, Hazarika A. Effect of leukoreduction on transfusion-related immunomodulation in patients undergoing cardiac surgery. Transfus Med. 2020;30:497–504. https://doi.org/10.1111/tme.12714.
49. McEver RP. Selectins: initiators of leucocyte adhesion and signalling at the vascular wall. Cardiovasc Res. 2015;107:331–9. https://doi.org/10.1093/cvr/cvv154.
50. Peterson JM, Smith TA, Rock EP, Magnani JL. Selectins in biology and human disease: opportunity in E-selectin antagonism. Cureus. 2024;16:e61996. https://doi.org/10.7759/cureus.61996.
51. Levine AJ, Parkes K, Rooney SJ, Bonser RS. The effect of adhesion molecule blockade on pulmonary reperfusion injury. Ann Thorac Surg. 2002;73:1101–6. https://doi.org/10.1016/s0003-4975(01)03380-x.
52. Huang J, Choudhri TF, Winfree CJ, McTaggart RA, Kiss S, Mocco J, et al. Postischemic cerebrovascular E-selectin expression mediates tissue injury in murine stroke. Stroke. 2000;31:3047–53.
53. Calvey CR, Toledo-Pereyra LH. Selectin inhibitors and their proposed role in ischemia and reperfusion. J Investig Surg. 2007;20:71–85. https://doi.org/10.1080/08941930701250212.
54. Stahli BE, Gebhard C, Duchatelle V, Cournoyer D, Petroni T, Tanguay JF, et al. Effects of the P-selectin antagonist inclacumab on myocardial damage after percutaneous coronary intervention according to timing of infusion: insights from the SELECT-ACS trial. J Am Heart Assoc. 2016;5:e004255. https://doi.org/10.1161/jaha.116.004255.
55. Yilmaz G, Granger DN. Cell adhesion molecules and ischemic stroke. Neurol Res. 2008;30:783–93. https://doi.org/10.1179/174313208X341085.
56. McKenzie ME, Gurbel PA. The potential of monoclonal antibodies to reduce reperfusion injury in myocardial infarction. BioDrugs. 2001;15:395–404. https://doi.org/10.2165/00063030-200115060-00005.
57. Yonekawa K, Harlan JM. Targeting leukocyte integrins in human diseases. J Leukoc Biol. 2005;77:129–40. https://doi.org/10.1189/jlb.0804460.
58. Nadkarni NA, Arias E, Fang R, Haynes ME, Zhang HF, Muller WA, et al. Platelet endothelial cell adhesion molecule (PECAM/CD31) blockade modulates neutrophil recruitment patterns and reduces infarct size in experimental ischemic stroke. Am J Pathol. 2022;192:1619–32. https://doi.org/10.1016/j.ajpath.2022.07.008.

59. Arias E, Nadkarni N, Fang R, Haynes M, Batra A, Muller W, et al. Inhibition of PECAM-1 significantly delays leukocyte extravasation into the subcortex post-stroke. FASEB J. 2022;36 Suppl 1. https://doi.org/10.1096/fasebj.2022.36.S1.R5646.
60. Dragun D, Tullius SG, Park JK, Maasch C, Lukitsch I, Lippoldt A, et al. ICAM-1 antisense oligodesoxynucleotides prevent reperfusion injury and enhance immediate graft function in renal transplantation. Kidney Int. 1998;54:590–602. https://doi.org/10.1046/j.1523-1755.1998.00026.x.
61. Enlimomab Acute Stroke Trial Investigators. Use of anti-ICAM-1 therapy in ischemic stroke: results of the Enlimomab Acute Stroke Trial. Neurology. 2001;57:1428–34. https://doi.org/10.1212/wnl.57.8.1428.
62. Rubin BB, Smith A, Liauw S, Isenman D, Romaschin AD, Walker PM. Complement activation and white cell sequestration in postischemic skeletal muscle. Am J Phys. 1990;259:H525–31.
63. Kyriakides C, Austen W, Wang Y, Favuzza J, Kobzik L, Moore FD, et al. Skeletal muscle reperfusion injury is mediated by neutrophils and the complement membrane attack complex. Am J Phys. 1999;277:C1263–8. https://doi.org/10.1152/ajpcell.1999.277.6.C1263.
64. Lindsay TF, Hill J, Ortiz F, Rudolph A, Valeri CR, Hechtman HB, et al. Blockade of complement activation prevents local and pulmonary albumin leak after lower torso ischemia-reperfusion. Ann Surg. 1992;216:677–83. https://doi.org/10.1097/00000658-199212000-00010.
65. Harkin DW, Marron CD, Rother RP, Romaschin A, Rubin BB, Lindsay TF. C5 complement inhibition attenuates shock and acute lung injury in an experimental model of ruptured abdominal aortic aneurysm. Br J Surg. 2005;92:1227–34. https://doi.org/10.1002/bjs.4938.
66. Schröppel B, Akalin E, Baweja M, Bloom RD, Florman S, Goldstein M, et al. Peritransplant eculizumab does not prevent delayed graft function in deceased donor kidney transplant recipients: results of two randomized controlled pilot trials. Am J Transplant. 2020;20:564–72. https://doi.org/10.1111/ajt.15580.
67. Zhao H, Perez JS, Lu K, George AJ, Ma D. Role of Toll-like receptor-4 in renal graft ischemia-reperfusion injury. Am J Physiol Renal Physiol. 2014;306:F801–11. https://doi.org/10.1152/ajprenal.00469.2013.
68. O'Neill S, Harrison EM, Ross JA, Wigmore SJ, Hughes J. Heat-shock proteins and acute ischaemic kidney injury. Nephron Exp Nephrol. 2014;126:167–74. https://doi.org/10.1159/000363323.
69. Wang Y, Abarbanell AM, Herrmann JL, Weil BR, Poynter J, Manukyan MC, et al. Toll-like receptor signaling pathways and the evidence linking toll-like receptor signaling to cardiac ischemia/reperfusion injury. Shock. 2010;34:548–57. https://doi.org/10.1097/SHK.0b013e3181e686f5.
70. Hartley B, Bassiouni W, Schulz R, Julien O. The roles of intracellular proteolysis in cardiac ischemia-reperfusion injury. Basic Res Cardiol. 2023;118:38. https://doi.org/10.1007/s00395-023-01007-z.
71. Fujimura M, Gasche Y, Morita-Fujimura Y, Massengale J, Kawase M, Chan PH. Early appearance of activated matrix metalloproteinase-9 and blood-brain barrier disruption in mice after focal cerebral ischemia and reperfusion. Brain Res. 1999;842:92–100. https://doi.org/10.1016/s0006-8993(99)01843-0.
72. Ziswiler R, Daniel C, Franz E, Marti HP. Renal matrix metalloproteinase activity is unaffected by experimental ischemia-reperfusion injury and matrix metalloproteinase inhibition does not Alter outcome of renal function. Exp Nephrol. 2001;9:118–24. https://doi.org/10.1159/000052602.
73. Cortes AL, Gonsalez SR, Rioja LS, Oliveira SSC, Santos ALS, Prieto MC, et al. Protective outcomes of low-dose doxycycline on renal function of Wistar rats subjected to acute ischemia/reperfusion injury. Biochim Biophys Acta Mol basis Dis. 2018;1864:102–14. https://doi.org/10.1016/j.bbadis.2017.10.005.
74. Barr TL, Latour LL, Lee KY, Schaewe TJ, Luby M, Chang GS, et al. Blood-brain barrier disruption in humans is independently associated with increased matrix metalloproteinase-9. Stroke. 2010;41:e123–8. https://doi.org/10.1161/STROKEAHA.109.570515.

75. Park W, Wei S, Kim BS, Kim B, Bae SJ, Chae YC, et al. Diversity and complexity of cell death: a historical review. Exp Mol Med. 2023;55:1573–94. https://doi.org/10.1038/s12276-023-01078-x.
76. Ketelut-Carneiro N, Fitzgerald KA. Apoptosis, pyroptosis, and necroptosis-oh my! The many ways a cell can die. J Mol Biol. 2022;434:167378. https://doi.org/10.1016/j.jmb.2021.167378.
77. Tang L, Zhang W, Liao Y, Wang W, Deng X, Wang C, et al. Autophagy: a double-edged sword in ischemia-reperfusion injury. Cell Mol Biol Lett. 2025;30:42. https://doi.org/10.1186/s11658-025-00713-x.
78. Shen S, Shao Y, Li C. Different types of cell death and their shift in shaping disease. Cell Death Discov. 2023;9:284. https://doi.org/10.1038/s41420-023-01581-0.
79. Lasorsa F, Rutigliano M, Milella M, d'Amati A, Crocetto F, Pandolfo SD, et al. Ischemia-reperfusion injury in kidney transplantation: mechanisms and potential therapeutic targets. Int J Mol Sci. 2024;25:4332. https://doi.org/10.3390/ijms25084332.
80. Knight KR, Messina A, Hurley JV, Zhang B, Morrison WA, Stewart AG. Muscle cells become necrotic rather than apoptotic during reperfusion of ischaemic skeletal muscle. Int J Exp Pathol. 1999;80:169–75. https://doi.org/10.1046/j.1365-2613.1999.00111.x.
81. Mojoudi M, Taggart MS, Kharga A, Chen H, Dinicu AT, Wilks BT, et al. Anti-apoptotic treatment of warm ischemic male rat livers in machine perfusion improves symptoms of ischemia-reperfusion injury. Heliyon. 2024;10:e29519. https://doi.org/10.1016/j.heliyon.2024.e29519.
82. Bertheloot D, Latz E, Franklin BS. Necroptosis, pyroptosis and apoptosis: an intricate game of cell death. Cell Mol Immunol. 2021;18:1106–21. https://doi.org/10.1038/s41423-020-00630-3.
83. Dugbartey GJ. Cellular and molecular mechanisms of cell damage and cell death in ischemia-reperfusion injury in organ transplantation. Mol Biol Rep. 2024;51:473. https://doi.org/10.1007/s11033-024-09261-7.
84. Maslov LN, Popov SV, Naryzhnaya NV, Mukhomedzyanov AV, Kurbatov BK, Derkachev IA, et al. The regulation of necroptosis and perspectives for the development of new drugs preventing ischemic/reperfusion of cardiac injury. Apoptosis. 2022;27:697–719. https://doi.org/10.1007/s10495-022-01760-x.
85. Zhang CH, Yan YJ, Luo Q. The molecular mechanisms and potential drug targets of ferroptosis in myocardial ischemia-reperfusion injury. Life Sci. 2024;340:122439. https://doi.org/10.1016/j.lfs.2024.122439.
86. Li N, Jiang W, Wang W, Xiong R, Wu X, Geng Q. Ferroptosis and its emerging roles in cardiovascular diseases. Pharmacol Res. 2021;166:105466. https://doi.org/10.1016/j.phrs.2021.105466.
87. Granger DN, Kvietys PR. Reperfusion therapy-What's with the obstructed, leaky and broken capillaries? Pathophysiology. 2017;24:213–28. https://doi.org/10.1016/j.pathophys.2017.09.003.
88. Yu H, Kalogeris T, Korthuis RJ. Reactive species-induced microvascular dysfunction in ischemia/reperfusion. Free Radic Biol Med. 2019;135:182–97. https://doi.org/10.1016/j.freeradbiomed.2019.02.031.
89. El Amki M, Glück C, Binder N, Middleham W, Wyss MT, Weiss T, et al. Neutrophils obstructing brain capillaries are a major cause of no-reflow in ischemic stroke. Cell Rep. 2020;33:108260. https://doi.org/10.1016/j.celrep.2020.108260.
90. Szabo A, Varga R, Keresztes M, Vizler C, Nemeth I, Razga Z, et al. Ischemic limb preconditioning downregulates systemic inflammatory activation. J Orthop Res. 2009;27:897–902. https://doi.org/10.1002/jor.20829.
91. Kharbanda RK, Nielsen TT, Redington AN. Translation of remote ischaemic preconditioning into clinical practice. Lancet. 2009;374:1557–65. https://doi.org/10.1016/S0140-6736(09)61421-5.
92. Stokfisz K, Ledakowicz-Polak A, Zagorski M, Zielinska M. Ischaemic preconditioning – current knowledge and potential future applications after 30 years of experience. Adv Med Sci. 2017;62:307–16. https://doi.org/10.1016/j.advms.2016.11.006.

93. Ali ZA, Callaghan CJ, Lim E, Ali AA, Nouraei SA, Akthar AM, et al. Remote ischemic preconditioning reduces myocardial and renal injury after elective abdominal aortic aneurysm repair: a randomized controlled trial. Circulation. 2007;116:I98–105. https://doi.org/10.1161/circulationaha.106.679167.
94. Botker HE, Kharbanda R, Schmidt MR, Bottcher M, Kaltoft AK, Terkelsen CJ, et al. Remote ischaemic conditioning before hospital admission, as a complement to angioplasty, and effect on myocardial salvage in patients with acute myocardial infarction: a randomised trial. Lancet. 2010;375:727–34. https://doi.org/10.1016/S0140-6736(09)62001-8.
95. Walsh SR, Boyle JR, Tang TY, Sadat U, Cooper DG, Lapsley M, et al. Remote ischemic preconditioning for renal and cardiac protection during endovascular aneurysm repair: a randomized controlled trial. J Endovasc Ther. 2009;16:680–9. https://doi.org/10.1583/09-2817.1.
96. Healy DA, Boyle E, McCartan D, Bourke M, Medani M, Ferguson J, et al. A multicenter pilot randomized controlled trial of remote ischemic preconditioning in major vascular surgery. Vasc Endovasc Surg. 2015;49:220–7. https://doi.org/10.1177/1538574415614404.
97. Kepler T, Kuusik K, Lepner U, Starkopf J, Zilmer M, Eha J, et al. The effect of remote ischaemic preconditioning on arterial stiffness in patients undergoing vascular surgery: a randomised clinical trial. Eur J Vasc Endovasc Surg. 2019;57:868–75. https://doi.org/10.1016/j.ejvs.2018.12.002.
98. De Freitas S, Hicks CW, Mouton R, Garcia S, Healy D, Connolly C, et al. Effects of ischemic preconditioning on abdominal aortic aneurysm repair: a systematic review and meta-analysis. J Surg Res. 2019;235:340–9. https://doi.org/10.1016/j.jss.2018.09.049.
99. Kepler T, Kuusik K, Lepner U, Starkopf J, Zilmer M, Eha J, et al. Remote ischaemic preconditioning attenuates cardiac biomarkers during vascular surgery: a randomised clinical trial. Eur J Vasc Endovasc Surg. 2020;59:301–8. https://doi.org/10.1016/j.ejvs.2019.09.502.
100. Zhao ZQ. Postconditioning in reperfusion injury: a status report. Cardiovasc Drugs Ther. 2010;24:265–79. https://doi.org/10.1007/s10557-010-6240-1.
101. Kaur S, Jaggi AS, Singh N. Molecular aspects of ischaemic postconditioning. Fundam Clin Pharmacol. 2009;23:521–36. https://doi.org/10.1111/j.1472-8206.2009.00733.x.
102. Wang Z, Wen J, Zhou C, Wang Z, Wei M. Gene expression profiling analysis to investigate the role of remote ischemic postconditioning in ischemia-reperfusion injury in rats. BMC Genomics. 2019;20:361. https://doi.org/10.1186/s12864-019-5743-9.
103. Gyurkovics E, Aranyi P, Stangl R, Onody P, Ferreira G, Lotz G, et al. Postconditioning of the lower limb—protection against the reperfusion syndrome. J Surg Res. 2011;169:139–47. https://doi.org/10.1016/j.jss.2009.10.014.
104. Sinay L, Kurthy M, Horvath S, Arato E, Shafiei M, Lantos J, et al. Ischaemic postconditioning reduces peroxide formation, cytokine expression and leukocyte activation in reperfusion injury after abdominal aortic surgery in rat model. Clin Hemorheol Microcirc. 2008;40:133–42.
105. Mockford KA, Girn HR, Homer-Vanniasinkam S. Postconditioning: current controversies and clinical implications. Eur J Vasc Endovasc Surg. 2009;37:437–42. https://doi.org/10.1016/j.ejvs.2008.12.017.
106. Schmidt CA, Rancic Z, Lachat ML, Mayer DO, Veith FJ, Wilhelm MJ. Hypothermic, initially oxygen-free, controlled limb reperfusion for acute limb ischemia. Ann Vasc Surg. 2015;29:560–72. https://doi.org/10.1016/j.avsg.2014.09.033.
107. Kerstens TP, Landman TRJ, Schoon Y, Meijer FJA, Warlé MC, de Leeuw FE, et al. The effect of remote ischemic postconditioning on quality of life and clinical events after an ischemic stroke. Curr Neurovasc Res. 2023;20:472–9. https://doi.org/10.2174/0115672026275008231120063757.
108. Pagel PS, Crystal GJ. The discovery of myocardial preconditioning using volatile anesthetics: a history and contemporary clinical perspective. J Cardiothorac Vasc Anesth. 2018;32:1112–34. https://doi.org/10.1053/j.jvca.2017.12.029.
109. Kalenka A, Maurer MH, Feldmann RE, Kuschinsky W, Waschke KF. Volatile anesthetics evoke prolonged changes in the proteome of the left ventricule myocardium: defining a

molecular basis of cardioprotection? Acta Anaesthesiol Scand. 2006;50:414–27. https://doi.org/10.1111/j.1399-6576.2006.00984.x.
110. Kalenka A, Gross B, Maurer MH, Thierse HJ, Feldmann RE Jr. Isoflurane anesthesia elicits protein pattern changes in rat hippocampus. J Neurosurg Anesthesiol. 2010;22:144–54. https://doi.org/10.1097/ANA.0b013e3181cb7cb8.
111. Xiao YY, Chang YT, Ran K, Liu JP. Delayed preconditioning by sevoflurane elicits changes in the mitochondrial proteome in ischemia-reperfused rat hearts. Anesth Analg. 2011;113:224–32. https://doi.org/10.1213/ANE.0b013e3182239b71.
112. Wang JK, Wu HF, Zhou H, Yang B, Liu XZ. Postconditioning with sevoflurane protects against focal cerebral ischemia and reperfusion injury involving mitochondrial ATP-dependent potassium channel and mitochondrial permeability transition pore. Neurol Res. 2015;37:77–83. https://doi.org/10.1179/1743132814y.0000000410.
113. Symons JA, Myles PS. Myocardial protection with volatile anaesthetic agents during coronary artery bypass surgery: a meta-analysis. Br J Anaesth. 2006;97:127–36. https://doi.org/10.1093/bja/ael149.
114. Bignami E, Biondi-Zoccai G, Landoni G, Fochi O, Testa V, Sheiban I, et al. Volatile anesthetics reduce mortality in cardiac surgery. J Cardiothorac Vasc Anesth. 2009;23:594–9. https://doi.org/10.1053/j.jvca.2009.01.022.
115. Guinot PG, Ellouze O, Grosjean S, Berthoud V, Constandache T, Radhouani M, et al. Anaesthesia and ICU sedation with sevoflurane do not reduce myocardial injury in patients undergoing cardiac surgery: a randomized prospective study. Medicine (Baltimore). 2020;99:e23253. https://doi.org/10.1097/md.0000000000023253.
116. Jahn N, Völker MT, Laudi S, Stehr S, Schneeberger S, Brandacher G, et al. Analysis of volatile anesthetic-induced organ protection in simultaneous pancreas-kidney transplantation. J Clin Med. 2022;11:3385. https://doi.org/10.3390/jcm11123385.
117. Abu-Amara M, Gurusamy KS, Hori S, Glantzounis G, Fuller B, Davidson BR. Pharmacological interventions versus no pharmacological intervention for ischaemia reperfusion injury in liver resection surgery performed under vascular control. Cochrane Database Syst Rev. 2009:CD007472. https://doi.org/10.1002/14651858.CD007472.pub2.
118. Abu-Amara M, Gurusamy KS, Glantzounis G, Fuller B, Davidson BR. Pharmacological interventions for ischaemia reperfusion injury in liver resection surgery performed under vascular control. Cochrane Database Syst Rev. 2009:CD008154. https://doi.org/10.1002/14651858.CD008154.
119. Laws PE, Spark JI, Cowled PA, Fitridge RA. The role of statins in vascular disease. Eur J Vasc Endovasc Surg. 2004;27:6–16. https://doi.org/10.1016/j.ejvs.2003.09.014.
120. Cowled PA, Khanna A, Laws PE, Field JB, Fitridge RA. Simvastatin plus nitric oxide synthase inhibition modulates remote organ damage following skeletal muscle ischemia-reperfusion injury. J Investig Surg. 2008;21:119–26. https://doi.org/10.1080/08941930802046501.
121. Stalenhoef AF. The benefit of statins in non-cardiac vascular surgery patients. J Vasc Surg. 2009;49:260–5. https://doi.org/10.1016/j.jvs.2008.11.070.
122. Kertai MD, Boersma E, Westerhout CM, van Domburg R, Klein J, Bax JJ, et al. Association between long-term statin use and mortality after successful abdominal aortic aneurysm surgery. Am J Med. 2004;116:96–103. https://doi.org/10.1016/j.amjmed.2003.08.029.
123. Pasupathy S, Tavella R, Grover S, Raman B, Procter NEK, Du YT, et al. Early use of N-acetylcysteine with nitrate therapy in patients undergoing primary percutaneous coronary intervention for ST-segment-elevation myocardial infarction reduces myocardial infarct size (the NACIAM Trial [N-acetylcysteine in Acute Myocardial Infarction]). Circulation. 2017;136:894–903. https://doi.org/10.1161/circulationaha.117.027575.
124. Hausenloy DJ, Botker HE, Engstrom T, Erlinge D, Heusch G, Ibanez B, et al. Targeting reperfusion injury in patients with ST-segment elevation myocardial infarction: trials and tribulations. Eur Heart J. 2017;38:935–41. https://doi.org/10.1093/eurheartj/ehw145.
125. Cung TT, Morel O, Cayla G, Rioufol G, Garcia-Dorado D, Angoulvant D, et al. Cyclosporine before PCI in patients with acute myocardial infarction. N Engl J Med. 2015;373:1021–31. https://doi.org/10.1056/NEJMoa1505489.

Key References

Dugbartey GJ. Cellular and molecular mechanisms of cell damage and cell death in ischemia-reperfusion injury in organ transplantation. Mol Biol Rep. 2024;51:473. https://doi.org/10.1007/s11033-024-09261-7.

Granger DN, Kvietys PR. Reperfusion therapy-what's with the obstructed, leaky and broken capillaries? Pathophysiology. 2017;24:213–28. https://doi.org/10.1016/j.pathophys.2017.09.003.

Lasorsa F, Rutigliano M, Milella M, d'Amati A, Crocetto F, Pandolfo SD, et al. Ischemia-reperfusion injury in kidney transplantation: mechanisms and potential therapeutic targets. Int J Mol Sci. 2024;25:4332. https://doi.org/10.3390/ijms25084332.

Li N, Jiang W, Wang W, Xiong R, Wu X, Geng Q. Ferroptosis and its emerging roles in cardiovascular diseases. Pharmacol Res. 2021;166:105466. https://doi.org/10.1016/j.phrs.2021.105466.

Lutz J, Thurmel K, Heemann U. Anti-inflammatory treatment strategies for ischemia/reperfusion injury in transplantation. J Inflamm (Lond). 2010;7:27. https://doi.org/10.1186/1476-9255-7-27.

Stokfisz K, Ledakowicz-Polak A, Zagorski M, Zielinska M. Ischaemic preconditioning – current knowledge and potential future applications after 30 years of experience. Adv Med Sci. 2017;62:307–16. https://doi.org/10.1016/j.advms.2016.11.006.

Chapter 4
Abdominal Compartment Syndrome and Open Abdomen Treatment

Arne Seternes and Martin Björck

> **SN Flashcards**
> Test your learning and check your understanding of this book's contents: use the "Springer Nature Flashcards" app to access questions using ▶ https://sn.pub/wppvze. To use the app, please follow the instructions in Chap. 1.

Key Learning Points

- Intra-abdominal hypertension (IAH) is the sustained or repeated pathological elevation of intra-abdominal pressure (IAP) >12 mmHg.
- Abdominal perfusion pressure (APP) is the mean arterial pressure (MAP) minus IAP.
- Abdominal compartment syndrome (ACS) is the sustained IAP >20 mmHg (with or without an APP <60 mmHg) which is associated with new organ dysfunction or failure.
- Intra-abdominal pressure is most commonly measured using the Foley manometer method, which can be performed in and out of the ICU environment.

A. Seternes (✉)
Trondheim University Hospital, Department of Circulation and Medical Imaging, Norwegian University of Science and Technology, Trondheim, Norway
e-mail: arne.seternes@ntnu.no

M. Björck
Department of Surgical Sciences, Vascular Surgery, Uppsala University, Uppsala, Sweden
e-mail: martin.bjorck@surgsci.uu.se

R. Fitridge et al. (eds.), *Pathophysiology of Vascular Disease*,
https://doi.org/10.1007/978-3-032-31459-8_4

- ACS occurs in up to 20% of cases of open and endovascular repair of ruptured AAA. A further cohort of patients managed with emergency ruptured AAA open repair will require prophylactic open abdomen treatment.
- Major risk factors for the development of ACS include fluid overload/ generalised oedema, post-operative bleeding, and bowel ischaemia.
- The duration of IAH before decompression laparotomy (DL) is associated with the frequency of development of acute renal failure and need for dialysis.
- Non-surgical management of IAH includes adequate pain relief, drainage of gastric contents, early enteral feeding, use of neuromuscular blockade, reducing fluid overload, and the early use of a massive transfusion protocol in patients suspected to require 10 or more units of blood.
- A major problem associated with DL is lateralisation of the abdominal wall, which occurs when the musculature and fascia of the abdominal wall move laterally away from the midline with time. Vacuum-assisted wound closure and mesh-mediated fascial traction (VACM) is widely used to manage ACS and is associated with high rates of primary delayed fascial closure.

4.1 Introduction

The appreciation that a tense abdomen is life-threatening has been first described in ancient Greece. In 1984, the vascular surgeon Irving Kron named the condition abdominal compartment syndrome (ACS). He described ACS following surgery for ruptured abdominal aortic aneurysm (RAAA) [1]. ACS is often a consequence of aggressive resuscitation after major bleeding, and thus it is partly an iatrogenic condition. The first international conference on Intra-Abdominal Hypertension (IAH) and the Abdominal Compartment Syndrome was held in 2004. The conference resulted in the publication of two important consensus documents describing the definitions, risk factors [2], and treatment guidelines [3]. These were later revised using the GRADE Methodology. The Updated Consensus Definitions and Clinical Practice Guidelines from the World Society of the Abdominal Compartment Syndrome were published in 2013 [4].

4.2 Definition of Intra-Abdominal Hypertension (IAH)/ Abdominal Compartment Syndrome (ACS)

"*IAH is defined by a sustained or repeated pathological elevation in intra-abdominal pressure (IAP) >12 mmHg.*" This is the definition of IAH, as first stated in the 2006 consensus document [2] and has been unaltered in the updated guidelines in 2013. It has been shown in both animal research and in clinical studies that an IAP above 12 mmHg negatively affects organ function, in particular renal function [5]. It is important to note that a single elevated value may be the result of the patient being in pain or passing stools. This threshold for negative effects on organ function is important to consider in patients operated on for RAAA, since multiple prospective clinical studies have shown that it is uncommon that the IAP is <12 mmHg in the early postoperative period after open surgical repair (OSR) [6–8]. If haemodynamically unstable patients are treated with endovascular aortic repair (EVAR), the situation is quite similar [9, 10].

Although the evidence-based approach used in the revision of the Guidelines [4] has not found support for a sub-definition of low abdominal perfusion pressure (APP = MAP-IAP <60 mmHg), it is a clinical observation that hypotensive patients are more sensitive to IAH.

"*ACS is defined as a sustained IAP >20 mmHg (with or without an APP <60 mmHg) that is associated with new organ dysfunction/failure* [4]". Again, the exact wording is important: "*a sustained IAP >20 mmHg*" means that the measurement has to be repeated at least once, and it needs to be associated with "*new organ dysfunction/failure*", with a temporally associated deterioration of vital organ function. ACS is defined as the combination of this high IAP and its effect on vital organ function, never as a mere measurement of the pressure!

There are many ways to measure IAP. Most commonly, IAP is measured in the bladder, intermittently or continuously. Our preferred method is the Foley Manometer method (Holtech Medical, Charlottenlund, Denmark) with the advantage that it can easily be applied outside of the intensive care unit (ICU), a great advantage especially after EVAR for RAAA, since some of those patients can be handled in a surgical ward (Fig. 4.1a, b).

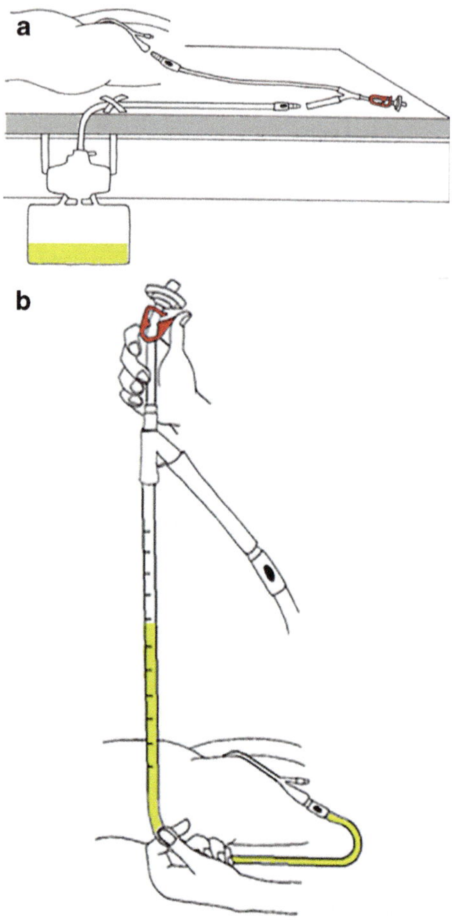

Fig. 4.1 (**a**) The Foley Manometer device is placed between the urinary catheter and the urine collecting bag. If the patient is anuric, the system is filled with saline, otherwise the urine from the patient serves as a measuring medium (**b**) When the IAP is measured, the "0 mmHg" mark of the manometer tube is placed at the mid-axillary line at the level of the iliac crest (mark for future reference). The filter is elevated vertically above the patient, and the bio-filter clamp is opened. Read the pressure in end-expiration, the tube is graded in mmHg (13.6 mm between each mark). Finally, the clamp is closed, and the system is replaced in its drainage position

4.3 How Common Is IAH/ACS After AAA Repair?

Although IAH and ACS occur in other clinical scenarios such as trauma, intestinal ischaemia, and aortic dissection, the situation that the vascular surgeon most often has to consider the possibility of IAH/ACS is after AAA repair, in particular after rupture [11]. The incidence of ACS will depend on several factors. The approach to resuscitation is of paramount importance. Balogh et al. showed that the administration of crystalloids is an independent risk factor for the development of ACS in abdominal trauma patients [12], and this is true in any bleeding patient. A policy of preoperative permissive hypotension in RAAA is likely to decrease the risk of developing post-operative IAH/ACS.

Mell et al. showed that patients who received less than one unit of plasma for every two units of red blood cells during RAAA repair had a four times higher mortality than those given more plasma [13], highlighting the importance of "massive transfusion" protocols. These protocols were introduced in most modern hospitals during the last decade, reducing both mortality and fluid overload, thereby decreasing the risk of ACS.

The introduction of endovascular aneurysm repair (EVAR) [14, 15] by Volodos in 1985 transformed aortic surgery. The application of EVAR in patients with RAAA has been first reported by Ohki and Veith in 2000 [16] and has become more frequently used over time worldwide [17]. In a contemporary nationwide study from the Swedish vascular registry (Swedvasc), ACS occurred as often after EVAR as after OSR (6.9% vs. 6.8%), although 10.7% of those operated on with OSR had been primarily left with an open abdomen (OA), thus preventing ACS [18, 19].

If measured consistently, IAP >20 mmHg occurs in about half the patients after OSR of a RAAA, and 20% develop ACS [5, 6]. In many older series, patients operated on for RAAA with EVAR were more haemodynamically stable, resulting in a lower incidence of IAH/ACS after EVAR [7]. The Zürich group who treated virtually all RAAA patients with EVAR and who monitored IAP reported a high incidence (20%, 20/102) of ACS [9], similar to the incidence after OSR. In a prospective cohort study in four Swedish hospitals, the risk of requiring treatment with open abdomen (OA) after aortic repair was higher after rupture, but similar after EVAR and OSR; in all, 28 of 1041 operations or 2.9% of cases [20].

4.4 Pathophysiology and Risk Factors for ACS After AAA Repair

Most risk factors for the development of ACS are associated with bleeding, shock, and resuscitation, and they are well described in the guidelines [4]. In the largest study published so far on ACS after AAA repair, 120 out of 8765 patients (1.4%) developed the complication [18]. In these 120 patients, all the case records, including all the data from the ICU and reoperations, were scrutinised and *three main pathophysiological mechanisms* were identified.

1. The most common cause was *fluid overload/general oedema*, which was the main cause in 55 patients (47%).
2. *Postoperative bleeding* was the cause of IAH/ACS in 34 (29%). As expected, those patients developed ASC most rapidly after the first operation of AAA repair.
3. Finally, in 27 patients (23%) *bowel ischaemia* was identified as the main cause of IAH/ACS, although a vicious circle was established when in most cases a gangrenous colon dilated, resulting in further increase of IAP, and more pronounced ischaemia. This mechanism had previously been studied in a prospective study after RAAA, when a direct association between IAH and colonic ischaemia was verified [8].

Ersryd et al [18] also reported that ACS developed early in most cases (and, in particular, after EVAR). Decompression laparotomy (DL) was performed within 24 h after completion of AAA repair in 56 (49%), between 24 and 48 h in 30 (26%), and after 48 h in 29 (25%). The duration of IAH before DL was associated with the likelihood of development of renal failure and need of renal replacement therapy (RRT). This association had previously been shown in a prospective multicentre study of patients treated with open abdomen (OA) for ACS, in a mixed ICU patient population which was dominated by trauma, but also included patients with RAAA [21].

4.5 Prevention of ACS and Medical Management

It is also possible to treat IAH in a proactive way, preventing further deterioration of the patient and development of ACS. This treatment is sometimes referred to as "medical management", or "conservative management", which is not an appropriate label since it can be quite aggressive. The aim is to prevent further increase of the IAP, as well as to support organ function.

There are two mechanisms through which the IAP can be reduced. One is volume reduction of the intra-abdominal cavity. Evacuation of the retroperitoneal haematoma after EVAR for RAAA has been attempted with lumbectomy (surgical approach through the lateral/dorsal part of the abdominal wall). Another alternative was described by Hörer et al., who inserted tissue plasminogen activator (tPA) through a 20F catheter placed in the haematoma with CT guidance in 13 patients [22]. None of these techniques are truly minimally invasive, and major (even fatal) bleeding complications have been reported. Decompression midline laparotomy seems both safer and more effective than these approaches.

Drainage of gastric content is important, but early enteral nutrition should not be halted [23], since bowel movements are of strategic importance. Enteral feeding can be initiated on the first postoperative day, even in the presence of IAH, but the gastric contents should be drained twice daily to avoid accumulation. However, enemas and other activities to stimulate the faecal flow are seldom effective after aortic repair. Early enteral nutrition and avoiding opioids are more effective and epidural anaesthesia is preferred (see below). It is common that the IAP increases hours before the first bowel action, after which the IAP drops substantially. Free drainable fluid in the abdominal cavity after AAA repair is uncommon.

Abdominal compliance (AC) measures the ease of abdominal expansion, expressed as a change (delta = Δ) in intra-abdominal volume (IAV) per change in intra-abdominal pressure (IAP): AC = ΔIAV/ΔIAP. This is a dynamic variable which is dependent on baseline IAV and IAP, as well as on reshaping and stretching capacity of the abdominal wall. The first phenomenon is that the abdomen transforms from an oval into a circular shape (reshaping), followed by stretching, and finally by a rapid increase in IAP. In a review of AC, the most important conclusion has been that patients with high IAP have a reduced AC, making the IAP very sensitive to small changes in IAV [24]. This phenomenon explains the often dramatically fast increase of IAP before the ACS develops, and why proactive early and frequent monitoring of IAP, and preventive actions, are so important.

One of the most effective ways of decreasing the IAP is pain relief, but it is also strategically important to avoid opioids, to prevent obstipation. During RAAA repair, there is seldom time to insert an epidural catheter prior to surgery, and after surgery the patient often has coagulopathy. We routinely discuss this with the anaesthesiologists, postpone the use of low molecular weight heparin (LMWH) medication, give platelets if necessary, and then use epidural analgesia whenever possible. This is quite effective in reducing IAP, can often increase urinary output, and become the turning point in the critical postoperative period. In an RCT, IAP was reduced from 16.82±4.56 to 6.30±3.11 mmHg after treatment with epidural analgesia in patients with IAH [25].

Neuro-muscular blockade (NMB) is an effective way of immediately reducing IAP when the patient is on the ventilator, which is often the case, especially after OSR of RAAA. It reduces IAP by 30–50%, which is often sufficient to improve renal function, reduce fluid overload, and reverse the situation of increasing IAP before ACS develops. In a study on 191 trauma patients undergoing damage control laparotomy, 92 who were on NMB during the first 24 h had higher primary fascial closure rate [26]. A large French RCT showed that NMB used for 48 h in 340 mixed ICU patients was safe and improved survival in patients with acute respiratory failure [27]. There are no published specific data on the effect of NMB in RAAA patients, but in our experience it works well.

Reducing fluid overload acts through reducing intra-abdominal volume. Intensivists have different opinions how fluid overload can be prevented, and this issue is highly controversial. Many argue that colloids are beneficial in this situation; others that they only leak into the extra-cellular space, adding further to the fluid overload and affecting renal function negatively. In our practice, plasma tends to be used in the early post-operative phase to correct coagulopathy. If the patient is on a ventilator, an increased Positive end-expiratory pressure (PEEP) may help to recruit fluid from the lungs, but be aware, PEEP has the potential to decrease the inflow to the right atrium with reduced preload and increased need for volume replacement. If a major fluid overload is present, often renal replacement therapy (RRT) is necessary.

Fluid overload is often more iatrogenic than is recognised. The Uppsala/Trondheim protocol is very restrictive with regard to the administration of crystalloids from early resuscitation. Not all are aware of the fact that when fractionated blood products (erythrocytes, plasma, and thrombocytes, 1:1:1) are given to compensate for one litre of blood loss, 4–500 ml of saline solution is also added. Thus, even if only blood products are given, the transfusion to compensate for 10 litres of blood loss will automatically result in a fluid overload of 4–5 litres of saline, making further administration of crystalloids dangerous [4, 13, 28].

4.6 Decompression Laparotomy (DL)

When ACS is developing or present, the only effective treatment is DL. It should preferably be performed in the midline, from the costal arch to the symphysis pubis. To not open the entire abdomen is a classical mistake. It is not only less effective, but also more difficult to close.

The timing of DL is important but a complex issue in clinical practice. Ideally, the two strategies of early or delayed DL should be compared in a randomised trial. It does not make sense to await until severe organ dysfunction/failure has developed before performing DL, but OA treatment itself is a morbid procedure associated with both morbidity and mortality. In a large Swedish cohort of 120 patients treated for ACS after AAA repair, timing of DL, i.e. the duration of IAP >15 mmHg, or >20 mmHg, was not associated with mortality, but was associated with need of RRT [18]. This lack of association with increased mortality is probably a result of confounding factors, since it makes sense to perform DL as soon as possible, once the decision has been made. This is another advantage of starting to monitor IAP and treat IAH early: if the patient fails to improve on intensive medical therapy, the decision to perform DL can be taken without further delay, since we already know that the patient has not responded to non-surgical treatment.

When a decision to perform DL has been taken, often in the middle of the night, there may be a waiting list for the operating theatre, and it is not possible to perform DL in the ICU [29]. Other patients may have high priorities, in which case NMB can reduce the ischaemic injury to the abdominal organs while waiting. It is important to inform the anaesthesiologist that the patient needs to have an extra bolus of fluid prior to DL, to avoid hypotension, which is common when you open or reopen the abdomen.

The effect of DL is often dramatic, reducing IAP and improving oxygenation and urinary output. Effects on multiple organ failure scores (SOFA, APACHE) are not as immediate, however, since multiple organ failure is not reversed quickly. In a multicentre study on 33 patients undergoing DL for overt ACS with different pathologies including RAAA, the IAP decreased from 23 mmHg (range 21–27) to 12 mmHg (9–15) after 2 h [21].

4.7 Prophylactic Open Abdomen Treatment

Is it better to leave all patients open as a routine after OSR of a RAAA, or is it better to close most patients (who do not have an obvious tense abdomen), and follow them closely in the postoperative period? In their experience, the Mayo Clinic reported having left 19% open after RAAA repair (43/223) [30], and in Trondheim, 52 out of 244 patients treated with RAAA were left open [31]. A similar experience was reported from Zürich [9], and in a Swedish national cohort study, this proportion was 10.7% after OSR [19]. It is obvious from all reports that a proportion needs to be left open primarily, but what proportion remains controversial.

Based on a systematic evidence-based medicine review of the literature, the Updated Consensus document favours primary closure and IAP measurement [4]. They recommend "*measuring IAP when any known risk factor for IAH/ACS is present in a critically ill or injured patient*", and "*use of protocolised monitoring and management of IAP versus not.*" Furthermore, they issued a strong negative recommendation: "*We could make **no** recommendation regarding the prophylactic use of the open abdomen*".

A recent paper compared 79 patients treated with a primarily OA after OSR for RAAA at a centre performing this as a routine, compared to a propensity score-matched control group of 148 patients treated at other centres in which 73% had the abdomen closed at the end of the procedure [32]. There was no difference in mortality or post-operative complications, thus no benefit associated with a routine practice of leaving all patients open could be demonstrated.

Our policy is to leave the patient open primarily after OSR of a RAAA only if the abdomen is tense and difficult to close, which occurs in approximately 5–10% of cases. However, most patients with RAAA nowadays are treated with EVAR. We monitor IAP in the OR (which is of particular importance after EVAR), every hour for 4 h, followed by every 4 h for the first 48 h. Monitoring is performed more frequently when there is IAH, and DL is performed on demand. In a review article adapting the World Society of the Abdominal Compartment Syndrome Guidelines to vascular surgery, this treatment algorithm was described in more detail [30]. For patients having their RAAA treated with an EVAR in local anaesthesia and transferred directly to the vascular ward, one should be suspicious of IAH/ACS if the patient deteriorates. The IAP could be difficult to interpret in patients in pain, and such a patient might need to be referred to the ICU for further workup.

4.8 Management of the Patient with Open Abdomen (OA)

How to care for the patient who needs a period of OA treatment is a complex issue. The first issue is how to manage the open abdomen itself: maintain a sterile environment, keep the intestines moist and protected from injury, protect the abdominal wall, and enable closure as soon as possible. A classification system of the open abdomen was developed in 2009, in order to facilitate training and research [33], and later updated in 2016 [34]. Preventing and controlling contamination, as well as lateralisation of the abdominal wall, are the key elements to enable closure of the abdomen as soon as possible [4, 33–35].

The problem of lateralisation was defined and highlighted in the Updated Consensus document [4]: "*Lateralisation of the abdominal wall is the phenomenon where the musculature and fascia of the abdominal wall, most exemplified by the rectus abdominis muscles and their enveloping fascia, move laterally away from the midline with time.*" It is also included in the classification system of OA [33, 34].

The importance of closing the abdomen as soon as possible to maintain a sterile environment was illustrated by the results from Helsinki, Finland [36]. They used a temporary abdominal closure (TAC) device including continuous negative pressure (the VACM method, see below). The OA was progressively colonised and 80% of the patients had positive bacterial cultures after 2 weeks of OA treatment.

The choice of TAC has attracted much attention, and multiple solutions have been developed, ever since the first report in the scientific literature of leaving the abdomen open, in 1897 [37]. An important innovation was developed by paediatric surgeons, who started to repair omphalocele in the 1940s, using silastic coverage of the intestines, a first generation of plastic. A similar system has been later popularised in trauma surgery by the Colombian invention of the Bogotá bag, using the plastic bag from a drip that is sutured to the skin or the fascia. This system works well for a few days, but during a more prolonged treatment (which is often necessary after AAA repair) three major problems develop. Two of those were solved by the later development of the vacuum pack technique, developed in 1995 by Barker et al. in Philadelphia [38]. The active suction prevented leakage of fluids from the OA, and the surgical towels covered with plastic prevented adhesions forming between the intestines and the abdominal wall. This system was further refined by a commercially available ready-made system, (V.A.C.® Abdominal Dressing System; KCI, USA). Later, other negative pressure systems were developed by different suppliers.

A third problem, the lateralisation of the abdominal wall, remained however, making it difficult to close patients who had been treated with OA for at least 5 days. This was the reason why a novel method was developed in Uppsala and Malmö, Sweden; the Vacuum-assisted wound closure and mesh-mediated fascial traction (VACM) method. The pilot experience of VACM was published in 2007 [39]. This is a combination of the commercially available VAC system (later replaced by the ABThera system) with a prolene mesh that is sutured to the fascial edges to permit an active traction towards the midline (details shown in Fig. 4.2). A multicentre study of this technique (including only patients requiring OA for at least 4 days) showed an 89% primary delayed fascial closure rate after a median time of 15 days

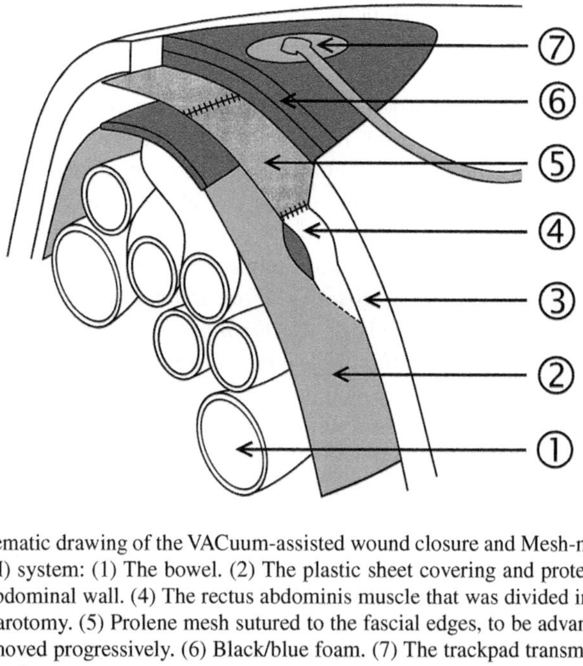

Fig. 4.2 A schematic drawing of the VACuum-assisted wound closure and Mesh-mediated fascial traction (VACM) system: (1) The bowel. (2) The plastic sheet covering and protecting the intestines. (3) The abdominal wall. (4) The rectus abdominis muscle that was divided in the midline at the primary laparotomy. (5) Prolene mesh sutured to the fascial edges, to be advanced toward the midline and removed progressively. (6) Black/blue foam. (7) The trackpad transmitting the negative pressure into the system

with OA [40], and in a sub-group analysis of those treated for aortic disease this figure was 100% [20]. These results have been repeated independently at other major centres [41, 42] as well as in a large multicentre study on patients treated for ACS after AAA repair [43] and are now the preferred TAC method in many centres worldwide. To reduce the burden on the operating theatre, one study found it safe and time-efficient to perform the dressing changes in the ICU [29].

4.9 Prognosis

The overall mortality in patients who develop ACS after AAA repair is high. In the national Swedish study of 6612 patients, the 30-day mortality rate after RAAA was 42% among those who developed ACS compared to 24% without ACS. At 1 year, mortality was 51% versus 32% [19]. After intact AAA repair, 30-day mortality was 12% with ACS versus 1.8% without. At 1 year, mortality was 28% versus 6%. When ACS developed, renal failure, multiple organ failure, intestinal ischaemia, and prolonged intensive care stay were all very much more frequent. Interestingly, morbidity and mortality were similar, regardless of the primary surgical technique (OSR or EVAR), if the patient developed ACS.

Those results are actually rather encouraging, since untreated ACS has a mortality approaching 100% [44]. Perhaps the fact that ACS has been recognised and treated for many years in Sweden is one of the explanations why survival after RAAA has increased over time [45].

4.10 Conclusion

In conclusion, IAH and ACS are common and life-threatening complications after aortic surgery. Preventing and treating this complication in a timely way, when it occurs despite prevention, are important parts of any strategy aiming at improving outcomes after aortic surgery, whether by an open or endovascular approach.

Multiple Choice Questions

1. Abdominal compartment syndrome (ACS):
   (a) Is rarely encountered when endovascular repair of a ruptured abdominal aortic aneurysm is performed
   (b) Is not associated with crystalloid fluid replacement in patients sustaining abdominal trauma
   (c) Can be defined as sustained intra-abdominal pressure of >20 mm Hg which is associated with new organ dysfunction or failure

(d) Is most commonly diagnosed by measuring intra-abdominal pressure using an intraperitoneal manometer
(e) Is rarely caused by post-operative bleeding.

Answer: (c) Can be defined as sustained intra-abdominal pressure of >20 mm Hg which is associated with new organ dysfunction or failure

2. Management of abdominal compartment syndrome (ACS) includes:

(a) Use of opioid pain relief
(b) Adequate pain relief, drainage of gastric contents, use of neuromuscular blockade and reducing fluid overload
(c) Elective decompression laparotomy (DL) once ACS is diagnosed
(d) Limited laparotomy is sufficient to treat ACS
(e) Following decompressive laparotomy, most patients can have their abdomen closed within 24 h

Answer: (b) Adequate pain relief, drainage of gastric contents, use of neuromuscular blockade and reducing fluid overload

References

1. Kron IL, Harman PK, Nolan SP. The measurement of intra-abdominal pressure as a criterion for abdominal re-exploration. Ann Surg. 1984;199:28–30.
2. Malbrain ML, Cheatham ML, Kirkpatrick A, Sugrue M, Parr M, De Waele J, et al. Results from the international conference of experts on intra-abdominal hypertension and abdominal compartment syndrome. I Definitions. Intensive Care Med. 2006;32:1722–32. https://doi.org/10.1007/s00134-006-0349-5.
3. Cheatham ML, Malbrain ML, Kirkpatrick A, Sugrue M, Parr M, De Waele J, et al. Results from the international conference of experts on intra-abdominal hypertension and abdominal compartment syndrome. II Recommendations. Intensive Care Med. 2007;33:951–62. https://doi.org/10.1007/s00134-007-0592-4.
4. Kirkpatrick AW, Roberts DJ, De Waele J, Jaeschke R, Malbrain ML, De Keulenaer B, et al. Intra-abdominal hypertension and the abdominal compartment syndrome: updated consensus definitions and clinical practice guidelines from the World Society of the Abdominal Compartment Syndrome. Intensive Care Med. 2013;39:1190–206. https://doi.org/10.1007/s00134-013-2906-z.
5. Platell C, Hall J, Dobb G. Impaired renal function due to raised intraabdominal pressure. Intensive Care Med. 1990;16:328–9. https://doi.org/10.1007/BF01706359.
6. Djavani K, Wanhainen A, Bjorck M. Intra-abdominal hypertension and abdominal compartment syndrome following surgery for ruptured abdominal aortic aneurysm. Eur J Vasc Endovasc Surg. 2006;31:581–4. https://doi.org/10.1016/j.ejvs.2005.12.007.
7. Makar RR, Badger SA, O'Donnell ME, Loan W, Lau LL, Soong CV. The effects of abdominal compartment hypertension after open and endovascular repair of a ruptured abdominal aortic aneurysm. J Vasc Surg. 2009;49:866–72. https://doi.org/10.1016/j.jvs.2008.11.027.
8. Djavani K, Wanhainen A, Valtysson J, Bjorck M. Colonic ischaemia and intra-abdominal hypertension following open repair of ruptured abdominal aortic aneurysm. Br J Surg. 2009;96:621–7. https://doi.org/10.1002/bjs.6592.

9. Mayer D, Rancic Z, Meier C, Pfammatter T, Veith FJ, Lachat M. Open abdomen treatment following endovascular repair of ruptured abdominal aortic aneurysms. J Vasc Surg. 2009;50:1–7. https://doi.org/10.1016/j.jvs.2008.12.030.
10. Improve Trial Investigators. Comparative clinical effectiveness and cost effectiveness of endovascular strategy v open repair for ruptured abdominal aortic aneurysm: three year results of the IMPROVE randomised trial. BMJ. 2017;359:j4859. https://doi.org/10.1136/bmj.j4859.
11. Wanhainen A, Van Herzeele I, Bastos Goncalves F, Bellmunt Montoya S, Berard X, Boyle JR, et al. Editor's choice – European Society for Vascular Surgery (ESVS) 2024 clinical practice guidelines on the management of abdominal aorto-iliac artery aneurysms. Eur J Vasc Endovasc Surg. 2024;67:192–331. https://doi.org/10.1016/j.ejvs.2023.11.002.
12. Balogh Z, McKinley BA, Cocanour CS, Kozar RA, Valdivia A, Sailors RM, et al. Supranormal trauma resuscitation causes more cases of abdominal compartment syndrome. Arch Surg. 2003;138:637–42. discussion 42–3. https://doi.org/10.1001/archsurg.138.6.637.
13. Mell MW, O'Neil AS, Callcut RA, Acher CW, Hoch JR, Tefera G, et al. Effect of early plasma transfusion on mortality in patients with ruptured abdominal aortic aneurysm. Surgery. 2010;148:955–62. https://doi.org/10.1016/j.surg.2010.02.002.
14. Volodos NL. The 30th anniversary of the first clinical application of endovascular stent-grafting. Eur J Vasc Endovasc Surg. 2015;49:495–7. https://doi.org/10.1016/j.ejvs.2015.02.012.
15. Volodos NL, Shekhanin VE, Karpovich IP, Troian VI, Gur'ev IA. A self-fixing synthetic blood vessel endoprosthesis. Vestn Khir Im I I Grek. 1986;137:123–5.
16. Ohki T, Veith FJ. Endovascular grafts and other image-guided catheter-based adjuncts to improve the treatment of ruptured aortoiliac aneurysms. Ann Surg. 2000;232:466–79. https://doi.org/10.1097/00000658-200010000-00002.
17. Beck AW, Sedrakyan A, Mao J, Venermo M, Faizer R, Debus S, et al. Variations in abdominal aortic aneurysm care: a report from the international consortium of vascular registries. Circulation. 2016;134:1948–58. https://doi.org/10.1161/CIRCULATIONAHA.116.024870.
18. Ersryd S, Djavani Gidlund K, Wanhainen A, Smith L, Bjorck M. Editor's choice - abdominal compartment syndrome after surgery for abdominal aortic aneurysm: subgroups, risk factors, and outcome. Eur J Vasc Endovasc Surg. 2019;58:671–9. https://doi.org/10.1016/j.ejvs.2019.04.007.
19. Ersryd S, Djavani-Gidlund K, Wanhainen A, Bjorck M. Editor's choice - abdominal compartment syndrome after surgery for abdominal aortic aneurysm: a nationwide population based study. Eur J Vasc Endovasc Surg. 2016;52:158–65. https://doi.org/10.1016/j.ejvs.2016.03.011.
20. Sorelius K, Wanhainen A, Acosta S, Svensson M, Djavani-Gidlund K, Bjorck M. Open abdomen treatment after aortic aneurysm repair with vacuum-assisted wound closure and mesh-mediated fascial traction. Eur J Vasc Endovasc Surg. 2013;45:588–94. https://doi.org/10.1016/j.ejvs.2013.01.041.
21. De Waele JJ, Kimball E, Malbrain M, Nesbitt I, Cohen J, Kaloiani V, et al. Decompressive laparotomy for abdominal compartment syndrome. Br J Surg. 2016;103:709–15. https://doi.org/10.1002/bjs.10097.
22. Hörer T, Skoog P, Pirouzram A, Larzon T. Tissue plasminogen activator-assisted hematoma evacuation to relieve abdominal compartment syndrome after endovascular repair of ruptured abdominal aortic aneurysm. J Endovasc Ther. 2012;19:144–8. https://doi.org/10.1583/11-3699.1.
23. Reintam Blaser A, Starkopf J, Alhazzani W, Berger MM, Casaer MP, Deane AM, et al. Early enteral nutrition in critically ill patients: ESICM clinical practice guidelines. Intensive Care Med. 2017;43:380–98. https://doi.org/10.1007/s00134-016-4665-0.
24. Blaser AR, Bjorck M, De Keulenaer B, Regli A. Abdominal compliance: a bench-to-bedside review. J Trauma Acute Care Surg. 2015;78:1044–53. https://doi.org/10.1097/TA.0000000000000616.
25. Hakobyan RV, Mkhoyan GG. Epidural analgesia decreases intraabdominal pressure in postoperative patients with primary intra-abdominal hypertension. Acta Clin Belg. 2008;63:86–92. https://doi.org/10.1179/acb.2008.63.2.005.

26. Abouassaly CT, Dutton WD, Zaydfudim V, Dossett LA, Nunez TC, Fleming SB, et al. Postoperative neuromuscular blocker use is associated with higher primary fascial closure rates after damage control laparotomy. J Trauma. 2010;69:557–61. https://doi.org/10.1097/TA.0b013e3181e77ca4.
27. Papazian L, Forel JM, Gacouin A, Penot-Ragon C, Perrin G, Loundou A, et al. Neuromuscular blockers in early acute respiratory distress syndrome. N Engl J Med. 2010;363:1107–16. https://doi.org/10.1056/NEJMoa1005372.
28. Björck M, Wanhainen A. Management of abdominal compartment syndrome and the open abdomen. Eur J Vasc Endovasc Surg. 2014;47:279–87. https://doi.org/10.1016/j.ejvs.2013.12.014.
29. Seternes A, Fasting S, Klepstad P, Mo S, Dahl T, Björck M, et al. Bedside dressing changes for open abdomen in the intensive care unit is safe and time and staff efficient. Crit Care. 2016;20:164. https://doi.org/10.1186/s13054-016-1337-y.
30. Oelschlager BK, Boyle EM Jr, Johansen K, Meissner MH. Delayed abdominal closure in the management of ruptured abdominal aortic aneurysms. Am J Surg. 1997;173:411–5. https://doi.org/10.1016/S0002-9610(97)00081-0.
31. Fagertun H, Klepstad P, Aldstedt Nyronning L, Seternes A. Increasing use of prophylactic open abdomen therapy with vacuum assisted wound closure and mesh mediated fascial traction after repair of ruptured abdominal aortic aneurysm. Eur J Vasc Endovasc Surg. 2024;67:603–10. https://doi.org/10.1016/j.ejvs.2023.10.032.
32. Smidfelt K, Nordanstig J, Wingren U, Bergstrom G, Langenskiold M. Routine open abdomen treatment compared with on-demand open abdomen or direct closure following open repair of ruptured abdominal aortic aneurysms: a propensity score-matched study. SAGE Open Med. 2019;7:2050312119833501. https://doi.org/10.1177/2050312119833501.
33. Björck M, Bruhin A, Cheatham M, Hinck D, Kaplan M, Manca G, et al. Classification–important step to improve management of patients with an open abdomen. World J Surg. 2009;33:1154–7. https://doi.org/10.1007/s00268-009-9996-3.
34. Björck M, Kirkpatrick AW, Cheatham M, Kaplan M, Leppäniemi A, De Waele JJ. Amended classification of the open abdomen. Scand J Surg. 2016;105:5–10. https://doi.org/10.1177/1457496916631853.
35. Bjorck M, D'Amours SK, Hamilton AE. Closure of the open abdomen. Am Surg. 2011;77(Suppl 1):S58–61.
36. Rasilainen SK, Juhani MP, Kalevi LA. Microbial colonization of open abdomen in critically ill surgical patients. World J Emerg Surg. 2015;10:25. https://doi.org/10.1186/s13017-015-0018-5.
37. McCosh AJ II. The treatment of general septic peritonitis. Ann Surg. 1897;25:687–97.
38. Brock WB, Barker DE, Burns RP. Temporary closure of open abdominal wounds: the vacuum pack. Am Surg. 1995;61:30–5.
39. Petersson U, Acosta S, Björck M. Vacuum-assisted wound closure and mesh-mediated fascial traction–a novel technique for late closure of the open abdomen. World J Surg. 2007;31:2133–7. https://doi.org/10.1007/s00268-007-9222-0.
40. Acosta S, Bjarnason T, Petersson U, Pålsson B, Wanhainen A, Svensson M, et al. Multicentre prospective study of fascial closure rate after open abdomen with vacuum and mesh-mediated fascial traction. Br J Surg. 2011;98:735–43. https://doi.org/10.1002/bjs.7383.
41. Seternes A, Myhre HO, Dahl T. Early results after treatment of open abdomen after aortic surgery with mesh traction and vacuum-assisted wound closure. Eur J Vasc Endovasc Surg. 2010;40:60–4. https://doi.org/10.1016/j.ejvs.2010.02.018.
42. Rasilainen SK, Mentula PJ, Leppäniemi AK. Vacuum and mesh-mediated fascial traction for primary closure of the open abdomen in critically ill surgical patients. Br J Surg. 2012;99:1725–32. https://doi.org/10.1002/bjs.8914.
43. Acosta S, Seternes A, Venermo M, Vikatmaa L, Sörelius K, Wanhainen A, et al. Open abdomen therapy with vacuum and mesh mediated fascial traction after aortic repair: an international multicentre study. Eur J Vasc Endovasc Surg. 2017;54:697–705. https://doi.org/10.1016/j.ejvs.2017.09.002.

44. Vidal MG, Ruiz Weisser J, Gonzalez F, Toro MA, Loudet C, Balasini C, et al. Incidence and clinical effects of intra-abdominal hypertension in critically ill patients. Crit Care Med. 2008;36:1823–31. https://doi.org/10.1097/CCM.0b013e31817c7a4d.
45. Mani K, Bjorck M, Wanhainen A. Changes in the management of infrarenal abdominal aortic aneurysm disease in Sweden. Br J Surg. 2013;100:638–44. https://doi.org/10.1002/bjs.9046.

Key References

Acosta S, Seternes A, Venermo M, Vikatmaa L, Sörelius K, Wanhainen A, Svensson M, Djavani K, Björck M. Open abdomen therapy with vacuum and mesh-mediated fascial traction after aortic repair – an international multi-centre study. Eur J Vasc Endovasc Surg. 2017;54:697–705. https://doi.org/10.1016/j.ejvs.2017.09.002.

Balogh Z, McKinley BA, Cocanour CS, Kozar RA, Valdivia A, Sailors RM, et al. Supra-normal trauma resuscitation causes more cases of abdominal compartment syndrome. Arch Surg. 2003;138:637–43. https://doi.org/10.1001/archsurg.138.6.637.

Björck M, Kirkpatrick AW, Cheatham M, Kaplan M, Leppäniemi A, De Waele JJ. Amended classification of the open abdomen. Scand J Surg. 2016;105:5–10. https://doi.org/10.1177/1457496916631853.

Djavani K, Wanhainen A, Valtysson J, Björck M. Colonic ischaemia and intra-abdominal hypertension following open repair of ruptured abdominal aortic aneurysm. Br J Surg. 2009;96:621–7. https://doi.org/10.1002/bjs.6592.

Ersryd S, Djavani Gidlund K, Wanhainen A, Smith L, Björck M. Abdominal compartment syndrome after surgery for abdominal aortic aneurysm: subgroups, risk factors and outcome. Eur J Vasc Endovasc Surg. 2019;58:671–9. https://doi.org/10.1016/j.ejvs.2019.04.007.

Kirkpatrick AW, Roberts DJ, De Waele J, Jaeschke R, Malbrain ML, De Keulenaer B, et al. Intra-abdominal hypertension and the abdominal compartment syndrome: updated consensus definitions and clinical practice guidelines from the World Society of the Abdominal Compartment Syndrome. Intensive Care Med. 2013;39:1190–206. https://doi.org/10.1007/s00134-013-2906-z.

Mell MW, O'Neil AS, Callcut RA, Acher CW, Hoch JR, Tefera G, Turnipseed WD. Effect of early plasma transfusion on mortality in patients with ruptured abdominal aortic aneurysm. Surgery. 2010;148:955–62. https://doi.org/10.1016/j.surg.2010.02.002.

Chapter 5
Pathophysiology and Management of Extremity Compartment Syndromes

Carl-Magnus Wahlgren and David Lindström

SN Flashcards
Test your learning and check your understanding of this book's contents: use the "Springer Nature Flashcards" app to access questions using ▶ https://sn.pub/wppvze. To use the app, please follow the instructions in Chap. 1.

Key Learning Points

- Acute extremity compartment syndrome is a surgical emergency associated with significant morbidity if not expeditiously managed.
- The most important tool in diagnostics is to maintain a high level of clinical suspicion.
- Patients with classical clinical signs of compartment syndrome do not need any further investigation and should undergo urgent fasciotomy.
- When further diagnostic testing is needed, particularly in unconscious patients, compartment pressure can be measured. The differential pressure (diastolic blood pressure—intracompartmental pressure), with a threshold of 30 mmHg, is commonly recommended as it offers a more accurate assessment of the potential for compartment syndrome than absolute compartment pressure.

C.-M. Wahlgren
Department of Vascular Surgery, Karolinska University Hospital and Karolinska Institutet, Stockholm, Sweden
e-mail: carl.wahlgren@regionstockholm.se

D. Lindström (✉)
Section of Vascular Surgery, Department of Clinical Science and Education, Karolinska Institutet, Södersjukhuset, Stockholm, Sweden
e-mail: David.lindstrom@regionstockholm.se

R. Fitridge et al. (eds.), *Pathophysiology of Vascular Disease*,
https://doi.org/10.1007/978-3-032-31459-8_5

- The rising compartment pressure initiates a cycle of impaired venous return, reduced perfusion, and cellular ischaemia. This ischaemia triggers anaerobic metabolism, ATP depletion, and ultimately cell death, further exacerbating compartmental swelling.
- Reperfusion injury after ischaemia triggers microvascular dysfunction, leading to impaired perfusion, increased permeability, and edema, which can further elevate compartment pressures and worsen compartment syndrome.
- Understanding the pathophysiological mechanisms underlying compartment syndrome emphasises the need for early diagnosis and prompt fasciotomy to prevent irreversible muscle and nerve damage.
- Incisions in skin and fascia need to be long enough to make tissues loose and allow for postoperative swelling.
- After compartment syndrome has resolved, delayed primary closure of the fasciotomy incisions is performed, with the recommended intracutaneous suture method.

5.1 Introduction

Acute extremity compartment syndrome is a surgical emergency associated with significant morbidity if not expeditiously managed. It requires prompt diagnosis and early treatment with compartment decompression for good clinical outcome.

The definition of acute extremity compartment syndrome is increased pressure within the compartmental space, leading to decreased perfusion pressure and hypoxaemia of the tissues. This may lead to irreversible ischaemic necrosis of the muscles and nerves in the compartment causing functional impairment, limb amputation, multiple organ failure, or death [1, 2].

Acute limb compartment syndrome (ACS) in vascular surgery is mostly related to ischaemia-reperfusion (I/R) injury associated with acute ischaemia, vascular trauma, or phlegmasia cerulea dolens [3–5]. Iatrogenic causes with accumulation of blood or contrast fluid within the compartment after endovascular catheter or wire perforation have been described [3, 5]. Extremity compartment syndromes may result from internal compartment expansion due to fractures or crush injuries but also external compression from burns, tight plaster cast, or bandage [6]. The aim of this chapter is to summarise the pathophysiology and management of upper and lower limb compartment syndromes.

5.2 Epidemiology

No comprehensive review of the prevalence of extremity compartment syndrome has been published due to the variation of causes [7]. The incidence of lower extremity compartment syndrome after revascularisation of acute ischaemic limbs is approximately 10%–20% [4, 8, 9], but in contrast, the need for fasciotomy after elective vascular surgery is very low, from 0.15% to 0.45% [10]. Patman found that 32% of extremities with arterial injuries and only 2% with embolic occlusions underwent fasciotomy. In a retrospective series of vascular surgery patients (107 patients; 113 limbs) undergoing lower extremity fasciotomy, 72% of limbs underwent revascularisation for acute limb ischaemia, 6.2% of limbs were related to acute aortic disease, and 20% of limbs had undergone elective vascular surgery [2]. In total, 57% of limbs had signs of ACS and a therapeutic fasciotomy was performed, while 43% of fasciotomies were prophylactic. Data from the US National Trauma Data Bank showed that patients sustaining lower extremity arterial trauma required a fasciotomy in up to 42% of cases [11].

5.3 Pathophysiology

Skeletal muscles, nerves, and vessels in the upper and lower extremities are arranged into compartments surrounded by fascia. The upper arm contains two compartments (anterior and posterior) and the forearm has three (volar, lateral, and dorsal) compartments. In the thigh, there are three compartments (anterior, medial, and posterior), whereas there are four in the lower leg (anterior, lateral, deep posterior, and superficial posterior) [6, 12]. Compartments within the forearm and lower leg are especially limited in their ability to accommodate tissue oedema and are therefore more prone to develop increased compartment pressures [13]. The lower leg is the most common location of acute extremity compartment syndrome, with the anterior and lateral compartments most frequently affected [12].

The pathophysiology of acute extremity compartment syndrome involves an external compression or an internal expansion within the compartment that leads to increased tissue pressure, reduced capillary blood flow, local tissue hypoxia, and local tissue necrosis (Fig. 5.1) [1, 14]. Intrinsic causes of acute extremity compartment syndrome are tissue injury caused by a direct traumatic event or tissue ischaemia and reperfusion [1, 15]. The most common cause of compartment syndrome in vascular surgery is tissue oedema due to ischaemia-reperfusion injury caused by limb revascularisation. A traumatic vascular injury is often accompanied by fractures, so that ischaemia–reperfusion and haematoma formation may both contribute to the limb compartment syndrome [16]. The rising tissue pressure impairs venous outflow by compressing the veins. This increase in venous pressure reduces the arteriovenous pressure gradient, resulting in diminished local perfusion [1, 15, 16].

The combination of increased pressure in the interstitial and intercellular fluid spaces shuts off transcapillary movement. The resultant cellular ischaemia leads to muscle and nerve damage. Interstitial oedema develops from tissue necrosis and further worsens hypoxaemia and compartmental swelling. During acute limb ischaemia, the combination of decreased oxygen supply and congestion of red blood cells within the capillaries triggers a complex cascade of metabolic, inflammatory, and prothrombotic pathways [17, 18]. The cell shifts energy metabolism from an

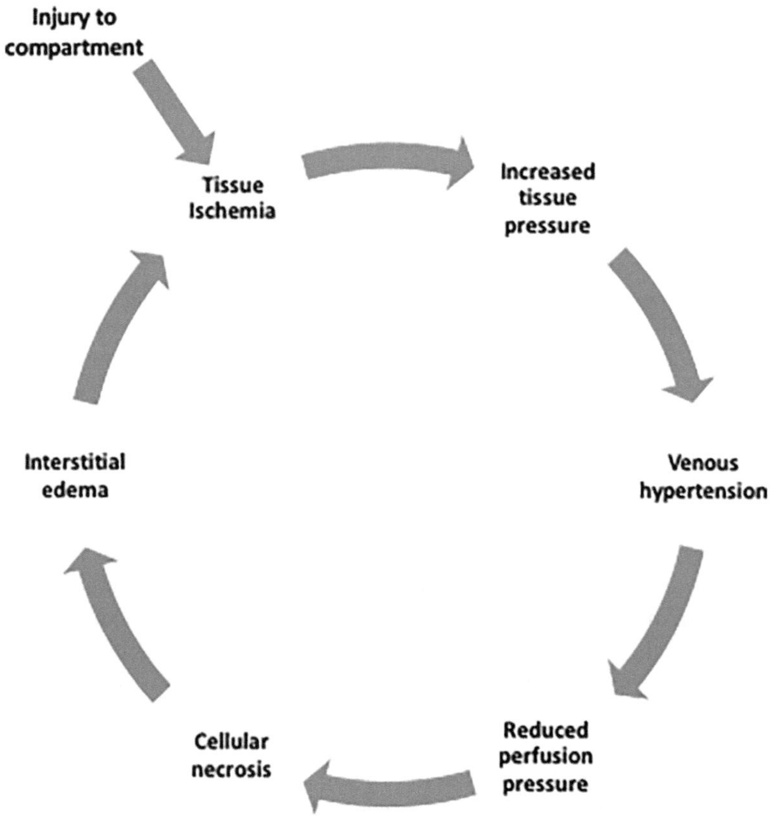

Fig. 5.1 Pathophysiology of acute extremity compartment syndrome [1, 14–16]

aerobic to anaerobic mechanism, producing lactic acid. Continued ischaemia causes depletion of energy-rich adenosine triphosphate (ATP), leading to leakage of extracellular calcium into the muscle cells, which ultimately results in dysfunction and cell death [19].

Reperfusion injury represents the response to tissue injury when the blood flow is restored after ischaemia. This contributes to a systemic inflammatory, metabolic, and thrombotic response. Microvascular dysfunction mediates many of the local and systemic consequences of ischaemia-reperfusion injury with a plethora of changes specific to arterioles, capillaries, and venules [17, 20]. This includes impaired vasodilation, decreased perfusion and fluid leakage, and increased permeability.

Ischaemia-reperfusion injury leads to microcirculatory changes due to activation of inflammatory mediators. Increased arterial resistance leads to decreased perfusion in the capillaries. The permeability results in an increased rate of transcapillary fluid leakage. Impaired tissue perfusion and oedema will further raise the intracompartmental pressure [17, 20]. The no-reflow phenomenon is another factor in this response relating to vascular congestion in the arterioles and capillaries [13, 20]. Reactive oxygen species cause damage including injury to DNA, oxidation of fatty acids and lipids, and oxidation of proteins and co-factors necessary for enzymatic function [21]. This leads to capillary leakage, resulting in additional oedema and rising compartment pressure (see Chap. 3).

The duration of ischaemia correlates with the onset of irreversible changes in various tissue types. The critical ischaemic time in different tissues at normal temperature can be defined as the maximum ischaemic time interval that a tissue can tolerate and still remain viable [22]. In the extremities, muscle tissue has the highest risk for ischaemia-reperfusion injury [17]. An ischaemic time of 4–6 h predisposes the patient to the development of a compartment syndrome [23]. Large-animal studies have demonstrated the neuromuscular ischaemic threshold of the limb to be less than 5 h, and similarly recommended restoration of flow within 3 h of injury for optimal functional recovery. Haemorrhagic shock also worsens the impact of ischaemia on the neuromuscular structures of the limb and reduces the ischaemic threshold to as little as 1 h [13].

5.4 Clinical Presentation

Acute limb compartment syndrome occurs after a precipitating causal event, most commonly trauma. In vascular surgery, compartment syndrome is also commonly seen following reperfusion after muscular ischaemia due to acute arterial occlusion or reduced distal perfusion during endovascular procedures or extracorporeal membrane oxygenation (ECMO) due to large catheters inserted into proximal arteries. Other contributing factors are fractures, haematomas, pressure injuries, and oedema. The time from insult to compartment syndrome development may vary from minutes to hours. The most sensitive tissues to ischaemia are unmyelinated nerve fibres followed by myelinated nerve fibres, skeletal muscle, skin, and then bone. As an example, the first sign might be an altered sensation between digit 1 and 2 in the foot—corresponding to deep peroneal nerve ischaemia in the anterior compartment. Pulses will generally be preserved for a long time into the syndrome, well beyond the indication for acute surgery. Patients who are alert and awake normally complain of severe pain, often resistant to analgesics, sometimes pain "out of proportion"—meaning that it does not correspond to the apparent severity of the injury sustained. Some of the other classical "P-signs" (pain, pain on passive stretch, paraesthesia, paralysis) of compartment syndrome might also be present. Commonly foot drop occurs in compartment syndrome affecting the lower leg, due to the involvement of anterior and lateral calf compartments. In general, the sensitivity of each symptom is low but the specificity quite high. The absence of symptoms should therefore not be used to rule out compartment syndrome. However, if three or more of the classical "4-P" symptoms are present, this increases the likelihood of the presence of a compartment syndrome [24].

Unfortunately, many patients are not fully awake and alert when the compartment syndrome occurs. This might be due to anaesthetics used in surgery, dementia, concomitant CNS or peripheral nerve injuries, or drugs and alcohol. For this group of patients, firmness/tenderness of the compartments relative to the unaffected limb might be a helpful observation. The assessment of distended muscles alone is not sufficient for diagnosing increased compartment pressure [25]. In children, the adult symptoms described above are unreliable; signs of increasing need for analgesics, agitation, and anxiety may be the clues to diagnosis and treatment [26, 27]. It should be noted that the syndrome usually evolves over some time, which is why repeated, serial clinical examinations over a short time sometimes make it easier to diagnose. A sensory deficit is sometimes the first sign of compartment syndrome, but, in vascular surgery, the preceding ischaemic event may already have caused sensory loss, reinforcing why it is important not to rely only on a single clinical sign.

Clinical signs suggestive of irreversible ischaemic damage include fixed, non-blanching skin staining or gangrene. In these cases, urgent amputation should be considered to prevent systemic complications. Factors associated with post-ischaemic compartment syndrome in non-traumatic acute limb ischaemia are inadequate backflow, high serum creatine kinase (CK) level, positive fluid balance after admission, and advanced-stage acute limb ischaemia [28]. In cases in which muscle swelling is highly likely, a prophylactic fasciotomy may be indicated. It may be reasonable to perform a prophylactic fasciotomy in severe acute ischaemia exceeding 4–6 h, especially if there is inadequate collateral flow, and also in association with vascular trauma [9, 28]. However, more recent research has cast doubt on the benefit of prophylactic fasciotomy, suggesting that careful observation and fasciotomy when required may reduce unnecessary surgery and morbidity [29, 30].

5.5 Diagnostic Testing

Any suspicion of acute limb compartment syndrome (both in conscious and unconscious patients) must lead to either prompt treatment or immediate further diagnostic testing. Clinical examination is recommended to diagnose post-reperfusion compartment syndrome in patients who have had revascularisation for acute limb ischaemia (European Society of Vascular Surgery [ESVS] Acute limb ischaemia guidelines Class I, Level B) [31]. Clinical assessment of suspected compartment syndrome is difficult; the majority of symptoms and signs are only reliably assessed in a fully conscious patient. Also, many patients may have some of these clinical signs present due to the injury that has caused the compartment syndrome such as the pulseless, painful, paraesthetic limb of acute ischaemia. The most important tool in diagnostics is to maintain a high level of clinical suspicion. A clinical situation with long-standing ischaemia, all the classical “P signs”, and a firm and tense calf does not need any further investigations and should undergo urgent fasciotomy. On the other hand, an unconscious patient in the intensive care unit with slightly firm calf after a short period of ischaemia should be worked-up more thoroughly before going ahead with immediate fascia release. The medicolegal and litigation situation in some parts of the world makes it wise to try to confirm the diagnosis if possible. The most commonly used method for confirmation of the diagnosis is pressure measurement in the respective compartment with multiple needle-sticks. All compartments in the affected limb should be measured. If any fracture is present, measurement should be done within five centimetres of the fracture. Some sedation or local anaesthetic might be helpful, especially in children. Most accurate results are reported with a side-port needle or a slit catheter connected to an arterial line or the Stryker manometer [32]. The normal compartment pressures in adults are around 8 mm Hg and in children 10–15 mm Hg [1]. As a diagnostic cut-off, the perfusion pressure has been proven to be more accurate than an absolute value. The differential pressure ($\Delta P =$ diastolic blood pressure − intracompartmental pressure) of 30 mm Hg is the most commonly used threshold [33, 34]. The ESVS acute limb ischaemia guidelines have a modest recommendation about compartment pressure measurement which *may be* considered to diagnose post-reperfusion compartment syndrome, when the clinical diagnosis is uncertain. (Class IIb, Level C) [31]. Collecting blood from the ipsilateral femoral vein and measuring lactate has also been shown to correlate with the risk of compartment syndrome but the clinical usefulness of this testing is not clear [35].

The dynamics of the syndrome is of importance; any measurement during surgery and anaesthesia should be repeated postoperatively if suspicion exists. Regional anaesthesia such as epidural catheters should be used with caution since they may mask symptoms and delay diagnosis [36]. Techniques with indwelling catheters allow continuous monitoring of limbs at risk, but these techniques are more complex and require prior training in their use [37].

Other methods to diagnose acute compartment syndrome have been proposed as well. Near-infrared spectroscopy (NIRS) has been useful in some case series [38] but, according to a recent review, the false-negative rate is too high to rely solely on NIRS in diagnosing a syndrome that needs timely treatment [39, 40]. In clinically advanced cases, the resulting inflammation may be associated with a leucocytosis or C-reactive protein (CRP) elevation. If tissue necrosis has developed, serum creatinine phosphokinase and myoglobin will be elevated, together with a metabolic acidosis. When rhabdomyolysis occurs, the urine will develop a brown discolouration, sometimes referred to as "tea-coloured". The colour stems from myoglobin in the urine which the kidneys are trying to excrete.

5.6 Management

5.6.1 Lower Extremity Operative Techniques

Acute limb compartment syndrome should be treated with fasciotomy of all affected compartments. In patients who present acutely (roughly within 12 h of onset of compartment syndrome), fasciotomy should be performed immediately. It is recommended that a fasciotomy should be performed as soon as possible once the diagnosis has been made, preferably within 2 h [31]. Fasciotomy performed longer than 12 h after the onset of compartment syndrome results in a significantly poorer functional outcome [40, 41]. If the presentation or diagnosis is delayed, consideration must be given as to whether the limb is unsalvageable. If so, a fasciotomy may lead to significant morbidity without improving functional outcome. Beyond 36 h after onset, rates of amputation, infection, neurological injury, and death increase. Early amputation rather than futile attempts at limb salvage should be considered [42, 43].

Preoperative non-surgical measures such as removal of casts and dressings and elevation of the affected limb should be performed during evaluation or waiting time for surgery. In the lower limb, the fasciotomy procedure should release any tissue that could constrict the respective compartment. The skin and fasciae should be released along the entire length of the compartments. The lower limb consists of the anterior, lateral (peroneal), superficial, and deep posterior compartments. The easiest and most common way to decompress the compartments is through two incisions (Fig. 5.2). One posteromedial incision (to open the superficial and deep posterior compartments) is performed two centimetres behind the medial border of the tibia; taking care not to injure the great saphenous vein. The superficial fascia is then opened along the length of the skin. Second, the soleus muscle attachment on the tibial border is sharply released to expose the deep posterior fascia which is then opened. The second anterolateral incision (to open the anterior and lateral compartments) is done one fingerbreadth anterior to the fibula from the fibular head to the ankle over the intermuscular septum between the anterior and lateral compartment, taking care not to injure the common and superficial peroneal nerves. The intermuscular septum can usually be seen as a white longitudinal line in the fascia. If any uncertainty exists, a short transverse incision can be used to confirm the location of the septum. The anterior and lateral compartments are then opened along the length of the incision. A single incision technique to treat lower limb compartments has also been used with similar outcomes but it is not recommended by the authors [44]. Irrespective of the techniques used, incisions in skin and fascia need to be long enough to make the tissues loose and allow for postoperative swelling [45]. Any dressing material should be sterile and loosely attached. A simple and cheap way to prepare for later closure is to suture

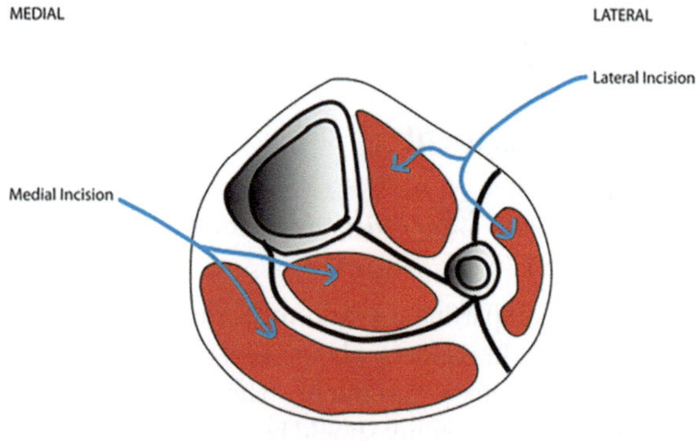

Fig. 5.2 Fasciotomy of the lower limb to decompress the four compartments (anterior; lateral; superficial; and deep posterior) with two incisions (anterolateral and posteromedial)

a running intracutaneous shoelace suture along the whole incision. The suture can be a 2/0 resorbable monofilament suture or a non-resorbable polypropelene suture. It is important to leave the sutures really loose; normally two sutures are needed to cover a lower limb incision.

Compartment syndrome in the thigh is rare, most commonly seen after blunt trauma. The thigh consists of three compartments (anterior, posterior, and medial) and is usually decompressed medially and/or laterally (Fig. 5.3). No good data on the optimal method are available, although a single-incision technique is reported more frequently [46].

5.6.2 *Upper Extremity Operative Technique*

In the upper extremity, the forearm is the most common site of development of compartment syndrome [1, 5]. Decompression of the volar and the lateral compartments is achieved through a curvilinear incision that begins proximal to the antecubital fossa, medial to the biceps tendon, extends to the radial side of the forearm, where it goes distally along the medial border of the brachioradial muscle, and finally across the carpal tunnel along the thenar crease (Fig. 5.4a) [3, 5, 6, 12]. The decompression of the dorsal compartment is achieved through an incision extending from just distal to the radial head to the midportion of the wrist (Fig. 5.4b). In the upper arm, the anterior compartment is incised just distal to the deltoid muscle to just above the elbow. The posterior compartment is incised over the triceps muscle in the midline to above the elbow [14].

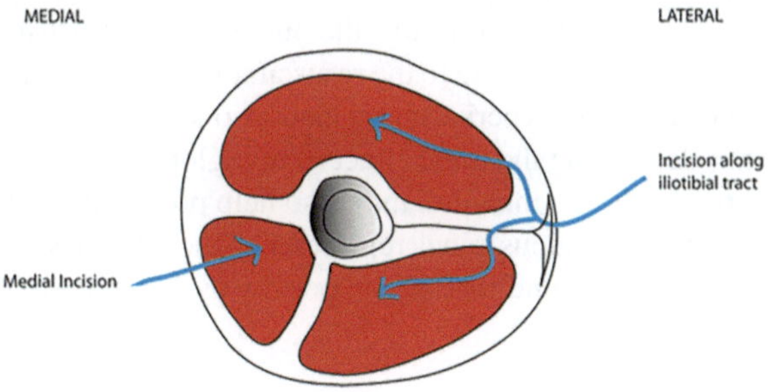

Fig. 5.3 Fasciotomy of the three compartments (anterior, posterior, and medial) in the thigh with decompression from a medial and lateral approach

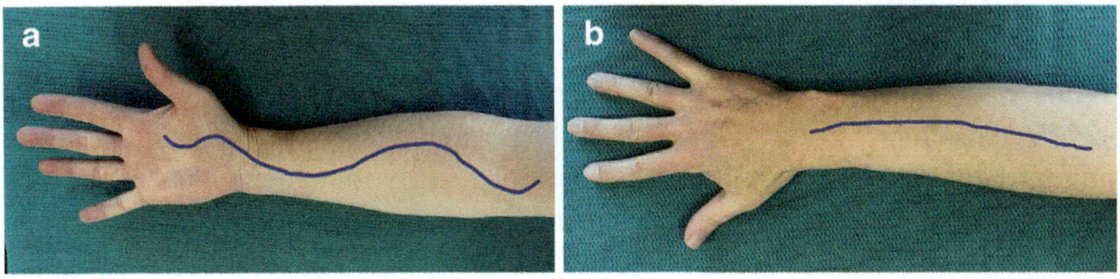

Fig. 5.4 Fasciotomy of the forearm with decompression of the volar and lateral compartments (**a**) and the dorsal compartment (**b**)

5.7 Postoperative Care

The postoperative lower limb should be held elevated, and a foot pump may be used after calf fasciotomy if available. Physiotherapy should be started immediately to activate dorsiflexion of the ankle. Pain medication should be administered as needed. There are a few options for dealing with the fasciotomy wounds after the compartment syndrome has resolved. Delayed primary closure, vacuum-assisted closure, secondary closure, skin grafts, and healing by secondary intention are all options. Delayed primary closure with the vessel loop shoelace technique is often referred to and can be used [47], but the authors recommend the pre-positioned intracutaneous suture method described above which is easier, quicker, and gives a better cosmetic outcome. Studies with vacuum-assisted closure have shown conflicting results, with low complication rates, but the need for skin grafting has been quite frequent, as well as high costs associated with the technique [48–50]. If the running sutures, described in the operative technique above, are used, the same sutures can be used to start closing and approximating the skin edges. If the fasciotomy has been done prophylactically and no swelling is present, complete skin closure can be performed within 24–48 h. If a true compartment exists with muscular swelling, the succeeding closure process can usually start after 48–72 h. This can normally be done in the ward without the need to go back to the surgical theatre unless there is a need for surgical debridement or haemostasis. Most patients tolerate careful pulling of the sutures every 24–48 h. When the skin edges are closed, the suture is tied on the outside and left in situ for 3 weeks.

Some adjunctive non-operative management methods have been described but there are no standard methods in use. Free radical scavengers such as mannitol [51] and hypertonic saline [13] have been shown to be of some benefit in compartment syndrome caused by ischaemia-reperfusion injury. Hyperbaric oxygen therapy has also been shown to improve the outcome of reperfusion injuries [52]. The addition of sodium bicarbonate to the resuscitation fluids is beneficial, as it will correct metabolic acidosis, hyperkalaemia, and also keeps the urine alkaline (urinary pH >6.5), thus decreasing the toxic effect of myoglobin on renal tubules. Forced diuresis with furosemide and mannitol may also help protect the kidneys [53]. If rhabdomyolysis occurs, continuous renal replacement therapy may be used, although a Cochrane analysis has found that the supporting evidence is weak [54].

5.8 Outcome

While fasciotomy wounds are associated with a moderate degree of morbidity [55, 56], fasciotomy does not appear to have any effect on long-term calf muscle pump function [57]. If fasciotomy is performed early for acute compartment syndrome, the outcome in terms of preventing limb loss, systemic complications, and long-term functional disability is good [34]. Failure to prevent and promptly treat compartment syndrome risks the development of systemic complications such as multi-organ failure (including hyperkalaemia, hypocalcaemia, coagulopathy, myoglobinuria, and renal failure) with a correspondingly high risk of death. One large study demonstrated that fasciotomy performed less than 12 h after the onset of the compartment syndrome resulted in normal function in 68% of the extremities. However, only 8% of those having late fasciotomy had normal function following decompression [41].

To study the outcome of compartment syndrome alone is difficult, since simultaneous vascular or traumatic injury may affect the outcome. The syndrome does have a high incidence of nerve deficit and foot drop (15%–32%) [2, 58], and mortality rates between 15% and 23% have been reported [2, 59]. In a retrospective study from 1980 to 1994, 53 patients had fasciotomies following surgical revascularisation [47]. At discharge, 11 (21%) patients had undergone amputation and six (11%) patients had died. In another retrospective review, lower extremity fasciotomies were performed for compartment syndrome after acute ischaemia and revascularisation in patients with vascular trauma or arterial occlusive disease [56]. Fourteen (11%) amputations were required for refractory limb ischaemia and eighteen (15%) patients died of cardiopulmonary or multisystem failure. After lower extremity trauma with compartment syndrome and fasciotomy, nearly 13% of patients required leg amputation [58]. In this study, 67% of amputees had associated vascular injuries. At long-term follow-up, 10% of patients reported moderate lower extremity pain and 69% had returned to work. Neuromuscular sequelae, as well as long-term functional outcome, have been emphasised as important factors for patient expectation and satisfaction [13, 23]. Most children experience full recovery after fasciotomy but the literature is limited [60]. In a case series, persistent Volkmann's contracture as a post-traumatic complication occurred in one of 23 children (4.2%) [60].

5.9 Conclusion

Extremity compartment syndrome in vascular surgery is a limb-threatening condition requiring emergent fasciotomy. The management strategy is to expeditiously decrease tissue pressure and minimise tissue damage and functional loss. There are significant complications related to lower extremity compartment syndrome including neuromuscular dysfunction and amputation. The fasciotomy wounds per se cause minimal morbidity and can normally be closed with a variety of techniques. The role of inflammatory and metabolic biomarkers for compartment syndrome and whether they can guide therapy need further evaluation. Future research should focus on early and improved diagnostics of compartment syndrome and refined treatment regimens for ischaemia-reperfusion injury.

Multiple Choice Questions

1. Diagnosis of limb compartment syndrome:

   (a) Is rarely made after revascularisation of acute limb ischaemia
   (b) Requires measurement of intracompartment pressure
   (c) Is not associated with duration and severity of ischaemia
   (d) Is most commonly caused by ischaemia/reperfusion injury
   (e) Distal pulses are usually lost as soon as compartment syndrome occurs

   Answers: (d) Is most commonly caused by ischaemia/reperfusion injury

2. Treatment of limb compartment syndrome (LCS):

   (a) Once diagnosed, LCS can be managed with elective compartment decompression
   (b) In the lower limb, release of the fascia throughout its length without extensive skin incision is effective
   (c) Only compartments in which raised pressure has been measured require decompression
   (d) If the fasciotomy was performed prophylactically and no post-operative swelling is present, complete skin closure can be performed within 24–48 h
   (e) Fasciotomy closure requires muscle swelling to completely resolve

   Answer: (d) If the fasciotomy was performed prophylactically and no post-operative swelling is present, complete skin closure can be performed within 24–48 h

References

1. von Keudell AG, Weaver MJ, Appleton PT, Bae DS, Dyer GSM, Heng M, et al. Diagnosis and treatment of acute extremity compartment syndrome. Lancet. 2015;386:1299–310. https://doi.org/10.1016/S0140-6736(15)00277-9.
2. Wesslen C, Wahlgren CM. Contemporary management and outcome after lower extremity fasciotomy in non-trauma-related vascular surgery. Vasc Endovasc Surg. 2018;52:493–7. https://doi.org/10.1177/1538574418773503.
3. McNally MM, Univers J. Acute limb Ischemia. Surg Clin North Am. 2018;98:1081–96. https://doi.org/10.1016/j.suc.2018.05.002.
4. Jensen SL, Sandermann J. Compartment syndrome and fasciotomy in vascular surgery. A review of 57 cases. Eur J Vasc Endovasc Surg. 1997;13:48–53.
5. Modrall GJ. Compartment syndrome. In: Cronenwett JL, Johnston KW, editors. Rutherfords vascular surgery and endovascular therapy, vol. 2. 7th ed. Saunders Elsevier; 2010. p. 2412–21.
6. Schmidt AH. Acute compartment syndrome. Orthop Clin North Am. 2016;47:517–25. https://doi.org/10.1016/j.ocl.2016.02.001.
7. Cone J, Inaba K. Lower extremity compartment syndrome. Trauma Surg Acute Care Open. 2017;2:e000094. https://doi.org/10.1136/tsaco-2017-000094.
8. Allenberg JR, Meybier H. The compartment syndrome from the vascular surgery viewpoint. Chirurg. 1988;59:722–7.

9. Papalambros EL, Panayiotopoulos YP, Bastounis E, Zavos G, Balas P. Prophylactic fasciotomy of the legs following acute arterial occlusion procedures. Int Angiol. 1989;8:120–4.
10. Patman RD. Compartmental syndromes in peripheral vascular surgery. Clin Orthop Relat Res. 1975;113:103–10.
11. Farber A, Tan TW, Hamburg NM, Kalish JA, Joglar F, Onigman T, et al. Early fasciotomy in patients with extremity vascular injury is associated with decreased risk of adverse limb outcomes: a review of the National Trauma Data Bank. Injury. 2012;43:1486–91. https://doi.org/10.1016/j.injury.2011.06.006.
12. Gourgiotis S, Villias C, Germanos S, Foukas A, Ridolfini MP. Acute limb compartment syndrome: a review. J Surg Educ. 2007;64:178–86. https://doi.org/10.1016/j.jsurg.2007.03.006.
13. Percival TJ, Rasmussen TE. Reperfusion strategies in the management of extremity vascular injury with ischaemia. Br J Surg. 2012;99(Suppl 1):66–74. https://doi.org/10.1002/bjs.7790.
14. Ledgerwood AM, Lucas CE. Management of extremity compartment syndrome. In: Cameron JL, Cameron AM, editors. Current surgical therapy. 11th ed. Elsevier; 2014. p. 1124–8.
15. Matsen FA 3rd. Compartmental syndromes. N Engl J Med. 1979;300:1210–1. https://doi.org/10.1056/NEJM197905243002108.
16. Janzing HM. Epidemiology, etiology, pathophysiology and diagnosis of the acute compartment syndrome of the extremity. Eur J Trauma Emerg Surg. 2007;33:576–83. https://doi.org/10.1007/s00068-007-7151-0.
17. Gillani S, Cao J, Suzuki T, Hak DJ. The effect of ischemia reperfusion injury on skeletal muscle. Injury. 2012;43:670–5. https://doi.org/10.1016/j.injury.2011.03.008.
18. Crawford RS, Watkins MT. Ischemia-reperfusion. In: Cronenwett JL, Johnston KW, editors. Rutherford's vascular surgery and endovascular therapy, vol. 1. 7th ed. Saunders; 2010. p. 89–100.
19. Santistevan JR. Acute limb ischemia: an emergency medicine approach. Emerg Med Clin North Am. 2017;35:889–909. https://doi.org/10.1016/j.emc.2017.07.006.
20. Seal JB, Gewertz BL. Vascular dysfunction in ischemia-reperfusion injury. Ann Vasc Surg. 2005;19:572–84. https://doi.org/10.1007/s10016-005-4616-7.
21. Yassin MM, Harkin DW, Barros D'Sa AA, Halliday MI, Rowlands BJ. Lower limb ischemia-reperfusion injury triggers a systemic inflammatory response and multiple organ dysfunction. World J Surg. 2002;26:115–21. https://doi.org/10.1007/s00268-001-0169-2.
22. Chafin B, Belmont MJ, Quraishi H, Clovis N, Wax MK. Effect of clamp versus anastomotic-induced ischemia on critical ischemic time and survival of rat epigastric fasciocutaneous flap. Head Neck. 1999;21:198–203. https://doi.org/10.1002/(sici)1097-0347(199905)21:3<198::aid-hed3>3.0.co;2-t.
23. Percival TJ, White JM, Ricci MA. Compartment syndrome in the setting of vascular injury. Perspect Vasc Surg Endovasc Ther. 2011;23:119–24. https://doi.org/10.1177/1531003511401422.
24. Ulmer T. The clinical diagnosis of compartment syndrome of the lower leg: are clinical findings predictive of the disorder? J Orthop Trauma. 2002;16:572–7. https://doi.org/10.1097/00005131-200209000-00006.
25. Shuler FD, Dietz MJ. Physicians' ability to manually detect isolated elevations in leg intracompartmental pressure. J Bone Joint Surg Am. 2010;92:361–7. https://doi.org/10.2106/JBJS.I.00411.
26. Bae DS, Kadiyala RK, Waters PM. Acute compartment syndrome in children: contemporary diagnosis, treatment, and outcome. J Pediatr Orthop. 2001;21:680–8.
27. Livingston KS, Glotzbecker MP, Shore BJ. Pediatric acute compartment syndrome. J Am Acad Orthop Surg. 2017;25:358–64. https://doi.org/10.5435/JAAOS-D-15-00655.
28. Orrapin S, Orrapin S, Arwon S, Rerkasem K. Predictive factors for post-ischemic compartment syndrome in non-traumatic acute limb ischemia in a lower extremity. Ann Vasc Dis. 2017;10:378–85. https://doi.org/10.3400/avd.oa.17-00055.

29. Moran BJ, Quintana MT, Michael Scalea T, DuBose J, Feliciano DV. Two urgency categories, same outcome: no difference after "therapeutic" vs. "prophylactic" fasciotomy. Am Surg. 2023;89:614–20. https://doi.org/10.1177/00031348211031860.
30. Keating JJ, Klingensmith N, Moren AM, Skarupa DJ, Loria A, Maher Z, et al. Dispelling dogma: American Association for Surgery of trauma prospective, multicenter trial of index vs delayed fasciotomy after extremity trauma. J Am Coll Surg. 2023;236:1037–44. https://doi.org/10.1097/XCS.0000000000000612.
31. Bjorck M, Earnshaw JJ, Acosta S, Bastos Goncalves F, Cochennec F, Debus ES, et al. Editor's choice - European Society for Vascular Surgery (ESVS) 2020 clinical practice guidelines on the management of acute limb ischaemia. Eur J Vasc Endovasc Surg. 2020;59:173–218. https://doi.org/10.1016/j.ejvs.2019.09.006.
32. Boody AR, Wongworawat MD. Accuracy in the measurement of compartment pressures: a comparison of three commonly used devices. J Bone Joint Surg Am. 2005;87:2415–22. https://doi.org/10.2106/JBJS.D.02826.
33. Whitesides TE, Haney TC, Morimoto K, Harada H. Tissue pressure measurements as a determinant for the need of fasciotomy. Clin Orthop Relat Res. 1975;113:43–51.
34. McQueen MM, Court-Brown CM. Compartment monitoring in tibial fractures. The pressure threshold for decompression. J Bone Joint Surg Br. 1996;78:99–104.
35. Mitas P, Vejrazka M, Hruby J, Spunda R, Pecha O, Lindner J, et al. Prediction of compartment syndrome based on analysis of biochemical parameters. Ann Vasc Surg. 2014;28:170–7. https://doi.org/10.1016/j.avsg.2012.12.006.
36. Klucka J, Stourac P, Stouracova A, Masek M, Repko M. Compartment syndrome and regional anaesthesia: critical review. Biomed Pap Med Fac Univ Palacky Olomouc Czech Repub. 2017;161:242–51. https://doi.org/10.5507/bp.2017.025.
37. Giannoudis PV, Tzioupis C, Pape HC. Early diagnosis of tibial compartment syndrome: continuous pressure measurement or not? Injury. 2009;40:341–2. https://doi.org/10.1016/j.injury.2009.02.010.
38. Steffen RJ, Sale S, Anandamurthy B, Cruz VB, Grady PM, Soltesz EG, et al. Using near-infrared spectroscopy to monitor lower extremities in patients on venoarterial extracorporeal membrane oxygenation. Ann Thorac Surg. 2014;98:1853–4. https://doi.org/10.1016/j.athoracsur.2014.04.057.
39. Boezeman RP, Moll FL, Unlu C, de Vries JP. Systematic review of clinical applications of monitoring muscle tissue oxygenation with near-infrared spectroscopy in vascular disease. Microvasc Res. 2016;104:11–22. https://doi.org/10.1016/j.mvr.2015.11.004.
40. Song W, Zhou D, Dong J. Predictors of secondary amputation in patients with grade IIIC lower limb injuries: a retrospective analysis of 35 patients. Medicine (Baltimore). 2017;96:e7068. https://doi.org/10.1097/MD.0000000000007068.
41. Sheridan GW, Matsen FA 3rd. Fasciotomy in the treatment of the acute compartment syndrome. J Bone Joint Surg Am. 1976;58:112–5.
42. Williams AB, Luchette FA, Papaconstantinou HT, Lim E, Hurst JM, Johannigman JA, et al. The effect of early versus late fasciotomy in the management of extremity trauma. Surgery. 1997;122:861–6. https://doi.org/10.1016/s0039-6060(97)90099-4.
43. Finkelstein JA, Hunter GA, Hu RW. Lower limb compartment syndrome: course after delayed fasciotomy. J Trauma. 1996;40:342–4. https://doi.org/10.1097/00005373-199603000-00002.
44. Bible JE, McClure DJ, Mir HR. Analysis of single-incision versus dual-incision fasciotomy for tibial fractures with acute compartment syndrome. J Orthop Trauma. 2013;27:607–11. https://doi.org/10.1097/BOT.0b013e318291f284.
45. Mathis JE, Schwartz BE, Lester JD, Kim WJ, Watson JN, Hutchinson MR. Effect of lower extremity fasciotomy length on intracompartmental pressure in an animal model of compart-

ment syndrome: the importance of achieving a minimum of 90% fascial release. Am J Sports Med. 2015;43:75–8. https://doi.org/10.1177/0363546514554601.
46. Ojike NI, Roberts CS, Giannoudis PV. Compartment syndrome of the thigh: a systematic review. Injury. 2010;41:133–6. https://doi.org/10.1016/j.injury.2009.03.016.
47. Janzing HM, Broos PL. Dermatotraction: an effective technique for the closure of fasciotomy wounds: a preliminary report of fifteen patients. J Orthop Trauma. 2001;15:438–41. https://doi.org/10.1097/00005131-200108000-00010.
48. Johnson LS, Chaar M, Ball CG, Perez S, Nicholas JM, Wyrzykowski AD, et al. Management of extremity fasciotomy sites prospective randomized evaluation of two techniques. Am J Surg. 2018;216:736–9. https://doi.org/10.1016/j.amjsurg.2018.07.033.
49. Kakagia D, Karadimas EJ, Drosos G, Ververidis A, Trypsiannis G, Verettas D. Wound closure of leg fasciotomy: comparison of vacuum-assisted closure versus shoelace technique. A randomised study. Injury. 2014;45:890–3. https://doi.org/10.1016/j.injury.2012.02.002.
50. Jauregui JJ, Yarmis SJ, Tsai J, Onuoha KO, Illical E, Paulino CB. Fasciotomy closure techniques. J Orthop Surg (Hong Kong). 2017;25:2309499016684724. https://doi.org/10.1177/2309499016684724.
51. Shah DM, Bock DE, Darling RC 3rd, Chang BB, Kupinski AM, Leather RP. Beneficial effects of hypertonic mannitol in acute ischemia–reperfusion injuries in humans. Cardiovasc Surg. 1996;4:97–100. https://doi.org/10.1016/0967-2109(96)83793-8.
52. Robins M, Falkson SR, Goldfarb J, et al. Hyperbaric treatment of ischemia reperfusion injury. [Updated 2024 Feb 12]. In: StatPearls [Internet]. Treasure Island: StatPearls Publishing; 2024. Available from: https://www.ncbi.nlm.nih.gov/books/NBK513221/.
53. Bocca G, van Moorselaar JA, Feitz WF, van der Staak FH, Monnens LA. Compartment syndrome, rhabdomyolysis and risk of acute renal failure as complications of the lithotomy position. J Nephrol. 2002;15:183–5.
54. Zeng X, Zhang L, Wu T, Fu P. Continuous renal replacement therapy (CRRT) for rhabdomyolysis. Cochrane Database Syst Rev. 2014:CD008566. https://doi.org/10.1002/14651858.CD008566.pub2.
55. Johnson SB, Weaver FA, Yellin AE, Kelly R, Bauer M. Clinical results of decompressive dermotomy-fasciotomy. Am J Surg. 1992;164:286–90. https://doi.org/10.1016/s0002-9610(05)81089-x.
56. Rush DS, Frame SB, Bell RM, Berg EE, Kerstein MD, Haynes JL. Does open fasciotomy contribute to morbidity and mortality after acute lower extremity ischemia and revascularization? J Vasc Surg. 1989;10:343–50. https://doi.org/10.1067/mva.1989.14338.
57. Ris HB, Furrer M, Stronsky S, Walpoth B, Nachbur B. Four-compartment fasciotomy and venous calf-pump function: long-term results. Surgery. 1993;113:55–8.
58. Lollo L, Grabinsky A. Clinical and functional outcomes of acute lower extremity compartment syndrome at a major trauma hospital. Int J Crit Illn Inj Sci. 2016;6:133–42. https://doi.org/10.4103/2229-5151.190648.
59. Heemskerk J, Kitslaar P. Acute compartment syndrome of the lower leg: retrospective study on prevalence, technique, and outcome of fasciotomies. World J Surg. 2003;27:744–7. https://doi.org/10.1007/s00268-003-6691-7.
60. Erdos J, Dlaska C, Szatmary P, Humenberger M, Vecsei V, Hajdu S. Acute compartment syndrome in children: a case series in 24 patients and review of the literature. Int Orthop. 2011;35:569–75. https://doi.org/10.1007/s00264-010-1016-6.

Key References

Bjorck M, Earnshaw JJ, Acosta S, Bastos Goncalves F, Cochennec F, et al. Editor's choice - European Society for Vascular Surgery (ESVS) 2020 clinical practice guidelines on the management of acute limb Ischaemia. Eur J Vasc Endovasc Surg. 2020;59:173–218. https://doi.org/10.1016/j.ejvs.2019.09.006.

Kakagia D, Karadimas EJ, Drosos G, Ververidis A, et al. Wound closure of leg fasciotomy: comparison of vacuum-assisted closure versus shoelace technique. A randomised study. Injury. 2014;45(5):890–3. https://doi.org/10.1016/j.injury.2012.02.002. [published Online First: 2012/03/02].

Percival TJ, Rasmussen TE. Reperfusion strategies in the management of extremity vascular injury with ischaemia. Br J Surg. 2012;99(Suppl 1):66–74. https://doi.org/10.1002/bjs.7790. [published Online First: 2012/03/28].

von Keudell AG, Weaver MJ, Appleton PT, Bae DS, et al. Diagnosis and treatment of acute extremity compartment syndrome. Lancet. 2015;386(10000):1299–310. https://doi.org/10.1016/S0140-6736(15)00277-9. [published Online First: 2015/10/16].

Chapter 6
Pathophysiology of Varicose Veins, Chronic Venous Insufficiency, and Venous Ulceration

Manjit S. Gohel and Guilherme Pena

SN Flashcards
Test your learning and check your understanding of this book's contents: use the "Springer Nature Flashcards" app to access questions using ▶ https://sn.pub/wppvze. To use the app, please follow the instructions in Chap. 1.

Key Learning Points

- Chronic venous disease (CVD) is a common global health issue with growing prevalence due to risk factors including ageing and obesity. While milder forms are frequent, advanced stages such as venous ulcers represent a major heath burden.
- The foundational cause of advanced skin changes and ulceration in chronic venous insufficiency is persistently elevated venous pressure, known as chronic venous hypertension.
- The modern understanding of CVD pathophysiology centres on inflammation as an important driver. Venous hypertension triggers endothelial dysfunction, leading to leukocyte adhesion, infiltration, and a chronic inflammatory state that cause tissue damage and disease progression.

M. S. Gohel
Cambridge University Hospitals & Imperial College, London, UK
e-mail: manjit.gohel@nhs.net

G. Pena (✉)
Discipline of Surgery, Adelaide University, Adelaide, SA, Australia

Vascular Surgery Unit, Flinders Medical Centre, Adelaide, Australia
e-mail: Guilherme.Pena@sa.gov.au

R. Fitridge et al. (eds.), *Pathophysiology of Vascular Disease*,
https://doi.org/10.1007/978-3-032-31459-8_6

- The CEAP system (**C**linical signs, a**E**tiology, **A**natomy, and **P**athophysiology) is the standard for describing and classifying the clinical signs, aetiology, and anatomy of venous disease. However, for tracking disease progression or treatment response, the Revised Venous Clinical Severity Score (r-VCSS) is a crucial evaluative tool.
- It is important to determine if CVD is primary or secondary. Secondary CVD, most commonly caused by a previous deep vein thrombosis (DVT), can lead to a more rapid and severe disease progression.
- The calf muscle pump is the primary mechanism for propelling blood towards the heart against gravity. Its failure, whether from immobility or other neuromuscular conditions, can significantly contribute to venous hypertension, even with minimal anatomical disease.
- Post-thrombotic syndrome (PTS) is a complex clinical condition that develops in 20%–50% of patients after a proximal DVT, usually within two years. It is caused by venous outflow obstruction and/or post-thrombotic valvular incompetence. Key risk factors include proximal DVT location, recurrent DVT, and obesity.
- The primary goal in managing venous disease is to reduce chronic venous hypertension. This involves identifying and, where feasible, correcting treatable causes like superficial venous reflux or venous outflow obstruction.
- Minimally invasive endovenous ablation procedures have revolutionised the treatment of superficial venous reflux. These interventions effectively improve quality of life, accelerate ulcer healing, and are cost-effective.
- Deep venous stenting is an evolving treatment reserved for carefully selected patients with significant symptoms and advanced disease due to iliac vein outflow obstruction. It is not indicated for asymptomatic or mildly symptomatic individuals, and the field requires more robust long-term data.

6.1 Introduction

Chronic venous disease (CVD) is a widespread and significant global health issue, encompassing a range of functional and morphological abnormalities in the venous system. It represents a wide clinical spectrum of disorders that are common, potentially disabling, and a considerable source of patient distress and healthcare expense [1–3]. Recognised for thousands of years, the impact of venous disease is set to grow, as risk factors such as advanced age and obesity become more prevalent.

As its core, CVD involves pathological and haemodynamic alterations that impair the return of blood from the lower limbs to the heart. The term covers a spectrum of conditions, while the related term, chronic venous insufficiency (CVI), typically denotes the more advanced stages. In CVI, impaired venous flow leads to persistent venous hypertension and subsequent complications such as oedema, skin changes, and ulceration [4].

The prevalence of CVD is high worldwide, though it varies geographically. A recent systematic review highlights the frequency of its milder forms, with telangiectasia or reticular veins (C1) affecting approximately 26% of people and varicose veins (C2) present in about 19%. While less common, the advanced stages still represent a major health burden; oedema (C3) occurs in 8% of the population, skin changes (C4) in 5%, healed venous ulcer (C5) in 1%, and active ulcers (C6) in approximately 0.4%. The prevalence of C2 stage, for instance, is highest in Western Europe (21%) compared to regions like Middle East and Africa (5.5%), though estimates vary considerably across individual studies [5].

A key challenge in managing CVD is the often-poor correlation between the anatomical patterns of venous reflux or occlusion and the clinical presentation. This complexity, combined with the high prevalence and significant impact in quality of life, underscores the importance of understanding and effectively managing this common condition.

6.1.1 Risk Factors for Chronic Venous Disease

The aetiology of CVD is recognised as multifactorial, involving a complex interplay between inherent patient susceptibility and cumulative environment exposures. Non-modifiable risk factors establish an individual's baseline vulnerability. Advanced age is a consistent predictor, likely reflecting the cumulative effects of haemodynamic stress alongside age-related structural degeneration within the vein wall, including alterations in collagen, and impaired valve function. Female sex is also strongly associated with increased prevalence, attributed largely to the effects of hormones (oestrogen and progesterone) which increase venous distensibility and potentially weaken wall structure, Furthermore, a positive family history underscores a genetic predisposition [4, 6, 7].

Modifiable and environmental factors also significantly contribute to CVD development and progression. Obesity is a major risk factor, exerting influence through both increased intra-abdominal pressure which impedes venous return and a pro-inflammatory state driven by adipose tissue, potentially causing CVD signs even without demonstrable reflux [8]. Pregnancy acts as significant physiological stressor via hormonal dilatation, increased blood volume, and mechanical compression of pelvic veins by the gravid uterus [9]. Occupations involving prolonged standing or sitting, along with general inactivity, lead to calf muscle pump dysfunction, venous stasis, and elevated venous pressure.

A history of DVT is the principal cause of secondary CVI, leading to post-thrombotic syndrome (PTS) characterised by valve destruction and/or persistent venous obstruction [6, 7]. The clinical manifestation and severity in any given patient often result from the cumulative impact and interaction of these diverse risk factors over time.

6.2 Clinical Spectrum of Venous Disease

Patients with venous disease of the lower extremity present with a wide range of symptoms and clinical signs. A useful descriptive classification is the CEAP system, which provides vital information based on **C**linical signs, a**E**tiology, **A**natomy, and **P**athophysiology. Its primary role is descriptive, offering a snapshot of the disease state [10]. The clinical (C) component is the most widely used aspect, categorising the visible manifestations from C0 (no signs) to C6 (active ulceration) (Fig. 6.1). Key signs include C1 (telangiectasias/reticular veins), C2 (varicose veins), C3 (oedema), and the more advanced C4 skin changes (including pigmentation/eczema—C4a, lipodermatosclerosis/atrohie blanche—C4b, and the prognostically significant corona phebectatica—C4c, added in the 2020 revision) [10]. C5 signifies healed ulcer, while C6 indicates an active one. The 2020 CEAP update also added the modifier 'r' to denote recurrent varicose veins (C2r) and ulcers (C6r). While these signs provide objective classification, patient symptoms (including aching, heaviness, itching) correlate poorly with the C class and should be assessed separately. Details of the CEAP system, including recent updates, are summarised in Table 6.1.

Because CEAP is descriptive and not designed to measure changes or severity quantitatively, complementary tools are essential. The Revised Venous Severity Score (r-VCSS) is particularly important as an evaluative instrument. It consists of several clinical descriptors (including pain, oedema, skin changes, ulcer characteristics) score on a 0–3 scale, providing a composite score reflecting overall clinical severity. Its main value lies in its ability to track changes longitudinally within patients over time or quantify the clinical response to treatment [11]. This makes the r-VCSS invaluable for clinical practice to monitor progress and also important in research for comparing outcomes of different interventions, addressing a key limitation of the CEAP system.

Furthermore, while the CEAP focusses on lower extremity venous disease, it does not adequately address Pelvic Venous Disorders (PeVD). For this, the SVP classification has been developed, considering Symptoms, Varices (type and location, including pelvic, vulvar, gluteal, thigh), and pathophysiology specific to pelvic venous incompetence or obstruction [12].

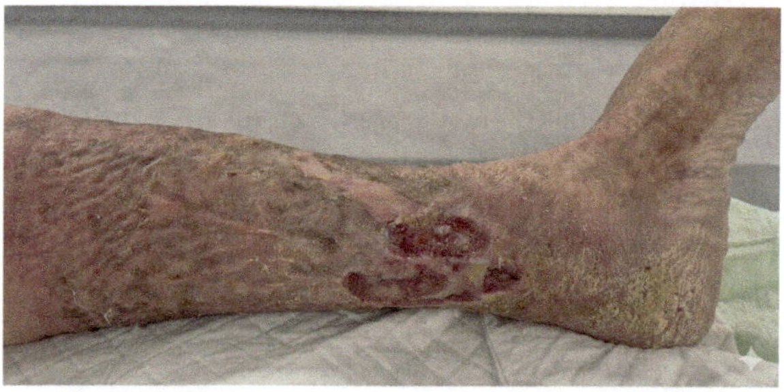

Fig. 6.1 Venous ulcer at ankle (CEAP classification C6)

Table 6.1 CEAP classification (modified from [10])

Component	Class	Description	Key 2020 updates
C-clinical	C0	No visible/palpable signs	
	C1	Telangiectasias/reticular veins	
	C2	Varicose veins	
	C2r	Recurrent varicose veins	Added ‘r’ modifier for recurrence
	C3	Oedema	
	C4a	Pigmentation/eczema	
	C4b	Lipodermatosclerosis/atrophie blanche	
	C4c	Corona phlebectatica	Added C4c category for Corona phlebectatica
	C5	Healed ulcer	
	C6	Active ulcer	
	C6r	Recurrent active ulcer	Added ‘r’ modifier for recurrence
	(modifier)	Add ‘s’ for symptomatic, ‘a’ for asymptomatic	
E-aetiology	Ec; ep; es; En	Aetiology: Congenital, primary, secondary, no cause found	Refined definitions; es subcategorised into Esi/ese
A-anatomy	As; ad; ap	Location: Superficial, deep, perforating veins	Replaced numeric codes with standard abbreviations for segments
P-Pathophys.	Pr; Po; pr,o; Pn	Mechanism: Reflux, obstruction, both, none identified	Uses new anatomy abbreviations for detailed reporting

6.3 Venous Anatomy

The lower extremity venous system consists of superficial, deep, and perforating veins. In general, deep veins accompany the associated arteries, whereas superficial veins do not usually have named arteries in the same distribution. Frequent and variable connections exist between the deep and superficial venous systems of the leg through a complex network of tributaries.

6.3.1 Superficial Veins

The superficial venous system of the lower limb is principally composed of the great saphenous vein (GSV) and small saphenous vein (SSV), which receive flow from numerous interconnecting tributaries. The GSV originates as a continuation of the medial marginal vein of the foot, ascending anterior to the medial malleolus and along the anteromedial aspect of the tibia and knee. The

GSV continues its course through the anteromedial thigh, contained within the saphenous compartment. Its confluence with the deep system occurs at the common femoral vein, just inferior to the inguinal ligament. The SSV originates from the lateral aspect of the venous arch of the foot, coursing subcutaneously posterior to the lateral malleolus. It ascends within the calf, penetrates the deep fascia, and travels between the heads of gastrocnemius muscle to typically join the popliteal vein posteriorly. However, the terminal anatomy of the SSV is highly variable; the saphenopopliteal junction may be absent, in which case the SSV continues on the posterior aspect of the thigh (Giacomini vein) and may drain into the GSV.

6.3.2 *Deep Veins*

Located deeper than the muscle fascia in the leg, deep veins usually accompany the associated artery and may exist in pairs, particularly below the knee. Below the knee, anterior and posterior tibial veins and the peroneal vein form the popliteal vein, which runs alongside the popliteal artery. Additionally, gastrocnemius and soleus veins are also considered below-knee deep veins. Frequently duplicated, the popliteal vein passes through the adductor hiatus to become the femoral vein (previously known as the superficial femoral vein). The common femoral vein is formed by the confluence of the femoral vein and the profunda vein (or deep femoral vein) in the groin. The common femoral vein terminates at the inferior margin of the inguinal ligament, where it becomes the external iliac vein, which in turn becomes the common iliac vein after the internal iliac vein confluence. Formed by the confluence of the right and left common iliac veins, the inferior vena cava (IVC) runs on the right of the aorta and drains into the right atrium. The IVC may be divided into infrarenal, suprarenal, and suprahepatic segments. This system of deep veins serves as the principal pathway for blood returning from the lower extremity.

6.3.3 *Perforating Veins*

A perforating vein (or perforator) in the lower extremity may be defined as a vein that pierces the muscle fascia to connect deep and superficial veins [13]. Perforator veins have unidirectional valves assuring flow from superficial to the deep system, except in the foot. Although enormous variation is present, perforators are commonly located along the medial lower leg (Boyd's & Cockett's perforators) or medial aspect of the thigh (Hunter's or Dodd's perforators). Incompetent perforator veins have been associated with chronic venous insufficiency [14, 15].

6.3.4 Valvular Anatomy

Venous valves, predominantly intimal folds, are essential anatomical structures ensuring unidirectional blood flow towards the heart. Their operation is passive, governed by pressure gradients generated through cardiac activity, respiration, and skeletal muscle pump. The anatomical distribution of these valves is notably heterogeneous. They are abundant and functionally critical in the veins of the limbs, particularly the lower extremities where they counteract substantial gravitational effects. In contrast, the inferior vena cava is typically avalvular, with only exceptional reports of sporadic monocuspid valves. The common iliac vein may occasionally feature a valve in a small percentage of the population, while the external iliac veins often exhibit more variability in valve presence, reflecting a transition from the densely valved femoral venous system [16].

Within the infrainguinal venous system, both superficial and deep veins are characterised by these unidirectional valves. The leaflets of these valves open to permit antegrade flow towards the heart and coapt towards the centre of the vein to prevent retrograde flow, a condition known as reflux or incompetence, which is commonly evaluated using duplex ultrasound (DUS). Cadaveric studies have consistently identified valves in certain key proximal locations, such as in the common femoral veins and the proximal femoral vein, particularly near the confluence with profunda femoris veins. Beyond these consistently valved proximal segments, the overall frequency of valves then typically increases more distally down the leg. Perforating veins may also contain valves which direct flow from the superficial to deep venous system [17]. Furthermore, research has highlighted the existence and potential incompetence of valves within very small veins (100 μm–2 mm) of the leg. This microvalve incompetence can occur independently from reflux in larger veins, such as the great saphenous vein. In scenarios involving GSV reflux, the incompetence of these microvalves in its tributaries, termed 'boundary' valves, is thought to significantly contribute to the progression of associated cutaneous manifestations [18].

6.4 Normal Venous Function

The primary role of the lower extremity venous system is to transport deoxygenated blood from the capillary beds back to the right atrium. Veins are distinct from arteries in that they are high-capacitance, high-volume, and low-resistance vessels. A significant portion of the circulating blood, approximately 60 to 75%, is held within the venous system at any time. Of this total volume, about 80% is contained in the veins that are less than 200 μm in diameter [19].

In healthy veins, the vast majority of the venous return is carried in the deep veins (over 80%), while the superficial veins drain only the skin and subcutaneous fat and tissues. However, superficial veins also have an important role in thermoregulation and may play a much more dominant role in venous return in the presence of deep venous occlusive disease [19].

The primary mechanism for propelling venous blood toward the right heart is the calf muscle pump, located in the posterior compartment of the lower leg. In addition to the calf muscle pump, a smaller but still significant foot muscle pump also exists. During ambulation or physical exertion, the contraction of the calf and foot muscles extrinsically compresses the deep veins, forcing the blood upwards towards the heart [20]. When at rest, venous sinusoids within the calf and foot muscles fill with blood. Subsequent muscle contraction during activities like walking compresses these veins, pushing the blood up the leg. This contraction also serves to close the perforating veins, which prevents the backflow (reflux) of blood into the superficial veins.

Unlike arterial pressure, which is generated by muscular contractions of the heart, pressure within the venous system is heavily influenced by gravity. In a supine position, the venous pressure in the lower extremities is comparable to that in the abdomen and chest. However, when an individual is standing still, the venous pressure in the foot can reach 90–100 mmHg. This pressure dramatically decreases to 20–30 mmHg with ambulation, only to return to the baseline levels when the activity stops (Fig. 6.2) [21].

The time taken for the venous pressure in the leg to return to its baseline after calf muscle has been active is a measurable value known as the venous refilling time (VRT). A very short VRTs (<20 s) indicate severe venous dysfunction. While several measures may be used to counter venous hypertension, elevation is the only method able to completely reverse raised venous pressure.

In summary, fully functional calf and foot muscle pumps along with competent valves are essential for reducing venous pressure and preventing the signs and symptoms of chronic venous hypertension [6, 22].

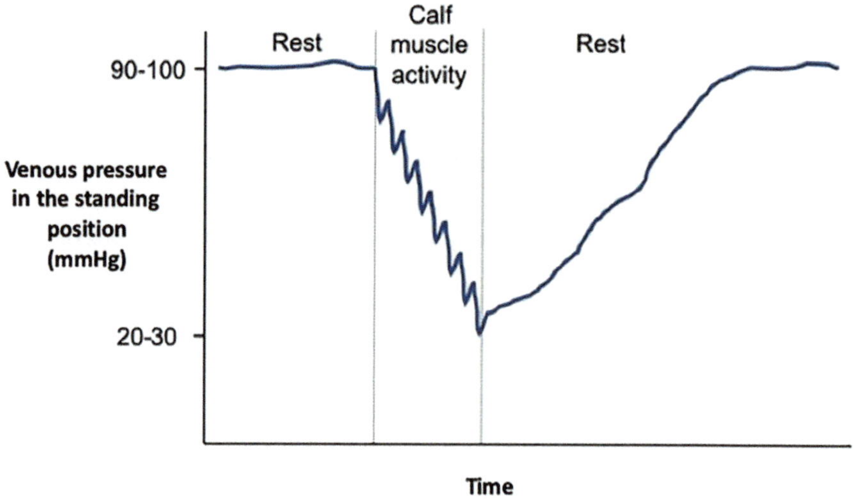

Fig. 6.2 Normal ambulatory venous pressure measurement

6.5 Pathophysiology of Chronic Venous Hypertension

Abnormally and persistently raised venous pressure in the leg as a result of venous dysfunction is termed 'chronic venous hypertension' and is widely accepted as the process leading to skin changes and eventually to venous ulceration. In most patients with chronic venous hypertension, there are pathological processes (most commonly venous reflux and/or outflow obstruction) that result in increased venous pressure and clinical symptoms and/or signs. However, any failure or dysfunction of the normal muscle pump mechanisms may lead to a deterioration in clinical status in patients with little superficial or deep venous disease on imaging. Factors such as poor mobility (with secondary calf muscle deconditioning), ankle stiffness (inhibiting effective calf muscle contraction), stroke, or neuromuscular conditions may all inhibit calf muscle pump effectiveness [23]. Venous hypertension may also be exacerbated by central causes of venous hypertension (such as right heart failure) or truncal obesity, which may act as a functional venous outflow obstruction [24] (Fig. 6.3).

6.5.1 *Microcirculatory Changes in Venous Hypertension and Inflammation*

The microcirculation is the smallest functional unit of the cardiovascular system, representing the direct interface between the blood and tissue. The association between chronic venous hypertension and microcirculatory changes that lead to venous ulceration is generally undisputed, though precise mechanisms are poorly understood. An early theory, postulated by Homans in 1917, suggests that the stagnation of venous blood caused local tissue hypoxia. However, the view that ulceration is due to simple hypoxia is likely too simplistic and has largely been abandoned. It is now understood that venous hypertension increases capillary endothelial permeability, leading to soft tissue oedema, haemosiderin deposition, white cell activation, and chronic inflammatory cascades that can culminate in skin ulceration [25]. Based predominantly on observed microcirculatory changes in patients with chronic venous hypertension, multiple theories for venous ulceration have been proposed.

An early microcirculatory theory was the 'Fibrin cuff theory', which hypothesised that fibrinogen leakage from permeable capillaries formed cuffs around them, acting as a barrier to oxygen and nutrient diffusion and causing skin breakdown [26]. However, this theory was later challenged by the fact that ulcer healing could be achieved even in the continued presence of these fibrin cuffs.

The current paradigm centres on inflammation as a critical driver of CVD onset and progression. This inflammatory cascade is not simply a response but a complex interplay between blood cells, vascular cells, and extracellular matrix, orchestrated by haemodynamic forces. The inflammatory process begins with endothelial dysfunction, triggered by altered shear stress and pressure of venous

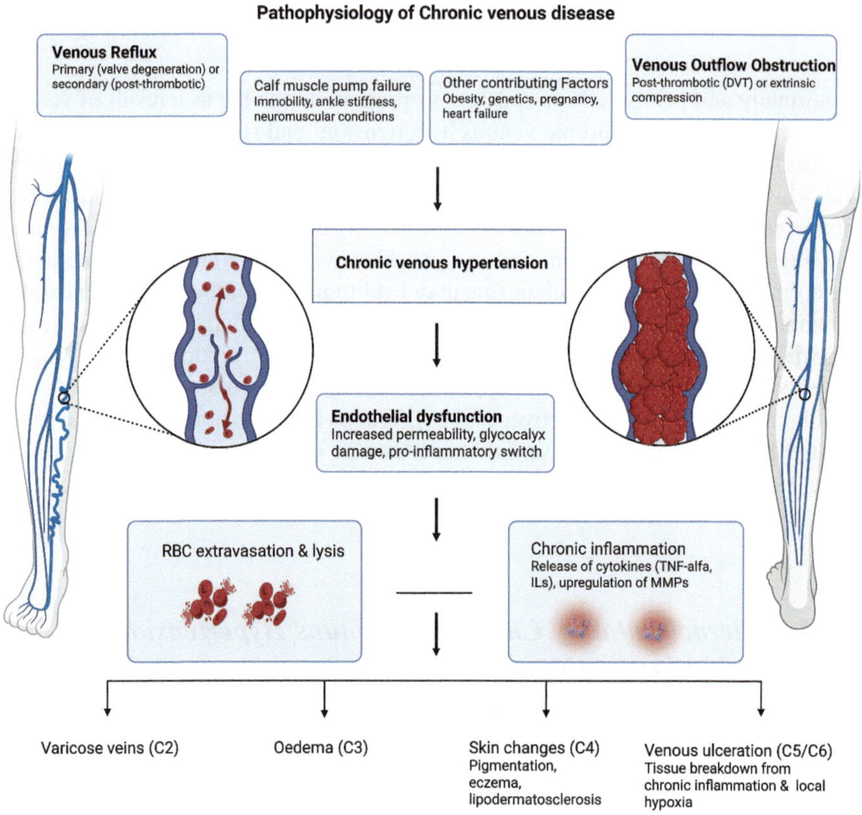

Fig. 6.3 Pathophysiology of chronic venous disease. Chronic venous hypertension (CVH), the central driver of chronic venous disease (CVD), is primarily caused by venous reflux and/or outflow obstruction, often exacerbated by factors like calf muscle pump failure. CVH initiates a cascade of microcirculatory damage, beginning with endothelial dysfunction. This dysfunction increases venous permeability and promotes a self-perpetuating cycle of chronic inflammation. This inflammatory state and increased permeability lead to red blood cell leakage (causing hemosiderin skin pigmentation) and enzymatic tissue degradation. These pathological processes manifest clinically as progressive signs including varicose veins (C2), oedema (C3), skin changes such as lipodermatosclerosis (C4), and ultimately, venous ulceration (C5/C6)

hypertension [27]. This stress induces a pro-inflammatory phenotypical switch in the endothelial cells and causes significant damage to the glycocalyx. The breakdown of the glycocalyx impairs the vascular barrier, allowing fluid to leak into the interstitium (causing oedema) and promoting the adhesion and infiltration of leukocytes [6]. The severity of this endothelial dysfunction correlates with the clinical severity of CVD.

The damaged endothelium upregulates adhesion molecules (e.g. ICAM-1, VCAM-1, selectins) and chemokines (e.g. MCP-1), which recruit a diverse population of leukocytes from the bloodstream into the vein wall and surrounding tissue [28].

Key immune cells involved include the following:

- *Monocytes/Macrophages*: These cells are central to the disease process. Critically, they are responsible for processing the red blood cells that extravasate due to high venous pressure. This process releases iron, which is stored as haemosiderin, causing the characteristic skin pigmentation and perpetuating local oxidative stress and inflammation [29].
- *Neutrophils*: As some of the first responders, neutrophils are key initiators of the inflammatory response. Venous hypertension and stasis cause a 'leukocyte trap' where neutrophils become caught in the microcirculation and infiltrate the tissue, contributing to local damage though the release of enzymes and reactive oxygen species [6, 30].
- *Lymphocytes*: Both T and B lymphocytes are important players. Memory T helper and cytotoxic T cells participate in the pathogenesis, releasing inflammatory cytokines that fuel the pro-inflammatory environment.

This cellular activity is coordinated by an uncontrolled release of proinflammatory cytokines, including TNF-α, TGF-β, and various interleukins (IL-1, IL-17, IL-18), which dominate the local environment, particularly in venous ulcers. These cytokines, in turn, upregulate the expression of matrix metalloproteinases (MMPs), which are enzymes that degrade the extracellular matrix. This degradation can lead to the weakening and fibrosis of the vein wall and valves, ultimately causing venous dilation and dysfunction [31].

Overall, the immune system's involvement in CVD is through complex feedback loops. It responds to the initial damage caused by venous stasis and haemodynamic changes, but the resulting proinflammatory environment it creates then becomes a primary driver of further endothelial dysfunction, tissue damage, and disease progression [6].

6.6 Genetic and Epigenetic Factors

CVD has a significant genetic component, with family history being a well-established risk factor. Studies have demonstrated that the risk of developing varicose veins can be as high as 90% when both parents are affected [32]. Early genetic insights came from congenital disorders with venous manifestations, such as lymphoedema-distichiasis syndrome, with mutations in the FOXC2 gene, and cerebral autosomal-dominant arteriopathy with subcortical infarcts and leukoencephalopathy (CADASIL), which pointed to the Notch3 gene [33–35]. More recent, large-scale genome-wide association studies (GWAS) have moved beyond single-gene disorders and identified numerous susceptibility loci for varicose veins, including EFEMP1, CASZ1, and PIEZO1 [34, 36, 37]. Furthermore, specific genetic variations have been linked to complications of CVD, such as venous leg ulcers. Mutations in genes involved in iron metabolism (HFE, SLC40A1) and tissue repair (F13A1, MTHFR) have been shown to increase the risk of ulcer development and impair healing, highlighting how genetic predisposition can influence disease progression and severity [33, 34].

The pathophysiology of CVD involves complex changes in gene expression within the vessel wall. Prolonged venous hypertension incites an inflammatory response that alters the cellular environment and gene activity [33, 34, 38]. Transcriptomic analyses comparing varicose veins with healthy tissue reveal significant changes in expression of genes responsible for extracellular matrix (ECM) organisation and vascular development. A key finding is the dysregulation of MMPs and their inhibitors (TIMPs), leading to excessive ECM degradation and weakening of the vein wall [34]. For example, the downregulation of the desmuslin gene has been observed in incompetent veins, which is thought to cause a loss of vascular tone by disrupting smooth muscle cell integrity [33]. While these changes in gene expression are consistently documented, it is often difficult to distinguish whether they are a cause or consequence of the disease [33, 34].

6.7 Aetiology of Chronic Venous Disease

The determination of underlying aetiology of CVD is important because it directly influences prognosis, guides treatment choices, and affects patient outcomes. The CEAP classification system broadly categorises the causes as either primary, caused by a degenerative process of the vein wall or its valves, or secondary, resulting from other intravenous of extravenous conditions. It is also important to recognise that combinations of these aetiological states can coexist [10].

In addition to primary and secondary causes, the CEAP classification includes two other aetiological categories. Congenital (Ec) causes refer to venous disorders resulting from conditions present at birth, even if they only become apparent later in life. This includes venous malformations, venous agenesis, or arteriovenous malformations (see Chap. 24). The final category, no venous cause identified (En), is a classification of exclusion. It is used for patients who present with clinical signs and symptoms consistent with venous disease, but in whom no primary, secondary, or congenital aetiology can be found through investigation [10].

6.7.1 Primary Chronic Venous Disease

Primary venous disease is defined as a degenerative process affecting the venous valve and/or venous wall, which leads to weakness and dilatation of the valve and/or vein wall weakness and dilatation that results in pathological reflux, as demonstrated by imaging [39]. This condition frequently manifests in the saphenous veins, where it is known as truncal insufficiency.

Our understanding of the mechanisms that result in venous valvular incompetence remains far from complete. Several researchers have evaluated a range of biological and histological features in patients with varicose veins. Features such as disruption of the extracellular matrix, imbalance of matrix metalloproteinases and tissue inhibitors of metalloproteinases, dysregulation of apoptosis (see Glossary), and reduction in venous tone have been observed in the vein wall [40]. It is debatable whether the vein wall changes precede valvular incompetence, or if the primary event is vein valvular reflux, leading to secondary vein wall changes. Usually, by the time patients present, multiple changes are present, making it impossible to separate the 'chicken' and the 'egg'. Venous stasis and hypertension may promote further vein wall stretch and lead to hypoxia. This hypoxia arises from two main factors: reduced oxygen flow caused by blood stagnation and compression of vasa vasorum as a reaction to venous dilatation [41, 42]. These conditions suggest that once vein wall and valvular function begin to fail, a vicious cycle of cellular damage is triggered [6, 43].

Interestingly, observational studies have evaluated patterns of venous reflux and showed that in some patients, the superficial reflux starts in the lower leg, before progressing up the leg (so-called 'ascending' theory), whereas in other patients, there is primary reflux at the saphenofemoral junction, which progresses down the leg ('descending' theory) [44, 45]. It is likely therefore that no single pathophysiological mechanism exists, and in reality, the precise processes leading to venous hypertension vary between patients. The 'self-perpetuating' nature of venous dysfunction may encourage early intervention with, for example, venoactive medications intended to reduce inflammation and increase venous tone. However, evidence showing that early treatment can prevent the development of varicose veins is lacking.

6.7.2 *Secondary Chronic Venous Disease*

Secondary chronic venous disease (CVD) occurs when venous pathology is attributable to a specific acquired condition that damages the venous system or impairs its function. The 2020 CEAP classification refines the aetiology into two main subcategories: intravenous (Esi) and extravenous (Ese). Intravenous causes involve direct damage to the vein wall and/or its valves [10]. The most common cause of secondary intravenous CVD is deep vein thrombosis (DVT), which can lead to post-thrombotic syndrome. Following a DVT, the vein can become either permanently obstructed, or the valves can be damaged during thrombus recanalisation, leading to deep venous reflux [46]. This combination of obstruction and reflux results in severe venous hypertension, a more rapid disease progression, and higher incidence of advanced clinical signs like venous ulcers compared to primary CVD [47].

Extravenous causes (Ese), on the other hand, lead to venous hypertension without direct damage to the venous structures. This condition affects venous haemodynamics either locally or systemically [10]. An example is extrinsic compression, where an external structure compresses a vein, such as in non-thrombotic iliac vein lesions (e.g. May-Thurner syndrome) or from an abdominal or pelvic mass. However, May-Thurner syndrome can also represent a combined aetiology. The chronic pulsatile compression of the left common iliac vein by the right common iliac artery can cause endothelial injury, which in turn leads to deposition of elastin and collagen, creating a secondary intraluminal obstruction [48].

Another important extravenous cause is the failure of the venous muscle pumps, particularly the calf muscle pump. This can result from motor disorders (e.g. paraplegia, chronic immobility), which lead to ineffective emptying of the deep veins and subsequent venous hypertension. Conditions causing elevated central venous pressure, such as obesity or right-sided heart failure, can also be categorised as extravenous causes of CVD [10].

6.8 Post-Thrombotic Syndrome

Post-thrombotic syndrome (PTS) is a complex and diverse clinical entity that occurs in 20%–50% of patients after proximal DVT, usually occurring within 2 years of the DVT [49, 50]. PTS is a significant public health concern due to its profound impact on quality of life and healthcare costs The diagnosis and assessment of PTS remains challenging and controversial, but the Villalta scale is the most widely accepted tool [51]. The score consists of 11 domains (each scoring 0, 1, 2, or 3) comprising of 5 patient-reported symptom domains (pain, cramps, leg heaviness, pruritus, and paraesthesia), 6 clinician-assessed domains based on clinical signs (oedema, induration, hyperpigmentation, venous ectasia, redness, calf tenderness), and assessment for the presence of a venous ulcer. A score ≥ 5 indicates the presence of PTS. The underlying cause of PTS is venous outflow obstruction, post-thrombotic valvular incompetence, or a combination of the two, resulting in a spectrum of clinical presentations and severities. Interestingly, the pattern of symptoms and signs may reflect the dominant underlying pathology. Pain and swelling, for example, may be more indicative of outflow obstruction, whereas ulcers may be more commonly associated with reflux. In reality, clinical presentations and patterns of disease are enormously varied, preventing easy classification of patients.

Several key factors have been identified that increase a patient's susceptibility to developing PTS. The location of the initial thrombus is important, with proximal DVTs, particularly those in the iliofemoral segment, conferring a higher risk than more distal thrombus, due to impairment of major collateral blood flow. Other significant predictors include history of recurrent DVT, obesity, and the presence of pre-existing chronic venous disease. Furthermore, the severity of symptoms during an acute DVT episode is also predictive of future PTS development [52]. While adequate anticoagulation is the cornerstone of management of acute DVT, the quality and type of anticoagulant therapy may play a crucial role in PTS. Subtherapeutic anticoagulation, especially with vitamin K antagonists such as warfarin, has been linked to a higher risk of PTS. Conversely, treatment with direct oral anticoagulants (DOACs) appears to be associated with lower risk of developing PTS, particularly severe forms, compared to warfarin [53].

6.8.1 Deep Vein Thrombosis and Thrombus Resolution

DVT is common, with an incidence of 0.5–1 per 1000 adults per year in western countries [54]. The thrombus may cause complete or partial occlusion of the deep vein and commonly leads to the typical clinical features including pain, swelling, redness, and tenderness [55]. For over a century, our understanding of venous thrombosis has focussed on Virchow's triad of venous stasis, vein wall changes, and pro-thrombotic changes in the blood constituents [56]. Although precise factors causing DVT may vary from individual to individual, it is likely that multiple contributory factors combine to result in thrombus formation. Ordinarily, the venous endothelial cells maintain a non-thrombogenic environment by expressing fibrinolytic and anti-inflammatory factors [57]. Conversely, at times of endothelial disturbance (e.g. after trauma), a pro-thrombotic environment is created by vasoconstriction and release of factors such as platelet activating factor (PAF), von Willebrand factor (vWF), and others. The early phase of thrombosis (up to 2–3 days) is driven largely by neutrophils, whereas the later phase (to 14 days) is dominated by monocytes as the thrombus reduces in size with a progressive increase in fibrosis. The processes of inflammation and thrombosis are intimately related, with the presence of one promoting the other. Another important group of mediators involved in thrombosis includes the selectins. P- and E-selectin are cell-adhesion molecules that are integral in the white cell and endothelial wall interaction. Genetic 'knockout' studies in mice have shown reduced thrombosis when selectin genes are deleted, and selectin-specific antibodies or receptor antagonists have also been shown to inhibit thrombosis [58].

As a counter to thrombosis, the fibrinolytic system is responsible for containing the extent of the thrombus. A proenzyme, plasminogen is converted to the active enzyme, plasmin, which is the primary enzyme responsible for breaking down fibrin. The fibrinolytic process is controlled by plasminogen activators (tissue-type and urokinase-type) which in turn are inhibited by plasminogen activator inhibitors (PAIs). PAI inhibitors have been proposed as a novel mechanism for reducing thrombosis [59]. There are several parallels between venous thrombus resolution and wound healing, with eventual fibrosis. After DVT and subsequent inflammation and remodelling, one of three eventual scenarios may result:

1. Total thrombus resolution with no significant residual outflow obstruction.
2. Limited thrombus resolution with partial venous outflow obstruction.
3. No thrombus resolution with total obliteration of venous channel.

Most of the measures to prevent or treat PTS presume the 'open-vein hypothesis', which simply states that an open and widely patent deep vein after DVT is less likely to result in PTS [60]. However, the severity of PTS symptoms doesn't consistently align with the degree of anatomical obstruction seen on imaging. Some individuals with significant obstruction may have mild symptoms, while others with less apparent obstruction may experience severe symptoms [61]. However, there remains a concern that patients with outflow obstruction will be at higher risk of developing symptomatic or advanced venous disease in the future. The anatomical disease may act as a 'permissive' pathology [62], remaining largely subclinical, but with patients becoming very symptomatic with only a small additional venous pathology. Reasons for variability in thrombus resolution after DVT between patients are poorly understood.

6.8.2 *Impact of Venous Outflow Obstruction*

Residual venous fibrosis after DVT results in increased outflow resistance and reduced compliance in a more rigid vein. Autologous resolution of thrombus is thought to be less effective for DVTs in the iliocaval segment, in comparison to infrainguinal DVT, which may explain the higher rate of PTS in this group [63]. The resultant impedance to normal venous drainage results in the symptoms and clinical signs associated with PTS. The impairment to effective venous drainage may be mitigated partially by the formation of venous collaterals as alternative draining channels. However, even florid venous collaterals are unlikely to ever match the venous drainage capacity and efficiency of an intact large deep vein. From Pouseille's law, flow is proportional to the fourth power of the radius of a tube. Therefore, it would require 16 1 cm diameter collateral veins to match the potential flow in a 2 cm deep vein.

6.9 Principles of Management of Venous Disease

As the underlying cause of advanced venous disease and ulceration is chronic venous hypertension, the principles of management focus on the identification and correction of the factors causing venous hypertension. A detailed description of the clinical management of patients with venous disease is beyond the remit of this chapter. For comprehensive evidence-based recommendations, readers should refer to recent guidelines, such as those from the European Society for Vascular Surgery (2022) [64] and the joint American Vascular Societies (2023) [65, 66].

6.9.1 *Clinical Evaluation*

A detailed clinical history should include the severity of symptoms and the impact on quality of life, as the decision to intervene may be largely driven by these considerations. Common symptoms of venous disease include pain, heaviness, swelling, restless legs, cramps, and itching [67]. Details of previous venous thromboembolism, previous venous interventions, and relevant medications (anticoagulation, immunosuppression, oestrogen-containing medications) should be recorded. In a clinical field renowned for a high level of litigation, careful documentation is essential and patient expectations from any interventions should be clearly established.

6.9.2 *Investigations*

The main goals of venous investigations are to identify potentially treatable superficial or deep venous disease and confirm the diagnosis. A wide variety of anatomical and haemodynamic venous assessments can be performed, but DUS is the first-line investigation. DUS is non-invasive and can offer an excellent, detailed map of venous incompetence and obstruction. In many cases, this is the only investigation necessary to plan intervention. If venous outflow obstruction is suspected, additional evaluation using computerised tomography (CT), magnetic resonance (MR), or conventional venography may be required.

6.9.3 *Treatment*

6.9.3.1 General Principles

The primary goal of treatment of venous disease is to reduce chronic venous hypertension. Treatable superficial reflux or venous outflow obstruction should be addressed where feasible. As chronic venous hypertension is usually multifactorial, there may be residual dysfunction despite superficial or deep venous intervention (or venous intervention may not be feasible or accepted by the patient). In such cases, compression and elevation are the mainstay of management.

6.9.3.2 Superficial Venous Interventions

The presence of incompetence in the GSV, SSV, associated tributaries, or perforating veins is commonly seen in patients with varicose veins and chronic venous insufficiency. Traditional treatment of superficial reflux involved surgical ligation and 'stripping' of incompetent veins. However, superficial venous interventions have been revolutionised by minimally invasive endovenous ablation procedures. These treatments utilise heat (laser, radiofrequency) or chemical (sclerotherapy, cyanoacrylate) ablation to close the incompetent superficial vein(s) [64]. Often performed under local anaesthesia in an outpatient setting, endovenous ablation procedures offer a well-tolerated and effective approach to address the usual underlying cause of venous hypertension. Endovenous interventions have been shown to improve patient quality of life [68] and accelerate venous ulcer healing and are cost effective [69, 70].

6.9.3.3 Deep Venous Interventions

Deep venous intervention is a rapidly evolving field primarily for patients suffering from significant symptoms of CVD. Indications for treatment are carefully considered, with a consensus against intervention in asymptomatic or mildly symptomatic individuals, regardless of the severity of outflow stenosis/obstruction [64]. The procedure is typically reserved for those with advanced disease, such as patients in clinical classes C4-C6 of the CEAP classification, or those with severe PTS as measured by the Vilalta scale. Venous claudication, characterised by pain and heaviness in the limb during exercise secondary to venous hypertension, is an important factor that may benefit from intervention. For these symptomatic patients with iliac vein outflow obstruction, endovascular treatment is the therapy of choice.

Despite its growing application, deep venous intervention is an area with limited evidence base and a need for more robust long-term data. While recent years have seen the development and approval of dedicated venous stents and the increased use of intravascular ultrasound (IVUS) to improve diagnostic accuracy and guide stent placement, challenges remain. Existing research suffers from significant methodological flaws such as patient and treatment selection bias. Consequently, while the procedure is considered beneficial for carefully selected patients, the long term-effectiveness and outcomes are still awaited. Careful consideration weighing the pros and cons for each individual case is recommended, acknowledging that the risks and benefits have not yet been fully quantified by high quality studies.

6.10 Conclusions

The venous system is a complex, highly dynamic component of the circulation. Low resistance, highly compliant venous channels effectively counter venous hypertension using intrinsic mechanisms such as calf and foot muscle pumps and vein valves. Venous dysfunction is often complex and multifactorial, resulting in a spectrum of venous disease. The underlying cause of chronic venous insufficiency and ulceration is venous hypertension. The precise mechanisms and pathways linking chronic venous hypertension to venous skin damage and ulceration are incompletely understood. The principles of managing chronic venous insufficiency are to identify treatable superficial venous reflux or venous outflow obstruction.

Multiple Choice Questions

1. In the microcirculatory changes induced by venous hypertension, what is the fate of extravasated red blood cells and the resultant product that is directly responsible for the characteristic skin pigmentation observed in advanced chronic venous disease?

(a) They are trapped by a perivascular fibrin cuff, leading to hypoxia.
(b) They are processed by monocytes/macrophages, releasing iron which is stored as haemosiderin.
(c) They are broken down by T lymphocytes, releasing iron and collagen.
(d) They spontaneously dissolve, accelerating venous reflux.
(e) They are pushed back into capillary by the calf pump.

Answer: (b) They are processed by monocytes/macrophages, releasing iron which is stored as haemosiderin

2. Advanced Chronic Venous Disease involves the degradation of the extracellular matrix in the vein wall and valves. Transcriptomic analyses consistently reveal the dysregulation of which specific family of enzymes and their inhibitor, leading to excessive extracellular matrix degradation?

(a) Plasminogen activators and Plasmin.
(b) Reactive Oxygen Species and Antioxidants.
(c) Cytokines (e.g. TNF-α, IL-18) and chemokines (e.g. MCP-1)).
(d) Iron metabolism genes (HFE, SLC40A1).
(e) Matrix metalloproteinases and their inhibitors (TIMPs).

Answer: (e) Matrix metalloproteinases and their inhibitors (TIMPs)

References

1. Robertson L, Evans C, Fowkes FG. Epidemiology of chronic venous disease. Phlebology. 2008;23:103–11. https://doi.org/10.1258/phleb.2007.007061.
2. Guest JF, Fuller GW, Vowden P. Venous leg ulcer management in clinical practice in the UK: costs and outcomes. Int Wound J. 2018;15:29–37. https://doi.org/10.1111/iwj.12814.
3. Davies AH. The seriousness of chronic venous disease: a review of real-world evidence. Adv Ther. 2019;36:5–12. https://doi.org/10.1007/s12325-019-0881-7.
4. Eberhardt RT, Raffetto JD. Chronic venous insufficiency. Circulation. 2014;130:333–46. https://doi.org/10.1161/CIRCULATIONAHA.113.006898.
5. Salim S, Machin M, Patterson BO, Onida S, Davies AH. Global epidemiology of chronic venous disease: a systematic review with pooled prevalence analysis. Ann Surg. 2021;274:971–6. https://doi.org/10.1097/SLA.0000000000004631.
6. Ortega MA, Fraile-Martínez O, García-Montero C, Álvarez-Mon MA, Chaowen C, Ruiz-Grande F, et al. Understanding chronic venous disease: a critical overview of its pathophysiology and medical management. J Clin Med. 2021;10:3239. https://doi.org/10.3390/jcm10153239.
7. Raffetto J, Mannello F. Pathophysiology of chronic venous disease. Int Angiol. 2014;33:212–21.
8. Davies HO, Popplewell M, Singhal R, Smith N, Bradbury AW. Obesity and lower limb venous disease–the epidemic of phlebesity. Phlebology. 2017;32:227–33. https://doi.org/10.1177/0268355516649333.
9. Ismail L, Normahani P, Standfield NJ, Jaffer U. A systematic review and meta-analysis of the risk for development of varicose veins in women with a history of pregnancy. J Vasc Surg Venous Lymphat Disord. 2016;4(518–24):e1. https://doi.org/10.1016/j.jvsv.2016.06.003.

10. Lurie F, Passman M, Meisner M, Dalsing M, Masuda E, Welch H, et al. The 2020 update of the CEAP classification system and reporting standards. J Vasc Surg Venous Lymphat Disord. 2020;8:342–52. https://doi.org/10.1016/j.jvsv.2016.06.003.
11. Vasquez MA, Rabe E, McLafferty RB, Shortell CK, Marston WA, Gillespie D, et al. Revision of the venous clinical severity score: venous outcomes consensus statement: special communication of the American Venous forum ad hoc outcomes working group. J Vasc Surg. 2010;52:1387–96. https://doi.org/10.1016/j.jvs.2010.06.161.
12. Meissner MH, Khilnani NM, Labropoulos N, Gasparis AP, Gibson K, Greiner M, et al. The symptoms-varices-pathophysiology classification of pelvic venous disorders: a report of the American Vein & Lymphatic Society international working group on pelvic venous disorders. Phlebology. 2021;36:342–60. https://doi.org/10.1177/0268355521999559.
13. Zukowski AJ, Nicolaides AN, Szendro G, Irvine A, Lewis R, Malouf GM, et al. Haemodynamic significance of incompetent calf perforating veins. Br J Surg. 1991;78:625–9. https://doi.org/10.1002/bjs.1800780532.
14. Delis KT, Ibegbuna V, Nicolaides AN, Lauro A, Hafez H. Prevalence and distribution of incompetent perforating veins in chronic venous insufficiency. J Vasc Surg. 1998;28:815–25. https://doi.org/10.1016/s0741-5214(98)70056-4.
15. Delis KT. Leg perforator vein incompetence: functional anatomy. Radiology. 2005;235:327–34. https://doi.org/10.1148/radiol.2351031598.
16. Caggiati A. The venous valves of the lower limbs. Phlebolymphology. 2013;20:87–95.
17. Moore HM, Gohel M, Davies AH. Number and location of venous valves within the popliteal and femoral veins: a review of the literature. J Anat. 2011;219:439–43. https://doi.org/10.1111/j.1469-7580.2011.01409.x.
18. Vincent JR, Jones GT, Hill GB, van Rij AM. Failure of microvenous valves in small superficial veins is a key to the skin changes of venous insufficiency. J Vasc Surg. 2011;54:62S-9S. e1-3. https://doi.org/10.1016/j.jvs.2011.06.085.
19. Bergan J, Pascarella L. Chapter 4: Venous anatomy, physiology, and pathophysiology. In: Bergan JJ, editor. The vein book. Elsevier; 2007. p. 39–45.
20. Williams KJ, Ayekoloye O, Moore HM, Davies AH. The calf muscle pump revisited. J Vasc Surg Venous Lymphat Disord. 2014;2:329–34. https://doi.org/10.1016/j.jvsv.2013.10.053.
21. Nicolaides AN, Hussein MK, Szendro G, Christopoulos D, Vasdekis S, Clarke H. The relation of venous ulceration with ambulatory venous pressure measurements. J Vasc Surg. 1993;17:414–9. https://doi.org/10.1067/mva.1993.37694.
22. Panny M, Ammer K, Kundi M, Katzenschlager R, Hirschl M. Severity of chronic venous disorders and its relationship to the calf muscle pump. Vasa. 2009;38:171–6. https://doi.org/10.1024/0301-1526.38.2.171.
23. Shiman MI, Pieper B, Templin TN, Birk TJ, Patel AR, Kirsner RS. Venous ulcers: a reappraisal analyzing the effects of neuropathy, muscle involvement, and range of motion upon gait and calf muscle function. Wound Repair Regen. 2009;17:147–52. https://doi.org/10.1111/j.1524-475X.2009.00468.x.
24. Vlajinac HD, Marinkovic JM, Maksimovic MZ, Matic PA, Radak DJ. Body mass index and primary chronic venous disease–a cross-sectional study. Eur J Vasc Endovasc Surg. 2013;45:293–8. https://doi.org/10.1016/j.ejvs.2012.12.011.
25. Raffetto JD. Pathophysiology of chronic venous disease and venous ulcers. Surg Clin North Am. 2018;98:337–47. https://doi.org/10.1016/j.suc.2017.11.002.
26. Burnand KG, Whimster I, Naidoo A, Browse NL. Pericapillary fibrin in the ulcer-bearing skin of the leg: the cause of lipodermatosclerosis and venous ulceration. Br Med J (Clin Res Ed). 1982;285:1071–2. https://doi.org/10.1136/bmj.285.6348.1071.
27. Zamboni P, Lanzara S, Mascoli F, Caggiati A, Liboni A. Inflammation in venous disease. Int Angiol. 2008;27:361–9.
28. Mosmiller LT, Steele KN, Shrader CD, Petrone AB. Evaluation of inflammatory cell biomarkers in chronic venous insufficiency. Phlebology. 2017;32:634–40. https://doi.org/10.1177/0268355517701806.

29. Caggiati A, Rosi C, Casini A, Cirenza M, Petrozza V, Acconcia MC, et al. Skin iron deposition characterises lipodermatosclerosis and leg ulcer. Eur J Vasc Endovasc Surg. 2010;40:777–82. https://doio.org/10.1016/j.ejvs.2010.08.015
30. Coleridge Smith PD, Thomas P, Scurr JH, Dormandy JA. Causes of venous ulceration: a new hypothesis. Br Med J (Clin Res Ed). 1988;296:1726–7. https://doi.org/10.1136/bmj.296.6638.1726.
31. Castro-Ferreira R, Cardoso R, Leite-Moreira A, Mansilha A. The role of endothelial dysfunction and inflammation in chronic venous disease. Ann Vasc Surg. 2018;46:380–93. https://doi.org/10.1016/j.avsg.2017.06.131.
32. Cornu-Thenard A, Boivin P, Baud J-M, de Vincenzi I, Carpentier PH. Importance of the familial factor in varicose disease: clinical study of 134 families. J Dermatol Surg Oncol. 1994;20:318–26. https://doi.org/10.1111/j.1524-4725.1994.tb01631.x.
33. Anwar MA, Georgiadis KA, Shalhoub J, Lim CS, Gohel MS, Davies AH. A review of familial, genetic, and congenital aspects of primary varicose vein disease. Circ Cardiovasc Genet. 2012;5:460–6. https://doi.org/10.1161/CIRCGENETICS.112.963439.
34. Baylis RA, Smith NL, Klarin D, Fukaya E. Epidemiology and genetics of venous thromboembolism and chronic venous disease. Circ Res. 2021;128:1988–2002. https://doi.org/10.1161/CIRCRESAHA.121.318322.
35. Mellor RH, Brice G, Stanton AW, French J, Smith A, Jeffery S, et al. Mutations in FOXC2 are strongly associated with primary valve failure in veins of the lower limb. Circulation. 2007;115:1912–20. https://doi.org/10.1161/CIRCULATIONAHA.106.675348.
36. Shadrina AS, Sharapov SZ, Shashkova TI, Tsepilov YA. Varicose veins of lower extremities: insights from the first large-scale genetic study. PLoS Genet. 2019;15:e1008110. https://doi.org/10.1371/journal.pgen.1008110.
37. Fukaya E, Flores AM, Lindholm D, Gustafsson S, Zanetti D, Ingelsson E, et al. Clinical and genetic determinants of varicose veins: prospective, community-based study of ~ 500,000 individuals. Circulation. 2018;138:2869–80. https://doi.org/10.1161/CIRCULATIONAHA.118.035584.
38. Ku KH, Subramaniam N, Marsden PA. Epigenetic determinants of flow-mediated vascular endothelial gene expression. Hypertension. 2019;74:467–76. https://doi.org/10.1161/HYPERTENSIONAHA.119.13342.
39. Eklof B, Rutherford RB, Bergan JJ, Carpentier PH, Gloviczki P, Kistner RL, et al. Revision of the CEAP classification for chronic venous disorders: consensus statement. J Vasc Surg. 2004;40:1248–52. https://doi.org/10.1016/j.jvs.2004.09.027.
40. Lim CS, Davies AH. Pathogenesis of primary varicose veins. Br J Surg. 2009;96:1231–42. https://doi.org/10.1002/bjs.6798.
41. Anwar MA, Shalhoub J, Lim CS, Gohel MS, Davies AH. The effect of pressure-induced mechanical stretch on vascular wall differential gene expression. J Vasc Res. 2012;49:463–78. https://doi.org/10.1159/000339151.
42. Lim C, Gohel M, Shepherd A, Paleolog E, Davies A. Venous hypoxia: a poorly studied etiological factor of varicose veins. J Vasc Res. 2011;48:185–94. https://doi.org/10.1159/000320624.
43. Jacobs BN, Andraska EA, Obi AT, Wakefield TW. Pathophysiology of varicose veins. J Vasc Surg Venous Lymphat Disord. 2017;5:460–7. https://doi.org/10.1016/j.jvsv.2016.12.014.
44. Qureshi MI, Gohel M, Wing L, MacDonald A, Lim CS, Ellis M, et al. A study to evaluate patterns of superficial venous reflux in patients with primary chronic venous disease. Phlebology. 2015;30:455–61. https://doi.org/10.1177/0268355514536384.
45. Labropoulos N, Giannoukas AD, Delis K, Mansour MA, Kang SS, Nicolaides AN, et al. Where does venous reflux start? J Vasc Surg. 1997;26:736–42. https://doi.org/10.1016/s0741-5214(97)70084-3.
46. Vedantham S. Valvular dysfunction and venous obstruction in the post-thrombotic syndrome. Thromb Res. 2009;123:S62–S5. https://doi.org/10.1016/S0049-3848(09)70146-X.
47. Labropoulos N, Gasparis AP, Pefanis D, Leon LR Jr, Tassiopoulos AK. Secondary chronic venous disease progresses faster than primary. J Vasc Surg. 2009;49:704–10. https://doi.org/10.1016/j.jvs.2008.10.014.

48. Poyyamoli S, Mehta P, Cherian M, Anand RR, Patil SB, Kalva S, et al. May-thurner syndrome. Cardiovasc Diagn Ther. 2021;11:1104. https://doi.org/10.21037/cdt.2020.03.07
49. Kahn SR. The post-thrombotic syndrome. Hematology Am Soc Hematol Educ Program. 2016;2016:413–8. https://doi.org/10.1182/asheducation-2016.1.413.
50. Galanaud J-P, Monreal M, Kahn SR. Epidemiology of the post-thrombotic syndrome. Thromb Res. 2018;164:100–9. https://doi.org/10.1016/j.thromres.2017.07.026.
51. Soosainathan A, Moore HM, Gohel MS, Davies AH. Scoring systems for the post-thrombotic syndrome. J Vasc Surg. 2013;57:254–61. https://doi.org/10.1016/j.jvs.2012.09.011.
52. Khider L, Planquette B, Smadja DM, Sanchez O, Rial C, Goudot G, et al. Acute phase determinant of post-thrombotic syndrome: a review of the literature. Thromb Res. 2024;238:11–8. https://doi.org/10.1016/j.thromres.2024.04.004.
53. Brown C, Tokessy L, Delluc A, Carrier M. Risk of developing post thrombotic syndrome after deep vein thrombosis with different anticoagulant regimens: a systematic review and pooled analysis. Thromb Res. 2024;240:109057. https://doi.org/10.1016/j.thromres.2024.109057.
54. White RH. The epidemiology of venous thromboembolism. Circulation. 2003;107:I4–8. https://doi.org/10.1161/01.CIR.0000078468.11849.66.
55. Kahn SR. The clinical diagnosis of deep venous thrombosis: integrating incidence, risk factors, and symptoms and signs. Arch Intern Med. 1998;158:2315–23. https://doi.org/10.1001/archinte.158.21.2315.
56. Kumar DR, Hanlin E, Glurich I, Mazza JJ, Yale SH. Virchow's contribution to the understanding of thrombosis and cellular biology. Clin Med Res. 2010;8:168–72. https://doi.org/10.3121/cmr.2009.866.
57. Wakefield TW, Myers DD, Henke PK. Mechanisms of venous thrombosis and resolution. Arterioscler Thromb Vasc Biol. 2008;28:387–91. https://doi.org/10.1161/ATVBAHA.108.162289.
58. Myers D Jr, Farris D, Hawley A, Wrobleski S, Chapman A, Stoolman L, et al. Selectins influence thrombosis in a mouse model of experimental deep venous thrombosis. J Surg Res. 2002;108:212–21. https://doi.org/10.1006/jsre.2002.6552.
59. Peng S, Xue G, Gong L, Fang C, Chen J, Yuan C, et al. A long-acting PAI-1 inhibitor reduces thrombus formation. Thromb Haemost. 2017;117:1338–47. https://doi.org/10.1160/TH16-11-0891.
60. Kuo WT. Optimizing catheter-directed thrombolysis for acute deep vein thrombosis: validating the open vein hypothesis. J Vasc Interv Radiol. 2013;24:24–6. https://doi.org/10.1016/j.jvir.2012.10.023.
61. Ashrani AA, Heit JA. Incidence and cost burden of post-thrombotic syndrome. J Thromb Thrombolysis. 2009;28:465–76. https://doi.org/10.1007/s11239-009-0309-3.
62. Raju S, Neglen P. High prevalence of nonthrombotic iliac vein lesions in chronic venous disease: a permissive role in pathogenicity. J Vasc Surg. 2006;44:136–43. https://doi.org/10.1016/j.jvs.2006.02.065.
63. Kearon C. Natural history of venous thromboembolism. Circulation. 2003;107:I22–30. https://doi.org/10.1161/01.CIR.0000078464.82671.78.
64. De Maeseneer MG, Kakkos SK, Aherne T, Baekgaard N, Black S, Blomgren L, et al. Editor's choice–European Society for Vascular Surgery (ESVS) 2022 clinical practice guidelines on the management of chronic venous disease of the lower limbs. Eur J Vasc Endovasc Surg. 2022;63:184–267. https://doi.org/10.1016/j.ejvs.2021.12.024.
65. Gloviczki P, Lawrence PF, Wasan SM, Meissner MH, Almeida J, Brown KR, et al. The 2022 Society for Vascular Surgery, American Venous Forum, and American Vein and Lymphatic Society clinical practice guidelines for the management of varicose veins of the lower extremities. Part I. Duplex scanning and treatment of superficial truncal reflux: endorsed by the Society for Vascular Medicine and the International Union of Phlebology. J Vasc Surg Venous Lymphat Disord. 2023;11(231–61):e6. https://doi.org/10.1016/j.jvsv.2022.09.004.
66. Gloviczki P, Lawrence PF, Wasan SM, Meissner MH, Almeida J, Brown KR, et al. The 2023 Society for Vascular Surgery, American Venous forum, and American vein and lymphatic soci-

ety clinical practice guidelines for the management of varicose veins of the lower extremities. Part II: Endorsed by the Society of Interventional Radiology and the Society for Vascular Medicine. J Vasc Surg Venous Lymphat Disord. 2024;12:101670. https://doi.org/10.1016/j.jvsv.2023.08.011.
67. Ruckley CV, Evans CJ, Allan PL, Lee AJ, Fowkes FG. Chronic venous insufficiency: clinical and duplex correlations. The Edinburgh vein study of venous disorders in the general population. J Vasc Surg. 2002;36:520–5. https://doi.org/10.1067/mva.2002.126547.
68. Brittenden J, Cotton SC, Elders A, Tassie E, Scotland G, Ramsay CR, et al. Clinical effectiveness and cost-effectiveness of foam sclerotherapy, endovenous laser ablation and surgery for varicose veins: results from the comparison of LAser, surgery and foam sclerotherapy (CLASS) randomised controlled trial. Health Technol Assess. 2015;19:1–342. https://doi.org/10.3310/hta19270.
69. Epstein DM, Gohel MS, Heatley F, Liu X, Bradbury A, Bulbulia R, et al. Cost-effectiveness analysis of a randomized clinical trial of early versus deferred endovenous ablation of superficial venous reflux in patients with venous ulceration. Br J Surg. 2019;106:555–62. https://doi.org/10.1002/bjs.11082.
70. Gohel MS, Heatley F, Liu X, Bradbury A, Bulbulia R, Cullum N, et al. Early versus deferred endovenous ablation of superficial venous reflux in patients with venous ulceration: the EVRA RCT. Health Technol Assess. 2019;23:1–96. https://doi.org/10.3310/hta23240.

Key References

Anwar MA, Georgiadis KA, Shalhoub J, Lim CS, Gohel MS, Davies AH. A review of familial, genetic, and congenital aspects of primary varicose vein disease. Circ Cardiovasc Genet. 2012;5:460–6. https://doi.org/10.1161/CIRCGENETICS.112.963439.

Eklof B, Perrin M, Delis KT, Rutherford RB, Gloviczki P, American Venous F, et al. Updated terminology of chronic venous disorders: the VEIN-TERM transatlantic interdisciplinary consensus document. J Vasc Surg. 2009;49:498–501. https://doi.org/10.1016/j.jvs.2008.09.014.

Gohel MS, Heatley F, Liu X, Bradbury A, Bulbulia R, Cullum N, et al. Early versus deferred endovenous ablation of superficial venous reflux in patients with venous ulceration: the EVRA RCT. Health Technol Assess. 2019;23:1–96. https://doi.org/10.3310/hta23240.

Lurie F, Passman M, Meisner M, Dalsing M, Masuda E, Welch H, et al. The 2020 update of the CEAP classification system and reporting standards. J Vasc Surg Venous Lymphat Disord. 2020;8:342–52. https://doi.org/10.1016/j.jvsv.2019.12.075.

Soosainathan A, Moore HM, Gohel MS, Davies AH. Scoring systems for the post-thrombotic syndrome. J Vasc Surg. 2013;57:254–61. https://doi.org/10.1016/j.jvs.2012.09.011.

Chapter 7
Pathophysiology of Wound Healing

Stuart J. Mills, Sparsh Tiwari, Guilherme Pena, and Allison J. Cowin

SN Flashcards
Test your learning and check your understanding of this book's contents: use the "Springer Nature Flashcards" app to access questions using ▶ https://sn.pub/wppvze. To use the app, please follow the instructions in Chap. 1.

Key Learning Points

- Wound healing is a dynamic process that progresses through four distinct yet interconnected stages: haemostasis, inflammation, proliferation, and remodelling. While these stages have a defined sequence, they often overlap, with one stage gradually transitioning into the next. Each stage of wound healing is char-

S. J. Mills (✉) · A. J. Cowin
Regenerative Medicine Group, Future Industries Institute, Adelaide University, Adelaide, SA, Australia
e-mail: stuart.mills@unisa.edu.au; Allison.Cowin@unisa.edu.au

S. Tiwari
Regenerative Medicine Group, Future Industries Institute, Adelaide University, Adelaide, SA, Australia

Faculty of Health and Medical Sciences, Adelaide University, Adelaide, SA, Australia
e-mail: sparsh.tiwari@student.adelaide.edu.au

G. Pena
Faculty of Health and Medical Sciences, Adelaide University, Adelaide, SA, Australia

Vascular Surgery Unit, Flinders Medical Centre, Bedford Park, SA, Australia
e-mail: guilherme.pena@sa.gov.au

R. Fitridge et al. (eds.), *Pathophysiology of Vascular Disease*,
https://doi.org/10.1007/978-3-032-31459-8_7

acterised by involvement of specific cell types that play crucial roles in orchestrating the repair process.

- The haemostasis stage primarily involves platelets and coagulation factors. Wound healing initiates with platelet degranulation, releasing growth factors (TGF-α, TGF-β, PDGF, VEGF) and triggering the coagulation cascade via complement activation. This culminates in fibrin clot formation, providing a provisional matrix for cellular migration.
- The Inflammation stage is dominated by neutrophils and macrophages. Chemotactic signals (PDGF, TGF-β, DAMPs, PAMPs) promote inflammatory cell recruitment. Neutrophils, followed monocytes/macrophages, infiltrate the wound, facilitated by adhesion molecules (E-selectin, Integrins, ICAM-1, VCAM-1).
- Neutrophils combat infection through ROS release and NET formation (netosis). Macrophages transition from a pro-inflammatory (M1) phenotype early in wound healing, which clears debris, to an anti-inflammatory (M2) phenotype, which promotes tissue repair.
- Proliferation involves the contribution of keratinocytes, fibroblasts, and endothelial cells. Keratinocytes migrate across the provisional matrix, facilitated by MMPs (MMP-9, MMP-1) and altered integrin expression. Fibroblasts and myofibroblasts synthesise collagen, elastin, and other ECM components and contribute to wound contraction.
- The remodelling phase, lasting up to 2 years, focuses on scar formation through ECM reorganisation. Collagen III is replaced by collagen I, and the balance between MMPs and TIMPs ensures controlled ECM remodelling and scar maturation.
- Angiogenesis, driven by FGF-2 and VEGF, provides essential nutrients and oxygen. Pericytes regulate vessel stability. Lymphangiogenesis, mediated by VGER3 and VEGFC/D, restores lymphatic drainage.
- Chronic wounds exhibit persistent inflammation, elevated levels of MMPs, and decrease in levels of TIMPs, leading to ECM degradation. Pressure ulcers, venous ulcers, and diabetes-related foot ulcers exemplify this imbalance.
- Biofilms, complex communities of microorganisms encased in a protective matrix, present a significant challenge in wound healing. These microbial communities exhibit heighted resistance to host immune responses and antimicrobial agents, making them difficult to eradicate. The presence of biofilm perpetuates inflammation, impairs re-epithelisation, and contributes to chronic infection, ultimately hindering the wound healing process.
- Venous hypertension, leading to microcirculatory dysfunction, perivascular fibrin cuff formation, and chronic inflammation, drives venous ulcer development.
- Diabetes-related foot ulcers are characterised by a complex interplay of factors that impair healing, including chronic inflammation, MMP dysregulation, biofilm formation, tissue hypoxia, and genetic/epigenetic influences. These factors

collectively contribute to a hostile wound environment, hindering tissue repair and increasing the risk of complications.
- Identification of biomarkers involved in wound behaviours and a deeper understanding of individual wound pathophysiology are paving the way for personalised wound care strategies.

7.1 Introduction

The skin is the largest organ of the body, which has a range of functions, including mechanical protection, temperature regulation, detecting external stimuli, preventing water loss, and acting as a physical barrier to repel any invading pathogens [1]. Depending on its severity, damage to the skin can be life-threatening. It is, therefore, imperative that the skin be repaired in as timely a manner as possible. Wound healing is a process made up of four sequential but overlapping stages that are haemostasis, inflammation, proliferation, and a remodelling phase. These stages involve the interaction of numerous cell types to restore the epithelial/dermal barrier and the nerve, lymphatic, and blood supply. Disruptions to the highly organised wound healing process can be caused by various factors such as age, nutrition, extrinsic factors, and co-morbidities, such as infection, chronic venous insufficiency (CVI), and diabetes. This can result in the formation of chronic wounds, which can take months to heal and frequently reoccur or, in the worst case, these wounds may even fail to heal entirely [2]. Understanding the key processes involved in normal wound healing and how co-morbidities can disrupt this intricate process is the key for creating more successful wound healing therapies and optimising treatments.

7.2 The Wound Healing Process

7.2.1 Haemostasis

The first stage of the wound healing process, haemostasis, begins immediately after the insult to the skin, to prevent further blood loss and limit infection into the wound site [1, 3]. To achieve this, the blood vessels vasoconstrict and a clot is formed to cover the wound [1]. This process begins when the platelets degranulate and release the contents of their α-granules, which includes transforming growth factor alpha and beta (TGF-α and TGF-β), platelet-derived growth factor (PDGF), vascular endothelial growth factor (VEGF), serotonin, thromboxane A_2, and cyclic AMP, though this has been shown to not be essential for skin repair [1]. Wounding also leads to the activation of complement, a group of serine proteases, which initiates

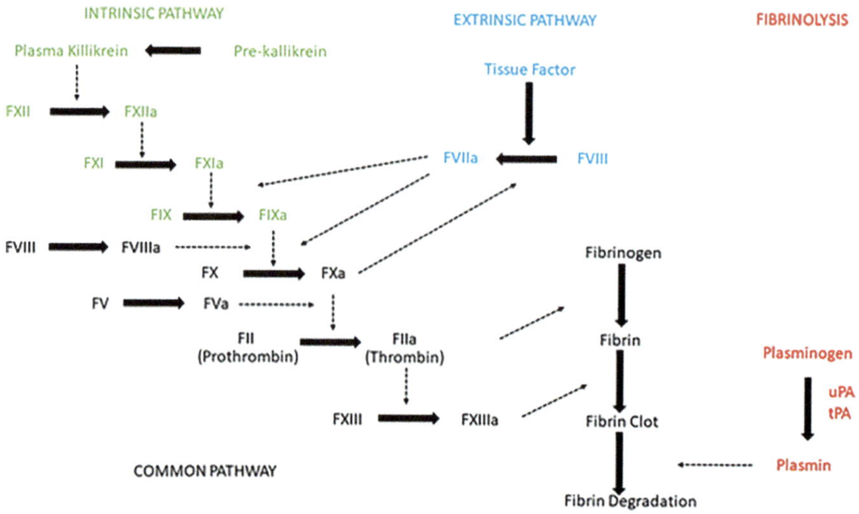

Fig. 7.1 Intrinsic and extrinsic pathways of the coagulation cascade

the coagulation cascade (Fig. 7.1). The coagulation cascade results in the cleavage of fibrinogen into fibrin and the formation of the fibrin clot. The clot not only acts as a plug, helping to prevent further blood loss, but also acts as a matrix, allowing skin cells to migrate into the wound site, to enable the repair/regeneration process (Fig. 7.2a) [4, 5]. Any deficiencies in the clotting process can lead to continued bleeding [6].

7.2.2 Inflammation

The main purpose of the inflammatory stage of wound healing is to remove damaged tissue and cells from the wound site and to kill any invading pathogens. This stage also begins immediately after wounding with the release of damage-associated molecular pathogens (DAMPs), pathogen-associated molecular pathogens (PAMPs), and chemotactic signals such as PDGF and TGF-β [5]. These factors initially attract neutrophils into the wound site within 30–45 minutes [7]. In the case of TGF-β, this is achieved via a rapid chemotaxis signal through the neutrophil cell surface serine/threonine receptors, which activates the Smad pathway. This enables the neutrophils to detect TGF-β concentration gradients, allowing them to direct their migration towards the wound site [8]. Other chemotactic signals work in a similar manner employing different signalling pathways.

An additional initiating signal of inflammation is a Ca^{2+} wave caused by a change in ion permeability in damaged cells at the wound edge, which results in an increasing cytoplasmic Ca^{2+} gradient. This increase in Ca^{2+} is also seen in adjacent, undamaged cells several layers deep and results in the formation of reactive oxygen species (ROS), which act as a further chemotactic signal for leukocyte recruitment [1].

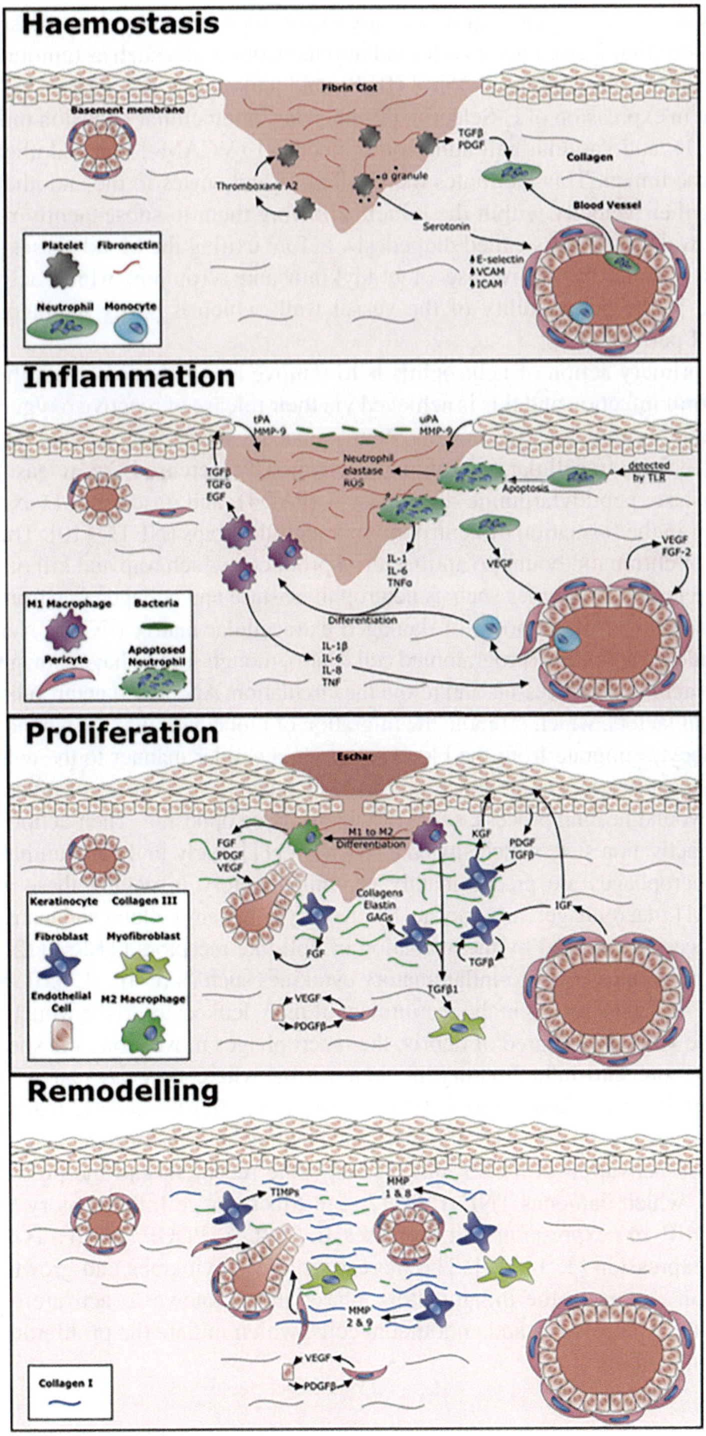

Fig. 7.2 The four phases of the wound healing process

Leukocyte recruitment requires their extravasation from the blood vessels to the wound site (Fig. 7.2b). Factors released into the wound site, such as tumour necrosis factor alpha (TNF-α), Interleukin-8 (IL-8), and leukotriene B4 (LTB4), result in an increase in expression of E-Selectin, β2-integrins, intercellular adhesion molecule-1 (ICAM-1), and vascular cell adhesion molecule-1 (VCAM-1) on endothelial cells within the lumen. This facilitates the binding of leukocytes to the endothelial cells slowing their velocity within the lumen, allowing them to subsequently roll along the cell walls, a process called diapedesis, before exiting the blood vessel [9]. This process is aided by the release of bradykinin and serotonin, which activates an increase in the permeability of the vessel wall, which is partly mediated by the action of pericytes [7].

The primary action of neutrophils is to remove any pathogens from the wound site to limit infection and this is achieved via their release of reactive oxygen species (ROS) and a process called netosis. Netosis occurs when neutrophils release their DNA into the extracellular environment, activated by increased Ca^{2+} release, neutrophil elastase, peptidylarginine deaminase 4 (PAD4), and gasdermin D expression, resulting in the formation of neutrophil extracellular traps (NETs) [10]. These traps consist of chromatin bound to antibacterial products, which trap and kill pathogens.

The release of proteases such as neutrophil elastase and collagenases from neutrophils also aids in the removal of damaged extracellular matrix (ECM). Neutrophils often undergo apoptosis (programmed cell death), though studies have shown that they can re-enter the blood vessels and rejoin the circulation. Apoptosed neutrophils release additional factors, which promote the migration of monocytes into the wound site.

Monocytes migrate from the blood stream in a similar manner to the neutrophils. Monocytes differentiate into macrophages, which can have a variety of functions during the wound healing process, some of which can be opposing. Their action depends on their activation state which sits on a spectrum [11]. Early in the inflammatory process, macrophages are predominantly pro-inflammatory in nature; these are often termed M1 macrophages, and they act by phagocytosing any cellular and matrix debris. This process is initiated by the activation of Toll-like receptors (TLRs) [12, 13] and results in the release of pro-inflammatory cytokines such as IL-1β, IL-6, IL-8, IL-12, and TNF-α, which results in the recruitment of more leukocytes to the wound site.

As the wound is cleared of debris, the macrophages move along the spectrum to become more anti-inflammatory in their action where they prevent any further release of the pro-inflammatory cytokines. These are often termed M2 macrophages, which form in response to IL-4 and IL-13. The mechanism for this change in state is through activation of TLR9 and A_2 adenosine receptors and the production of lipoxins, which dampens TNF-α, IL-12, and Macrophage Inflammatory Protein 1 alpha (MIP-1α) expression and increases IL-2, IL-4, PDGF, VEGF, TGF-α, and TGF-β expression [1, 14, 15]. The increase in these cytokines and growth factors signals an ending to the inflammatory phase and is known to activate other cell types such as fibroblasts and endothelial cells, which initiate the proliferation stage of wound healing.

7.2.3 *Proliferation*

The proliferative stage is when many of the main structures of the skin are reformed such as the epidermis, the extracellular matrix of the dermis, and the nerve, blood, and lymphatic vessels.

7.2.3.1 Re-Epithelialisation

Re-epithelialisation is the process through which the epidermal barrier is reformed to prevent infection and water loss and to help regulate temperature. For this process to occur, matrix metalloproteinases (MMPs) are expressed at the leading edge of the epidermal tongue. MMP-9 is highly expressed by epithelial cells and acts to cleave basal lamina collagen (type IV) and anchoring fibril collagen (type VII). This enables keratinocytes to become detached from the basal lamina to initiate migration. MMP-1 is also expressed by keratinocytes as they migrate past the leading edge, which degrades collagen I and III, creating a space for the keratinocytes to migrate into [16]. As the ECM at this point of the wound healing process is predominantly made of fibrin, fibronectin, and vitronectin, keratinocytes shift their integrin expression from collagen-laminin ($\alpha 2\beta 1$) to fibronectin-tenascin ($\alpha 5\beta 1$ and $\alpha v\beta 6$) and vitronectin ($\alpha v\beta 1$), allowing them to interact with the provisional matrix and migrate over it. Interestingly, proliferation of epidermal cells is not the key factor in reforming the epidermis, but migration appears to play a much more important role. This is highlighted by the change in integrin expression, which is normally reserved to the basal layer of the skin, but at a wound edge all layers of the skin change their integrin expression and migrate to help reform the epidermis [1]. To prevent excessive re-epithelialisation once the epidermis is re-established, the filopodia at the leading edges interacts with the opposing leading epidermal keratinocytes and this interaction leads to a “zippering up” of the wound [17–19].

7.2.3.2 Matrix Formation

Matrix formation is the process where the provisional matrix is gradually replaced with collagen and elastin and involves fibroblasts and their subpopulation, myofibroblasts. Fibroblasts, like epidermal cells, alter their integrin expression, to $\alpha 3$ and $\alpha 5$ integrins in response to PDGF, so that they too can migrate across the provisional ECM. Once in the wound, they begin to produce collagen, proteoglycans, glycosaminoglycans, and elastin.

Myofibroblasts help to promote wound contraction, which acts to bring the two migrating epithelial tongues into closer proximity, thus reducing the degree of re-epithelialisation that must occur. For this process to happen, fibroblasts express α-smooth muscle actin and generate contractile forces in response to TGF-$\beta 1$ [20].

Once wound contraction is no longer required, fibroblasts release cyclic adenosine monophosphate (cAMP) and there is an influx of calcium into the cells, which desensitises cell surface PDGF and EGF receptors resulting in quiescent cells [21].

7.2.3.3 Angiogenesis and Lymphangiogenesis

Angiogenesis is the process of new blood vessel growth from already existing vessels and is distinct from vasculogenesis, which involves recruitment of endothelial progenitor cells (EPCs) from the bone marrow. This process supplies nutrition and oxygen to the wound site, enabling cells to metabolise, proliferate, and migrate within the wound site.

Initially during angiogenesis, pericytes on the blood vessel migrate away from damaged vessels (Fig. 7.2c), allowing endothelial cells to initiate proliferation in response to FGF-2 and VEGFA [7]. Degradation of the ECM by proteinases uncovers matricryptic sites (see Glossary), some of which allow adhesion with endothelial cells, enabling them to proliferate and migrate into the wound. Pericytes play a key role by producing tissue inhibitors of matrix metalloproteinases 3 (TIMP-3), which not only regulate matrix turnover by MMPs, but also prevent capillary tube regression in response to MMP-1 and MMP-10 expression [7]. Once the endothelial cells have formed new blood vessels, the pericytes return in response to PDGFβ expression, and they then bind to the outside of the vessel which stabilises it and prevents its degradation.

Lymphatic vessels, which are crucial for tissue haemostasis and immune surveillance, are also reformed in a similar manner to blood vessels in that they sprout from pre-existing lymphatic vessels in response to VEGF receptor 3 (VEGFR3), VEGFC, and VEGFD. Reformation of the lymphatic system is often overlooked in wound healing; but its reformation leads to faster clearance of oedema and conversely any interruption in its formation results in a delayed resolution of oedema [22].

7.2.4 Remodelling

Remodelling in the skin is a process that can continue for up to 2 years. It involves the formation of collagen, its degradation, remodelling, and its reorientation into bundles to form a mature scar. In general, collagen III is replaced by collagen I; hyaluronan is replaced by heparan sulphate in the basement membrane and by dermatan and chondroitin sulphate in the interstitium [23]. This process is tightly controlled by the expression of MMPs, which act to degrade the provisional matrix allowing the deposition of new matrix, and TIMPs, which act as inhibitors of MMPs, thus preventing excessive breakdown of the ECM (Fig. 7.2d).

In most adult healing, a wound results in the formation of a hypertrophic scar, which lies within the original boundaries of the wound. Studies have revealed that the degree of scarring can be dependent on mechanotransduction (see Glossary) forces and inflammation. Increased mechanotransduction forces have been shown to increase inflammation and the formation of myofibroblasts within the wound, resulting in greater numbers of macrophages present and an increase in the degree of scarring [1]. Interestingly, it has been shown that when macrophages are absent from a wound, scar-free healing can occur in adults [24].

Overall, this intricate, multistage process is designed to heal the skin in as timely a manner as possible to help restore its function and prevent any pathogenic infection. The multitude of factors, cell types, interactions, and the timing of the different events make wound healing a complex process to study and fully understand. Any disruption to this sophisticated process can lead to delays in healing or the formation of chronic wounds, which can take months to heal or fail to heal completely. As our understanding of this process advances, and also what factors can result in its disruption, improved diagnoses and the production of advanced therapies should be more achievable.

7.3 Factors that Can Disrupt the Wound Healing Processes

7.3.1 Inflammation and Proteolytic Activity

Inflammation and proteolysis are two of the key mediators of the wound healing process, acting as checkpoints, which either promote or prevent the progression of the wound healing process. These processes exist in a balance. Too much or too little inflammation and/or proteolysis can stall the wound healing process and can result in the formation of a slow healing or chronic wound. Examples of wounds that form from this imbalance include pressure ulcers, venous ulcers, arterial ulcers, and diabetes-related ulcers.

One of the main causes for these non-healing wounds is that the inflammatory phase of healing fails to resolve and results in a continuing escalation of inflammatory cells invading the wound, with a subsequent increase in ECM destruction. Neutrophil activity in these wounds is elevated with increased production of ROS, neutrophil elastase, and MMP-8, which result in the degradation of growth factors (PDGF and TGF-β) and ECM [25]. The effect of this is twofold; not only is there destruction of the ECM but the cells present in the wound cannot respond to make more ECM due to the concurrent breakdown in growth factor signalling, resulting in excessive damage to the ECM [26]. The decreased availability of key growth factors also results in the reduced regulation of macrophage and neutrophil expression of pro-inflammatory cytokines such as IL-1β, IL-6, IL-8, and TNF-α. This exacerbates the inflammatory response by recruiting more activated neutrophils and macrophages, which in turn produce more pro-inflammatory cytokines, creating a self-feeding loop, resulting in persistent inflammation.

This exacerbation of the inflammatory response also has a direct effect on proteinase production within the wound by unbalancing the MMP:TIMP ratio, leading to increased MMP and decreased TIMP expression [27]. Consequently, further degradation of the ECM occurs, which impairs cell migration and reduces collagen deposition, strengthening the self-perpetuating cycle of ECM degradation and inflammation [28].

Pressure ulcers show this imbalance of the MMP-TIMP ratio. They occur over bony prominences such as the heels, ankles, and toes and are caused by pressure on the soft tissue, which restricts local blood flow. This type of wound has elevated levels of MMP-1, MMP-2, MMP-8, and MMP-9 and decreased levels of TIMPs due to breakdown from neutrophil elastase. This is also accompanied by shearing forces, which together results in an increase in hypoxia and tissue necrosis. This imbalance of proteinases along with the hypoxia and necrosis increases the ECM breakdown and results in incomplete healing.

7.3.2 *Infection and Biofilms in Wound Healing*

7.3.2.1 Wound Healing and Infection

Chronic wounds often exhibit persistent infection once the wound has developed, which promotes chronicity, morbidity and potentially, mortality [26]. Some of the most common bacteria that infect wounds and are known to delay the wound healing process when present in excess of 10^5 per gram of wound tissue include *Staphylococcus aureus, Pseudomonas aeruginosa,* and β-haemolytic *Streptococcus* [25]. Infection may be clinically obvious, but biofilm formation can occur in the absence of these signs. Optimal treatment ideally should occur before the onset of clinical infection (Fig. 7.3). If this opportunity is missed, the wound becomes much more difficult to treat [29].

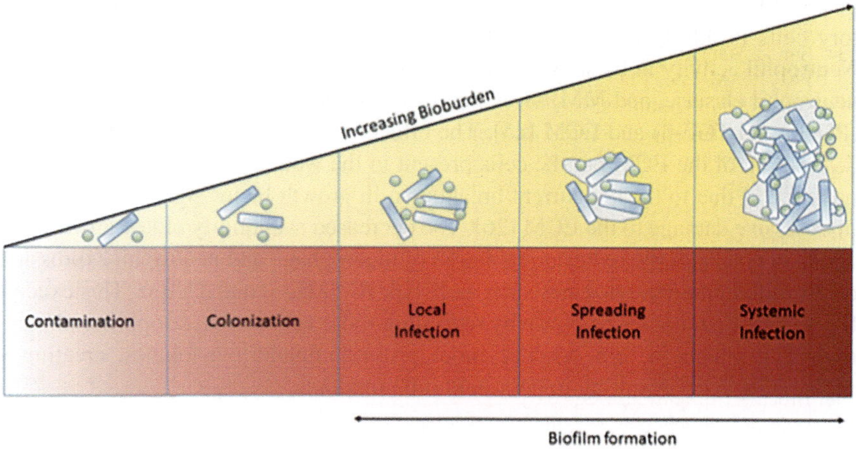

Fig. 7.3 Increasing bioburden seen in diabetes-related foot ulcers

Within infected wounds, there is an increase in inflammatory infiltrate due to activation of TLRs by infectious agents such as bacteria, viruses, and fungi. In an infected wound, there is also the production of ROS and proteases from bacteria, which breakdown the ECM and initiate the inflammatory response. Therefore, the exacerbation of the inflammatory reaction is twofold from both the host and the invading bacteria. In a chronic infection, the immune cells infiltrating the wound are unable to sufficiently clear the infection and debris from the wound, and there is a continuing escalation of the inflammatory response and breakdown of the ECM, which prevents the resolution of the inflammatory phase. Interestingly, it is still unclear whether these changes are due to the infection or because of the chronicity of the wound and, therefore, the full influence of infection on the wound healing process is still to be determined.

7.3.2.2 Wound Healing and Biofilms

Microorganisms in wounds can form polymicrobial communities, which encase themselves in polysaccharide and lipid envelopes, called biofilms. These envelopes enable them to mask themselves from immune surveillance [26]. Biofilms are resistant to penetration by large protein antibodies, antibiotics, silver ions, and even neutralisation of highly oxidising solutions such as bleach. This makes the bacteria more resistant to immunological responses, antibiotics, antiseptics, and chemical treatments [30]. Due to these factors, biofilms can lead to a range of pathologies, including periodontal disease, prosthetic/ graft infections, and osteomyelitis.

Biofilms are more than just an envelope protecting the bacteria inside from host immune attack. They are highly organised structures, more akin to a microcolony, with channels for nutrient transfer and exchange of signalling molecules for communication between bacteria. There can be a range of pH and oxygen concentrations throughout the biofilm, which make it an ideal environment to host a wider range of bacteria, with differing metabolic states, including both aerobic and anaerobic bacteria [29]. The variation in the microenvironment also affects the bacteria directly. For example, aerobic bacteria which are found in low oxygen areas of the biofilm become dormant and are called "persister cells".

The presence of a biofilm can severely impede wound re-epithelialisation, but it also provides a constant inflammatory stimulus, which promotes an excessive influx of immune cells to remove the biofilm. This floods the wound with further ROS and proteases, which act to breakdown the ECM and degrade the wound further. The presence of the biofilm also leads to higher rates of chronic, recurring infection. Identification of biofilm formation, particularly in its early stages, is difficult due to a lack of routine diagnostic tests. However, microscopy can be used to detect biofilm formation. Interestingly, a study by Johani et al. investigated biofilm formation in 65 DRFU patients, using in situ hybridisation and scanning electron microscopy, and found that all 65 had biofilm formation present [31].

7.3.2.3 The Infection Challenge

The significant challenge of infected wounds is the increasing prevalence of antimicrobial resistance (AMR) to treatment. It is estimated that, by 2050, AMR will result in 10 million deaths globally, which is higher than the current number of deaths from cancer annually [32]. The main resistant bacteria in skin soft tissue injuries and surgical site infections are *Staphylococcus aureus*, *Escherichia coli*, *Klebsiella pneumoniae*, *Pseudomonas aeruginosa,* and *Acinetobacter baumannii* [32].

Despite recent advances in the treatment of infection, the role that bacteria play in the wound environment, and how this can lead to complications, is still relatively unknown. There are still questions around whether bacterial bioburden or the interaction between different bacteria is more important in the context of healing. Others cite the presence of anaerobic bacteria as one of the main causes of poor healing outcomes. It has previously been difficult to identify all the bacteria present in a wound as the gold standard has been to isolate and grow up the bacteria in culture. Recent advances in gene sequencing technologies have allowed the sequencing of the 16S ribosomal RNA region of bacteria, which is a much more powerful technique for the identification of specific strains of bacteria. This technique also allows the analysis of microbial load, microbial diversity, and the presence of pathogens, which provides a much fuller picture of wound infection. However, the technique is limited as it does not differentiate between live and dead bacteria, and it does not distinguish how the pathogens are interacting [33].

There is a clear need for new advanced therapeutics and to better manage our current diagnostics and treatment regimens of infection, to help alleviate our dependence on the currently available antimicrobial treatments.

7.3.3 Wound Healing in Chronic Venous Disease

Chronic venous disease (CVD) is a prevalent condition that significantly impacts patient wellbeing and healthcare resources. An important feature of CVD is its progressive nature, often leading to the formation of venous leg ulcers (VLUs), a severe manifestation classified as CEAP (see Glossary) clinical class C6 [34]. VLUs affect approximately 1% of general population, with prevalence increasing to 3% in those over 80 years of age [35].

VLUs arise from a complex interplay of factors, with chronic venous hypertension as the central driver. Venous reflux, outflow obstruction, calf pump failure, and obesity all contribute to elevated venous pressure, affecting the microcirculation in the lower extremity and ultimately leading to ulceration [36]. The key pathological mechanisms include the following:

- Microcirculatory dysfunction: Venous hypertension leads to venous stasis, endothelial cell activation, and increased vascular permeability. This results in extravasation of erythrocytes and leukocytes into the surrounding tissues, creating a chronic inflammatory environment [37].

- Perivascular fibrin cuff formation: Fibrin leakage, triggered by venous hypertension, polymerises into fibrin and accumulates around blood vessels. This fibrin cuff impairs oxygen and nutrient diffusion, leading to tissue hypoxia and contributing to persistence of ulceration [38].
- Chronic inflammation: Chronic inflammation is a hallmark of CVD and a key aspect of VLU formation and chronicity. This persistent inflammatory state is characterised by leukocyte activation, cytokine cascade, and increased MMP activity, leading to cellular dysfunction and tissue damage. Overexpression of MMPs and cytokines contributes to the destruction of the vein wall, valve leaflet, endothelium, and surrounding tissue. High MMP levels in VLUs correlate with poor wound healing, and their regulation is linked to cytokines, urokinase-type plasminogen activator (uPA), extracellular MMP inducer (EMMPRIN), and decreased activity of TIMPs. Cytokines play a crucial role throughout the various stages of CVD, influencing inflammation and tissue remodelling [37].

Compression therapy is a cornerstone of VLU treatment, offering benefits beyond simply improving venous blood flow. It actively modulates the inflammatory response, creating an environment more favourable for healing. This is achieved by reducing levels of pro-inflammatory cytokines such as interleukins TNF-α and IFN-γ, while simultaneously increasing levels of the anti-inflammatory cytokine TGF-β. Furthermore, compression therapy helps control excessive degradation of the extracellular matrix by reducing levels of MMP-1, MMP-2, and MMP-3, ultimately promoting healing [39, 40].

VLUs typically appear as shallow wounds with irregular edges and significant amounts of exudate. They are most commonly found around the medial malleolus and lower calf, the area where venous hypertension is often more pronounced. These ulcers can occur as single or multiple lesions, varying in shape but usually possessing well-defined margins. The wound bed often shows signs of healing with granulation and fibrinous tissue present. Necrotic tissue is less common. Pain associated with ulceration can range from non-existent to severe. In addition to the ulcer itself, patients often exhibit other signs of CVD, such as leg swelling and eczema. Skin changes including haemosiderin staining and lipodermatosclerosis may be present, accompanied by varicose veins [34, 37]. Compression therapy remains essential for reducing venous hypertension and promoting healing. However, addressing the underlying venous incompetence, often through endovenous ablation, is crucial to accelerate wound healing and prevent recurrence [34, 41, 42].

7.3.4 Diabetes and Diabetes-Related Foot Ulcers (DRFU)

The global prevalence of diabetes mellitus has increased from 200 million in 1990 to 830 million in 2022 [43]. Since 2000, the mortality rates of diabetes have been increasing, whereas the rates of death from cardiovascular disease, cancer, and chronic respiratory disease have decreased [43]. Hyperglycaemia can affect the immune function of the host in a variety of ways resulting in poor chemotaxis and phagocytosis of pathogens within the wound. In addition to this, the reaction between sugars and amino groups can lead to the formation of advanced glycation end-products (AGEs) [30]. This inhibits nicotinamide adenine dinucleotide phosphate (NADPH) and antioxidant production, which protect the cells from ROS. The cellular damage leads to increased leukocyte infiltration and an exacerbation of the inflammatory response as well as an increase in ECM breakdown. These conditions can help promote the formation of diabetes-related foot ulcers.

7.3.4.1 Diabetes-Related Foot Ulcers

Diabetes-related foot ulcers (DRFU) are a highly morbid complication of diabetes mellitus (DM), affecting approximately 34% of people with diabetes over their lifetime [44]. Among those who develop DRFUs, 15% will require major amputation after which the 5-year mortality risk rises to 50–68% [2]. The poor healing of DRFUs presents a significant clinical challenge, with approximately 60–70% of DRFUs remaining refractory to clinical management after 12 weeks [45]. In patients with diabetes, the normal continuum of healing is disrupted by a combination of intrinsic (tissue hypoxia, neuropathy, local and systemic complication of diabetes) and extrinsic factors (infection, callus formation, ongoing pressure onto wound), leading to chronic wounds that stall in the inflammatory phase of wound healing [46, 47] (for a more detailed exploration of the pathophysiology of DRFUs, please refer to Chap. 8). It is important to recognise that DRFUs are heterogeneous, with the clinical presentation and underlying pathophysiology varying depending on the predominant abnormality.

7.3.4.2 Chronic Wound Characteristics and Impaired Healing in DRFUs

DRFUs, like most chronic wounds, are characterised by a chronically inflamed wound milieu and a persistent overproduction of pro-inflammatory cytokines, which delay the resolution of the inflammatory stage of wound healing. This sustained inflammatory response creates a hostile environment for healing, preventing the proper formation of granulation tissue and re-epithelialisation [48].

DRFUs also display elevated levels of MMP-1, MMP-8, and MMP-9, which, coupled with low TIMP levels, are associated with non-healing wounds [49]. Recent therapies, such as sucrose octasulfate dressings, which inhibit excess MMP activity, offer promising results in improving wound healing in neuroischaemic ulcers [50].

Biofilms are frequently implicated in DRFUs and significantly impede healing [51, 52]. The extracellular polymeric substance (EPS) matrix shields bacteria, making biofilm infections particularly difficult to treat. Differentiating biofilms from slough (dead host tissue) is crucial, as biofilms consist of living bacteria within the EPS matrix [53]. The presence of biofilms in DRFUs contributes to antibiotic resistance and evades the host's immune response by hindering the function of neutrophils and macrophages. This results in a chronic inflammatory state that promotes bacterial growth and delays healing. While visual cues may suggest the presence of a biofilm, definitive diagnosis often requires advanced imaging techniques or biomarkers [53].

7.3.4.3 Tissue Hypoxia and Impaired Angiogenesis in DRFUs

Tissue hypoxia, a common feature of DRFUs, arises from a combination of factors. Peripheral artery disease, prevalent in individuals with diabetes, restricts blood flow to the extremities [54]. Furthermore, microcirculatory deficiencies, including reduced capillary size, thickened basement membranes, and arteriolar hyalinosis, disrupt oxygen delivery to the tissues [55]. Impaired endothelial function, potentially involving reduced nitric oxide synthase activity, further compromises blood flow. Shunts in the microcirculation, coupled with sympathetic nerve denervation and autonomic neuropathy, lead to the maldistribution of blood flow. Diabetic neuropathy impairs the neurovascular response, also contributing to tissue hypoxia leading to defects in the secretion of vasodilators like substance P, calcitonin gene-related peptide, and histamine. This impaired vasodilation, particularly in response to trauma or pressure, further compromises tissue perfusion. Despite reduced oxygen levels, the expression of hypoxia-inducible factor-1α (HIF-1α) and its target genes is paradoxically reduced in DRFUs, impairing cellular responses to hypoxia, particularly angiogenesis, and further delaying wound healing [56, 57].

7.3.4.4 Genetic and Epigenetic Factors in DRFUs

Recent research has highlighted the role of genetic and epigenetic factors in DRFU. Studies in diabetic mice and patient samples have identified epigenetic modifications, such as the demethylation of repressive histone markers on the IL-12 promoter by the enzyme JMJD3, leading to increased inflammatory gene expression in various cell types [58]. MicroRNAs (miRNAs) also appear to play a role in DRFUs. Studies in animals and humans have revealed differential expression of miRNAs in diabetic versus non-diabetic wound healing. For example, miR-146b, a modulator of inflammation in monocytes and fibroblasts, is significantly upregulated in diabetic wounds [59]. These findings suggest that miRNAs may contribute to the dysregulated inflammatory response and impaired healing observed in DRFUs.

7.3.4.5 Cellular Senescence in DRFUs

Resident cells within DRFUs can exhibit phenotypic alterations. Fibroblasts isolated from DRFUs often display characteristics of senescence, including decreased proliferative responses to growth factors [47, 60]. This cellular senescence may contribute to the impaired healing capacity of these wounds. The complex pathophysiology of diabetes-related foot ulcers underscores the need for continued research to elucidate the mechanisms underlying impaired wound healing. A recent systematic review has critically assessed the current evidence for various interventions [61]. This knowledge is essential not only for optimising existing therapies, but also for guiding the development of innovative strategies to address this significant clinical challenge.

7.3.4.6 Nutrition and DRFU Healing

Patients with diabetes face a heightened risk and prevalence of malnutrition, partly due to factors such as antihyperglycemic medications, dietary restrictions aimed at blood glucose control, and diabetes-related autonomic neuropathy, which presents as anorexia or gastroparesis [62]. Indeed, studies within European and Asian cohorts have demonstrated a high prevalence of malnutrition or high risk for malnutrition among DRFU patients [63–67]. As wound healing is an energy-intensive process, adequate intake of fluids and essential micronutrients is crucial for optimal repair. Malnutrition has been implicated in perturbed inflammatory phase resolution, decreasing fibroblast proliferation and collagen synthesis, as well as increasing infection risk by decreasing T-cell function, phagocytic activity, and complement and antibody levels [68]. Nevertheless, robust evidence for the effectiveness of nutritional supplementation for improving DRFU healing is lacking, with studies for the most part illustrating no clear benefit or harm [69]. Updated Australian guidelines on interventions to improve wound healing, therefore, assert meeting adequate daily nutritional needs as part of the best standard of care, but fall short of recommending using nutritional interventions solely to improve healing of diabetes-related foot ulcers [70].

7.4 Advances in Wound Healing

There have been consistent improvements in wound healing research allowing a greater understanding of what is occurring at the cellular, protein, and epigenetic levels during the wound healing process. Initially, wound research tended to look at one cell type or one protein in isolation. More recently, 3D skin equivalent models have been utilised employing multiple cell types, which has allowed a greater insight into how cells interact and how the different populations contribute to the wound healing process [71]. These skin equivalents are now incorporating skin structures such as glands, hair follicles, and even a vascular network. There has also been an increase in the number of genetic models and models of disease available for research, particular in rodent models, which can help in further understanding of how co-morbidities such as diabetes and infection can alter the wound healing response. While these models can be a great source of information, they must be used with caution as they often don't always translate to the human scenario [71].

Recently, there have been significant advances in imaging technologies such as confocal and multiphoton microscopy and photoacoustic imaging. These technologies, used with fluorescent staining of the different cell lineages, allow deeper imaging of the skin/wound for greater lengths of time. This enables the study of how the different cell types are contributing to healing, at the different stages of the wound healing process [1].

Another advancement in our understanding of the pathophysiology of wound healing is in the field of 'omics'. Transcriptomics, epigenomic, proteomic, and 16S sequencing now allow us to interrogate the changes at the RNA, DNA, and protein levels in different types of wounds at different stages of the process, and together with 16S genomic sequencing, it is now possible to determine the pathogens present within the wound and their bioburden [1]. Studies utilising 16S sequencing have led to a much fuller picture of which types of pathogens are more prevalent in wounds and which are more resistant to the specific antimicrobials used for treatment [1]. These new techniques have led to the production of huge quantities of data, the analysis of which is now becoming the rate limiting step of this research, though recent advances in AI are helping to overcome this issue.

These types of analyses continue to add to our knowledge of what is occurring in the wound at each stage of wound healing. The identification of specific biomarkers during this process could potentially lead to more accurate prediction of wound healing outcomes and identification of future therapeutics. Together, these advances are potentially leading to an era of greater personalised medicine.

7.5 Conclusions

The study of wound healing in skin is a complex and multifaceted area due to the significant number of factors involved. Recent advances in our understanding, brought about by improvement in technologies, have led to a better identification of the main mechanisms that can profoundly affect the healing process. This is leading to a more personalised approach to diagnosis and treatment. There is still, however, a significant lack of successful therapeutics available for the treatment of chronic wounds, which actively address some of the imbalances found in these wounds.

Multiple Choice Questions

1. The wound healing process is composed of four stages. During the inflammation phase, which specific pro-inflammatory cytokines are known to be produced by M1 macrophages after activation of toll-like receptors, leading to recruitment of more leucocytes?

   (a) IL-1β, IL-6, IL8, IL12, and TNF-α
   (b) TGF-α, PDGF, and VEGF
   (c) IL-4 and IL-13
   (d) Lipoxins and TGF-β
   (e) MMP-9 and collagenase

   Answer: (a) IL-1β, IL-6, IL8, IL12, and TNF-α

2. Chronic wounds, such as venous ulcers and diabetes-related foot ulcers, are characterised by a persistent imbalance in proteolytic activity. What is the molecular consequence of the unresolved inflammatory phase that results in the excessive destruction of the extracellular matrix?

   (a) Conversion of M1 macrophages to M2 macrophages
   (b) Increase in TIMP expression and decrease in MMP expression
   (c) Unbalancing of the MMP:TIMP ratio, leading to increased MMP and decreased TIMP expression
   (d) Paradoxical reduction in HIF-1α expression
   (e) Increased production of NADPH and antioxidants

   Answer: (c) Unbalancing of the MMP:TIMP ratio, leading to increased MMP and decreased TIMP expression

References

1. Pena OA, Martin P. Cellular and molecular mechanisms of skin wound healing. Nat Rev Mol Cell Biol. 2024;25:599–616. https://doi.org/10.1038/s41580-024-00715-1.
2. Edmonds M, Manu C, Vas P. The current burden of diabetic foot disease. J Clin Orthop Trauma. 2021;17:88–93. https://doi.org/10.1016/j.jcot.2021.01.017.
3. Sorg H, Sorg CGG. Skin wound healing: of players, patterns, and processes. Eur Surg Res. 2023;64:141–57. https://doi.org/10.1159/000528271.
4. Gailit J, Welch MP, Clark RA. TGF-beta 1 stimulates expression of keratinocyte integrins during re-epithelialization of cutaneous wounds. J Invest Dermatol. 1994;103:221–7. https://doi.org/10.1111/1523-1747.ep12393176.
5. Li J, Chen J, Kirsner R. Pathophysiology of acute wound healing. Clin Dermatol. 2007;25:9–18. https://doi.org/10.1016/j.clindermatol.2006.09.007.
6. Berntorp E, Fischer K, Hart DP, Mancuso ME, Stephensen D, Shapiro AD, et al. Haemophilia. Nat Rev Dis Primers. 2021;7:45. https://doi.org/10.1038/s41572-021-00278-x.
7. Thomas H, Cowin AJ, Mills SJ. The importance of pericytes in healing: wounds and other pathologies. Int J Mol Sci. 2017;18:1129. https://doi.org/10.3390/ijms18061129.

8. Wahl SM, Hunt DA, Wakefield LM, McCartney-Francis N, Wahl LM, Roberts AB, et al. Transforming growth factor type beta induces monocyte chemotaxis and growth factor production. Proc Natl Acad Sci USA. 1987;84:5788–92. https://doi.org/10.1073/pnas.84.16.5788.
9. Ley K, Laudanna C, Cybulsky MI, Nourshargh S. Getting to the site of inflammation: the leukocyte adhesion cascade updated. Nat Rev Immunol. 2007;7:678–89. https://doi.org/10.1038/nri2156.
10. Vorobjeva NV, Chernyak BV. NETosis: molecular mechanisms, role in physiology and pathology. Biochemistry (Mosc). 2020;85:1178–90. https://doi.org/10.1134/S0006297920100065.
11. Murray PJ. Macrophage polarization. Annu Rev Physiol. 2017;79:541–66. https://doi.org/10.1146/annurev-physiol-022516-034339.
12. Chen L, DiPietro LA. Toll-like receptor function in acute wounds. Adv Wound Care (New Rochelle). 2017;6:344–55. https://doi.org/10.1089/wound.2017.0734.
13. Mills SJ, Ahangar P, Thomas HM, Hofma BR, Murray RZ, Cowin AJ. Flightless I negatively regulates macrophage surface TLR4, delays early inflammation, and impedes wound healing. Cells. 2022;11:2192. https://doi.org/10.3390/cells11142192.
14. Falanga V. Growth factors and wound healing. Dermatol Clin. 1993;11:667–75.
15. Pinhal-Enfield G, Ramanathan M, Hasko G, Vogel SN, Salzman AL, Boons GJ, et al. An angiogenic switch in macrophages involving synergy between Toll-like receptors 2, 4, 7, and 9 and adenosine A(2A) receptors. Am J Pathol. 2003;163:711–21. https://doi.org/10.1016/S0002-9440(10)63698-X.
16. Saarialho-Kere UK, Pentland AP, Birkedal-Hansen H, Parks WC, Welgus HG. Distinct populations of basal keratinocytes express stromelysin-1 and stromelysin-2 in chronic wounds. J Clin Invest. 1994;94:79–88. https://doi.org/10.1172/JCI117351.
17. Ashcroft GS, Dodsworth J, van Boxtel E, Tarnuzzer RW, Horan MA, Schultz GS, et al. Estrogen accelerates cutaneous wound healing associated with an increase in TGF-beta1 levels. Nat Med. 1997;3:1209–15. https://doi.org/10.1038/nm1197-1209.
18. Cavani A, Zambruno G, Marconi A, Manca V, Marchetti M, Giannetti A. Distinctive integrin expression in the newly forming epidermis during wound healing in humans. J Invest Dermatol. 1993;101:600–4. https://doi.org/10.1111/1523-1747.ep12366057.
19. Millard TH, Martin P. Dynamic analysis of filopodial interactions during the zippering phase of Drosophila dorsal closure. Development. 2008;135:621–6. https://doi.org/10.1242/dev.014001.
20. Desmouliere A, Geinoz A, Gabbiani F, Gabbiani G. Transforming growth factor-beta 1 induces alpha-smooth muscle actin expression in granulation tissue myofibroblasts and in quiescent and growing cultured fibroblasts. J Cell Biol. 1993;122:103–11. https://doi.org/10.1083/jcb.122.1.103.
21. Lin YC, Grinnell F. Decreased level of PDGF-stimulated receptor autophosphorylation by fibroblasts in mechanically relaxed collagen matrices. J Cell Biol. 1993;122:663–72. https://doi.org/10.1083/jcb.122.3.663.
22. Kataru RP, Jung K, Jang C, Yang H, Schwendener RA, Baik JE, et al. Critical role of CD11b+ macrophages and VEGF in inflammatory lymphangiogenesis, antigen clearance, and inflammation resolution. Blood. 2009;113:5650–9. https://doi.org/10.1182/blood-2008-09-176776.
23. Singer AJ, Clark RA. Cutaneous wound healing. N Engl J Med. 1999;341:738–46. https://doi.org/10.1056/NEJM199909023411006.
24. Martin P, D'Souza D, Martin J, Grose R, Cooper L, Maki R, et al. Wound healing in the PU.1 null mouse–tissue repair is not dependent on inflammatory cells. Curr Biol. 2003;13:1122–8. https://doi.org/10.1016/s0960-9822(03)00396-8.
25. Zhao R, Liang H, Clarke E, Jackson C, Xue M. Inflammation in chronic wounds. Int J Mol Sci. 2016;17:2085. https://doi.org/10.3390/ijms17122085.
26. Demidova-Rice TN, Hamblin MR, Herman IM. Acute and impaired wound healing: pathophysiology and current methods for drug delivery, part 1: normal and chronic wounds: biology, causes, and approaches to care. Adv Skin Wound Care. 2012;25:304–14. https://doi.org/10.1097/01.ASW.0000416006.55218.d0.

27. Yager DR, Zhang LY, Liang HX, Diegelmann RF, Cohen IK. Wound fluids from human pressure ulcers contain elevated matrix metalloproteinase levels and activity compared to surgical wound fluids. J Invest Dermatol. 1996;107:743–8. https://doi.org/10.1111/1523-1747.ep12365637.
28. Mast BA, Schultz GS. Interactions of cytokines, growth factors, and proteases in acute and chronic wounds. Wound Repair Regen. 1996;4:411–20. https://doi.org/10.1046/j.1524-475X.1996.40404.x.
29. Kalan LR, Brennan MB. The role of the microbiome in nonhealing diabetic wounds. Ann N Y Acad Sci. 2019;1435:79–92. https://doi.org/10.1111/nyas.13926.
30. Alavi A, Sibbald RG, Mayer D, Goodman L, Botros M, Armstrong DG, et al. Diabetic foot ulcers: part I. Pathophysiology and prevention. J Am Acad Dermatol. 2014;70:1 e–18. https://doi.org/10.1016/j.jaad.2013.06.055.
31. Johani K, Malone M, Jensen S, Gosbell I, Dickson H, Hu H, et al. Microscopy visualisation confirms multi-species biofilms are ubiquitous in diabetic foot ulcers. Int Wound J. 2017;14:1160–9. https://doi.org/10.1111/iwj.12777.
32. Monk EJM, Jones TPW, Bongomin F, Kibone W, Nsubuga Y, Ssewante N, et al. Antimicrobial resistance in bacterial wound, skin, soft tissue and surgical site infections in Central, Eastern, Southern and Western Africa: a systematic review and meta-analysis. PLOS Glob Public Health. 2024;4:e0003077. https://doi.org/10.1371/journal.pgph.0003077.
33. Misic AM, Gardner SE, Grice EA. The wound microbiome: modern approaches to examining the role of microorganisms in impaired chronic wound healing. Adv Wound Care (New Rochelle). 2014;3:502–10. https://doi.org/10.1089/wound.2012.0397.
34. De Maeseneer MG, Kakkos SK, Aherne T, Baekgaard N, Black S, Blomgren L, et al. Editor's choice – European Society for Vascular Surgery (ESVS) 2022 clinical practice guidelines on the management of chronic venous disease of the lower limbs. Eur J Vasc Endovasc Surg. 2022;63:184–267. https://doi.org/10.1016/j.ejvs.2021.12.024.
35. Harrison MB, Graham ID, Friedberg E, Lorimer K, Vandevelde-Coke S. Regional planning study. Assessing the population with leg and foot ulcers. Can Nurse. 2001;97:18–23.
36. Raffetto JD. Pathophysiology of chronic venous disease and venous ulcers. Surg Clin North Am. 2018;98:337–47. https://doi.org/10.1016/j.suc.2017.11.002.
37. Raffetto JD, Ligi D, Maniscalco R, Khalil RA, Mannello F. Why venous leg ulcers have difficulty healing: overview on pathophysiology, clinical consequences, and treatment. J Clin Med. 2020;10:29. https://doi.org/10.3390/jcm10010029.
38. Burnand KG, Whimster I, Naidoo A, Browse NL. Pericapillary fibrin in the ulcer-bearing skin of the leg: the cause of lipodermatosclerosis and venous ulceration. Br Med J (Clin Res Ed). 1982;285:1071–2. https://doi.org/10.1136/bmj.285.6348.1071.
39. Beidler SK, Douillet CD, Berndt DF, Keagy BA, Rich PB, Marston WA. Multiplexed analysis of matrix metalloproteinases in leg ulcer tissue of patients with chronic venous insufficiency before and after compression therapy. Wound Repair Regen. 2008;16:642–8. https://doi.org/10.1111/j.1524-475X.2008.00415.x.
40. Beidler SK, Douillet CD, Berndt DF, Keagy BA, Rich PB, Marston WA. Inflammatory cytokine levels in chronic venous insufficiency ulcer tissue before and after compression therapy. J Vasc Surg. 2009;49:1013–20. https://doi.org/10.1016/j.jvs.2008.11.049.
41. Barwell JR, Davies CE, Deacon J, Harvey K, Minor J, Sassano A, et al. Comparison of surgery and compression with compression alone in chronic venous ulceration (ESCHAR study): randomised controlled trial. Lancet. 2004;363:1854–9. https://doi.org/10.1016/S0140-6736(04)16353-8.
42. Gohel MS, Heatley F, Liu X, Bradbury A, Bulbulia R, Cullum N, et al. A randomized trial of early Endovenous ablation in venous ulceration. N Engl J Med. 2018;378:2105–14. https://doi.org/10.1056/NEJMoa1801214.
43. World Health Organisation. https://www.who.int/news-room/fact-sheets/detail/diabetes. Accessed 20 Nov 2024.

44. Reardon R, Simring D, Kim B, Mortensen J, Williams D, Leslie A. The diabetic foot ulcer. Aust J Gen Pract. 2020;49:250–5. https://doi.org/10.31128/AJGP-11-19-5161.
45. Fu K, Zheng X, Chen Y, Wu L, Yang Z, Chen X, et al. Role of matrix metalloproteinases in diabetic foot ulcers: potential therapeutic targets. Front Pharmacol. 2022;13:1050630. https://doi.org/10.3389/fphar.2022.1050630.
46. Falanga V. Wound healing and its impairment in the diabetic foot. Lancet. 2005;366:1736–43. https://doi.org/10.1016/S0140-6736(05)67700-8.
47. Loot MA, Kenter SB, Au FL, van Galen WJ, Middelkoop E, Bos JD, et al. Fibroblasts derived from chronic diabetic ulcers differ in their response to stimulation with EGF, IGF-I, bFGF and PDGF-AB compared to controls. Eur J Cell Biol. 2002;81:153–60. https://doi.org/10.1078/0171-9335-00228.
48. Davis FM, Kimball A, Boniakowski A, Gallagher K. Dysfunctional wound healing in diabetic foot ulcers: new crossroads. Curr Diab Rep. 2018;18:2. https://doi.org/10.1007/s11892-018-0970-z.
49. Lobmann R, Ambrosch A, Schultz G, Waldmann K, Schiweck S, Lehnert H. Expression of matrix-metalloproteinases and their inhibitors in the wounds of diabetic and non-diabetic patients. Diabetologia. 2002;45:1011–6. https://doi.org/10.1007/s00125-002-0868-8.
50. Edmonds M, Lazaro-Martinez JL, Alfayate-Garcia JM, Martini J, Petit JM, Rayman G, et al. Sucrose octasulfate dressing versus control dressing in patients with neuroischaemic diabetic foot ulcers (explorer): an international, multicentre, double-blind, randomised, controlled trial. Lancet Diabetes Endocrinol. 2018;6:186–96. https://doi.org/10.1016/S2213-8587(17)30438-2.
51. Mamdoh H, Hassanein KM, Eltoony LF, Khalifa WA, Hamed E, Alshammari TO, et al. Clinical and bacteriological analyses of biofilm-forming staphylococci isolated from diabetic foot ulcers. Infect Drug Resist. 2023;16:1737–50. https://doi.org/10.2147/IDR.S393724.
52. Percival SL, Hill KE, Williams DW, Hooper SJ, Thomas DW, Costerton JW. A review of the scientific evidence for biofilms in wounds. Wound Repair Regen. 2012;20:647–57. https://doi.org/10.1111/j.1524-475X.2012.00836.x.
53. Goswami AG, Basu S, Banerjee T, Shukla VK. Biofilm and wound healing: from bench to bedside. Eur J Med Res. 2023;28:157. https://doi.org/10.1186/s40001-023-01121-7.
54. Fitridge R, Chuter V, Mills J, Hinchliffe R, Azuma N, Behrendt CA, et al. The intersocietal IWGDF, ESVS, SVS guidelines on peripheral artery disease in people with diabetes mellitus and a foot ulcer. J Vasc Surg. 2023;78:1101–31. https://doi.org/10.1016/j.jvs.2023.07.020.
55. Sharma S, Schaper N, Rayman G. Microangiopathy: is it relevant to wound healing in diabetic foot disease? Diabetes Metab Res Rev. 2020;36(Suppl 1):e3244. https://doi.org/10.1002/dmrr.3244.
56. Catrina SB, Okamoto K, Pereira T, Brismar K, Poellinger L. Hyperglycemia regulates hypoxia-inducible factor-1alpha protein stability and function. Diabetes. 2004;53:3226–32. https://doi.org/10.2337/diabetes.53.12.3226.
57. Catrina SB, Zheng X. Disturbed hypoxic responses as a pathogenic mechanism of diabetic foot ulcers. Diabetes Metab Res Rev. 2016;32(Suppl 1):179–85. https://doi.org/10.1002/dmrr.2742.
58. Gallagher KA, Joshi A, Carson WF, Schaller M, Allen R, Mukerjee S, et al. Epigenetic changes in bone marrow progenitor cells influence the inflammatory phenotype and alter wound healing in type 2 diabetes. Diabetes. 2015;64:1420–30. https://doi.org/10.2337/db14-0872.
59. Madhyastha R, Madhyastha H, Nakajima Y, Omura S, Maruyama M. MicroRNA signature in diabetic wound healing: promotive role of miR-21 in fibroblast migration. Int Wound J. 2012;9:355–61. https://doi.org/10.1111/j.1742-481X.2011.00890.x.
60. Berlanga-Acosta JA, Guillen-Nieto GE, Rodriguez-Rodriguez N, Mendoza-Mari Y, Bringas-Vega ML, Berlanga-Saez JO, et al. Cellular senescence as the pathogenic hub of diabetes-related wound chronicity. Front Endocrinol (Lausanne). 2020;11:573032. https://doi.org/10.3389/fendo.2020.573032.

61. Chen P, Vilorio NC, Dhatariya K, Jeffcoate W, Lobmann R, McIntosh C, et al. Guidelines on interventions to enhance healing of foot ulcers in people with diabetes (IWGDF 2023 update). Diabetes Metab Res Rev. 2024;40:e3644. https://doi.org/10.1002/dmrr.3644.
62. Thaenpramun R, Komolsuradej N, Buathong N, Srikrajang S. Association between glycaemic control and malnutrition in older adults with type 2 diabetes mellitus: a cross-sectional study. Br J Nutr. 2024;131:1497–505. https://doi.org/10.1017/S0007114524000175.
63. Eneroth M, Larsson J, Oscarsson C, Apelqvist J. Nutritional supplementation for diabetic foot ulcers: the first RCT. J Wound Care. 2004;13:230–4. https://doi.org/10.12968/jowc.2004.13.6.26627.
64. Gau BR, Chen HY, Hung SY, Yang HM, Yeh JT, Huang CH, et al. The impact of nutritional status on treatment outcomes of patients with limb-threatening diabetic foot ulcers. J Diabetes Complicat. 2016;30:138–42. https://doi.org/10.1016/j.jdiacomp.2015.09.011.
65. Rouland A, Fourmont C, Sberna AL, Aho Glele LS, Mouillot T, Simoneau I, et al. Malnutrition in type 2 diabetic patients does not affect healing of foot ulcers. Acta Diabetol. 2019;56:171–6. https://doi.org/10.1007/s00592-018-1233-9.
66. Xie Y, Zhang H, Ye T, Ge S, Zhuo R, Zhu H. The geriatric nutritional risk index independently predicts mortality in diabetic foot ulcers patients undergoing amputations. J Diabetes Res. 2017;2017:5797194. https://doi.org/10.1155/2017/5797194.
67. Zhang SS, Tang ZY, Fang P, Qian HJ, Xu L, Ning G. Nutritional status deteriorates as the severity of diabetic foot ulcers increases and independently associates with prognosis. Exp Ther Med. 2013;5:215–22. https://doi.org/10.3892/etm.2012.780.
68. Barchitta M, Maugeri A, Favara G, San Lio RM, Evola G, Agodi A, et al. Nutrition and wound healing: an overview focusing on the beneficial effects of curcumin. Int J Mol Sci. 2019;20:1119. https://doi.org/10.3390/ijms20051119.
69. Moore ZE, Corcoran MA, Patton D. Nutritional interventions for treating foot ulcers in people with diabetes. Cochrane Database Syst Rev. 2020;7:CD011378. https://doi.org/10.1002/14651858.CD011378.pub2.
70. Chen P, Carville K, Swanson T, Lazzarini PA, Charles J, Cheney J, et al. Australian guideline on wound healing interventions to enhance healing of foot ulcers: part of the 2021 Australian evidence-based guidelines for diabetes-related foot disease. J Foot Ankle Res 2022;15:40. https://doi.org/10.1186/s13047-022-00544-5
71. Wilkinson HN, Hardman MJ. Wound healing: cellular mechanisms and pathological outcomes. Open Biol. 2020;10:200223. https://doi.org/10.1098/rsob.200223.

Key References

Demidova-Rice TN, Hamblin MR, Herman IM. Acute and impaired wound healing: pathophysiology and current methods for drug delivery, part 1: normal and chronic wounds: biology, causes, and approaches to care. Adv Skin Wound Care. 2012;25:304–14. https://doi.org/10.1097/01.ASW.0000416006.55218.d0.

Li J, Chen J, Kirsner R. Pathophysiology of acute wound healing. Clin Dermatol. 2007;25:9–18. https://doi.org/10.1016/j.clindermatol.2006.09.007.

Singer AJ, Clark RA. Cutaneous wound healing. N Engl J Med. 1999;341:738–46. https://doi.org/10.1056/NEJM199909023411006.

Zhao R, Liang H, Clarke E, Jackson C, Xue M. Inflammation in Chronic Wounds. Int J Mol Sci. 2016;17:2085. https://doi.org/10.3390/ijms17122085.

Chapter 8
Pathophysiology and Principles of Management of Diabetes-Related Foot Complications

Guilherme Pena, Vivienne Chuter, David G. Armstrong, Joseph L. Mills, and Robert Fitridge

SN Flashcards
Test your learning and check your understanding of this book's contents: use the "Springer Nature Flashcards" app to access questions using ▶ https://sn.pub/wppvze. To use the app, please follow the instructions in Chap. 1.

G. Pena (✉)
Faculty of Health and Medical Sciences, Adelaide University, Adelaide, SA, Australia

Vascular Unit, Flinders Medical Centre, Bedford Park, SA, Australia
e-mail: guilherme.pena@sa.gov.au

V. Chuter
Discipline of Podiatry | School of Health Sciences, Western Sydney University, Sydney, NSW, Australia
e-mail: V.Chuter@westernsydney.edu.au

D. G. Armstrong
Department of Surgery, Keck School of Medicine of University of Southern California, Los Angeles, CA, USA

J. L. Mills
Division of Vascular Surgery and Endovascular Therapy, Michael E. DeBakey Department of Surgery, Baylor College of Medicine, Houston, TX, USA
e-mail: Joseph.Mills@bcm.edu

R. Fitridge
Faculty of Health and Medical Sciences, Adelaide University, Adelaide, SA, Australia

Vascular and Endovascular Service, Central Adelaide Local Health Network, Adelaide, SA, Australia
e-mail: robert.fitridge@adelaide.edu.au

R. Fitridge et al. (eds.), *Pathophysiology of Vascular Disease*,
https://doi.org/10.1007/978-3-032-31459-8_8

Key Learning Points

- Diabetes-related foot complications (DRFCs) are the most common cause of non-traumatic lower limb amputation; 85% of these amputations are preceded by foot ulceration.
- Diabetes-related peripheral neuropathy (DPN) is the most prevalent chronic complication of diabetes, affecting at least half of all patients with diabetes during their lifetime. The pathogenesis of DPN is complex, multifactorial, and not fully understood. Metabolic abnormalities that are implicated in the pathogenesis of DPN include non-enzymatic glycosylation of neural structures, malfunction of polyol metabolism, activation of the hexosamine pathway, and protein kinase C (PKC) isoforms.
- Approximately 50% of patients with a diabetes-related foot ulcer (DRFU) have coexisting PAD. PAD in diabetes tends to occur more distally than smoking-related PAD and is particularly common below the knee. These atherosclerotic lesions tend to be multilevel with a high prevalence of long occlusions.
- Conventional methods of assessing tissue perfusion in the peripheral circulation are frequently unreliable in patients with diabetes, and, therefore, it is challenging to determine the presence and extent of perfusion deficit in people with foot ulceration.
- WIfI classification should be used for limb staging of foot complications in diabetes and is based on grading Wound, Ischaemia and foot Infection on a scale from 0 to 3. WIfI can be used to assess the risk of major limb amputation at one year and also the need for, and expected benefit of, revascularisation.
- The principles of management of diabetes-related foot ulcers include offloading, wound management, management of infection, assessment of perfusion, and revascularisation, if required.
- Infection severity guides the choice of the empiric antibiotic regimen and its route of administration. The presence of osteomyelitis has important diagnostic, therapeutic, and prognostic implications.
- Assessment of perfusion in the foot in diabetes can be challenging. The level of perfusion required to heal a foot ulcer depends on multiple factors such as ulcer size and location, and the presence/extent of gangrene and infection. A combination of assessments including pulse palpation, ABIs, and TPs is recommended as a baseline in all patients with DFU to detect the presence and severity of PAD. The Global Vascular Guidelines on the management of chronic limb-threatening ischaemia and the Intersocietal IWGDF, ESVS, SVS (International Working Group on the Diabetic Foot, European Society for Vascular Surgery and Society for Vascular Surgery) guidelines on peripheral artery disease in people with diabetes mellitus and a foot ulcer recommend an evidence-based approach to assessment and treatment of patients with diabetes and a foot ulcer.
- Charcot neuroarthropathy is a serious but frequently missed condition of the foot in people with DPN. It is an inflammatory process that results in significant musculoskeletal injury, including soft tissue and bone injury, which contributes to joint destruction due to fractures, dislocations, and subsequent permanent foot deformity. The hallmark of acute Charcot is a warm, swollen, and erythematous

foot with intact skin (in the presence of DPN), which can easily be misinterpreted as acute infection, gout, or osteomyelitis. The initial management of active Charcot foot includes early diagnosis, offloading and immobilisation. These are essential to minimise long-term consequences of the condition, which include significant foot deformity and associated risk of secondary DRFU, osteomyelitis, and amputation.

8.1 Introduction

Diabetes is a major public health challenge worldwide, which is associated with a variety of complications including cardiovascular, kidney, eye, and foot disease. It is an important cause of mortality, morbidity, cost (to health systems and the patient), and disability worldwide. The number of adults living with diabetes worldwide has quadrupled over the last 35 years and will continue to rise [1]. In 2024, an estimated 589 million adults aged 20–70, representing 11.1% of this age group, were living with diabetes. This number is projected to rise to 852.5 million by 2050. While the global population is expected to grow by 25% over the next 25 years, the number of individuals with diabetes is forecast to increase by a more significant 45%. Notably, an estimated 95% of this increase will occur in low- and middle-income countries, which are also anticipated to experience greater population growth than high-income countries [2]. This rising disease prevalence is also accompanied by an increase in associated comorbidities [3].

Diabetes-related foot ulcer (DRFU) is defined as a foot ulcer in a person with current or previously diagnosed diabetes mellitus and is usually accompanied by diabetes-related peripheral neuropathy (DPN) and/or peripheral artery disease (PAD) in the lower extremity [4]. It is estimated that patients with diabetes have a nearly 25% lifetime risk of developing a foot ulcer. Approximately 50% of these ulcers become infected, and a significant portion require hospitalisation [5, 6]. The cost of care for patients with diabetes and a DRFU is a major economic burden for both society and individual patients [7]. These costs are significantly increased when ulcers become infected or when patients need prolonged inpatient treatment or amputation [8].

Diabetes-related foot complications (DRFCs) are the most common cause of non-traumatic lower limb amputation (major and minor) internationally and it is believed that every 30 seconds, a lower limb is lost somewhere in the world as a consequence of diabetes [9]. Individuals with diabetes experience a substantially increased risk of major amputation, with the risk being 9.5 to over 30 times higher compared to those without diabetes [10].

A history of DRFU is significantly associated with negative outcomes. The risk of death at 5 years for a patient with DRFU is 2.5 times as high as the risk for a patient with diabetes who does not have a foot ulcer [11]. Of all amputations in patients with diabetes, 85% are preceded by foot ulceration, which subsequently deteriorates to gangrene or infection [12]. Mortality after diabetes-related major amputation is notoriously high; 70% at 5 years for all patients with diabetes and 74% at 2 years for those undergoing dialysis [13, 14]. Even minor amputations carry a substantial risk of mortality [15]. A recent meta-analysis revealed mortality rates following these procedures, reaching 20% at 1 year, 28% at 3 years, and 44.1% at 5 years. These findings emphasise that even seemingly minor amputations represent a critical turning point in the lives of these patients, with profound long-term consequences [16].

More than three-quarters of patients with DRFU can achieve primary healing within 1 year [13]. Unfortunately, patients with a DRFU history have a high risk of re-ulceration [17]. Approximately 40% of patients will suffer from a recurrence within 1 year after ulcer healing, almost 60% within 3 years, and 65% within 5 years [13]. Thus, it may be more useful to think of patients who have achieved wound closure as being in remission rather than being cured or healed.

8.2 Pathophysiology of Diabetes-Related Foot Complications

The pathogenesis of foot ulceration in diabetes is complex and requires an appreciation of the role of several contributory factors, including DPN, PAD, limited joint mobility (and other biomechanical problems), and susceptibility to infection [6, 18].

8.2.1 Neuropathy and Biomechanical Abnormalities

DPN is a highly prevalent complication, affecting approximately 50% of individuals with diabetes throughout their lives and resulting in significant morbidity [19]. Interestingly, individuals with type 2 diabetes exhibit a higher prevalence of DPN than those with type 1 diabetes [20]. While glycaemic control impacts the progression of DPN in type 1 diabetes, its effect on the onset and progression of DPN in type 2 diabetes is less pronounced, suggesting the involvement of other risk factors. Notably, conventional cardiovascular risk factors such as obesity, hypertension, dyslipidaemia, elevated triglycerides, and smoking independently elevate the risk of developing DPN [21, 22].

The pathogenesis of DPN is not fully understood but it is likely to be multifactorial. Factors such as metabolic abnormalities related to non-enzymatic glycosylation of neural structures (formation of advanced glycation end-products—AGEs), dysfunction of polyol and myo-inositol pathways; microvascular insufficiency (disease of the vasa nervorum); mitochondrial dysfunction, and oxidative/ nitrosative stress are considered important in the pathogenesis of this complication. Furthermore, dyslipidaemia and hyperglycaemia stimulate the release of pro-inflammatory cytokines and chemokines, leading to inflammatory and immune-mediated neurotoxicity [21, 22].

DPN typically manifests as a symmetrical, sensorimotor polyneuropathy, initially affecting the toes bilaterally and progressing proximally in a "stocking distribution." Once established in the lower limbs, it can also involve the upper limbs. Motor manifestations typically follow sensory loss, initially affecting the intrinsic muscles of the foot [21].

Key Clinical Manifestations of DPN

- *Sensory Neuropathy*: Loss of protective sensation (LOPS), predisposing to undetected injuries and repetitive trauma.
- *Motor Neuropathy*: Foot muscle weakness and atrophy leading to foot deformities (hammer toes, claw toes, prominent metatarsal heads, pes cavus) and altered foot biomechanics.
- *Autonomic Neuropathy*: Sudomotor dysfunction contributing to dry inelastic skin, increased vulnerability to wounds, and microcirculatory dysfunction.

Sensory neuropathy with loss of protective sensation is particularly relevant to the development of DRFUs. The inability to detect pain signals leads to delayed recognition of minor injuries, allowing them to progress in severity due to reinjury or repetitive trauma. This creates a vicious cycle of increased forces and impaired sensation, further exacerbating the ulcer. Furthermore, the insensate foot fails to initiate appropriate vascular neuroregulatory changes, hindering the supply of oxygen and nutrients necessary for wound healing and compounding the existing microvascular insufficiency [21, 23].

Motor neuropathy contributes to foot deformities and biomechanical abnormalities through atrophy of the intrinsic foot muscles. This imbalance between flexors and extensors, particularly atrophy of the small muscles responsible for metatarsophalangeal plantar flexion, results in structural deformities and restricted joint mobility, commonly associated with areas of elevated plantar pressures [21, 24].

The interplay of sensory, motor, and autonomic neuropathy contributes to a cascade of biomechanical abnormalities that significantly increase the risk of foot ulceration. These abnormalities can be further assessed through gait analysis and plantar pressure mapping.

Studies have shown that people with DRFUs exhibit specific gait abnormalities, including reduced joint range of motion, increased ground reaction forces, slower walking speed, and higher plantar pressures [25]. These findings underscore the importance of pressure offloading in the prevention and management of DRFUs.

8.2.2 *Peripheral Artery Disease*

Diabetes is a significant risk factor for the development of PAD [26], and approximately 50% of patients with DRFUs have coexisting PAD [27, 28]. PAD in diabetes occurs predominantly in the infra-inguinal vasculature, and its anatomic distribution differs from that in patients without diabetes, with distinct characteristics, treatment, and outcomes. The atherosclerotic lesions tend to be multilevel and particularly severe in the below-knee vessels, such as the tibial and peroneal arteries, with a high prevalence of long occlusions [26, 29]. The predilection for crural and pedal vessel involvement combined with extensive arterial calcification increases the technical challenges associated with revascularisation using either open bypass or endovascular techniques [30, 31]. Furthermore, in patients with diabetes, a similar degree of anatomical arterial disease can result in a more severe perfusion deficit than in those without diabetes because of a paucity of collateral vessels as well as the influence of physiological factors associated with diabetes, such as arteriolar shunting [32]. The presence of PAD among patients with DRFU is associated with worse outcomes, including poor wound healing, higher rates of lower extremity amputation and higher mortality [17, 33].

Assessing foot perfusion is challenging in patients with diabetes. These patients commonly lack typical symptoms of vascular insufficiency such as claudication or rest pain [34]. However, assessing perfusion is a crucial step in managing patients with DRFUs, as it helps to estimate the risk of amputation, predict the likelihood of wound healing, and determine the potential benefits of revascularisation.

Perfusion assessment needs to be assessed in terms of global and regional perfusion deficits rather than as an absolute measurement. The amount of blood flow required to heal a foot lesion depends on several factors including the presence of infection, extent of tissue loss, abnormal mechanical loading of the foot during walking and co-morbidities such as renal failure [35–37]. Conventional methods of assessing tissue perfusion in the peripheral circulation may be unreliable in patients with diabetes (see below).

In addition to PAD, numerous studies have identified microvascular abnormalities in the skin and subcutaneous tissues of individuals with diabetes. These encompass both structural changes, such as thickening of the capillary basement membrane, reduced capillary luminal size and density, and pericyte degeneration, as well as functional impairments, including endothelial dysfunction with diminished vasodilatory responses and the presence of arteriovenous shunting, which can divert blood flow away from capillaries, compromising tissue nutrition [38]. However, despite the critical role of the microcirculation in delivering oxygen and nutrients essential for wound healing, the contribution of these microvascular abnormalities to impaired healing in DRFU remains incompletely understood [31].

In summary, the combination of foot deformity, loss of protective sensation, dry skin, inadequate off-loading, repetitive minor trauma, and perfusion deficit can lead to tissue damage and ulceration. Once an ulcer has formed, healing may be delayed or not occur.

8.3 Clinical Assessment of Diabetes-Related Foot Complications

8.3.1 History and Physical Examination

A thorough history and physical examination of each patient presenting with diabetes-related foot pathology should include a history of duration of diabetes and adequacy of control, significant medical co-morbidities, a history of pedal wounds, prior amputations, and lower extremity vascular interventions.

Physical examination should follow a systematic approach, and the patient should be examined, including both feet. Foot deformities (e.g. claw toes, hammer toes), bony prominences and limited joint mobility should be noted as they increase the risk of ulceration. Footwear must be inspected for appropriate design and fit. Any wounds must be carefully assessed, and accurate documentation made regarding wound location; size; depth; characteristic of the wound base and margins; exudate (amount and type); and the presence and severity of infection.

The possibility of DPN and vascular insufficiency must be assessed. A history of paraesthesia, including foot tingling, burning, and/or numbness allodynia (pain due to a stimulus that doesn't normally cause pain), or dysesthesia can help to identify those patients with neuropathy. Sensory examination involves assessing for loss of protective sensation using the 10 g (5.07 Semmes-Weinstein) monofilament. In addition, loss of vibration perception may also predict DRFU, and vibration perception should be assessed using a tuning fork (128 Hz) or biothesiometer/neurothesiometer [39]. When a monofilament or tuning fork is not available, the light touch test (also known as the Ipswich Touch test) can be used to assess tactile sensation. This is performed by lightly touching the tips of the toes of the patient with the tip of the index finger for 1–2 seconds [39]. A history of claudication or other walking impairment, ischaemic rest pain, and non-healing wounds are suggestive of PAD. Lower extremity vascular examination should begin with palpation of lower extremity pulses (i.e. femoral, popliteal, dorsalis pedis, and posterior tibial), auscultation for femoral bruits, and inspection of the legs and feet [40].

8.3.2 Assessment of Foot Perfusion

While pulse palpation remains a valuable clinical tool for identifying the presence of PAD in individuals with diabetes, its accuracy in this population is not well-established [31]. Clinicians should interpret palpation findings with caution and consider them alongside other potential indicators of PAD such as hair loss, muscle wasting, and cool skin. However, it is important to acknowledge the subjective nature of these clinical observations. Bedside testing techniques, offering objective measurements of lower limb blood flow, can enhance diagnostic accuracy of assessment for PAD and provide critical insights into the perfusion status of patients with diabetes.

8.3.2.1 Ankle-Brachial Index (ABI)

ABI is the ratio of systolic pressure at the ankle to that in the arm. It is a quick, simple, and non-invasive test used to document PAD [41]. In addition to PAD, the ABI is also an indicator of generalised atherosclerosis [42]. Historically, the ABI has been calculated based on the higher ankle pressure; however, recent guidelines recommend the lower ankle pressure should be used for diagnosis of PAD as it improves diagnostic accuracy of the test [31, 43]. An ABI of 0.90 or lower is generally accepted as indicative of PAD. Values >1.30 indicate that the arteries were not able to be compressed, which is more common among individuals with diabetes and/or advanced chronic kidney disease [43]. Individuals with diabetes and/or renal disease frequently have calcium depositions in the arterial media; a condition known as medial arterial calcification (MAC) or Mönckeberg medial sclerosis (MMS), which most commonly affects the calf arteries [44]. This condition causes arterial wall stiffness, which results in vessels that are more difficult or impossible to occlude in the calf and ankle.

However, it should be noted that incompressibility in the presence of significant PAD can also falsely elevate the ABI to values that are within a normal or near-normal range. In such circumstances, other abnormal findings may be present, including monophasic pedal Doppler waveforms. Therefore, in the setting of definite or suspected incompressible ABI values, additional testing should be undertaken and, in some populations, for example people living with diabetes, use of multiple vascular tests is recommended.

Research has not established a clear ABI threshold to predict wound healing outcomes. While an ABI below 0.5 is suggestive of a higher chance of non-healing (30% to 45% increase in pretest probability of non-healing of DRFU) or major amputation (>45% increase in pretest probability of major amputation for ABI < 0.4), values above 0.9 do not necessarily guarantee successful healing or rule out major amputation [45].

8.3.2.2 Toe Pressure and Toe-Brachial Index

An alternative to ABI is to measure toe pressures and the toe-brachial pressure index (TBI). These may be more useful measures of the presence of PAD and perfusion in the patient with diabetes because MAC frequently spares the pedal arteries [46]. Toe pressures are obtained by placing cuffs around the base of the toe, ideally the hallux, with a digital flow sensor beyond the cuff. Toe pressures may be measured by photoplethysmography (detecting pulsatile flow and producing a pulse wave curve) or laser Doppler (detecting changes in wavelength when the laser encounters red blood cells) [47]. TBI is the ratio between toe pressure and the highest of the two brachial pressures. A TBI ≥ 0.70 is generally considered within the normal range, whilst a TBI <0.25 is consistent with severe PAD [43, 48].

In the context of DRFU management, the current evidence is insufficient to establish the predictive capacity of TBI for outcomes such as DRFU healing, healing post-minor amputation, or the necessity for minor versus major amputation. Findings suggest that a toe pressure ≥ 30 mmHg may be associated with an elevated pretest probability of both DRFU resolution and successful healing following minor amputation, with an estimated increase of at least 30%. Conversely, a toe pressure below 30 mmHg appears to confer a modest increase (approximately 15%) in the pretest probability of major amputation [45].

8.3.2.3 Doppler Waveform Assessment

Audio and visual analyses of Doppler waveforms are useful tools for assessment of the presence of PAD. A normal Doppler waveform in the lower extremities has a characteristic triphasic pattern, composed primarily of a systolic forward-flow phase, a late-systolic reverse flow phase, and a smaller, diastolic forward-flow phase. However, a biphasic waveform, in which there is loss of the final diastolic forward flow component, may also be considered a normal finding [49, 50]. The detection of an abnormal or normal pedal Doppler arterial waveform using a handheld Doppler device offers moderate to high accuracy in both confirming and excluding, respectively, the presence of PAD [45, 51].

8.3.2.4 Transcutaneous Oxygen Pressure and Skin Perfusion Pressure

Transcutaneous oxygen tension ($TcPO_2$) measures the transfer of oxygen molecules to the skin surface, allowing objective quantification of the degree of perfusion in the proximity of the anatomical location of testing [52]. $TcPO_2$ maps the actual oxygen supply available for the skin tissue cells, and it also responds to microcirculatory events. The measured $TcPO_2$ in the dermis is displayed in millimetres of mercury, with a normal healthy value in the foot for an individual breathing normobaric air being >50 mmHg [53].

Skin perfusion pressure (SPP) is the blood pressure that is required to restore capillary flow to capillaries following controlled occlusion and subsequent flow return. This provides a quantitative measure of systolic pressure in the microcirculation at specific anatomical sites (e.g. at a wound edge) with normal SPP values for a healthy adult ranging from 50 to 100 mmHg [54–56].

$TcPO_2$ and SPP values can be used to predict the presence of vascular disease and the likely success of healing an ulcer and major/minor amputations with or without revascularisation. $TcPO_2$ measurements with an oxygen challenge are also utilised as an indicator of whether or not hyperbaric therapy will likely be beneficial in wound healing [48].

A recent systematic review on the performance of non-invasive bedside tests for assessment of perfusion found that in individuals with DRFU, a $TcPO_2 \geq 25$ mmHg or higher appears to significantly enhance the likelihood of DRFU healing, potentially increasing the pretest probability of healing by up to 45%. Conversely, a $TcPO_2 < 20$ mmHg may slightly elevate the risk of minor amputation but does not seem to impact the likelihood of major amputation. Additionally, a skin perfusion pressure of >40 mmHg shows promise in improving the odds of both DRFU healing and successful healing after minor amputation, with a potential increase in pretest probability of up to 45% [45].

8.3.3 Diagnosis of Osteomyelitis

The accurate diagnosis of foot sepsis and in particular osteomyelitis (OM) in the foot in diabetes is important for planning adequate treatment. Prevalence of bone involvement is variable, depending on the context. It is found in approximately 60% of patients hospitalised for a diabetes-related foot infection (DRFI) and 10%–20% of apparently less severe infections presenting in an outpatient setting [57]. The differentiation of bone infection from soft tissue infection may be challenging, as can be the differentiation of bone infection from non-infectious bone disorders [58]. Conditions such as acute gout and acute Charcot neuroarthropathy present significant diagnostic challenges and may co-exist with OM or foot sepsis.

A definitive diagnosis of OM ideally requires both the presence of histological findings consistent with bone infection (acute or chronic inflammatory cells, necrosis) and the isolation of bacteria from an aseptically obtained bone sample [59]. However, bone biopsy is not widely performed (most frequently due to commencement of antibiotics prior to review of the foot), and the clinician may rely on clinical, laboratory and imaging findings for diagnosis. The presence of visible exposed bone; bone palpable with a probe ("probe-to-bone test"); erythematous and indurated ("sausage") toe, especially with an ulcer; an ulcer that is deep, fails to heal despite offloading or is located over a bony prominence; and the presence of a soft tissue sinus are suggestive of osteomyelitis [57, 60].

The probe-to-bone test (PBT) is a useful clinical diagnostic tool for diagnosing osteomyelitis. PBT is conducted by using a sterile probe to gently explore the wound. If the probe encounters a hard or gritty substance that is presumed to be bone or joint space, the test is considered positive, and this greatly increases the likelihood of osteomyelitis in a high-risk population. The test can also be useful to rule out OM, as a negative probe-to-bone test in a patient at low risk strongly argues against the diagnosis of osteomyelitis [61]. Occasionally, a viscous exudate (joint fluid) may be found in a sinus, also supporting a diagnosis of joint infection. A systematic review of the PTB test found that, for detecting diabetes-related foot osteomyelitis (DRFO), the sensitivity was 0.87 and specificity 0.83 [62].

Imaging diagnosis of osteomyelitis usually begins with plain X-rays. X-ray provides an inexpensive, widely available tool for initial evaluation, and it is often adequate for imaging the foot in patients with suspicion of DRFO. Radiographic signs of osteomyelitis include decreased density of bone, lytic changes and cortical erosion, trabecular destruction, bone necrosis, Brodie's abscess, sclerosis, and periosteal reaction. X-ray has low sensitivity, especially in the early stages of osteomyelitis, as radiological changes may be delayed for up to four weeks following infection. Comparison with previous X-ray or a repeat X-ray at 2–6 weeks may be useful. A combination of a probe-to-bone test, plain X-ray, and biomarkers (ESR, CRP) can be considered as part of the initial investigation for DRFO [57]. If X-ray is negative and clinical suspicion remains high, the patient will need additional imaging. MRI is the preferred advanced imaging modality for diagnosing osteomyelitis due to good sensitivity and specificity and good spatial resolution for assessment of both soft tissues and bone. In situations where MRI is contraindicated or unavailable, a nuclear medicine scan such as a leukocyte scan, preferably combined with a bone scan, is the best alternative. Other imaging modalities may also be helpful in the diagnosis of OM [57, 59] (Table 8.1).

Table 8.1 Imaging modalities for diagnosis of osteomyelitis [57]

Imaging modality	Advantages	Disadvantages
Plain radiography	Readily available and inexpensive	Low sensitivity in early stages of osteomyelitis
	May be used to monitor response to antibiotic treatment	Specificity is limited by difficulty differentiating infection from Charcot's arthropathy and other pathologies (e.g. gout)
	Can reveal the presence of radio-opaque foreign bodies, gas in soft tissues, calcified arteries, fractures, or bony abnormalities	
MRI	Preferred advanced imaging modality for diagnosing osteomyelitis	Reduced performance with severe ischaemia
	Does not use radiation	Not all patients are suitable for MRI (e.g. pacemaker)
	Excellent spatial resolution and is very useful for evaluation of bone marrow as well as of soft tissue structures. Good for detection of sinus tracts, deep tissue necrosis, abscesses and other inflammatory changes	
Nuclear medicine scan	More sensitive than radiographs for detecting osteomyelitis during early stages of the disease.	Poor specificity and low resolution of images

(Continued)

Table 8.1 (Continued)

Imaging modality	Advantages	Disadvantages
	Labelled leucocyte scintigraphy with either indium-111 (^{111}In) or technetium-99 (^{99}mTc), improves specificity	Includes a 24-hour waiting period before imaging can begin as well as low resolution of the images
	White blood cell-labelled single-photon emission computed tomography can be combined with computed tomography (^{99}mTc WBC labelled-SPECT/CT) imaging to provide good spatial resolution	Limited availability
PET (PET/CT)	Excellent spatial resolution	Limited availability
	Does not require blood processing	High costs

8.4 Staging and Risk Stratification of Diabetes-Related Foot Complications

Based on a thorough history, physical examination, and ABI/ toe pressures, each patient should be classified and assigned to a specific foot risk category. Staging is important to provide risk stratification of patients with respect to disease natural history and allow meaningful comparison of different treatment strategies.

Various classification systems have been used to stratify patients with diabetes-related foot complications in an attempt to predict outcomes in terms of likelihood of healing and risk of lower limb amputation and thus help planning treatment strategies.

The Meggitt-Wagner wound classification system is based on assessment of ulcer depth and the presence of osteomyelitis or gangrene [63]. The drawback of the Wagner classification system is that it does not specifically address two critically important parameters in a foot with diabetes: ischaemia and infection [64].

The University of Texas classification grades the ulcer based on depth. Each grade is then staged according to the presence of infection, ischaemia or both. However, this classification lacks adequate assessment of infection and ischaemia as they are included only as dichotomised variables [65].

The SINBAD wound classification system is recommended to classify severity of DRFU based on six key factors: the wound **S**ite (anatomical location), presence of **I**schaemia, presence or absence of **N**europathy, clinical signs of **B**acterial Infection, and the **A**rea (size), and **D**epth (including involvement of deeper tissue structures. A score is assigned to each factor (a score of 0 for normal or 1 for abnormal), with these added to give a total SINBAD score between 0 and 6, with higher score indicative of greater DRFU severity [66]. SINBAD's simplicity, using only clinical exam, makes it universally applicable for triaging DRFU, especially in resource-limited settings lacking specialised equipment like those required for TP and $TcPO_2$ assessment.

8.4.1 WIfI Threatened Limb Classification

In 2014, the Society for Vascular Surgery developed a Lower Extremity Threatened Limb Classification System which represents a synthesis of multiple previously published classification schemes that focused on DRFU and pure ischaemia (CLTI) models. This classification is referred to as WIfI (Wound, Ischaemia, and Foot Infection) and is based on grading each of the three major factors on a scale from 0 to 3, where 0 represents none, 1 mild, 2 moderate, and 3 severe [67].

Wounds are classified from grade 0 through grade 3 based on size, depth, severity, and anticipated difficulty achieving wound healing (Table 8.2). Ischaemia classification is based on ABI, ankle pressure, Toe pressure (TP) or transcutaneous oxygen saturation ($TcPO_2$) (Table 8.3). Since patients with diabetes may have falsely elevated ABIs due to MAC, toe waveform and TP are preferred. SPP or

Table 8.2 WIfI wound grading [67]

Grade	Ulcer	Gangrene
0	No ulcer	No gangrene
	Ischaemic rest pain (requires typical symptoms + ischaemia grade 3); no wound	
1	Small, shallow ulcer(s) on distal leg or foot; no exposed bone, unless limited to distal phalanx	No gangrene
	Minor tissue loss. Salvageable with simple digital amputation (1 or 2 digits) or skin coverage	
2	Deeper ulcer with exposed bone, joint or tendon: generally not involving the heel; shallow heel ulcer, without calcaneal involvement	Gangrenous changes limited to digits
	Major tissue loss salvageable with multiple (≥3) digital amputations or standard transmetatarsal amputation +/− skin coverage	
3	Extensive deep ulcer involving forefoot and/or midfoot; deep, full thickness heel ulcer +/− calcaneal involvement	Extensive gangrene involving forefoot and / or midfoot; full thickness heel necrosis +/− calcaneal involvement
	Extensive tissue loss salvageable only with complex foot reconstruction or non-traditional TMA (Chopart or Lisfranc); flap coverage or complex management needed for large soft tissue defect	

Table 8.3 WIfI ischaemia grading [67]

Grade	ABI	Ankle systolic pressure	TP, $TcPO_2$
0	≥0.80	>100 mmHg	≥60 mmHg
1	0.6–0.79	70–100 mmHg	40–59 mmHg
2	0.4–0.59	50–70 mmHg	30–39 mmHg
3	≤0.39	<50 mmHg	<30 mmHg

TP toe pressure, $TcPO_2$ transcutaneous oxygen pressure
If TP and ABI measurements result in different grades, TP will be the primary determinant of ischaemia grade

Table 8.4 WIfI infection grading [67]

Grade	Clinical manifestation of infection
0	No symptoms or signs of infection
1	Infection present, as defined by the presence of at least 2 of the following items: (a) local swelling or induration. (b) Erythema >0.5 to ≤2 cm around the ulcer. (c) Local tenderness or pain. (d) Local warmth. (e) Purulent discharge (thick, opaque to white, or sanguineous secretion). Local infection involving only skin and the subcutaneous tissue (without involvement of deeper tissues and without systemic signs as described below). Exclude other causes of inflammatory response of the skin (e.g. trauma, gout, acute Charcot neuro-osteoarthropathy, fracture, thrombosis, venous stasis)
2	Local infection (as described above) with erythema extending >2 cm from wound edge, or involving structures deeper than skin and subcutaneous tissues (e.g. abscess, osteomyelitis, septic arthritis, fasciitis), and no signs or symptoms of systemic inflammatory response syndrome (SIRS)
3	Local infection (as described above) with the signs of SIRS, as manifested by two or more of the following: (a) Temperature >38 °C or <36 °C (b) Heart rate >90 beats/min (c) Respiratory rate >20 breaths/min or $PaCO_2$ <33 mmHg (d) White cell count >12,000 or <4000/mm^3 or 10% immature (band) forms.

$TcPO_2$ measurements are also useful for assessment of perfusion and are used in some units instead of TP. Patients with TP < 30 mmHg have severe ischaemia and are likely to require revascularisation to achieve wound healing and limb salvage. The WIfI classification incorporates the scheme proposed by the Infectious Diseases Society of America (IDSA) to assess severity of infection (Table 8.4).

The three categories (wound, ischaemia, and foot infection) with four grades of severity produce a grid with 64 theoretically possible clinical combinations (WIfI classes). A Delphi consensus of the members of the Society of Vascular Surgery Lower Extremity Guidelines Committee assigned a risk category to each of the combinations with regard to risk of limb amputation at 1 year (very low risk, low risk, moderate risk, or high risk) and benefit of revascularisation (very low benefit, low benefit, moderate benefit, or high benefit) for each of the possible combinations. (Table 8.5). Each risk category is related to the clinical staging of the limb which is assigned from the combined scores of the three categories (wound, infection, and ischaemia). Clinical stages 1–4 relate to risk categories very low through to high. Advanced gangrene or infection with an unsalvageable foot is excluded from the standard classification (WIfI clinical stage 5). Limbs should be restaged following treatment, for example, revascularisation, treatment of infection or wound improvement/deterioration.

Several reported series have been published with analysis of outcomes of patients with threatened limbs, including patients with DRFCs, based on WIfI clinical stage validating this model [33, 36, 68, 69]. Research indicates a strong correlation between WIfI clinical stage and one-year amputation risk. Patients classified as WIfI stage 1 demonstrate a minimal risk of amputation, with rates consistently below 5%. Those in stages 2 and 3 face an intermediate risk, with amputation rates typically falling between 5% and 10%. Notably, stage 4 patients exhibit a significantly elevated risk, exceeding 20%, underscoring the severity of this clinical presentation [70]. Within the WIfI classification, it seems that wound status is the strongest predictor of

Table 8.5 WIfI clinical stages

(a) Estimated risk of amputation at 1 year

	Ischaemia 0				Ischaemia 1				Ischaemia 2				Ischaemia 3			
Wound 0	VL	VL	L	M	VL	L	M	H	L	L	M	H	L	M	M	H
Wound 1	VL	VL	L	M	VL	L	M	H	L	M	H	H	M	M	H	H
Wound 2	L	L	M	H	M	M	H	H	M	H	H	H	H	H	H	H
Wound 3	M	M	H	H	H	H	H	H	H	H	H	H	H	H	H	H
	fI 0	fI1	fI2	fI3	fI 0	fI1	fI2	fI3	fI 0	fI1	fI2	fI3	fI 0	fI1	fI2	fI3

(b). Estimated likelihood of benefit of revascularization (assuming infection can be controlled first)

	Ischaemia 0				Ischaemia 1				Ischaemia 2				Ischaemia 3			
Wound 0	VL	VL	VL	VL	VL	L	L	M	L	L	M	M	M	H	H	H
Wound 1	VL	VL	VL	VL	L	M	M	M	M	H	H	H	H	H	H	H
Wound 2	VL	VL	VL	VL	M	M	H	H	H	H	H	H	H	H	H	H
Wound 3	VL	VL	VL	VL	M	M	H	H	H	H	H	H	H	H	H	H
	fI 0	fI1	fI2	fI3	fI 0	fI1	fI2	fI3	fI 0	fI1	fI2	fI3	fI 0	fI1	fI2	fI3

VL = Very low benefit

L = Low benefit

M = Moderate benefit

H = High benefit

Very Low (VL) risk of amputation = Clinical Stage 1

Low (L) risk of amputation = Clinical Stage 2

Moderate (M) risk of amputation = Clinical Stage 3

High (H) risk of amputation = Clinical Stage 4

Unsalvageable limb = Clinical Stage 5

Unsalvageable limb = Clinical Stage 5

fI, foot Infection

amputation risk. This is likely because, unlike infection or ischaemia which can often be treated directly, wound healing is complex and depends on controlling these other factors, along with offloading and proper wound care [33].

8.5 Principles of Management of Diabetes-Related Foot Complications

The goals of treatment of the patient with a DRFU are to achieve wound healing, improve quality of life, avoid amputations and prevent ulcer recurrence. In order to achieve these goals, establishment of a multidisciplinary team is considered to be the best practice strategy [12, 71]. This integrated approach acknowledges that no one specialist possesses all the expertise and knowledge to manage the patient. In particular, the management of patients with chronic and complex wounds requires input from a number of healthcare professionals. The multidisciplinary team may include, but is not limited to, podiatrists, vascular specialists, orthopaedic surgeons, endocrine specialists, infectious disease specialists, diabetes educator, wound care nurses, orthotists, and radiologists.

At initial clinical assessment of a patient with a DRFU, a decision needs to be made whether the patient is suitable for outpatient management or if admission to hospital is required for intravenous antibiotics, surgical debridement and/or revascularisation. The principles of management of patients with diabetes and foot ulcers include offloading, wound management, management of infection and revascularisation if required.

8.5.1 Offloading

Patients with diabetes should wear appropriate footwear that fits, protects and accommodates the shape of their feet in order to prevent ulceration [40]. For patients with a plantar DRFU, prescription of appropriate offloading devices to heal the ulcer is recommended. There are numerous products available to assist in redistributing pressure over a larger weight-bearing area, thus providing offloading.

The gold standard for treating neuropathic plantar ulcers is the use of non-removable, knee-high offloading devices [40, 72]. Evidence supports that these devices, which patients cannot remove, are associated with faster ulcer healing compared to removable options [73]. However, in situations where frequent wound care or wound review is required (such as ischaemic or heavily exudating ulcers) or when active infection is present, non-removable offloading devices are not suitable, and a removable knee-high walker may be considered. When knee-high devices are contraindicated or not tolerated by people with DRFU, other offloading devices such as an ankle-high offloading device, cast shoe, or custom-made temporary shoe should be considered [40, 72]. When removable offloading devices are prescribed, potential issues with patient adherence must be anticipated and strategies put in place to improve patient compliance [13].

Elective foot surgery can be considered for recalcitrant forefoot plantar ulcers and to prevent ulcer recurrence in high-risk patients. Procedures may include Achilles tendon lengthening (for plantar metatarsal head ulcers), digital flexor tenotomy (for toe apical ulcers with flexible toe deformity), joint arthroplasty (for neuropathic hallux ulcers), or metatarsal head resection (for plantar metatarsal head ulcers) [40].

Once a plantar ulcer is healed, the use of footwear that has a demonstrated plantar pressure relieving effect during walking is indicated to reduce the risk of re-ulceration. Offloading for non-plantar ulcer depends on the type and location of the wound and various modalities can be considered, including shoe modifications, temporary footwear, toe spacers and orthoses [40].

8.5.2 *Wound Management*

In individuals with diabetes, wound healing challenges arise from a complex interplay of pathophysiological factors. These include perfusion deficit due to macrovascular and microvascular disease, neuropathic dysfunction, immunological compromise and the presence of critical colonisation/infection [74]. More details about the pathophysiology of wound healing are described in Chap. 7 (Pathophysiology of Wound Healing).

The basic principle of wound management involves regular cleaning with sterile water or saline, debridement if necessary to remove debris, slough, necrotic and infected matter from the wound surface, and dressings with the aim of controlling exudate and creating a clean wound bed to promote wound healing. Debridement may be undertaken using physical (e.g. surgical, sharp or hydrodebridement), biological (larvae), autolytic (hydrogels) or biochemical (enzymes) methods [75, 76].

Depending on the severity of the foot wound, urgent surgical debridement may be required for drainage of necrotic tissue and/or pus. This also permits adequate assessment of the extent of infection and enables deep specimen(s) to be obtained for culture to determine the causative organisms and their antibiotic sensitivities. As a general rule, all necrotic and infected tissue should be removed, ensuring that no bone is left exposed, while leaving part of the wound open to allow drainage [74].

Bone resection and minor amputation are often necessary when osteomyelitis, extensive soft tissue necrosis, and/or deep abscess are present. Minor amputation may consist of simple removal of a toe, ray amputation (toe and metatarsal), or transmetatarsal amputation. Once the infection is under control and the necessary surgical drainage/debridement has been performed, attention to the long-term function of the foot is a key issue. Patients who have undergone previous surgeries or amputations may have biomechanical consequences that can potentially result in an unstable foot or lead to a foot prone to re-ulceration [77]. A previous systematic review of re-amputation following partial first ray amputation found that 1 in 5 participants had undergone a subsequent amputation due to neuropathic DRFU in the 26-month follow-up time. Approximately 40% of amputations involved the lesser digits [78]. This is consistent with evidence of increased plantar pressures under the lesser metatarsals following hallux amputation, with development of lesser digital deformity contributing to increased risk of ulceration and amputation of the second and third digits and metatarsophalangeal joints [79]. These changes are proposed to occur as a result of transference of weight-bearing to the lesser metatarsophalangeal joints (MTPJs), subsequent structural changes, and biomechanical changes to foot function that develop as a result of the index amputation or are pre-existing [80–82]. For example, limited ankle dorsiflexion has previously been associated with increased forefoot plantar pressures and neuropathic DRFU in diabetes populations [83]. Transmetatarsal amputation has been found to be associated with increased forefoot plantar pressures compared to the unaffected limb, with participants walking with restricted maximum dynamic ankle dorsiflexion [84]. These findings highlight the critical need to address biomechanical consequences of amputation to prevent a need for re-amputation. To this end, surgical and conservative interventions to reduce pre-existing and post-surgical risk factors for post-amputation DRFU and re-amputation have been suggested to minimise the risk of complications and improve long-term outcomes [85]. Such interventions, including digital flexor tenotomy for DRFU secondary to flexible digital deformity, are currently recommended for neuropathic DRFU where non-surgical offloading therapies have failed.

Wound care is an essential aspect in the management of DRFUs and post-operative wounds. There are several types of dressings available from basic wound contact dressings to more advanced gels, films, and antimicrobial dressings. Dressings serve multiple purposes: managing wound exudate, maintaining a warm, moist environment for healing, controlling microbial growth, protecting the wound and promoting healing [86].

Research suggests that sucrose octasulphate dressings, when applied to non-infected neuro-ischaemic foot ulcers, can enhance wound healing compared to non-interactive dressings. The potassium salt in these dressings interacts with the wound environment, inhibiting excessive matrix metalloproteinases (MMPs) and restoring the biological activity of growth factors [87]. Based on this evidence, the IWGDF recommends considering these dressings for neuro-ischaemic foot ulcers showing insufficient improvement with standard care [75].

Negative pressure wound therapy (NPWT) is commonly used for complex wounds, as it is thought to promote healing via physical and biological mechanisms [75]. While previous reports have suggested NPWT offers benefits in both healing time and the proportion of healed post-operative wounds in the foot with diabetes [88], a recent randomised controlled trial presented a contrasting view. This trial, which assessed healing by secondary intention for surgical wounds (predominantly in patients with diabetes and foot wounds), found no evidence that NPWT reduced wound healing time compared to standard dressings selected by the clinical care team [89].

Hyperbaric oxygen therapy (HBOT) has been suggested to improve oxygen supply to wounds and therefore has been used as an adjunctive therapy to normal wound care in DRFCs. Treatment involves placing the patient in a compression chamber, increasing the environmental pressure within the chamber, and administering 100% oxygen for respiration. In this way, it is possible to deliver an increased partial pressure of oxygen to the tissues. Although some evidence suggests HBOT may offer benefits in promoting wound healing and reducing ulcer size, conclusive evidence of its effectiveness in preventing amputations is still lacking [76, 90, 91]. The

IWGDF recommends that HBOT might be considered as adjunct therapy where standard of care alone has failed [75].

Topical oxygen therapy (TOT) is emerging as a promising therapeutic approach for enhancing wound healing, with a growing body of evidence supporting its efficacy [92, 93]. This treatment modality works by increasing oxygen levels directly at the wound site, thereby creating an environment that promotes tissue repair [94]. Unlike HBOT, TOT offers the significant advantage of being easily administered by patients in their own homes, improving accessibility.

Poor nutritional status is common among patients with diabetes and foot ulcers. A recent study demonstrated that most individuals with DRFU do not meet dietary consensus guidelines for nutrients such as protein, fibre, zinc, vitamins E and A, which all potentially impact wound healing capacity [95]. In addition, reports have demonstrated very high levels of micronutrient deficiencies, including vitamin C, in this population [96]. Despite the known importance of nutrition for wound healing, the role of nutrition therapy in promoting wound healing in DRFUs is still not clear due to lack of good quality RCTs [76, 97].

8.5.3 Management of Infection

While most DRFIs are relatively superficial at presentation, microorganisms can spread contiguously to subcutaneous tissues, including fascia, tendons, muscle, joints and bone, and infection can become limb- or life-threatening [98].

The system proposed by the Infectious Diseases Society of America, which is incorporated into the WIfI classification, categorises the severity of infection in the foot with diabetes. Infection severity guides the choice of the empiric antibiotic regimen and its route of administration and helps the clinician to determine the need for hospitalisation, the requirement and timing for surgery and influence the likelihood of amputation. Table 8.6 describes features associated with more serious foot infection and a potential need for admission to hospital. Mild infections are usually treated with oral antibiotics while limb- and life-threatening infections requires intravenous antibiotic therapy and may need surgical debridement.

The empirical antibiotic regimen should be based on the anticipated spectrum of infecting organisms and local protocol. *S. aureus* and beta-haemolytic streptococci are widely recognised as common pathogens in acute DRFIs. In chronic wounds, especially in the setting of prior antimicrobial therapy, infections are more frequently polymicrobial and the causative pathogens are more diverse, often including aerobic gram-negative bacilli and obligate anaerobic bacteria [99]. A major problem in treating DRFIs has been the increased rate of isolation of antibiotic-resistant pathogens, particularly methicillin-resistant *S. aureus* (MRSA). Therefore, depending on patient risk and local prevalence of MRSA, an antimicrobial agent active against these bacteria should be added to the empirical regimen.

It is of paramount importance to collect and process specimens for culture appropriately. Superficial wound swabs are easy to obtain; however, they frequently grow contaminants and are less likely to yield the true pathogens. Specimens should be

Table 8.6 Characteristics suggesting a more serious diabetes-related foot infection and potential need for hospital admission

Wound specific	
Wound	Penetrates to subcutaneous tissues (e.g. fascia, tendon, muscle, joint or bone)
Cellulitis	Extensive, >2 cm distant from ulceration or rapidly progressive
Local signs	Severe inflammation or induration, crepitus, bullae, discoloration, necrosis, or gangrene, ecchymoses or petechiae, new anaesthesia
General	
Presentation	Acute onset/worsening or rapidly progressive
Systemic signs	Leukocytosis, very high C-reactive protein or erythrocyte sedimentation rate, severe/worsening hyperglycaemia, acidosis, deterioration of renal function, electrolyte abnormalities
Complicating features	Presence of a foreign body, puncture wound, deep abscess, arterial or venous insufficiency, lymphoedema, immunosuppressive illness or treatment, lack of home support, and unable to comply with the required outpatient treatment regimen
Current treatment	Progression while on apparently appropriate antibiotic and appropriate supportive therapy

Adapted from IWGDF—Guidelines on the diagnosis and treatment of diabetes-related foot infections (2023) [57]

obtained only after cleansing and debriding the wound and ideally should include tissue obtained by curettage or biopsy [57, 99].

In some chronic infections, such as osteomyelitis, if it is safe, it is advisable to discontinue antibiotic therapy for a period of time (for at least a few days, and ideally for at least 2 weeks) before obtaining deep cultures because prior antibiotic therapy can cause false-negative results [57, 100].

Surgery remains a cornerstone of treatment for many deep infections. Bone resection and minor amputations are often required when there is osteomyelitis or extensive soft tissue infection. The 2023 IWGDF/IDSA guidelines recommend utilising cultures obtained from "marginal" or "proximal" bone tissue to inform the duration of antibiotic therapy following minor amputations in cases of diabetes-related foot infections [57]. However, the clinical utility of this recommendation has been questioned. Concerns have been raised regarding the lack of standardisation in obtaining bone specimens, the potential for false-positive results due to contamination of the surgical field, the possibility of false-negative results due to prior antibiotic administration, and the absence of a clear correlation between positive cultures and patient outcomes. While some advocate for the use of bone biopsies for histological examination, there is currently no robust evidence demonstrating a clear benefit of bone biopsy results on patient outcomes in the context of diabetes-related foot osteomyelitis treatment. Furthermore, the potential delay in obtaining biopsy results and the documented low inter-rater agreement among pathologists in diagnosing osteomyelitis based on histopathology limit its practical application in routine clinical practice [57, 101].

Table 8.7 summarises the IWGDF recommendations for the duration of antibiotic treatment according to the clinical presentation.

Table 8.7 Suggested route, setting, and duration of antibiotic therapy, by clinical presentation

Site of infection, by severity or extent	Route of administration	Setting	Duration of therapy
Soft tissue only			
Mild	Oral	Outpatient	1–2 weeks
Moderate/severe	Oral/initial parenteral	Outpatient / inpatient	2–4 weeks
Bone or joint			
No residual infected tissue (e.g. post-amputation)	Oral/initially IV	Inpatient, then outpatient	2–5 days
Residual infected soft tissue (but not bone)	Oral/initially IV	Inpatient, then outpatient	1–2 weeks
Positive culture or histology of bone margin after bone resection	Oral/initially IV	Inpatient, then outpatient	3 weeks
No surgery, or residual dead bone post-operatively	Oral/initially IV	Inpatient, then outpatient	6 weeks

Adapted from 2023 IWGDF/IDSA guidelines on the diagnosis and treatment of diabetes-related foot infections [57]

Management of osteomyelitis has been an area of controversy, particularly in relation to selection of patients for non-operative management and duration of antibiotic treatment if surgery is not performed. Traditionally, osteomyelitis has been treated with a prolonged (≥ 3 months) course of antibiotics. However, more recent trials have demonstrated that a shorter period of treatment (6 weeks) may be as effective and associated with significantly fewer adverse effects related to antibiotics such as diarrhoea [102]. As a result, the IWGDF guidelines recommend 6 weeks of antibiotic therapy for patients who do not undergo resection of infected bone [57]. A key issue is to appropriately select patients for non-operative management. Patients in whom infection is confined to a small, forefoot lesion; without severe or necrotising soft-tissue infections or peripheral arterial disease are more likely to benefit from non-surgical treatment. Other factors such as fitness for surgery, likely foot function if surgery is undertaken and patient preference needs to be considered when deciding treatment [103].

8.5.4 Lower Limb Arterial Revascularisation

All patients with DRFU should be evaluated for the presence of PAD at the time of presentation by clinical assessment and basic non-invasive perfusion testing. Subsequently, it is important to determine if PAD is of sufficient severity to contribute to delayed wound healing and increased risk of amputation. The WIfI classification system helps the clinician in estimating the potential benefit of revascularisation. If revascularisation is being considered, anatomical information on the arteries of the lower limb should be obtained to assess the presence, severity, and distribution of arterial stenoses or occlusions. Modalities that can be used to obtain anatomical information include arterial duplex ultrasound, computed tomographic angiography, magnetic resonance angiography, or intra-arterial digital subtraction angiography.

The aim of revascularisation in the patient with DRFU is to treat the perfusion deficit by restoring direct flow to at least one of the foot arteries. If an endovascular approach is undertaken, the target artery should preferably be the one supplying the specific anatomical region (angiosome) where the wound is located [31]. The level of perfusion required to heal a foot ulcer depends on multiple factors such as ulcer size and location, presence/extent of gangrene and infection [104]. A patient with a shallow, uninfected toe ulcer may need less perfusion to heal the foot, while a patient with extensive tissue necrosis is likely to require a much better perfusion to achieve wound healing [104]. As a general rule, revascularisation should aim to provide in-line flow to the foot whenever possible.

The decision regarding the revascularisation technique is complex and the clinician must take into consideration morphology and length of the arterial lesion, availability of autogenous venous conduit, patient comorbidities and team expertise.

Patients with Chronic Limb-Threatening Ischaemia (CLTI)—which includes patients with diabetes-related foot ulcer and perfusion deficit—are a heterogeneous group with varying degrees of limb threat, comorbidities and anatomical complexities of occlusive disease. Recent landmark trials, BEST-CLI and BASIL-2, offer important insights into optimal treatment strategies [105, 106]. BEST-CLI demonstrated that in patients with infra-inguinal disease suitable for both surgical and endovascular interventions, surgery using the single segment of great saphenous vein (GSV) conduit surpasses endovascular approaches. However, when a single segment of usable GSV is unavailable, outcomes are comparable [105]. Conversely, BASIL-2 showed that, in CLTI cases secondary to infrapopliteal disease, endovascular treatment outperforms vein bypass in reducing mortality and major amputations [106]. These trial results underscore the critical importance for vascular specialists to develop and maintain expertise in both bypass and endovascular techniques, enabling them to tailor treatment plans to individual patient needs.

In addition to revascularisation, aggressive medical therapy and cardiovascular risk management, including support for cessation of smoking, treatment of hypertension and prescription of a statin and antiplatelets, should be ensured in patients with diabetes and PAD [31, 37]. A detailed assessment and treatment algorithm of managing patients with CLTI can be found on the Global Vascular Guidelines on management of Chronic Limb-Threatening Ischaemia [37] and the intersocietal IWGDF, ESVS, SVS guidelines on peripheral artery disease in people with diabetes mellitus and a foot ulcer [31]. Figure 8.1 illustrates a suggested approach to assessment and initial management of patients with DRFUs.

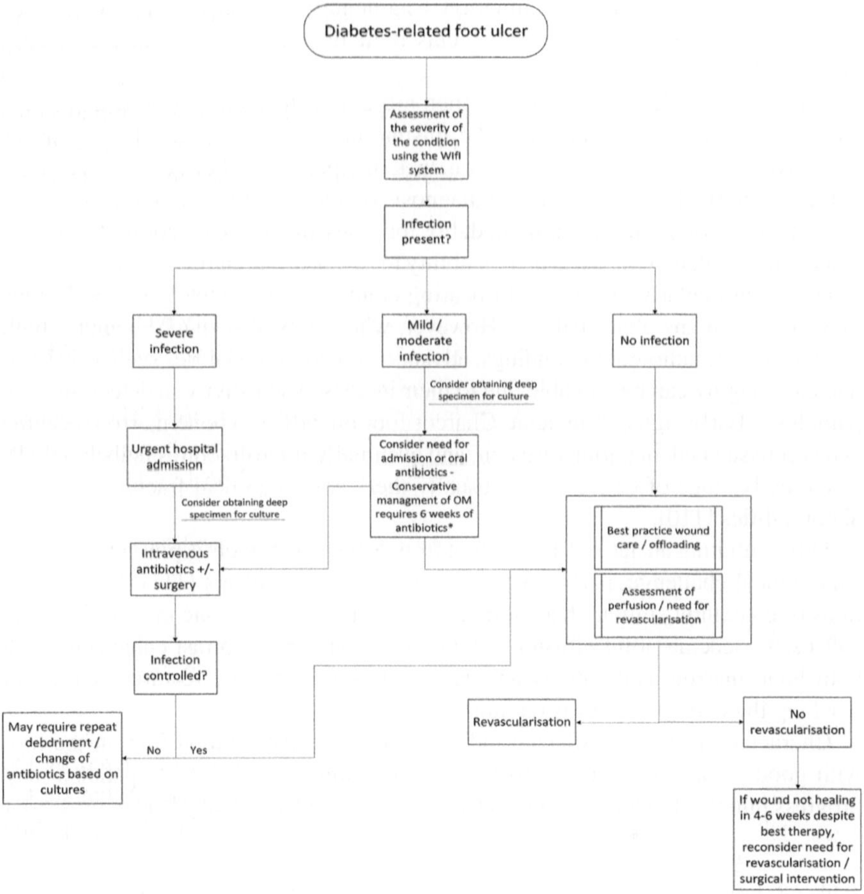

Fig. 8.1 A systematic approach to the assessment and management of diabetes related foot complications. (Modified from Jeffcoate et al. [18], *according to Senneville É et al. [57])

8.6 Charcot Neuroarthropathy (CNO)

Charcot neuroarthropathy is a relatively common complication occurring in 1–2% of patients with diabetes and neuropathy. It is most often unilateral (80% of cases) and is characterised by pathological fractures, joint dislocation, deformity and severe destruction of the foot [107]. It has serious implications for the patient as it may result in significant deformity, ulceration, and subsequent limb loss. The presence of ulceration in a patient with CNO dramatically elevates the risk of limb loss, increasing it by a factor of six [108].

The pathogenesis of CNO appears to be multifactorial, with a genetic predisposition, altered levels of neuropeptides (calcitonin gene-related peptide and nitric oxide) in the foot, an increase in inflammatory cytokines, and a disorder of bone turnover all contributing [109]. The natural progression of Charcot foot is marked by distinct stages: inflammation, fragmentation, coalescence, and consolidation. These stages can be further classified into active and inactive disease phases [110].

A patient with acute Charcot foot often presents with a warm, swollen, and erythematous foot and this can easily be misinterpreted as acute infection, gout, or osteomyelitis. The absence of ulceration, lack of other signs of infection and a WCC within the normal range favours the diagnosis of acute CNO over an infective process. X-ray is the initial imaging modality for assessment of Charcot foot. The primary value of plain X-rays lies in their ability to assess the alignment and relationship of bones, particularly under weight-bearing conditions. In the early stages, X-rays may not reveal any abnormalities. However, when clinical suspicion remains high despite normal radiographic findings, advanced imaging modalities such as MRI or nuclear imaging can be valuable due to their increased sensitivity in detecting bone pathology. Early signs of an acute Charcot foot on MRI are bone marrow oedema and soft tissue oedema, joint effusion, and eventually microfractures (subchondral). In the early stage of Charcot foot, usually there are no cortical fractures or gross abnormalities [110].

Differentiating an active Charcot foot from acute osteomyelitis presents a significant clinical challenge, particularly in patients with foot ulcers [111]. Both conditions often exhibit similar characteristics on MRI, including bone marrow oedema, soft tissue oedema, joint effusions, fluid collections, and contrast enhancement in both bone marrow and soft tissues. However, some imaging features can aid in reaching the correct diagnosis (summarised in Table 8.8) [110].

Characteristically, the affected individual has preserved blood flow in the foot with good pedal pulses. Repetitive cumulative injuries to insensate patients may progress into the destructive stage of Charcot arthropathy and may lead to gross foot

Table 8.8 Features on MRI to help differentiate active Charcot from osteomyelitis

	Active Charcot	Osteomyelitis
Location of bone abnormality	Tends to be periarticular Usually involves several joints and bones (most commonly Tarso-metatarsal joints and metatarsophalangeal joints)	Tends to involve a single bone with diffuse marrow involvement Typically develops through the continuous spread of infection from existing skin ulceration and sinus tracts.
Sinus tract	Usually not present	Usually present
Ghost sign (bones that "disappear" on T1-weighted images and "reappear" after contrast administration (or T2-weighted images)	Negative	Positive
Other features	Presence of subchondral cysts and intra-articular bodies	Subchondral cysts and intra-articular bodies tend to disappear in the setting of infection

deformity. The hallmark deformity of this condition is midfoot collapse, described as a "rocker-bottom" foot. The process leading to gross deformities of the foot and/or ankle is relatively painless given the neuropathy [110].

The most important strategies for management of active Charcot foot are early diagnosis, offloading and immobilisation. The use of a non-removable knee-high device to immobilise and offload the foot and prevent foot deformity is considered the treatment of choice. This can be achieved with a total contact cast (TCC) or a knee-high walker rendered non-removable. A removable knee-high device should be considered when a non-removable device is contraindicated or not tolerated. In addition, use of assistive devices can be helpful to reduce weight bearing in the affected limb [112].

Patients with active CNO should be informed that remission may take several months. Clinical experience suggests that offloading be continued for four to six weeks after the clinical signs of active CNO have resolved and the patient is deemed to be in remission [112].

While antiresorptive therapies such as bisphosphonates and calcitonin have been explored in the acute phase of CNO, conclusive evidence supporting their benefit remains elusive. IWGDF advises against the use of alendronate, pamidronate, zoledronate, calcitonin, parathyroid hormone, or methylprednisolone in the treatment of active CNO in individuals with diabetes and intact skin. They also suggest against the use of denosumab in this patient population. However, the IWGDF does recommend evaluating the need for vitamin D and calcium supplementation during the fracture healing phase in patients with diabetes and active CNO. The suggested dosages should align with established guidelines for individuals at risk for vitamin D deficiency or with insufficient calcium intake [112].

After the TCC has been removed, different offloading modalities can be used, including the Charcot restraint orthotic walker (CROW). Surgical procedures may be performed to correct bone alignment, excise exostoses and relieve area of high pressure. The goal for treatment for patients with chronic Charcot changes is to maintain a stable foot free from ulceration and infection, which frequently requires significant orthopaedic, podiatry, and orthotics input [113].

8.7 Prevention

Diabetes-related foot complications are potentially preventable, and every effort should be made to ensure that high-risk patients are identified and receive early treatment of foot complications. The IWGDF emphasises the importance of prevention of foot problems [39]. Successful efforts to prevent and treat foot complications in diabetes depend upon a well-organised multidisciplinary approach. Ideally, a foot care programme should provide the following:

1. Education for people with diabetes, their caregivers and for healthcare staff.
2. A system to detect all high-risk patients.

3. Measures to reduce risk of foot ulceration, such as podiatric maintenance care and appropriate footwear.
4. Prompt and effective treatment of any foot complication.
5. Focussed care of patients in remission to maximise ulcer-free, hospital-free and activity-rich days.
6. Auditing all aspects of DRFU care to identify problems and ensure that local practice meets accepted standards of care.

DRFU should be seen as a chronic potentially limb-threatening condition and strategies should be designed to meet the needs of patients requiring chronic care, rather than simply responding to acute problems when they occur. Responsive preventive strategies should aim to provide an efficient and cost-effective solution to a challenging and costly disease process.

8.8 Conclusion

Foot complications in diabetes are a major public health challenge worldwide and one of the 15 major causes of disability worldwide [114]. Unfortunately, the number of people with diabetes affected by foot pathology is likely to continue to rise due to the epidemiologic factors of population ageing and the globally increasing incidence of diabetes.

The prevention of DRFU is essential to reduce the risks to the patient and the resultant economic burden to society. Once an ulcer has developed, the management is complex and requires a multidisciplinary team approach to optimise outcomes. Treatment should be evidence-based and may include offloading, wound management, management of infection and revascularisation.

Significant and exciting advances in the management of diabetes-related foot complications have occurred in the past decades. There has been the development and implementation of international treatment guidelines for the foot with diabetes, such as the IWGDF guidelines, and growing implementation of diabetes foot care programs across the globe. There is now a better understanding of the pathophysiology of DRFCs, which allows the development of therapeutic interventions.

There are innovative technologies, such as negative pressure wound therapy and endovascular interventions, that have been adopted and have changed the management of DRFCs. This is an evolving field and there are several new technologies which have the potential to improve outcomes of patients with foot complications.

Despite all the recent advances, much remains to be done. Continuous investment in prevention, management, and research of the DRFC syndrome is of paramount importance.

Multiple Choice Questions

1. According to the WIfI criteria, a Toe pressure (TP) measurement <30 mmHg corresponds to which grade of ischaemia?

   (a) Grade 0
   (b) Grade1
   (c) Grade 3
   (d) Grade 3
   (e) Grade 4

   Answer: (d) Grade 3

2. The pathogenesis of diabetes-related peripheral neuropathy is complex and multifactorial. Which of the following is a metabolic abnormality implicated in its development?

   (a) Up-regulation of adhesion molecules such as VCAM-1
   (b) Arteriolar shunting in the peripheral circulation
   (c) Microvascular disease in the vasa vasorum
   (d) De-activation of the hexosamine pathway and protein kinase C (PKC) isoforms
   (e) Malfunction of polyol metabolism

   Answer: (e) Malfunction of polyol metabolism

References

1. NCD Risk Factor Collaboration. Worldwide trends in diabetes since 1980: a pooled analysis of 751 population-based studies with 4·4 million participants. Lancet. 2016;387:1513–30. https://doi.org/10.1016/S0140-6736(16)00618-8.
2. International Diabetes Federation. IDF Diabetes Atlas 2025. Available from: https://diabetesatlas.org
3. NCD Risk Factor Collaboration. Worldwide trends in diabetes prevalence and treatment from 1990 to 2022: a pooled analysis of 1108 population-representative studies with 141 million participants. Lancet. 2024;404:2077–93. https://doi.org/10.1016/s0140-6736(24)02317-1.
4. Van Netten JJ, Bus SA, Apelqvist J, Chen P, Chuter V, Fitridge R, et al. Definitions and criteria for diabetes-related foot disease (IWGDF 2023 update). Diabetes Metab Res Rev. 2024;40:e3654. https://doi.org/10.1002/dmrr.3654.
5. Singh N, Armstrong DG, Lipsky BA. Preventing foot ulcers in patients with diabetes. JAMA. 2005;293:217–28. https://doi.org/10.1001/jama.293.2.217.
6. Armstrong DG, Tan T-W, Boulton AJ, Bus SA. Diabetic foot ulcers: a review. JAMA. 2023;330:62–75. https://doi.org/10.1001/jama.2023.10578.
7. Driver VR, Fabbi M, Lavery LA, Gibbons G. The costs of diabetic foot: the economic case for the limb salvage team. J Am Podiatr Med Assoc. 2010;100:335–41. https://doi.org/10.7547/1000335.

8. Petrakis I, Kyriopoulos IJ, Ginis A, Athanasakis K. Losing a foot versus losing a dollar; a systematic review of cost studies in diabetic foot complications. Expert Rev Pharmacoecon Outcomes Res. 2017;17:165–80. https://doi.org/10.1080/14737167.2017.1305891.
9. Boulton AJ, Vileikyte L, Ragnarson-Tennvall G, Apelqvist J. The global burden of diabetic foot disease. Lancet. 2005;366:1719–24. https://doi.org/10.1016/s0140-6736(05)67698-2.
10. Kamitani F, Nishioka Y, Noda T, Myojin T, Kubo S, Higashino T, et al. Incidence of lower limb amputation in people with and without diabetes: a nationwide 5-year cohort study in Japan. BMJ Open. 2021;11:e048436. https://doi.org/10.1136/bmjopen-2020-048436.
11. Walsh JW, Hoffstad OJ, Sullivan MO, Margolis DJ. Association of diabetic foot ulcer and death in a population-based cohort from the United Kingdom. Diabet Med. 2016;33:1493–8. https://doi.org/10.1111/dme.13054.
12. Apelqvist J, Larsson J. What is the most effective way to reduce incidence of amputation in the diabetic foot? Diabetes Metab Res Rev. 2000;16(Suppl 1):S75–83. https://doi.org/10.1002/1520-7560(200009/10)16:1+<::aid-dmrr139>3.0.co;2-8.
13. Armstrong DG, Boulton AJM, Bus SA. Diabetic foot ulcers and their recurrence. N Engl J Med. 2017;376:2367–75. https://doi.org/10.1056/NEJMra1615439.
14. Meshkin DH, Zolper EG, Chang K, Bryant M, Bekeny JC, Evans KK, et al. Long-term mortality after nontraumatic major lower extremity amputation: a systematic review and meta-analysis. J Foot Ankle Surg. 2021;60:567–76. https://doi.org/10.1053/j.jfas.2020.06.027.
15. Armstrong DG, Swerdlow MA, Armstrong AA, Conte MS, Padula WV, Bus SA. Five year mortality and direct costs of care for people with diabetic foot complications are comparable to cancer. J Foot Ankle Res. 2020;13:16. https://doi.org/10.1186/s13047-020-00383-2.
16. Yammine K, Hayek F, Assi C. A meta-analysis of mortality after minor amputation among patients with diabetes and/or peripheral vascular disease. J Vasc Surg. 2020;72:2197–207. https://doi.org/10.1016/j.jvs.2020.07.086.
17. Ghanassia E, Villon L, Thuan Dit Dieudonne JF, Boegner C, Avignon A, Sultan A. Long-term outcome and disability of diabetic patients hospitalized for diabetic foot ulcers: a 6.5-year follow-up study. Diabetes Care. 2008;31:1288–92. https://doi.org/10.2337/dc07-2145.
18. Jeffcoate W, Boyko EJ, Game F, Cowled P, Senneville E, Fitridge R. Causes, prevention, and management of diabetes-related foot ulcers. Lancet Diabetes Endocrinol. 2024;12:472–82. https://doi.org/10.1016/S2213-8587(24)00110-4.
19. Hicks CW, Selvin E. Epidemiology of peripheral neuropathy and lower extremity disease in diabetes. Curr Diab Rep. 2019;19:86. https://doi.org/10.1007/s11892-019-1212-8.
20. Sun J, Wang Y, Zhang X, Zhu S, He H. Prevalence of peripheral neuropathy in patients with diabetes: a systematic review and meta-analysis. Prim Care Diabetes. 2020;14:435–44. https://doi.org/10.1016/j.pcd.2019.12.005.
21. Sloan G, Selvarajah D, Tesfaye S. Pathogenesis, diagnosis and clinical management of diabetic sensorimotor peripheral neuropathy. Nature Rev Endocrinol. 2021;17:400–20. https://doi.org/10.1038/s41574-021-00496-z.
22. Elafros MA, Andersen H, Bennett DL, Savelieff MG, Viswanathan V, Callaghan BC, et al. Towards prevention of diabetic peripheral neuropathy: clinical presentation, pathogenesis, and new treatments. Lancet Neurol. 2022;21:922–36. https://doi.org/10.1016/S1474-4422(22)00188-0.
23. Dinh TL, Veves A. A review of the mechanisms implicated in the pathogenesis of the diabetic foot. Int J Low Extrem Wounds. 2005;4:154–9. https://doi.org/10.1177/1534734605280130.
24. van Schie CH, Vermigli C, Carrington AL, Boulton A. Muscle weakness and foot deformities in diabetes: relationship to neuropathy and foot ulceration in caucasian diabetic men. Diabetes Care. 2004;27:1668–73. https://doi.org/10.2337/diacare.27.7.1668.
25. Alam U, Riley DR, Jugdey RS, Azmi S, Rajbhandari S, D'Août K, et al. Diabetic neuropathy and gait: a review. Diabetes Ther. 2017;8:1253–64. https://doi.org/10.1007/s13300-017-0295-y.

26. Jude EB, Oyibo SO, Chalmers N, Boulton AJ. Peripheral arterial disease in diabetic and nondiabetic patients: a comparison of severity and outcome. Diabetes Care. 2001;24:1433–7. https://doi.org/10.2337/diacare.24.8.1433.
27. Prompers L, Huijberts M, Apelqvist J, Jude E, Piaggesi A, Bakker K, et al. High prevalence of ischaemia, infection and serious comorbidity in patients with diabetic foot disease in Europe. Baseline results from the Eurodiale study. Diabetologia. 2007;50:18–25. https://doi.org/10.1007/s00125-006-0491-1.
28. Prompers L, Schaper N, Apelqvist J, Edmonds M, Jude E, Mauricio D, et al. Prediction of outcome in individuals with diabetic foot ulcers: focus on the differences between individuals with and without peripheral arterial disease. The EURODIALE Study. Diabetologia. 2008;51:747–55. https://doi.org/10.1007/s00125-008-0940-0.
29. Graziani L, Silvestro A, Bertone V, Manara E, Andreini R, Sigala A, et al. Vascular involvement in diabetic subjects with ischemic foot ulcer: a new morphologic categorization of disease severity. Eur J Vasc Endovasc Surg. 2007;33:453–60. https://doi.org/10.1016/j.ejvs.2006.11.022.
30. Hinchliffe RJ, Brownrigg JR, Andros G, Apelqvist J, Boyko EJ, Fitridge R, et al. Effectiveness of revascularization of the ulcerated foot in patients with diabetes and peripheral artery disease: a systematic review. Diabetes Metab Res Rev. 2016;32(Suppl 1):136–44. https://doi.org/10.1002/dmrr.2705.
31. Fitridge R, Chuter V, Mills J, Hinchliffe R, Azuma N, Behrendt C-A, et al. The intersocietal IWGDF, ESVS, SVS guidelines on peripheral artery disease in people with diabetes mellitus and a foot ulcer. J Vasc Surg. 2023;78:1101–31. https://doi.org/10.1016/j.jvs.2023.07.020.
32. Forsythe RO, Brownrigg J, Hinchliffe RJ. Peripheral arterial disease and revascularization of the diabetic foot. Diabetes Obes Metab. 2015;17:435–44. https://doi.org/10.1111/dom.12422.
33. Pena G, Kuang B, Edwards S, Cowled P, Dawson J, Fitridge R. Factors associated with key outcomes in diabetes related foot disease: a prospective observational study. Eur J Vasc Endovasc Surg. 2021;62:233–40. https://doi.org/10.1016/j.ejvs.2021.04.002.
34. Dolan NC, Liu K, Criqui MH, Greenland P, Guralnik JM, Chan C, et al. Peripheral artery disease, diabetes, and reduced lower extremity functioning. Diabetes Care. 2002;25:113–20. https://doi.org/10.2337/diacare.25.1.113.
35. Mills JL Sr. Update and validation of the Society for Vascular Surgery wound, ischemia, and foot infection threatened limb classification system. Semin Vasc Surg. 2014;27:16–22. https://doi.org/10.1053/j.semvascsurg.2014.12.002.
36. Zhan LX, Branco BC, Armstrong DG, Mills JL Sr. The Society for Vascular Surgery lower extremity threatened limb classification system based on Wound, Ischemia, and foot Infection (WIfI) correlates with risk of major amputation and time to wound healing. J Vasc Surg. 2015;61:939–44. https://doi.org/10.1016/j.jvs.2014.11.045.
37. Conte MS, Bradbury AW, Kolh P, White JV, Dick F, Fitridge R, et al. Global vascular guidelines on the management of chronic limb-threatening ischemia. J Vasc Surg. 2019;69:3S–125S.e40. https://doi.org/10.1016/j.jvs.2019.02.016.
38. Sharma S, Schaper N, Rayman G. Microangiopathy: is it relevant to wound healing in diabetic foot disease? Diabetes Metab Res Rev 2020;36:e3244. https://doi.org/10.1002/dmrr.3244
39. Schaper NC, van Netten JJ, Apelqvist J, Bus SA, Fitridge R, Game F, et al. Practical guidelines on the prevention and management of diabetes-related foot disease (IWGDF 2023 update). Diabetes Metab Res Rev. 2024;40:e3657. https://doi.org/10.1002/dmrr.3657.
40. Bus SA, Armstrong DG, Crews RT, Gooday C, Jarl G, Kirketerp-Moller K, et al. Guidelines on offloading foot ulcers in persons with diabetes (IWGDF 2023 update). Diabetes Metab Res Rev. 2024;40:e3647. https://doi.org/10.1002/dmrr.3647.
41. Carter SA. Indirect systolic pressures and pulse waves in arterial occlusive diseases of the lower extremities. Circulation. 1968;37:624–37. https://doi.org/10.1161/01.cir.37.4.624.

42. Fowkes FG, Murray GD, Butcher I, Heald CL, Lee RJ, Chambless LE, et al. Ankle brachial index combined with Framingham risk score to predict cardiovascular events and mortality: a meta-analysis. JAMA. 2008;300:197–208. https://doi.org/10.1001/jama.300.2.197.
43. Nordanstig J, Behrendt C-A, Baumgartner I, Belch J, Bäck M, Fitridge R, et al. European Society for Vascular Surgery (ESVS) 2024 clinical practice guidelines on the management of asymptomatic lower limb peripheral arterial disease and intermittent claudication. Eur J Vasc Endovasc Surg. 2024;67:9–96. https://doi.org/10.1016/j.ejvs.2023.08.067.
44. Everhart JE, Pettitt DJ, Knowler WC, Rose FA, Bennett PH. Medial arterial calcification and its association with mortality and complications of diabetes. Diabetologia. 1988;31:16–23. https://doi.org/10.1007/BF00279127.
45. Chuter V, Schaper N, Hinchliffe R, Mills J, Azuma N, Behrendt CA, et al. Performance of non-invasive bedside vascular testing in the prediction of wound healing or amputation among people with foot ulcers in diabetes: a systematic review. Diabetes Metab Res Rev. 2024;40:e3701. https://doi.org/10.1002/dmrr.3701.
46. Brooks B, Dean R, Patel S, Wu B, Molyneaux L, Yue DK. TBI or not TBI: that is the question. Is it better to measure toe pressure than ankle pressure in diabetic patients? Diabet Med. 2001;18:528–32. https://doi.org/10.1046/j.1464-5491.2001.00493.x.
47. Widmer LW, Vikatmaa P, Aho P, Lepantalo M, Venermo M. Reliability and repeatability of toe pressures measured with laser Doppler and portable and stationary photoplethysmography devices. Ann Vasc Surg. 2012;26:404–10. https://doi.org/10.1016/j.avsg.2011.10.011.
48. Andersen CA. Noninvasive assessment of lower extremity hemodynamics in individuals with diabetes mellitus. J Vasc Surg. 2010;52:76s–80s. https://doi.org/10.1016/j.jvs.2010.06.012.
49. Kim ES, Sharma AM, Scissons R, Dawson D, Eberhardt RT, Gerhard-Herman M, et al. Interpretation of peripheral arterial and venous doppler waveforms: a consensus statement from the Society for Vascular Medicine and Society for Vascular Ultrasound. Vasc Med. 2020;25:484–506. https://doi.org/10.1177/1358863x20937665.
50. Strandness DE Jr, Schultz RD, Sumner DS, Rushmer RF. Ultrasonic flow detection. A useful technic in the evaluation of peripheral vascular disease. Am J Surg. 1967;113:311–20. https://doi.org/10.1016/0002-9610(67)90272-3.
51. Alavi A, Sibbald RG, Nabavizadeh R, Valaei F, Coutts P, Mayer D. Audible handheld Doppler ultrasound determines reliable and inexpensive exclusion of significant peripheral arterial disease. Vascular. 2015;23:622–9. https://doi.org/10.1177/1708538114568703.
52. Quigley FG, Faris IB. Transcutaneous oxygen tension measurements in the assessment of limb ischaemia. Clin Physiol. 1991;11:315–20. https://doi.org/10.1111/j.1475-097x.1991.tb00660.x.
53. Fife CE, Smart DR, Sheffield PJ, Hopf HW, Hawkins G, Clarke D. Transcutaneous oximetry in clinical practice: consensus statements from an expert panel based on evidence. Undersea Hyperb Med. 2009;36:43–53.
54. Belcaro G, Labropoulos N, Laurora G, Cesarone MR, De Sanctis MT, Incandela L. Laser Doppler skin perfusion pressure in normal and vascular subjects with rest pain: an universal measurement? J Cardiovasc Surg. 1994;35:7–9.
55. Castronuovo JJ Jr, Adera HM, Smiell JM, Price RM. Skin perfusion pressure measurement is valuable in the diagnosis of critical limb ischemia. J Vasc Surg. 1997;26:629–37. https://doi.org/10.1016/s0741-5214(97)70062-4.
56. Castronuovo JJ. Diagnosis of critical limb ischemia with skin perfusion pressure measurements. J Vasc Ultrasound. 1997;21:175–9.
57. Senneville É, Albalawi Z, van Asten SA, Abbas ZG, Allison G, Aragón-Sánchez J, et al. IWGDF/IDSA guidelines on the diagnosis and treatment of diabetes-related foot infections (IWGDF/IDSA 2023). Diabetes Metab Res Rev. 2024;40:e3687. https://doi.org/10.1002/dmrr.3687.

58. Cortes-Penfield NW, Armstrong DG, Brennan MB, Fayfman M, Ryder JH, Tan TW, et al. Evaluation and management of diabetes-related foot infections. Clin Infect Dis. 2023;77:e1–e13. https://doi.org/10.1093/cid/ciad255.
59. Berendt AR, Peters EJ, Bakker K, Embil JM, Eneroth M, Hinchliffe RJ, et al. Diabetic foot osteomyelitis: a progress report on diagnosis and a systematic review of treatment. Diabetes Metab Res Rev. 2008;24(Suppl 1):S145–61. https://doi.org/10.1002/dmrr.836.
60. Grayson ML, Gibbons GW, Balogh K, Levin E, Karchmer AW. Probing to bone in infected pedal ulcers. A clinical sign of underlying osteomyelitis in diabetic patients. JAMA. 1995;273:721–3.
61. Lavery LA, Armstrong DG, Peters EJ, Lipsky BA. Probe-to-bone test for diagnosing diabetic foot osteomyelitis: reliable or relic? Diabetes Care. 2007;30:270–4. https://doi.org/10.2337/dc06-1572.
62. Lam K, Van Asten SA, Nguyen T, La Fontaine J, Lavery LA. Diagnostic accuracy of probe to bone to detect osteomyelitis in the diabetic foot: a systematic review. Clin Infect Dis. 2016;63:944–8. https://doi.org/10.1093/cid/ciw445.
63. Wagner FW Jr. The dysvascular foot: a system for diagnosis and treatment. Foot Ankle. 1981;2:64–122.
64. Oyibo SO, Jude EB, Tarawneh I, Nguyen HC, Harkless LB, Boulton AJ. A comparison of two diabetic foot ulcer classification systems: the Wagner and the University of Texas wound classification systems. Diabetes Care. 2001;24:84–8. https://doi.org/10.2337/diacare.24.1.84.
65. Armstrong DG, Lavery LA, Harkless LB. Validation of a diabetic wound classification system. The contribution of depth, infection, and ischemia to risk of amputation. Diabetes Care. 1998;21:855–9. https://doi.org/10.2337/diacare.21.5.855.
66. Ince P, Abbas ZG, Lutale JK, Basit A, Ali SM, Chohan F, et al. Use of the SINBAD classification system and score in comparing outcome of foot ulcer management on three continents. Diabetes Care. 2008;31:964–7. https://doi.org/10.2337/dc07-2367.
67. Mills JL Sr, Conte MS, Armstrong DG, Pomposelli FB, Schanzer A, Sidawy AN, et al. The Society for Vascular Surgery Lower Extremity Threatened Limb Classification System: risk stratification based on wound, ischemia, and foot infection (WIfI). J Vasc Surg. 2014;59:220–34.e1–2. https://doi.org/10.1016/j.jvs.2013.08.003.
68. Darling JD, McCallum JC, Soden PA, Guzman RJ, Wyers MC, Hamdan AD, et al. Predictive ability of the Society for Vascular Surgery Wound, Ischemia, and foot Infection (WIfI) classification system after first-time lower extremity revascularizations. J Vasc Surg. 2017;65:695–704. https://doi.org/10.1016/j.jvs.2016.09.055.
69. Hicks CW, Canner JK, Karagozlu H, Mathioudakis N, Sherman RL, Black JH, et al. The Society for Vascular Surgery Wound, Ischemia, and foot Infection (WIfI) classification system correlates with cost of care for diabetic foot ulcers treated in a multidisciplinary setting. J Vasc Surg. 2018;67:1455–62. https://doi.org/10.1016/j.jvs.2017.08.090.
70. Cook IO, Mayor JM, Mills JL Sr. A review of WIfI clinical staging to predict outcomes in patients with threatened limbs. Ann Vasc Surg. 2024;107:146–53. https://doi.org/10.1016/j.avsg.2024.01.024.
71. Reiber GE, Raugi GJ. Preventing foot ulcers and amputations in diabetes. Lancet. 2005;366:1676–7. https://doi.org/10.1016/s0140-6736(05)67674-x.
72. Fernando ME, Horsley M, Jones S, Martin B, Nube VL, Charles J, et al. Australian guideline on offloading treatment for foot ulcers: part of the 2021 Australian evidence-based guidelines for diabetes-related foot disease. J Foot Ankle Res. 2022;15:31. https://doi.org/10.1186/s13047-022-00538-3
73. Lazzarini P, Armstrong D, Crews R, Gooday C, Jarl G, Kirketerp-Moller K, et al. Effectiveness of offloading interventions for people with diabetes-related foot ulcers: a systematic review and meta-analysis. Diabetes Metab Res Rev. 2024;40:e3650. https://doi.org/10.1002/dmrr.3650.

74. Dayya D, O'Neill OJ, Huedo-Medina TB, Habib N, Moore J, Iyer K. Debridement of diabetic foot ulcers. Adv Wound Care. 2022;11:666–86. https://doi.org/10.1089/wound.2021.0016.
75. Chen P, Vilorio NC, Dhatariya K, Jeffcoate W, Lobmann R, McIntosh C, et al. Guidelines on interventions to enhance healing of foot ulcers in people with diabetes (IWGDF 2023 update). Diabetes Metab Res Rev. 2024;40:e3644. https://doi.org/10.1002/dmrr.3644.
76. Chen P, Vilorio NC, Dhatariya K, Jeffcoate W, Lobmann R, McIntosh C, et al. Effectiveness of interventions to enhance healing of chronic foot ulcers in diabetes: a systematic review. Diabetes Metab Res Rev. 2024;40:e3786. https://doi.org/10.1002/dmrr.3786.
77. Lázaro-Martínez JL, Aragón-Sánchez J, Álvaro-Afonso FJ, García-Morales E, García-Álvarez Y, Molines-Barroso RJ. The best way to reduce reulcerations: if you understand biomechanics of the diabetic foot, you can do it. Int J Low Extrem Wounds. 2014;13:294–319. https://doi.org/10.1177/1534734614549417.
78. Borkosky SL, Roukis TS. Incidence of re-amputation following partial first ray amputation associated with diabetes mellitus and peripheral sensory neuropathy: a systematic review. Diabet Foot Ankle. 2012;3 https://doi.org/10.3402/dfa.v3i0.12169.
79. Lavery LA, Lavery DC, Quebedeax-Farnham TL. Increased foot pressures after great toe amputation in diabetes. Diabetes Care. 1995;18:1460–2. https://doi.org/10.2337/diacare.18.11.1460.
80. Boyko EJ, Ahroni JH, Cohen V, Nelson KM, Heagerty PJ. Prediction of diabetic foot ulcer occurrence using commonly available clinical information: the Seattle diabetic foot study. Diabetes Care. 2006;29:1202–7. https://doi.org/10.2337/dc05-2031.
81. Boffeli TJ, Bean JK, Natwick JR. Biomechanical abnormalities and ulcers of the great toe in patients with diabetes. J Foot Ankle Surg. 2002;41:359–64. https://doi.org/10.1016/s1067-2516(02)80081-3.
82. Oliver NG, Attinger CE, Steinberg JS, Evans KK, Vieweger D, Kim PJ. Influence of hallux rigidus on Reamputation in patients with diabetes mellitus after partial hallux amputation. J Foot Ankle Surg. 2015;54:1076–80. https://doi.org/10.1053/j.jfas.2015.06.007.
83. Searle A, Spink MJ, Ho A, Chuter VH. Association between ankle equinus and plantar pressures in people with diabetes. A systematic review and meta-analysis. Clin Biomech. 2017;43:8–14. https://doi.org/10.1016/j.clinbiomech.2017.01.021.
84. Garbalosa JC, Cavanagh PR, Wu G, Ulbrecht JS, Becker MB, Alexander IJ, et al. Foot function in diabetic patients after partial amputation. Foot Ankle Int. 1996;17:43–8. https://doi.org/10.1177/107110079601700110.
85. Lázaro-Martínez JL, Aragón-Sánchez J, Alvaro-Afonso FJ, García-Morales E, García-Álvarez Y, Molines-Barroso RJ. The best way to reduce reulcerations: if you understand biomechanics of the diabetic foot, you can do it. Int J Low Extrem Wounds. 2014;13:294–319. https://doi.org/10.1177/1534734614549417.
86. Hilton JR, Williams DT, Beuker B, Miller DR, Harding KG. Wound dressings in diabetic foot disease. Clin Infect Dis. 2004;39(Suppl 2):S100–3. https://doi.org/10.1086/383270.
87. Edmonds M, Lázaro-Martínez JL, Alfayate-García JM, Martini J, Petit J-M, Rayman G, et al. Sucrose octasulfate dressing versus control dressing in patients with neuroischaemic diabetic foot ulcers (explorer): an international, multicentre, double-blind, randomised, controlled trial. Lancet Diabetes Endocrinol. 2018;6:186–96. https://doi.org/10.1016/S2213-8587(17)30438-2.
88. Armstrong DG, Lavery LA. Negative pressure wound therapy after partial diabetic foot amputation: a multicentre, randomised controlled trial. Lancet. 2005;366:1704–10. https://doi.org/10.1016/s0140-6736(05)67695-7.
89. Arundel C, Mandefield L, Fairhurst C, Baird K, Gkekas A, Saramago P, et al. Negative pressure wound therapy versus usual care in patients with surgical wound healing by secondary intention in the UK (SWHSI-2): an open-label, multicentre, parallel-group, randomised controlled trial. Lancet. 2025;405:1689–99. https://doi.org/10.1016/S0140-6736(25)00143-6.

90. Santema KTB, Stoekenbroek RM, Koelemay MJW, Reekers JA, van Dortmont LMC, Oomen A, et al. Hyperbaric oxygen therapy in the treatment of ischemic lower- extremity ulcers in patients with diabetes: results of the DAMO2CLES Multicenter Randomized Clinical Trial. Diabetes Care. 2018;41:112–9. https://doi.org/10.2337/dc17-0654.
91. Kranke P, Bennett MH, Martyn-St James M, Schnabel A, Debus SE, Weibel S. Hyperbaric oxygen therapy for chronic wounds. Cochrane Database Syst Rev. 2015;2015:Cd004123. https://doi.org/10.1002/14651858.CD004123.pub4.
92. Carter MJ, Frykberg RG, Oropallo A, Sen CK, Armstrong DG, Nair HK, et al. Efficacy of topical wound oxygen therapy in healing chronic diabetic foot ulcers: systematic review and meta-analysis. Adv Wound Care. 2023;12:177–86. https://doi.org/10.1089/wound.2022.0041.
93. Frykberg RG, Franks PJ, Edmonds M, Brantley JN, Téot L, Wild T, et al. A multinational, multicenter, randomized, double-blinded, placebo-controlled trial to evaluate the efficacy of cyclical topical wound oxygen (TWO2) therapy in the treatment of chronic diabetic foot ulcers: the TWO2 study. Diabetes Care. 2020;43:616–24. https://doi.org/10.2337/dc19-0476.
94. Frykberg R, Andersen C, Chadwick P, Haser P, Janssen S, Lee A, et al. Use of topical oxygen therapy in wound healing. J Wound Care. 2023;32:S1–S32. https://doi.org/10.12968/jowc.2023.32.Sup8b.S1.
95. Donnelly HR, Clarke ED, Collins CE, Collins RA, Armstrong DG, Mills JL, et al. Most individuals with diabetes-related foot ulceration do not meet dietary consensus guidelines for wound healing. Int Wound J. 2024;21:e14483. https://doi.org/10.1111/iwj.14483.
96. Pena G, Kuang B, Cowled P, Howell S, Dawson J, Philpot R, et al. Micronutrient status in diabetic patients with foot ulcers. Adv Wound Care. 2020;9:9–15. https://doi.org/10.1089/wound.2019.0973.
97. Da Porto A, Miranda C, Brosolo G, Zanette G, Michelli A, Da Ros R. Nutritional supplementation on wound healing in diabetic foot: what is known and what is new? World J Diabetes. 2022;13:940. https://doi.org/10.4239/wjd.v13.i11.940.
98. Lipsky BA, Aragon-Sanchez J, Diggle M, Embil J, Kono S, Lavery L, et al. IWGDF guidance on the diagnosis and management of foot infections in persons with diabetes. Diabetes Metab Res Rev. 2016;32(Suppl 1):45–74. https://doi.org/10.1002/dmrr.2699.
99. Spichler A, Hurwitz BL, Armstrong DG, Lipsky BA. Microbiology of diabetic foot infections: from Louis Pasteur to 'crime scene investigation'. BMC Med. 2015;13:2. https://doi.org/10.1186/s12916-014-0232-0.
100. Berthol N, Robineau O, Boucher A, Blondiaux N, Beltrand E, Valette M, et al. Two-step sequential approach for concomitant skin and soft tissue infection and osteomyelitis complicating the diabetic foot. Diabetes Care. 2017;40:e170–1. https://doi.org/10.2337/dc17-1471.
101. Senneville E, Joulie D, Blondiaux N, Robineau O. Surgical techniques for bone biopsy in diabetic foot infection, and association between results and treatment duration. J Bone Jt Infect. 2020;5:198–204. https://doi.org/10.7150/jbji.45338.
102. Tone A, Nguyen S, Devemy F, Topolinski H, Valette M, Cazaubiel M, et al. Six-week versus twelve-week antibiotic therapy for nonsurgically treated diabetic foot osteomyelitis: a multicenter open-label controlled randomized study. Diabetes Care. 2015;38:302–7. https://doi.org/10.2337/dc14-1514.
103. Lipsky BA. Treating diabetic foot osteomyelitis primarily with surgery or antibiotics: have we answered the question? Diabetes Care. 2014;37:593–5. https://doi.org/10.2337/dc13-2510.
104. Mills JL. Lower limb ischaemia in patients with diabetic foot ulcers and gangrene: recognition, anatomic patterns and revascularization strategies. Diabetes Metab Res Rev. 2016;32(Suppl 1):239–45. https://doi.org/10.1002/dmrr.2753.

105. Farber A, Menard MT, Conte MS, Kaufman JA, Powell RJ, Choudhry NK, et al. Surgery or endovascular therapy for chronic limb-threatening ischemia. New Engl J Med. 2022;387:2305–16. https://doi.org/10.1056/NEJMoa2207899.
106. Bradbury AW, Moakes CA, Popplewell M, Meecham L, Bate GR, Kelly L, et al. A vein bypass first versus a best endovascular treatment first revascularisation strategy for patients with chronic limb threatening ischaemia who required an infra-popliteal, with or without an additional more proximal infra-inguinal revascularisation procedure to restore limb perfusion (BASIL-2): an open-label, randomised, multicentre, phase 3 trial. Lancet. 2023;401:1798–809. https://doi.org/10.1016/S0140-6736(23)00462-2.
107. Armstrong DG, Peters EJG. Charcot's arthropathy of the foot. J Am Podiatr Med Assoc. 2002;92:390–4. https://doi.org/10.7547/87507315-92-7-390.
108. Wukich DK, Sadoskas D, Vaudreuil NJ, Fourman M. Comparison of diabetic Charcot patients with and without foot wounds. Foot Ankle Int. 2017;38:140–8. https://doi.org/10.1177/1071100716673985.
109. Johnson-Lynn SE, McCaskie AW, Coll AP, Robinson AHN. Neuroarthropathy in diabetes: pathogenesis of Charcot arthropathy. Bone Joint Res. 2018;7:373–8. https://doi.org/10.1302/2046-3758.75.Bjr-2017-0334.R1.
110. Rosskopf AB, Loupatatzis C, Pfirrmann CW, Böni T, Berli MC. The Charcot foot: a pictorial review. Insights Imaging 2019;10:1–13. https://doi.org/10.1186/s13244-019-0768-9
111. Ahmadi ME, Morrison WB, Carrino JA, Schweitzer ME, Raikin SM, Ledermann HP. Neuropathic arthropathy of the foot with and without superimposed osteomyelitis: MR imaging characteristics. Radiology. 2006;238:622–31. https://doi.org/10.1148/radiol.2382041393.
112. Wukich DK, Schaper NC, Gooday C, Bal A, Bem R, Chhabra A, et al. Guidelines on the diagnosis and treatment of active Charcot neuro-osteoarthropathy in persons with diabetes mellitus (IWGDF 2023). Diabetes Metab Res Rev. 2024;40:e3646. https://doi.org/10.1002/dmrr.3646.
113. Trepman E, Nihal A, Pinzur MS. Current topics review: Charcot neuroarthropathy of the foot and ankle. Foot Ankle Int. 2005;26:46–63. https://doi.org/10.1177/107110070502600109.
114. Lazzarini PA, Raspovic KM, Meloni M, van Netten JJ. A new declaration for feet's sake: halving the global diabetic foot disease burden from 2% to 1% with next generation care. Diabetes Metab Res Rev. 2024;40:e3747. https://doi.org/10.1002/dmrr.3747.

Chapter 9
Pathophysiology and Principles of Management of Vascular Malformations

Iris Baumgartner

SN Flashcards
Test your learning and check your understanding of this book's contents: use the "Springer Nature Flashcards" app to access questions using ▶ https://sn.pub/wppvze. To use the app, please follow the instructions in Chap. 1.

Key Learning Points

- Vascular development and homeostasis are complex processes, and disruption can lead to congenital vascular malformation.
- Congenital vascular malformations are classified based on the type of vessels involved (i.e. capillary, venous, arteriovenous, lymphatic) and their flow characteristics (low flow or high flow).
- Endothelial dysfunction, endothelial-to-mesenchymal transition (EndMT) and altered interactions between endothelial cells, smooth muscle cells, and pericytes play a central role in vascular malformation formation and progression.
- Disruption of signalling pathways such as Transforming growth factor-beta (TGF-β), Vascular endothelial growth factor (VEGF), and Notch contributes to abnormal vessel development and instability, which are key in vascular malformations' pathophysiology.
- Congenital vascular malformations have a complex genetic basis. Understanding the molecular and cellular mechanisms behind haemodynamic and structural abnormalities is essential for developing targeted therapies.

I. Baumgartner (✉)
Internal Medicine and Vascular Medicine, Bern Center for Vascular Medicine and Interventions, Bern, Switzerland

R. Fitridge et al. (eds.), *Pathophysiology of Vascular Disease*, https://doi.org/10.1007/978-3-032-31459-8_9

- Classical treatment strategies vary based on the lesion type, location, and symptoms. Options range from conservative management and supportive care to more invasive treatments such as sclerotherapy, laser therapy, embolisation, and surgery.
- Targeted therapies are a promising area in treating congenital vascular malformations. Some therapies, like bevacizumab and sirolimus, are already in clinical use. Other therapies, such as alpelisib, trametinib, and gene therapy, are still under investigation. Ongoing research is needed to refine dosing, assess long-term efficacy, and improve patient outcomes.
- A multidisciplinary team is often necessary to create an individualised treatment plan for each patient.
- Regular follow-up is essential to monitor for recurrence or complications, especially in cases with large or complex malformations.

9.1 Introduction

Congenital vascular malformations (CVMs) represent a diverse group of disorders that involve abnormal growth of blood vessels. Unlike tumours, vascular malformations are not neoplastic, meaning they do not involve uncontrolled cell division and metastatic spread. Rather, these malformations are congenital, arising from errors in the development or patterning of the vascular system during embryogenesis. Malformations can involve various vessel types, including arteries, veins, capillaries, and lymphatic vessels. Clinically, CVM may present as visible cutaneous lesions or as deeper, more complicated vascular anomalies, which can lead to functional or life-threatening complications [1, 2].

To understand how these malformations arise, it is important to understand the complexity of normal blood vessel development. Vascular development is a highly regulated process that involves the formation of blood vessels from endothelial progenitor cells through a process known as vasculogenesis (formation of new vessels) and angiogenesis (formation of new branches from existing vessels). During embryogenesis, blood vessels are formed from endothelial cells (ECs), which then interact with surrounding smooth muscle cells (SMCs) and extracellular matrix components to form mature and functional blood vessels. In normal vascular development, ECs form tight junctions and are surrounded by SMCs that regulate blood flow [3, 4]. This process is tightly regulated by a balance of pro-angiogenic and anti-angiogenic signals, including vascular endothelial growth factor (VEGF), transforming growth factor-beta (TGF-β), and the Notch signalling pathway [5]. Vascular homeostasis, the maintenance of stable vessel function, requires continuous remodelling of the vasculature, responding to physiological cues such as shear stress, blood flow, and oxygen demand [6]. Disruptions in any of these processes can lead to structural and functional abnormalities in blood vessels, which are characteristic of vascular malformations [7].

9.2 Types of Vascular Malformations

CVMs are classified based on their haemodynamic properties (fast-flow and slow-flow lesions) and the type of vessels involved. They are typically divided into capillary malformation (CM), venous malformation (VM), arteriovenous malformation (AVM) and lymphatic malformation (LM). Some individuals may present with a combination of various types of vessels involved, leading to a more complex pathophysiological profile. For example, a person may have both AVM and VM, which complicates treatment and management. Moreover, vascular malformations can be associated with other anomalies such as tissue overgrowth or may present as part of a broader clinical manifestation, such as Proteus Syndrome or Hereditary Hemorrhagic Telangiectasia (HHT) [8].

For precise classification, refer to the International Society for the Study of Vascular Anomalies (ISSVA) classification (Table 9.1). This authoritative system provides standardised definitions and categorisation for vascular anomalies, ensuring accurate diagnosis and treatment [9].

Table 9.1 Classification of vascular malformations

Flow classification	Vessel/lesion type	Clinical category
Fast-flow	Arteriovenous/ arterial	Isolated
		Multifocal
		Syndromic
Slow-flow	Capillary (CM)	Nevus simplex, salmon patch
		Port-wine CM (isolated/syndromic)
		Reticulate/telangiectatic CM (isolated/ syndromic)
		Geographic pattern CM (isolated/syndromic)
		Low-resistance CM/CM with faster flow
		Cutis marmorata telangiectatic congenita
		Telangiectasias and spider angiomas
	Lymphatic (LM)	Isolated
		Complex
		Lymphoedemas
	Venous (VM)	Isolated
		Multifocal
		Syndromic
	Combined	Isolated
		Syndromic
Developmental anomalies of named vessels	Vena cava	
	Aorta	
	Vein of Galen	
	Others	

Classification of vascular anomalies based on 2025 International Society for the Study of Vascular Anomalies (ISSVA) (https://www.issva.org/classification)

9.2.1 Capillary Malformations

CM are characterised by the presence of dilated capillaries and usually present as flat, red or purple lesions on the skin and are often referred to as port-wine stains (PWS). Pathophysiologically, CM are caused by abnormal endothelial cell proliferation and dilation of capillaries [10]. While CM can occur in isolation, they are also frequently seen as part of broader vascular syndromes. One such syndrome, CM-AVM Syndrome, is linked to inherited mutations in the *RASA1* (RAS p21 protein activator 1) or *EPHB4* (Ephrin type-B receptor 4) genes. Another key genetic factor involved in the development of certain types of CM is *GNAQ* (G protein subunit alpha q), a gene encoding the G protein subunit Gαq. Mutations in *GNAQ* have been identified as the underlying cause of various syndromes that feature CM, particularly in Sturge-Weber Syndrome (SWS) as well as in simple PWS.

9.2.2 Venous Malformations

VM are the most common type of CVM, characterised by abnormal development and dilation of venous structures and slow venous blood flow [11]. Lesions often become more prominent with increased blood flow during activities such as exercise, or in response to pressure and can cause pain and swelling in the affected area. The combination of venous stasis, tortuous venous anatomy, missing venous valves, and localised intravascular coagulopathy (LIC) elevates the risk of thrombotic events in affected individuals. VM are believed to arise due to defects in venous development during embryogenesis, with a failure of venous smooth muscle to mature or contract properly. These veins lack a normal smooth muscle layer and do not function as typical veins, leading to blood pooling within the malformation. Both *PIK3CA* (phosphatidylinositol-4,5-bisphosphate 3-kinase catalytic subunit alpha) and *TEK* (TEK receptor tyrosine kinase) genes play critical roles in the regulation of vascular development and endothelial cell function, and mutations in these genes have been linked to the development of VM. Truncal VM represents a distinct subtype characterised by abnormal development or dilation of larger central veins. This may occur in isolation as a persistent sciatic vein or may be associated with conditions like Klippel-Trenaunay Syndrome (KTS) as a marginal vein on the lateral aspect of the limb. Large truncal veins typically lack valves and are prone to thrombosis and potentially pulmonary embolism. Additionally, they are often linked to an aplastic or hypoplastic deep vein system, which makes treatment particularly challenging.

9.2.3 Arteriovenous Malformations

The pathological features of AVM include abnormal vascular morphogenesis, disrupted high blood flow dynamics, and the absence of a normal capillary network within the lesion [12]. The abnormal connection between arteries and veins disrupts normal blood flow and oxygen exchange. High-pressure arterial blood flows directly into the low-pressure venous system, potentially leading to cardiac overload. This shunting also dilates the veins, making them tortuous and susceptible to rupture. Arterial vessels in AVMs are often thin-walled, because the media is poorly developed or not developed at all. Irregular walls and little to no SMCs are present, which contribute to the fragility of AVM and their propensity for rupture. Venous vessels are often overstretched and have an irregular, fibrous wall structure. The normal elastic lamellae of the arteries are often missing. The endothelial cells are often atypically organised and express other surface markers (e.g. increased VEGF receptor expression).

The lack of capillaries in an AVM means that blood bypasses the normal sites of oxygen exchange and can lead to ischaemia in the surrounding tissue and organs. This "steal phenomenon" can lead to tissue damage, particularly in organs or tissues that rely on a rich network of capillaries for nutrient and gas exchange. In the brain, this can result in neurological deficits, while in the limbs, it may cause pain or ulcers. One of the key molecular pathways implicated in the development and progression of sporadic AVM is the RAS/MAPK (mitogen-activated protein kinase) signalling pathway. Some of these mutations occur in genes directly involved in the pathway, while others affect genes that interact with RAS/MAPK signalling. The *ENG* (Endoglin), *ACVRL1* (Activin A Receptor Type II-like 1), *GDF2/BMP9* (Growth Differentiation Factor 2/Bone Morphogenetic Protein 9), and *SMAD4* genes are associated with HHT, an autosomal dominant genetic disorder that increases the risk of developing AVM.

9.2.4 Lymphatic Malformations

LM arise from abnormal growth of lymphatic vessels, leading to fluid-filled cysts or masses. These are categorised by cyst size: microcystic LM consist of small lymphatic channels, while macrocystic LM have larger, more distinct cysts easily identified on imaging. Macrocysts can cause significant swelling and compress surrounding structures. Cystic hygromas, a common form of LM, typically occur in the neck, axilla, and head, presenting as large, multiloculated cysts.

Clinical presentation varies depending on the location. In the neck, LM often manifest as a soft, compressible mass, characteristic of cystic hygromas. LM in the extremities can cause localised swelling, deformity, or restricted movement. Additionally, they can be prone to recurrent infections or bleeding, potentially causing significant discomfort or disability. LM located in the oral cavity or around the eyes can cause cosmetic deformities, pain, and functional impairments. In rare cases, LM can involve internal organs such as the lungs, liver, or gastrointestinal tract, causing obstructive symptoms, organ dysfunction, and protein-losing enteropathy. While most LMs are congenital and grow proportionally with the child, they may also become symptomatic or present as rapidly enlarging masses, particularly if they become infected or undergo bleeding. The haemodynamic disturbances in LMs are related to impaired lymphatic drainage, leading to fluid accumulation and swelling. Dilated lymphatic channels fail to transport lymph effectively, promoting oedema, inflammation, and sometimes tissue fibrosis. These vessels, often lined by thin, abnormal lymphatic ECs, are susceptible to rupture and fluid leakage. LMs arise from defects in the development of lymphatic vessels, and genetic dysregulation in genes such as *VEGFR3* (FMS Related Receptor Tyrosine Kinase 4) or *PROX1* (Prospero Homeobox 1) and/or mutations in the *PIK3CA* gene have been identified [13].

9.3 Endothelial Dysfunction and Vascular Remodelling in Vascular Malformations

The pathogenesis of CVM is multifactorial, with EC dysfunction, altered endothelial-to-mesenchymal transition (EndMT), and aberrant interactions with SMCs and pericytes playing critical roles.

9.3.1 Altered Endothelial Cell Signalling

ECs are integral to the formation and maintenance of the vasculature. In healthy blood vessels, ECs regulate key processes such as vascular tone, permeability, blood coagulation, and inflammatory responses. Under normal conditions, ECs form tight junctions and communicate with underlying SMCs and pericytes to maintain vessel stability and integrity. However, in CVM, altered EC signalling can disrupt these functions and contribute to abnormal vessel development. A variety of genetic mutations and molecular signals lead to altered EC function in CVM. One of the most well-known examples is the involvement of the *PIK3CA* gene. Mutations in this gene result in the activation of the PI3K/AKT/mTOR signalling pathway, which promotes excessive EC proliferation and survival, contributing to the formation of abnormal blood vessels. Overactivation of this pathway can lead to vascular hyperplasia, vessel dilation, and tortuosity. Similarly, mutations in the *VEGFR2* gene (vascular endothelial growth factor receptor 2) or *ENG* gene (linked to HHT, a vascular disorder that leads to abnormal capillary and arteriovenous connections) can induce comparable changes. *VEGFR2* and its associated signalling pathways are crucial for EC proliferation, migration, and tube formation during angiogenesis. Dysregulation of these signalling pathways can lead to malformed vessels with improper EC coverage and inadequate vessel maturation. In addition to genetic mutations, the altered signalling of growth factors is a hallmark of endothelial dysfunction in CVM. For instance, VEGF plays a pivotal role in angiogenesis by promoting EC proliferation and survival. In CVM, dysregulated VEGF signalling can contribute to excessive angiogenesis, resulting in the formation of dilated and leaky blood vessels. Similarly, the TGF-β pathway is often implicated in vascular malformations. TGF-β regulates endothelial cell growth, differentiation, and extracellular matrix production. Overexpression of TGF-β can lead to abnormal vessel remodelling, fibrosis, and vessel wall thickening, all features commonly seen in CVM. Additionally, the Notch signalling pathway is crucial for EC differentiation and vessel maturation. Abnormal Notch signalling has been implicated in several types of CVM, particularly in the formation of AVM, where the differentiation of ECs into mature, stable vessels is impaired.

9.3.2 Endothelial-to-Mesenchymal Transition in Vascular Malformations

Endothelial-to-mesenchymal transition (EndMT) is a process where ECs, which line blood vessels, lose their characteristic properties and acquire mesenchymal traits, such as increased migratory capacity, enhanced extracellular matrix production, and the ability to differentiate into SMCs, fibroblasts, or other mesodermal lineages. In vascular malformations, ECs undergo dysregulated EndMT in response to molecular signals like inflammatory cytokines, growth factors (such as TGF-β), and hypoxia. This transition results in blood vessels exhibiting features of both endothelial and mesenchymal cells. TGF-β signalling, a key pathway in EndMT, is particularly important in this process. Elevated TGF-β levels activate Smad and non-Smad pathways, leading to the upregulation of mesenchymal markers (e.g. α-SMA, fibronectin) and downregulation of endothelial markers (e.g. VE-cadherin, CD31). This switch promotes the migration and proliferation of transformed ECs, contributing to the formation of abnormal blood vessels. In conditions like VM, CM, and AVM, EndMT drives abnormal vascular remodelling. ECs undergoing EndMT secrete extracellular matrix proteins, leading to fibrosis and vessel wall thickening, which can impair normal blood vessel function and sustain the malformations. EndMT also affects angiogenesis, with abnormal angiogenesis in vascular malformations resulting in poorly formed, leaky, and dysfunctional vessels that contribute to the pathophysiology of these disorders.

9.3.3 Role of Smooth Muscle Cells and Pericytes in Malformation Formation

SMCs and pericytes are key regulators of vascular structure and function, playing significant roles in the development and pathogenesis of vascular malformations. Pericytes, which surround ECs in capillaries and small venules, are critical for vascular stabilisation, angiogenesis, and maintaining blood-brain barrier integrity. In vascular malformations, pericyte dysfunction or loss is a major contributing factor. In VM and CM, pericyte loss leads to vessel instability and increased permeability. Without proper pericyte coverage, ECs become prone to abnormal growth, resulting in dilated, tortuous, and leaky vessels. Pericytes also affect EndMT, a process where

ECs acquire mesenchymal traits. In malformations, pericytes may promote EndMT in nearby ECs, leading to vessel wall thickening, fibrosis, and disrupted vascular function.

SMCs provide structural integrity and regulate vascular tone in larger vessels. In vascular malformations, abnormal SMC behaviour contributes to vessel remodelling and impaired blood flow. In AVM, excessive SMC recruitment leads to the formation of abnormal arteriovenous shunts and thickened vessel walls instead of a mature capillary bed, disrupting normal blood flow. In VM, insufficient SMC coverage around veins causes vessel dilation and weakness, contributing to the characteristic vulnerability to rupture. SMCs can undergo phenotypic switching to a synthetic state, producing extracellular matrix proteins and contributing to vascular fibrosis.

The interactions between ECs, SMCs, and pericytes are crucial for maintaining vascular integrity. In vascular malformations, disrupted signalling between these cell types leads to abnormal vessel formation. Signalling pathways like Notch, TGF-β, and Angiopoietin-Tie2 regulate SMC recruitment and vessel stabilisation. Disruption of these pathways in malformations can lead to excessive SMC proliferation and/or vessel instability. Proper pericyte-EC communication is necessary for maintaining vessel integrity and regulating angiogenesis. In malformations, impaired interactions contribute to vascular leakage and dilated, dysfunctional vessels.

9.4 Inflammatory and Mechanical Stress-Induced Dysfunction in Vascular Malformations

ECs respond to mechanical forces such as shear stress from blood flow. In vascular malformations, altered haemodynamics or turbulent flow can activate ECs, triggering inflammation and vascular remodelling. Chronic inflammatory stimuli, such as cytokines (e.g. TNF-α, IL-1β), promote endothelial dysfunction by increasing adhesion molecule expression (e.g. intercellular adhesion molecule-1 (ICAM-1), vascular cell adhesion molecule-1 (VCAM-1)), facilitating immune cell recruitment and exacerbating the inflammatory response. Oxidative stress, caused by an imbalance between reactive oxygen species (ROS) and antioxidants, further damages ECs, leading to apoptosis, increased permeability, and immune cell infiltration, driving the pathogenesis of CM and VM.

Persistent release of cytokines (e.g. TNF-α, IL-6, IL-1β) and growth factors (e.g. VEGF, fibroblast growth factor (FGF)) fosters EC proliferation, angiogenesis, and disorganised vessel growth. In AVM, these mediators exacerbate endothelial dysfunction, increasing permeability and vessel dilation. In VM and LM, inflammatory signals promote abnormal dilation, remodelling, congestion, and fluid retention. Inflammatory mediators also activate fibroblasts and SMCs, leading to extracellular matrix deposition and fibrosis. In VM, extracellular matrix (ECM) alterations contribute to vessel wall disruption. Immune cells play pivotal roles in progressing and sustaining CVM. Macrophages are key mediators of inflammation and remodelling; they secrete cytokines (e.g. TNF-α, IL-1β), growth factors (e.g. VEGF, TGF-β), and matrix metalloproteinases. CD4+ helper T cells (T lymphocytes) modulate inflammation and remodelling. Neutrophils are early responders to inflammation; they amplify cytokine release, perpetuating the inflammatory cycle. Hypoxia-induced factors, such as HIFs, further attract immune cells and perpetuate inflammation. Immune responses exacerbate vessel remodelling and dysfunction, with cytokines and matrix metalloproteinases (MMPs) driving abnormal growth and destabilisation. Infections within malformations, particularly cystic lymphatic spaces, amplify inflammation, risking sepsis, or systemic complications.

9.5 Genetics of Congenital Vascular Malformations

Genetic mutations and dysregulation are central to the pathophysiology of CVM. Genetic mutations affect vascular development at various levels such as angiogenesis, endothelial cell differentiation, and smooth muscle cell function [14]. Key molecular pathways involved include the PI3K/AKT/mTOR, TGF-β signalling, and RAS/MAPK pathway, respectively. Advances in genetic research have identified several key genes that play important roles in the development of CVM.

9.5.1 Key Genes Involved in Vascular Malformations

The *EPHB4* gene plays a critical role in blood and lymphatic vascular development by regulating EC function. Unlike classical growth factor receptors, *EPHB4* dampens Ras-MAPK pathway activation induced by other growth factor receptors [15, 16]. It achieves this by interacting with *RASA1*. The *RASA1* gene plays a critical role in regulating vascular development through its effects on Ras signalling. Mutations in *RASA1* can cause the development of CM and AVM, often as part of a broader CM-AVM Syndrome [17].

Somatic mutations in the *GNAQ* gene are associated with CVM, most notably simple PWS or SWS. SWS, also called encephalotrigeminal angiomatosis, is a rare neurocutaneous disorder marked by PWS, leptomeningeal angiomas, glaucoma, and various neurological symptoms such as seizures and developmental delays [18]. Most cases of SWS are caused by mutations in the *GNAQ* gene, particularly the Q209 mutation, which triggers the uncontrolled activation of Gαq signalling. One of the key effects of Gαq activation is the promotion of endothelial cell proliferation. In a normal vascular system, ECs divide and migrate in response to specific signals to form new blood vessels. However, when *GNAQ* is mutated and Gαq remains constitutively active, ECs proliferate excessively, leading to the formation of abnormally dilated capillaries. These new blood vessels often fail to mature properly and may lack the structural integrity and stability of normal vessels, leading to their dilation and dysfunction. In addition to promoting endothelial cell proliferation, Gαq activation can impair the normal functioning of ECs. This dysfunction can lead to increased vascular permeability, allowing fluid and inflammatory cells to leak from the capillaries into the surrounding tissues. In conditions like SWS, this endothelial dysfunction may also contribute to the formation of leptomeningeal angiomas in the brain, which can lead to neurological complications.

Both *PIK3CA* and *TEK* play key roles in vascular development, and mutations in these genes are associated with VM [19]. *PIK3CA* mutations typically affect the PI3K/Akt signalling pathway, leading to endothelial cell hyperproliferation, vessel dilation, and abnormal vascular remodelling. These mutations are usually somatic and are often found in the ECs of affected veins. The mutations, particularly in exons 9 and 20, result in constitutive activation of PI3K signalling, which causes dilated, unstable, and poorly organised blood vessels prone to leakage and swelling. *TEK* mutations affect the TIE2 receptor, which regulates EC function and vascular integrity. Gain-of-function mutations lead to hyperactivation of TIE2, causing endothelial dysfunction, abnormal angiogenesis, and vessel dilation, resulting in malformed veins. Mutations in *PIK3CA* and *TEK* can overlap in their presentations, with both contributing to vascular and lymphatic abnormalities. Somatic mutations in *PIK3CA* can manifest as PIK3CA-related overgrowth spectrum (PROS), congenital lipomatous overgrowth, vascular malformations, epidermal nevi, and scoliosis (CLOVES Syndrome), isolated macrodactyly and other segmental overgrowth syndromes, as well as simple LMs [20].

The RAS/MAPK signalling pathway plays a critical role in EC behaviour, vascular development, and angiogenesis. Dysregulation of this pathway often contributes to the abnormal vessel formation seen in AVM. The pathway is activated by growth factors binding to receptor tyrosine kinases (RTKs), leading to the activation of RAS, which triggers a cascade of kinases, including MAPKs such as ERK1/2, to regulate cellular responses. Key components of the RAS/MAPK pathway include growth factor receptors (e.g. EGFR, VEGFR), RAS proteins (e.g. KRAS, NRAS), RAF kinases (e.g. BRAF), MEK1/2, and ERK1/2 [21]. Mutations in these components, such as KRAS and BRAF, can lead to constitutive activation of the pathway, promoting abnormal endothelial cell proliferation and the formation of AVM [22]. Overexpression of EGFR and VEGFR in ECs can also cause excessive activation of the RAS/MAPK pathway, contributing to vascular malformations. RAS/MAPK signalling interacts with other pathways, such as PI3K/Akt and TGF-β, which also influence endothelial function and angiogenesis. For example, PIK3CA mutations that activate the PI3K/Akt pathway are often found in VM and may also play a role in AVM [23]. Dysregulated RAS/MAPK signalling contributes to increased blood flow and high-pressure shunting in AVMs, which can weaken vessel walls and lead to larger, more fragile vessels. This increases the risk of haemorrhage and exacerbates AVM pathology. In cases of familial or sporadic AVM, genetic testing for mutations in RAS/MAPK pathway genes (e.g. KRAS, BRAF, EGFR) can help identify the underlying genetic causes and inform personalised treatment strategies.

The *ENG, ACVRL1, GDF2/BMP9,* and *SMAD4* genes are vital for vascular remodelling and endothelial function. Mutations in these genes are linked to HHT, an autosomal dominant disorder characterised by telangiectasias, visceral AVM, and epistaxis [24]. *ENG* encodes endoglin, a TGF-β co-receptor that regulates Smad1/5/8 pathways essential for stable blood vessel formation. *ENG* mutations disrupt TGF-β signalling, causing abnormal vascular remodelling and AVM (HHT1). These AVMs affect organs such as the lungs, liver, brain, and gastrointestinal tract. *ACVRL1* encodes a receptor for Activin A and BMP9, crucial for endothelial signalling, angiogenesis, and vascular maintenance. *ACVRL1* mutations impair Smad1/5 pathways, leading to larger, more complex AVMs (HHT2) in the lungs, brain, liver, and other organs, resembling *ENG* mutation phenotypes. GDF2/BMP9, a TGF-β/BMP ligand, binds ACVRL1 and BMPR2 to activate Smad1/5/8 pathways. *GDF2* (Growth Differentiation Factor 2), also known as BMP9 (Bone Morphogenetic Protein 9), is a gene that encodes a protein in the TGF-β (Transforming Growth Factor-beta) superfamily.

Mutations in *GDF2/BMP9* disrupt vascular integrity, causing familial AVM, especially in the liver and lungs, and recurrent bleeding. *SMAD4* encodes a mediator of TGF-β signalling, essential for vascular integrity. Mutations in *SMAD4* cause vascular malformations and overlap with HHT and Juvenile Polyposis Syndrome (JPS). These defects often lead to bleeding, polyps, and fragile vessels in organs like the brain, liver, and gastrointestinal tract. Mutations in these genes disrupt TGF-β/BMP signalling, impair endothelial function, and promote AVM development, with overlapping clinical manifestations centred on vascular abnormalities and bleeding risk [25].

9.5.2 Key Genes in Specific Types of Vascular Malformation

9.5.2.1 Capillary Malformations

Somatic mutations in *GNA11* (e.g. c.548G>A, p.R183Q) are frequently associated with CM, particularly in disorders like PHACE Syndrome (posterior fossa malformations, haemangiomas, arterial anomalies, cardiac defects, and eye abnormalities) [26]. Germline mutations in *RASA1* are linked to CM-AVM, characterised by multiple small CM and AVM, inherited in an autosomal dominant pattern. *EPHB4* encodes a receptor tyrosine kinase critical for separating the venous and lymphatic vascular systems. Mutations in *EPHB4* cause CM-AVM2, leading to capillary and arteriovenous anomalies, due to deregulated RAS-MAPK signalling. Somatic mutations in *PIK3CA* are implicated in the pathogenesis of PROS, a disorder encompassing a range of vascular anomalies, including capillary and venous malformations. The *KRIT1* (*Krev/Ras Interaction Trafficking Protein 1*) *CCM1* (Cerebral Cavernous Malformation 1), *CCM2 (Cerebral Cavernous Malformation 2)*, and *PDCD10 (Programmed Cell Death 10)* genes contribute to the development of cerebral cavernous malformations (CCMs) in the brain. These mutations may also cause CM on the skin, particularly in CCM1 (*KRIT1*). Most isolated CM, such as PWS, result from somatic mutations in *GNAQ* or *GNA11* [27]. Syndromic forms (e.g. CM-AVM, CCMs) are usually inherited in an autosomal dominant manner [10].

Syndromic Associations

- Sturge-Weber Syndrome (SWS): associated with somatic *GNAQ* mutations, characterised by facial port-wine stains, glaucoma, and leptomeningeal angiomas [28].
- PHACE Syndrome: complex genetic aetiology involving *GNA11* mutations, linked to large facial haemangiomas and structural anomalies [29].
- CM-AVM Syndromes (1 and 2): caused by autosomal dominant *RASA1* (CM-AVM1) and *EPHB4* (CM-AVM2) mutations, resulting in mixed vascular anomalies [30].
- CLOVES Syndrome: associated with *PIK3CA* mutations, characterised by overgrowth and mixed vascular malformations [31].

9.5.2.2 Venous Malformations

Most isolated VMs are caused by somatic mutations in *TEK, PIK3CA,* or rarely *KRAS* (KRAS proto-oncogene), arising during development and leading to mosaicism [32]. Somatic mutations in *TEK* are a major cause of sporadic VM, leading to hyperactivation of TIE2 signalling and aberrant venous growth. *PIK3CA*, a key regulator of the PI3K-AKT pathway involved in cell growth and vascular maintenance, is associated with sporadic VM and VM in syndromic conditions like CLOVES Syndrome and PROS disorders, which include venous and mixed vascular anomalies. *EPHB4* encodes a receptor tyrosine kinase critical for venous development and separation from the lymphatic system, with germline mutations causing CM-VM2 (autosomal dominant). *RASA1* encodes a RAS GTPase-activating protein that regulates endothelial function and angiogenesis. Germline mutations are linked to CM-AVM1, which may involve venous anomalies (autosomal dominant). *KRAS*, a small GTPase in the RAS-MAPK pathway that regulates cell proliferation and differentiation, is implicated in certain rare sporadic VMs through somatic mutations that contribute to abnormal endothelial proliferation.

Syndromic Associations (Table 9.2)

- Cutaneomucosal venous malformation (VMCM): somatic mutations in *TEK* (TIE2 receptor gene), characterised by familial VM affecting skin and mucous membranes. Can involve internal organs, such as the gastrointestinal tract [33].
- Blue Rubber Bleb Nevus Syndrome (BRBNS): *TEK* (TIE2 receptor gene) mutations in some cases. Characterised by multiple VMs in the skin and internal organs, especially the gastrointestinal (GI) tract. Lesions appear as blue or rubbery nodules that may bleed easily. GI involvement often leads to chronic anaemia or gastrointestinal bleeding [34].
- Klippel-Trenaunay Syndrome (KTS): the genetic basis remains incompletely understood, though mutations in the VEGFR-3 receptor and somatic mutations in *PIK3CA* have been proposed. KTS is characterised by a triad of CM, VM, and soft tissue/bone overgrowth, typically affecting one extremity and resulting in limb asymmetry [35].

Table 9.2 Vascular malformations associated with other anomalies

Syndrome	Vascular malformation(s)	Associated anomalies	Gene(s) involved
Klippel-Trenaunay syndrome (KTS)	CM + VM ± LM	Limb overgrowth	PIK3CA
Parkes Weber syndrome (PWS)	CM + AVF	Limb overgrowth	RASA1
Servelle-Martorell syndrome	Limb VM	Bone undergrowth	
Sturge-Weber syndrome (SWS)	Facial + leptomeningeal CM	Eye anomalies ± bone and/or soft tissue overgrowth	GNAQ
	Limb CM	Congenital non-progressive limb overgrowth	GNA11
Maffucci syndrome	VM ± spindle-cell haemangioma	Enchondroma	IDH1/IDH2
Macrocephaly-CM (M-CM/MCAP)	CM	Macrocephaly	PIK3CA
Microcephaly-CM (MICCAP)	CM	Microcephaly	STAMBP
CLOVES syndrome	LM + VM + CM ± AVM	Lipomatous overgrowth	PIK3CA
Proteus syndrome	CM, VM and/or LM	Asymmetrical somatic overgrowth	AKT1
Bannayan-Riley-Ruvalcaba syndrome	AVM + VM	Macrocephaly, lipomatous overgrowth	PTEN
CLAPO syndrome	Lower lip CM + face and neck LM	Asymmetry and partial/generalised overgrowth	PIK3CA

CM capillary malformation, *LM* lymphatic malformation, *VM* venous malformation, *AVM* arteriovenous malformation, *AVF* Arteriovenous fistula

- CLOVES Syndrome: somatic mosaic mutations in *PIK3CA*, characterised by congenital lipomatous overgrowth, vascular malformations, epidermal nevi, and scoliosis.
- Generalised Lymphatic Anomaly (GLA) with VM: somatic mutations in *PIK3CA*. Coexistence of lymphatic and venous anomalies with bone involvement (osteolysis) and soft tissue overgrowth [36].
- PIK3CA-Related Overgrowth Spectrum (PROS): refers to a group of rare, genetic (somatic, not inherited), and often complex disorders caused by mutations in the *PIK3CA* gene. These conditions are characterised by overgrowth of various tissues in the body and abnormalities in vascular, skeletal, and other organ systems. The PROS spectrum encompasses several overlapping syndromes, including CLOVES Syndrome, KTS, vascular malformations with overgrowth and varicosities, Megalencephaly-CMs Syndrome (MCAP), and fibroadipose hyperplasia [37].
- CM-VM2 Syndrome: characterised by the presence of CM, AVM and VM, which are prominent features in this syndrome. CM-VM2 Syndrome and CM-

AVM2 Syndrome refer to the same condition and are used interchangeably. Both terms describe the vascular malformation syndrome caused by pathogenic variants in the *EPHB4* gene inherited in an autosomal dominant manner.

- Proteus Syndrome: somatic activating mutations in the *AKT1* (Glutamate to Lysine at position 17) gene, characterised by overgrowth of bones, skin, and other tissues. VM and other vascular anomalies are common [38].
- Maffucci Syndrome: somatic mutations in *IDH1* (Isocitrate Dehydrogenase 1) or *IDH2* (Isocitrate Dehydrogenase 2) gene, characterised by VM combined with multiple enchondromas (benign cartilage tumours). Risk of malignant transformation of enchondromas [39].

9.5.2.3 Arterio-Venous Malformations

The genetic basis of AVM involves both inherited and somatic mutations. Inherited mutations in genes such as *ENG*, *ACVRL1*, and *RASA1* are associated with conditions like HHT and CM-AVM, typically following an autosomal dominant inheritance pattern. In certain cases, somatic mutations in RAS-related genes (including *KRAS, NRAS*, and *HRAS*) lead to mosaicism, contributing to localised vascular malformations. These mutations are often seen in RASopathies, such as Noonan Syndrome, Costello Syndrome, and Cardiofaciocutaneous Syndrome, where AVMs are a common feature. Additionally, somatic mutations in genes like *PIK3CA* and *TEK* are seen in sporadic AVM, often in the context of overgrowth syndromes such as PROS and PWS.

Syndromic Associations

- Hereditary Haemorrhagic Telangiectasia (HHT): autosomal dominant, inherited mutations of *ENG, ACVRL1, SMAD4* or *BMP9/GDF2*. Characterised by recurrent epistaxis, mucocutaneous telangiectasias, AVM in lungs, liver, brain, and gastrointestinal tract [40].
- Capillary Malformation-Arteriovenous Malformation Syndrome (CM-AVM): inherited mutations of *RASA1* (CM-AVM1) and *EPHB4* (CM-AVM2) genes, characterised by multiple small AVM and CM.
- Parkes Weber Syndrome (PWS): somatic mutations in the *TEK* or *RASA1* genes [41]. This mosaic pattern leads to asymmetrical manifestations, such as asymmetrical limb enlargement, tissue hyperplasia, and localised AVM. AVM are the most prominent feature. In addition to AVM and overgrowth, patients may also have other vascular anomalies such as VM and CM.
- Sturge-Weber Syndrome (SWS): associated with mutations in the *GNAQ* gene, characterised by port-wine stain birthmarks and leptomeningeal AVM in the brain. SWS can also present with other vascular malformations, including AVM in the eye.
- Klippel-Trenaunay Syndrome (KTS): the genetic basis of KTS remains incompletely understood, though mutations of the VEGFR-3 receptor and somatic mutations in *PIK3CA* have been proposed. While not always associated with AVM, some patients with KTS may have microfistular arteriovenous shunts.

9.5.2.4 Lymphatic Malformations

LM can result from both inherited and somatic mutations. Inherited mutations are passed down through families and can follow autosomal dominant, autosomal recessive, or X-linked inheritance patterns (e.g. Milroy disease and FOXC2-related syndromes). These mutations occur in genes such as *CCBE1* (Collagen and calcium-binding EGF domains 1), *FLT4* (Fms-like tyrosine kinase 4; also known as VEGFR3), *GJC2* (Gap junction protein, gamma 2), *SOX18* (SRY-box transcription factor 18) and *FOXC2* (Forkhead box protein C2), and are linked to various syndromic conditions affecting the lymphatic system. *VEGFR3* (FLT4) encodes a receptor critical for lymphangiogenesis. Mutations in this gene lead to Milroy disease, a hereditary form of lymphoedema characterised by lower limb swelling due to impaired lymphatic vessel development. The *FOXC2* gene encodes the FOXC2 transcription factor essential for lymphatic valve development and vessel integrity. Mutations cause Lymphedema-Distichiasis Syndrome, marked by lower-limb lymphoedema and additional eyelashes (distichiasis). *GJC2* encodes connexin 47, a protein involved in lymphatic endothelial cell communication. Mutations can result in lymphoedema and possibly lymphatic malformations. *SOX18* is involved in early lymphatic endothelial differentiation. Mutations in this gene lead to Hypotrichosis-Lymphedema-Telangiectasia Syndrome, characterised by sparse hair, lymphoedema, and vascular abnormalities. *CCBE1* enhances VEGF-C activity, which is essential for lymphatic vessel formation. Mutations in *CCBE1* lead to Hennekam Syndrome, which includes generalised lymphoedema, lymphangiectasia, and intellectual disability. *GATA2*, encoding GATA2 a transcription factor crucial for haematopoiesis and lymphatic vessel maintenance, has mutations that cause Emberger Syndrome, which involves lymphoedema, immunodeficiency, and a predisposition to myelodysplastic syndrome.

Somatic mutations arise sporadically during development, leading to mosaic disorders and are often associated with genes like *PIK3CA, TEK, NRAS,* and *KRAS*. *PIK3CA* mutations are involved in PROS disorders, which include lymphatic malformations and overgrowth syndromes, due to their role in the PI3K-AKT pathway that regulates cell growth and vascular development. *TEK* encodes a receptor critical for vascular development, and mutations. *TEK* mutations are generally not associated with pure lymphatic malformations, although combined venous-lymphatic malformations can occur. Central Conducting Lymphatic Anomalies (CCLA) can also be associated with *RAS* mutations, particularly KRAS mutations. While *PIK3CA* mutations are the most commonly known genetic changes in CCLA, mutations in the RAS signalling pathway, including *KRAS*, have also been linked to this condition. Noonan syndrome is associated with mutations in several genes of the RAS/MAPK signalling pathway. The most commonly affected genes are *PTPN11, KRAS, SOS1, RAF1, BRAF*, and *NRAS*. These mutations lead to overactivation of the signalling pathway, resulting in a variety of symptoms, such as heart defects, developmental delay, characteristic facial features, and lymphatic anomalies.

Syndromic Associations

- CLOVES Syndrome: somatic mutations in *PIK3CA*, characterised by congenital lipomatous overgrowth, vascular malformations, epidermal nevi, and skeletal/spinal anomalies.
- Generalised Lymphatic Anomaly (GLA): mutations in *PIK3CA* and other genes are implicated in lymphangiogenesis. Characterised by diffuse lymphatic malformations involving multiple organs (e.g. bones, lungs, liver). Bone lesions can lead to fractures and deformities. GLA may be associated with chylothorax or lymphoedema.
- Gorham-Stout Disease (GSD): mutations in *PIK3CA* and other pathways are implicated. Characterised by progressive osteolysis (bone loss) with lymphatic and vascular malformations. Commonly affects ribs, spine, pelvis, and skull and can lead to life-threatening complications such as chylothorax [42].
- Proteus Syndrome: somatic mutations in *AKT1* are characterised by overgrowth of multiple tissues, including lymphatic malformations, disproportionate growth of limbs, vascular malformations, and connective tissue anomalies.
- Noonan Syndrome: mutations in several genes of the RAS/MAPK signalling pathway, most commonly affected *PTPN11*, *KRAS,* or *SOS1*. Characterised by short stature, facial dysmorphisms, congenital heart defects, and lymphoedema. Lymphatic malformations often involve the neck, chest, or abdomen [43].
- Capillary-Lymphatic-Venous Malformation: mutations in *PIK3CA* or *TEK* (TIE2 receptor gene), characterised by combined vascular anomalies involving capillaries, lymphatics, and veins. May present as diffuse swelling, pain, or functional impairment.
- Hennekam Syndrome: mutations in *CCBE1*, *FAT4,* or *ADAMTS3*, characterised by generalised lymphatic dysplasia leading to lymphoedema, lymphatic malformations, and facial dysmorphisms. May involve intestinal lymphangiectasia and protein-losing enteropathy [44].

Understanding the genetic basis of vascular malformations aids in accurate diagnosis, counselling, and potential therapeutic interventions, such as targeted therapies for the PI3K/AKT/mTOR pathway (e.g. sirolimus) or PI3K-AKT pathway (e.g. alpelisib).

9.6 Principles of Management of Vascular Malformations

9.6.1 General Treatment Options

Management strategies depend on the type, size, location, and symptoms of the malformation. Many vascular malformations are asymptomatic and do not require immediate intervention. Regular monitoring of lesion progression, particularly in paediatric cases, where growth may be expected, is important. Monitoring should be undertaken for complications such as bleeding, infection, or thrombosis. Chronic pain is a common symptom in VM and AVM. Use of analgesics, including non-steroidal anti-inflammatory drugs (NSAIDs), opioids (for severe pain), or topical therapies may be needed. Compression garments for VM and LM can help reduce swelling and discomfort. Counselling, support groups, or psychiatric care may be needed to address the psychological burden of visible lesions, particularly on the face or extremities [45]. Table 9.3 provides a summary of general treatment options for CVM.

Among treatment modalities, embolisation plays a crucial role in managing various vascular malformations, particularly when deep or complex lesions are involved. Before performing embolisation, a comprehensive assessment of the flow dynamics of the malformation must be determined to reduce the risk of complications, particularly in high-flow AVM. Vascular access points and the potential for collateral vessel involvement must be considered. Ethanol embolisation, which involves injecting absolute ethanol into blood vessels under general anaesthesia, is a highly effective procedure. However, it can be risky if the interventionalist is not familiar with the technique or the substance. In contrast to other embolic agents, ethanol causes EC damage through direct toxicity. The main mechanisms by which ethanol induces vessel occlusion and subsequent malformation regression include EC injury

Table 9.3 Summary of general treatment options for CVM

Treatment	Mechanism of action	Indications	Advantages	Disadvantages	Potential complications
Sclerotherapy	Injection of a sclerosing agent to induce endothelial damage and fibrosis, obliterating the malformation. Sclerosing agents include STS, polidocanol, and bleomycin [46, 53, 55, 98]	VM, LM, and sometimes CM.	Minimally invasive; can be effective for various types of VM and LM.	Pain, swelling, bruising at the injection site; skin ulceration or nerve injury (rare); may require multiple sessions.	Infection, tissue necrosis, embolism, recurrence of the malformation.
Laser therapy	Uses a specific wavelength of light to coagulate blood vessels, leading to their reabsorption [48–51]	Primarily for superficial VM and CM (e.g. PWS)	Effective for superficial lesions; minimal side effects	Effectiveness varies based on lesion depth, size, and location; hyperpigmentation, hypopigmentation, and scarring are possible side effects	

(Continued)

Table 9.3 (Continued)

Treatment	Mechanism of action	Indications	Advantages	Disadvantages	Potential complications
Embolisation	Injection of embolic agents (e.g. ethanol, polyvinyl alcohol (PVA) particles, coils, glue (N-butyl cyanoacrylate)) to block blood flow to the malformation [55–57, 60–66]	AVM (often pre-surgery or as a stand-alone treatment) [99]; deep, large, or complex VM	Can shrink the malformation and prevent further symptoms; useful for lesions in challenging anatomical locations	Potential for bleeding, infection, or damage to surrounding tissues; risk of non-target embolisation; may require multiple sessions	Recanalisation, tissue ischaemia, non-target organ embolisation
Surgical excision	Complete removal of the malformation	Isolated, well-defined, symptomatic VM or AVM; CM not responsive to other treatments	Potential for a permanent cure; prevents recurrence	Can be challenging for extensive lesions; risk of significant morbidity, including bleeding, infection, and nerve damage	
Cryotherapy	Freezing the tissue, leading to necrosis and reabsorption	Superficial VMs, CMs, and haemangiomas	Minimally invasive; lower complication rates compared to surgery	Limited to superficial lesions; risk of scarring, hypopigmentation, or changes in skin texture	

STS sodium tetradecyl sulphate, *CM* capillary malformation, *LM* lymphatic malformation, *VM* venous malformation, *AVM* rteriovenous malformation, *PVA* polyvinyl alcohol, *PWS* port-wine stains

(EC apoptosis and disruption of the integrity of the vascular endothelium), coagulation (injection of ethanol causes rapid coagulation of blood within the vessel), and fibrosis (over time, the area of tissue necrosis caused by ethanol embolisation is replaced by fibrous tissue, effectively obliterating the malformation). Multiple studies confirm the ability of ethanol not only to significantly reduce the size of AVMs, but also to heal AVM. Similarly, ethanol embolisation often successfully treats venous malformations (VM) by reducing swelling, pain, and bleeding, which leads to a better quality of life for patients. In large CVM, ethanol embolisation is combined with coils to reduce the amount of ethanol needed.

Ethanol is a potent tissue irritant and can cause unintended damage to surrounding healthy tissues. This may lead to necrosis, especially if the ethanol spreads to unintended areas. Inadvertent infusion of ethanol into normal vessels can cause damage, leading to complications such as vessel rupture, haemorrhage, or thrombosis. Careful targeting and monitoring are required to avoid such risks. While ethanol is primarily intended to act locally, systemic absorption can lead to alcohol toxicity, which may cause symptoms such as confusion, hypotension, respiratory depression, or even coma in severe cases. Patients need to be closely monitored after the procedure. Successful embolisation requires high levels of technical skill, as the procedure must be carefully controlled to avoid affecting adjacent structures, especially when treating CVM near critical vascular or neural structures.

Ethanol is often compared with other embolising agents such as coils, particles, or glue. Each agent has its advantages and disadvantages. Coils and particles are typically used in larger, more well-defined vessels, and they may be preferred in certain clinical situations. However, they do not offer the same degree of tissue necrosis and fibrosis that ethanol provides. While N-butyl cyanoacrylate (glue) can be effective in treating AVM and VM, it does not have the same destructive and sclerosing properties as ethanol, which makes ethanol more suitable for certain high-flow malformations. Other agents such as OK-432 or doxycycline are often preferred for LM [46]. However, ethanol has the advantage of being readily available and highly effective in the appropriate clinical settings [47].

9.6.2 *Management of Specific Vascular Malformations*

9.6.2.1 Management of Capillary Malformations (CM, Non-Syndromic)

While CM are not life-threatening, they can cause cosmetic concerns, especially if they are large or located in visible areas. The goal of treatment is primarily cosmetic improvement, symptom relief, and prevention of complications like bleeding or secondary infections. Pulsed dye laser (PDL) and intense pulsed light laser (IPL) are the most effective and commonly used treatments for CMs, particularly for lesions that are visible and cause cosmetic concern. Cryotherapy or topical treatments may be used in certain cases, though they are generally less effective. Surgical excision is typically reserved for smaller, isolated lesions or those not responsive to other treatments. Regular follow-up is necessary, as multiple treatments may be required for optimal results. Ultimately, the treatment plan should be tailored to the size, location, and nature of the CM, as well as the patient's age, overall health, and cosmetic concerns.

(a) *Pulsed Dye Laser*

The most commonly used laser for CM is the PDL, which targets the blood vessels in the lesion using a specific wavelength of light (585–595 nm). The laser is absorbed by the blood vessels, causing them to coagulate and shrink, ultimately leading to their reabsorption by the body. PDL is considered the first-line treatment for CM, particularly those on the face or visible areas. It is most effective in treating superficial, red or purple lesions. It can significantly reduce the size and colour intensity of the CM, often with minimal side effects. The treatment is usually done in an outpatient setting and is generally well-tolerated. Multiple sessions (typically 3–5) are required, spaced several weeks apart, to achieve optimal results. Some temporary side effects may include redness, swelling, bruising, or blistering at the treatment site, but these typically resolve within a few days to weeks [48–50].

(b) *Intense Pulsed Light (IPL) Therapy*

IPL uses broad-spectrum light to target haemoglobin in the blood vessels, similar to PDL, but with a broader range of wavelengths. It helps to reduce the redness and discoloration of the CMs. IPL can be an alternative to PDL in cases where PDL is ineffective or not available. It may be less effective on deeper lesions or in cases with larger, more widespread malformations. IPL is non-invasive and may be suitable for patients who are not candidates for lasers, or for those who prefer a less invasive approach. IPL typically requires multiple sessions to achieve the best results, though the treatment tends to have less downtime than laser therapy. Mild redness or swelling may occur after treatment but usually resolves quickly [51].

(c) *Cryotherapy*

Cryotherapy is more commonly used for superficial or localised lesions, but it may not be as effective as laser treatments for CM, especially larger or deeper lesions. It is a relatively simple and quick procedure, and it can be done under local anaesthesia, but there may be significant cosmetic concerns. It provides immediate removal of the malformation and may be suitable for patients with a small, well-defined lesion. Surgery carries the risks of scarring, infection, and longer recovery time compared to non-invasive treatments.

(d) *Monitoring and Long-Term Care*

While treatment of CM can improve their appearance, long-term follow-up is often necessary to monitor for recurrence, especially in cases where the malformation is large or persistent. In rare cases, CM may be associated with other anomalies (e.g. Sturge-Weber syndrome), requiring additional monitoring or treatment.

9.6.2.2 Management of Venous Malformations (VMs)

Treatment options should be tailored to the individual patient's needs, considering factors such as the lesion's size, location, and associated symptoms. VM are abnormal clusters of dilated veins that can occur in any part of the body, often causing cosmetic, functional, or pain-related issues. VM are usually congenital, but their symptoms may not become apparent until later in life. They are typically slow-flow lesions, which means that they do not present the same risk of rupture or bleeding as high-flow AVM lesions, but they can cause pain, swelling, LIC, and thromboembolism. Sclerotherapy and compression therapy are commonly used for superficial and mild to moderate cases. Laser therapy can also be effective for superficial VM. For larger, deeper, or more complex VMs, embolisation or surgical excision may be required. Endovenous thermoablation is an emerging therapy that can be useful for reducing malformation size and symptoms. Pain management and compression are helpful for symptom control in symptomatic VM. A multidisciplinary approach, often involving vascular specialists, interventionalists, and surgeons, is essential to determine the most appropriate course of action for each patient [52].

(a) *Compression Therapy*

This is a non-invasive treatment that involves using compression garments or bandages to apply pressure to the affected area, helping reduce swelling and discomfort associated with VM. Compression therapy is useful for superficial VM or in cases where the VM is located in an area prone to swelling or fluid buildup (e.g. the limbs). It can reduce symptoms such as pain, swelling, and heaviness, and prevent further deterioration of the veins.

(b) *Surgery*

In some cases, especially with large or localised VM (e.g. marginal vein), surgery may be required to remove the affected veins or tissue. This can involve excising the malformation or removing portions of it to alleviate symptoms and improve appearance. Surgical excision is considered when the VM is accessible, causes significant functional impairment, or if other treatments have been ineffective. It is particularly useful for smaller, localised VMs. Surgery can provide a more permanent solution and offers immediate results in terms of reducing the size of the malformation. Risks of surgery include scarring, infection, nerve damage, or recurrence of the malformation.

(c) *Sclerotherapy, Endovenous Thermoablation, and Embolisation*

Sclerotherapy is particularly effective for superficial VMs and those that are localised or in accessible areas. It can provide significant symptom relief, reduce the size of the lesion, and improve cosmetic outcomes. Sclerotherapy may be a first-line treatment in many cases. Common side effects include pain, swelling, and bruising at the injection site. In rare cases, more serious complications such as skin ulceration or nerve injury can occur. It often requires multiple sessions for optimal results, spaced several weeks apart [53, 54]. Endovenous thermoablation is typically used for larger VMs or those in deeper tissues. Side effects include temporary pain, bruising, and swelling. Rarely, there may be skin burns or nerve injury.

Embolisation using coils, glue, ethanol, or particles injected to block the abnormal veins is often used for deep, large, or complex VMs that are difficult to treat with surgery or sclerotherapy. Embolisation can be particularly useful for VM in challenging anatomical areas (e.g. deep tissues, organs, or joints). It can shrink the malformation and prevent further symptoms. Potential complications include bleeding, infection, or damage to surrounding tissues. There may also be a risk of embolisation affecting normal vessels [55–57].

(d) *Pain Control and Supportive Care*

For painful VM or those causing functional impairment, supportive treatments such as pain management (e.g. NSAIDs, acetaminophen, or opioids for severe pain) and anti-inflammatory medications may be used to control symptoms. Pain management is often necessary for larger or more symptomatic VMs that are not amenable to other treatments. Pain control improves quality of life, especially in cases where other treatments have not yet provided relief. Medications may have side effects, including gastrointestinal irritation or dependency with prolonged use of opioids.

Localised intravascular coagulopathy (LIC) associated with VM is a complex phenomenon that involves abnormal coagulation in the vessels due to altered blood flow or vessel wall abnormalities. Patients with LIC may have a tendency to form painful microthrombi within the affected VM. In cases of active thrombosis or risk of thromboembolism, low-dose anticoagulants (direct oral anticoagulants or low-molecular-weight heparin) may be indicated to manage coagulopathy, reduce pain, and prevent further clot formation. In rare and severe cases, if LIC evolves into a more generalised, disseminated intravascular coagulopathy (DIC), treatment may require the use of blood products such as fresh frozen plasma, platelets, or cryoprecipitate, depending on the specific coagulation profile. Regular assessment of the coagulation profile (including PT, aPTT, fibrinogen, and D-dimer) is important to guide treatment, particularly if there are signs of evolving coagulopathy. Given the complexity of VM and the potential for associated coagulopathy, a multidisciplinary approach is often required [58, 59].

9.6.2.3 Management of Arterio-Venous Malformations (AVM)

Treatment for AVM depends on their size, location, symptoms, and the risk of complications such as bleeding. The primary goals are to prevent bleeding and high-output heart failure, alleviate symptoms often related to steal-related ischaemia, and improve the patient's quality of life. Multidisciplinary care, often involving interventionalists, neurosurgeons, and vascular surgeons, is essential for selecting the most appropriate treatment strategy. The optimal treatment strategy varies for each individual. While some cases may require a combination of therapies (e.g. embolisation and surgery), others may be managed conservatively with regular monitoring to avoid unnecessary interventions.

(a) *Surgical Resection*

Surgery is considered the most effective treatment for superficial or easily accessible AVMs. It is particularly useful in cases where the AVM has caused symptoms like bleeding or pain, or when other treatments have failed. Surgical resection offers the potential for a permanent cure by completely removing the AVM. It can prevent recurrence or future complications, particularly in high-risk AVMs. Surgery carries risks such as bleeding, infection, and potential damage to surrounding healthy tissue, especially if the AVM is located in sensitive areas (e.g. brain, spinal cord). Post-surgical complications may include neurological deficits.

(b) *Embolisation*

Catheter-based and/or direct percutaneous embolisation are the treatment of choice in patients with AVM. Embolisation can be used as a preoperative adjunct to shrink the AVM before surgery, or as the primary treatment for inoperable AVM. Extracranial AVM can be treated by directly puncturing the AVM nidus and using a combination of coils and sclerosing agents. However, for AVM located in hard-to-reach areas, such as the deep brain or spinal cord, treatment typically involves direct intra-arterial or retrograde trans-venous catheter-based techniques. Potential complications include the formation of clots (which may dislodge), stroke, or damage to surrounding blood vessels. There is also the risk that the embolisation may not fully occlude the AVM, stimulating angiogenic growth and making further procedures challenging [60–66].

(c) *Supportive and Medical Management*

Small, asymptomatic AVMs, or those with a low risk of bleeding, may be managed conservatively with watchful waiting. This involves regular imaging (e.g. MRI or angiography) to monitor the AVM over time. This approach is appropriate for small, asymptomatic AVMs that have a low risk of bleeding or other complications, particularly in older patients or those who are not candidates for surgery. There are no direct side effects to observation, but the risk of bleeding or other complications remains. If symptoms develop or if the AVM increases in size, more aggressive treatment may be necessary.

9.6.2.4 Management of Lymphatic Malformations (LM)

The treatment of LM is highly individualised and depends on factors such as lesion size, location, symptoms, and the presence of complications. A multidisciplinary approach is often required, involving vascular specialists, interventionalists, surgeons, and sometimes paediatricians. The goal is to minimise symptoms, reduce lesion size, prevent recurrence, and improve both cosmetic and functional outcomes.

(a) *Sclerotherapy*

Sclerotherapy is a minimally invasive treatment for LM, especially macrocystic or localised types. Common sclerosing agents include OK-432 (Picibanil©), which stimulates an immune response leading to inflammation and fibrosis, and doxycycline, an antibiotic used for cystic LM. In some cases, ethanol, sodium tetradecyl sulfate, or polidocanol may be used to induce fibrosis. Mild pain, swelling, or bruising at the injection site can occur, while rare complications include skin ulceration, infection, or injury to nearby structures such as nerves or blood vessels. The procedure may require multiple sessions, spaced several weeks apart, and can be performed under local or general anaesthesia, depending on the agent used.

(b) *Surgical Excision*

Surgical resection is considered for lymphatic malformations that are symptomatic, causing significant functional impairment, or located in areas where other treatments (such as sclerotherapy) are not effective. Surgical resection can be challenging, especially when the malformation is large or located in a critical area, such as the neck or airway. In cases where complete excision is not possible, debulking procedures may be performed to reduce the size of the lesion and alleviate symptoms. Risks of surgery include bleeding, infection, scarring, nerve damage, or recurrence of the LM. For large or deeply located LM, complete excision may be challenging, and recurrence rates can be high.

(c) *Intra-Lesional Steroid Injection*

Steroid injections, such as triamcinolone, may be used to reduce inflammation and help shrink the LM. This works by suppressing the inflammatory response and inducing fibrotic changes in the lesion. Steroids are often used in conjunction with sclerotherapy or for small LM, particularly those that are painful or inflamed.

(d) *Endoscopic or Image-Guided Drainage*

For large, symptomatic LM, image-guided drainage (using ultrasound, CT, or MRI for guidance) can be performed to aspirate the cystic fluid, thereby temporarily reducing the size of the lesion and relieving symptoms. This approach may be used in cases where the LM is causing functional obstruction (e.g. difficulty breathing, swallowing) or in the case of significant fluid buildup. It is often considered in emergency situations or as a preparatory step before further treatment. Minimally invasive, providing immediate symptom relief (e.g. alleviating pressure on surrounding structures), and can be used as a temporary solution while other long-term treatments are being planned. Recurrence is common as drainage does not address the underlying malformation. There are risks of infection or bleeding, though minimal with proper technique.

(e) *Antibiotics (for complicated LM)*

If the LM becomes infected (a common complication in large, cystic LM), antibiotics are prescribed to treat the infection. In some cases, antibiotics may also be used to prevent infection during invasive procedures such as sclerotherapy or surgery. Antibiotics are necessary when infection is suspected or confirmed, particularly if there is redness, warmth, or drainage from the lesion.

(f) *Combination Therapy*

In some cases, a combination of therapies (e.g. sclerotherapy and surgery) may be necessary to optimise treatment outcomes. For example, sclerotherapy may reduce the size of the lesion before surgery to facilitate easier excision. This approach is typically used for complex or large LMs that cannot be fully treated with one modality. Combining different modalities can address various aspects of the malformation, such as symptom relief, size reduction, and cosmetic improvement. Potential risks are associated with each modality used (e.g. scarring, infection, or swelling), but combination therapy can be tailored to minimise these risks.

The prognosis for LM depends on several factors, including the size and location of the lesion, the type of treatment used, and the patient's overall health. Many small or superficial malformations that are treated early have a good prognosis, with a reduction in size and resolution of symptoms. However, there is a risk of recurrence, particularly in cases where the lesion is only partially treated or incompletely excised. Regular follow-up with imaging is essential to monitor for any changes or recurrence of the malformation. For more extensive or complicated malformations, particularly those involving vital structures (such as the airway or vital organs), the prognosis can be more challenging, and a multidisciplinary approach may be necessary for optimal management.

9.6.3 *Targeted Therapy of Vascular Malformations*

Given the genetic nature of many vascular malformations, genetic counselling can be crucial, especially in familial cases like HHT. Genetic testing for mutations in genes such as *TEK, RASA1, ENG, ALK1*, or *SMAD4* can help guide treatment decisions and anticipate disease progression.

While traditional treatments such as compression therapy, surgery, sclerotherapy, embolisation and laser therapy remain the mainstay for managing CVM, targeted therapies are an emerging and promising approach in the treatment of these conditions (Fig. 9.1). Targeted therapies aim to block or modulate the molecular pathways involved in vascular development, focusing on specific genes, proteins, or receptors that contribute to malformation growth [67]. Often, targeted therapies are combined with other modalities, such as surgery, embolisation, or sclerotherapy, to optimise clinical outcomes.

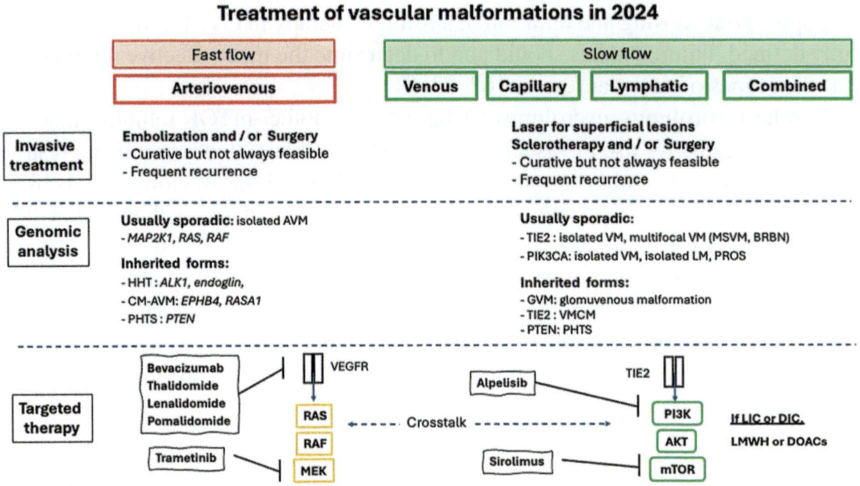

Fig. 9.1 Targeted therapy in patients with congenital vascular malformations [97]

(a) *Anti-VEGF Therapy (Bevacizumab)*

Bevacizumab (Avastin©) is a monoclonal antibody that binds to VEGF-A and prevents its interaction with VEGF receptors on ECs. This inhibits angiogenesis and reduces the size of abnormal blood vessels. It has been used off-label to treat AVM and other vascular malformations, showing promising results in some studies [68–72]. Common side effects of anti-VEGF therapy include hypertension, proteinuria, and an increased risk of bleeding. Anti-VEGF therapies have shown promise in treating certain types of vascular malformations, such as CM, haemangiomas, and even some AVM. They help reduce vascular proliferation, alleviate symptoms, and prevent complications like bleeding or ulceration.

(b) *PI3K/AKT/mTOR Pathway Inhibitors (Sirolimus and Everolimus)*

Sirolimus (Rapamycin©) is a macrolide immunosuppressant that exerts its therapeutic effects by inhibiting the mTOR pathway and represents a promising therapy for PIK3CA-related VM and LM, which are caused by activating mutations in the PI3K/Akt/mTOR signalling pathway. In these cases, sirolimus can reduce the size of the malformation, alleviate symptoms such as pain and swelling, and improve quality of life. Several studies have demonstrated the benefit of sirolimus in treating VM in both paediatric and adult populations. In these studies, patients treated with sirolimus showed significant reductions in lesion size, improved skin texture, and decreased symptoms of pain and swelling. In LM, sirolimus has been shown to shrink macrocystic lesions, reduce fluid accumulation, and improve clinical outcomes, including pain reduction and improved mobility. The response to sirolimus is often gradual, with clinical improvement observed over several months. Therefore, it is important for patients to be monitored regularly to assess the effectiveness of treatment and to adjust dosages as needed. While short-term studies have demonstrated efficacy, the long-term impact of sirolimus on vascular malformations, particularly with regard to recurrence and side effects, requires further investigation. The appropriate dosing and duration of sirolimus therapy in CVM have not yet been fully defined. Future studies should aim to determine the most effective regimen for different types of vascular lesions [67, 73–81].

Similar to sirolimus, everolimus (Afinitor©) is another mTOR inhibitor that has been investigated for use in vascular malformations. It has shown promising results in reducing the size and symptoms of vascular malformations in clinical trials [82]. mTOR inhibitors are generally well tolerated but are associated with potential side effects such as mouth ulcers, rash, diarrhoea, fatigue, increased risk of infections, and hyperlipidaemia. More serious, but rarer, side effects include pulmonary toxicity, haematologic abnormalities (e.g. thrombocytopenia), and kidney dysfunction. Close monitoring of renal function, blood cell counts, and lipid levels is necessary during treatment. Patients should also be monitored for signs of infection, as the drug suppresses immune function [83].

(c) *PI3K Inhibitors (Alpelisib)*

Alpelisib (Piqray©) is a PI3K inhibitor that selectively targets the p110α catalytic subunit of PI3K, making it a promising treatment option for vascular malformations associated with PIK3CA mutations, such as the PIK3CA-related overgrowth spectrum, VM and LM. Mouse models of PIK3CA-mutant vascular malformations have demonstrated that alpelisib can reduce vascular lesion size and improve vascular function by inhibiting endothelial cell proliferation and abnormal vascular growth [73]. Studies in PIK3CA-mutant mice showed that alpelisib not only inhibited the growth of vascular lesions but also led to vascular normalisation, a process by which malformed blood vessels become more structured and less prone to haemorrhage. Some case studies and early-phase clinical trials have reported positive outcomes in patients with PIK3CA-related overgrowth spectrum and PIK3CA-mutated vascular malformations [73]. These studies have shown that alpelisib can help reduce the size of VM and LM and improve symptoms such as pain and swelling. Overall, alpelisib has a manageable safety profile, but close monitoring for adverse effects, particularly hyperglycaemia and diarrhoea, is necessary. Its ability to target the PI3K/Akt/mTOR pathway, which is dysregulated in many vascular malformations, makes it an attractive option for patients who have not responded to conventional therapies. Although early preclinical and clinical data are promising, further studies are required to fully establish its role in vascular malformation management and optimise its use in clinical practice. As research progresses, alpelisib could become a cornerstone in the targeted treatment of PIK3CA-driven vascular malformations.

(d) *MAPK/ERK Signalling Pathway Inhibitors (Trametinib)*

Trametinib (Mekinist©) is an oral, selective inhibitor of MEK1/2 (Mitogen-Activated Protein Kinase Kinase 1 and 2), which are part of the MAPK/ERK signalling pathway. In the context of vascular malformations, mutations in genes upstream of MEK can result in constitutive activation of this pathway, contributing to EC proliferation and abnormal vascular remodelling. In various mouse models of vascular malformations, MEK inhibitors like trametinib have been shown to reduce vascular proliferation, lesion size, and symptoms related to abnormal vascular growth. In some models of AVM, trametinib has demonstrated the ability to reduce lesion volume and improve the overall vascular architecture [84, 85]. The clinical efficacy of trametinib in CVM has been evaluated in several small cohort studies and case reports. While results are still early, trametinib has shown promise in reducing the size and improving the clinical symptoms [86–89]. There is also interest in combining trametinib with other targeted therapies (e.g. PI3K inhibitors or mTOR inhibitors). The connection between trametinib and PIK3CA mutations lies in the potential cross-talk between the PI3K/Akt/mTOR and MAPK/ERK signalling pathways. Given the complexity of these signalling networks, a dual-targeted approach may offer improved therapeutic outcomes for patients with diseases driven by both pathways [90]. In terms of safety, trametinib is generally well tolerated, though side effects are possible. The most common adverse effects of trametinib include rash, diarrhoea, fatigue, oedema, and decreased left ventricular ejection fraction. Serious side effects, though rare, include cardiac toxicity and ocular toxicity, which necessitate regular monitoring during treatment. Given its mechanism of action in the MAPK pathway, trametinib's use in certain vascular malformations should be considered on a case-by-case basis, with appropriate monitoring for potential adverse effects [91].

(e) *Thalidomide*

Thalidomide is a drug known for its teratogenic effects in pregnancy. Despite its history, recent research into the anti-inflammatory, anti-angiogenic, and immunomodulatory properties of thalidomide has spurred its exploration as a treatment for vascular anomalies, such as gastrointestinal vascular malformation or AVM [92–95]. In several case reports, thalidomide has been used as an off-label therapy in patients with recurrent AVM. In one notable case, a patient with a large AVM experienced significant reduction in lesion size and symptom relief (e.g. reduction in swelling and pain) after several months of thalidomide [96].

(f) *Anti-TGF-β Therapy*

TGF-β is a key regulator of endothelial cell function, and mutations in the TGF-β signalling pathway are associated with the development of vascular malformations, particularly in HHT. Pamrevlumab (FG-3019) is a monoclonal antibody targeting TGF-β, which has shown promise in modulating fibrosis and abnormal vascular remodelling. TGF-β inhibitors are being explored for conditions such as VM, CM, and AVM, where TGF-β signalling may play a critical role in vessel abnormality and growth. Luspatercept is a fusion protein that modulates TGF-β signalling and has been explored in the treatment of HHT-associated vascular malformations. Early clinical trials have shown that it can reduce the frequency of bleeding in HHT patients, though further studies are needed to confirm its long-term efficacy. SB-431542 is a small molecule inhibitor of TGF-β receptor signalling which has shown promise in preclinical models of vascular malformations, particularly in reducing abnormal vessel growth in AVM. Targeting TGF-β signalling can lead to immune modulation, and the long-term effects of these therapies are still under investigation.

(g) *Gene Therapy*

Gene therapy is an emerging area in the treatment of vascular malformations, particularly those caused by inherited mutations. The goal is to correct the underlying genetic defect or modulate gene expression to restore normal vascular function. Gene editing technologies such as CRISPR-Cas9 have been used in preclinical studies to edit the genes responsible for vascular malformations. Gene delivery techniques using viral vectors to deliver therapeutic genes to ECs are also under investigation. These therapies could potentially restore normal endothelial function and prevent the formation of abnormal vessels. Gene therapy remains in the experimental phase, and challenges include efficient delivery to the affected tissues, long-term expression of the therapeutic gene, and potential off-target effects.

In many cases, a combination of targeted therapies is necessary to achieve optimal outcomes, particularly in complex or large vascular malformations. For example, combining anti-VEGF therapy with sirolimus or embolisation may provide synergistic effects in reducing vessel size and improving clinical symptoms. A multimodal approach that combines molecular therapies with traditional treatments (surgery, embolisation, or sclerotherapy) is often the most effective strategy for managing CVM. While some therapies, like anti-VEGF agents and mTOR inhibitors, are already in clinical use, others are still in experimental stages or clinical trials. These treatments hold significant promise in offering more targeted, effective, and minimally invasive options for managing vascular malformations, either alone or in combination with traditional approaches such as surgery and embolisation.

9.7 Conclusion

Congenital vascular malformations are developmental anomalies driven by specific genetic mutations that disrupt key cellular signalling pathways, such as the PI3K/AKT/mTOR and RAS/MAPK cascades. This molecular dysregulation is the root cause of the endothelial dysfunction, aberrant cell growth, and flawed vessel architecture that characterise these lesions. This understanding has been pivotal, reframing CVMs as genetic disorders rather than simple structural defects.

This new perspective is transforming clinical management, moving the field beyond purely procedural interventions. While established treatments like surgery, sclerotherapy and embolisation remain essential for managing symptoms, they are now being augmented by targeted molecular therapies. By directly inhibiting the specific overactive pathways, these novel agents offer a personalised approach that addresses the underlying cause of the malformation, heralding a new era where combined molecular and procedural strategies can achieve more comprehensive and lasting patient outcomes.

Multiple Choice Questions

1. Congenital vascular malformations are categorised based on which two fundamental characteristics, according to the International Society for the study of Vascular Anomalies classification?

   (a) Genetic mutation and patient age (paediatric vs. adult)
   (b) Surgical approach and size of the malformation
   (c) Type of vessels involved and their flow characteristics
   (d) Severity of pain and risk of haemorrhage
   (e) Response to sirolimus and bevacizumab

   Answer: (c) Type of vessels involved and their flow characteristics
2. What is the mechanism of action of the targeted therapy Sirolimus in treating PIK3CA-related vascular malformations?

   (a) It is a monoclonal antibody that binds to VEGF-A

(b) It is an immunosuppressant that inhibits the mTOR pathway
(c) It selectively targets the p110-alpha catalytic subunit of PI3K
(d) It is an inhibitor of MEK1/2, part of the RAS/MAPK pathway
(e) It modulates TGF-beta signalling to reduce vessel proliferation

Answer: (b) It is an immunosuppressant that inhibits the mTOR pathway

3. Endothelial-to-mesenchymal transition in vascular malformations:

(a) Does not result in increased angiogenesis
(b) Results in an increase in normal blood vessel formation
(c) Is a process where endothelial cells which line blood vessels lose their characteristic properties and acquire mesenchymal traits, such as increased migratory capacity and enhanced extracellular matrix production
(d) Can be inhibited by hyperbaric oxygen therapy
(e) Is only found in high flow vascular malformations

Answer: (c) Is a process where endothelial cells which line blood vessels lose their characteristic properties and acquire mesenchymal traits, such as increased migratory capacity and enhanced extracellular matrix production

References

1. Tuleja A, Bernhard S, Hamvas G, Andreoti TA, Rössler J, Boon L, et al. Clinical phenotype of adolescent and adult patients with extracranial vascular malformation. J Vasc Surg Venous Lymphat Disord. 2023;11:1034–44.e3. https://doi.org/10.1016/j.jvsv.2023.03.012.
2. Vuillemin N, Bernhard S, Haine A, Schindewolf M, Häberli D, Hügel U, et al. Capillary-venule malformation is a microfistulous variant of arteriovenous malformation. J Vasc Surg Venous Lymphat Disord. 2021;9:220–5. https://doi.org/10.1016/j.jvsv.2020.05.012.
3. Ajoolabady A, Pratico D, Ren J. Endothelial dysfunction: mechanisms and contribution to diseases. Acta Pharmacol Sin. 2024;45:2023–31. https://doi.org/10.1038/s41401-024-01295-8.
4. Bréchot N, Rutault A, Marangon I, Germain S. Blood endothelium transition and phenotypic plasticity: a key regulator of integrity/permeability in response to ischemia. Semin Cell Dev Biol. 2024;155:16–22. https://doi.org/10.1016/j.semcdb.2023.07.004.
5. Cuervo H, Mühleder S, García-Gónzalez I, Benedito R. Notch-mediated cellular interactions between vascular cells. Curr Opin Cell Biol. 2023;85:102254. https://doi.org/10.1016/j.ceb.2023.102254.
6. Aitken C, Mehta V, Schwartz MA, Tzima E. Mechanisms of endothelial flow sensing. Nat Cardiovasc Res. 2023;2:517–29. https://doi.org/10.1038/s44161-023-00276-0.
7. Frey S, Cantieni T, Vuillemin N, Haine A, Kammer R, von Tengg-Kobligk H, et al. Angioarchitecture and hemodynamics of microvascular arterio-venous malformations. PLoS One. 2018;13:e0203368. https://doi.org/10.1371/journal.pone.0203368.
8. Bernhard SM, Tuleja A, Laine JE, Haupt F, Häberli D, Hügel U, et al. Clinical presentation of simple and combined or syndromic arteriovenous malformations. J Vasc Surg Venous Lymphat Disord. 2022;10:705–12. https://doi.org/10.1016/j.jvsv.2021.10.002.
9. Kunimoto K, Yamamoto Y, Jinnin M. ISSVA classification of vascular anomalies and molecular biology. Int J Mol Sci. 2022;23:2358. https://doi.org/10.3390/ijms23042358.
10. Escobar K, Pandher K, Jahnke MN. Capillary malformations. Dermatol Clin. 2022;40:425–33. https://doi.org/10.1016/j.det.2022.06.005.

11. Bernhard SM, Kammer FR, Roumet MC, Haupt F, Tuleja A, Schindewolf M, et al. A proposal for a revision of the phlebographic classification of congenital venous malformations. Cardiovasc Diagn Ther. 2024;14:283–93. https://doi.org/10.21037/cdt-23-378.
12. Frey S, Haine A, Kammer R, von Tengg-Kobligk H, Obrist D, Baumgartner I. Hemodynamic characterization of peripheral arterio-venous malformations. Ann Biomed Eng. 2017;45:1449–61. https://doi.org/10.1007/s10439-017-1821-9.
13. Mäkinen T, Boon LM, Vikkula M, Alitalo K. Lymphatic malformations: genetics, mechanisms and therapeutic strategies. Circ Res. 2021;129:136–54. https://doi.org/10.1161/circresaha.121.318142.
14. Queisser A, Seront E, Boon LM, Vikkula M. Genetic basis and therapies for vascular anomalies. Circ Res. 2021;129:155–73. https://doi.org/10.1161/circresaha.121.318145.
15. Hume E, Cossio ML, Vargas P, Cubillos MP, Maccioni A, Lay-Son G. Another face of RASA1: report of familial germline variant in RASA1 with dysmorphic features. Am J Med Genet A. 2024;194:e63711. https://doi.org/10.1002/ajmg.a.63711.
16. Chen D, Van der Ent MA, Lartey NL, King PD. EPHB4-RASA1-mediated negative regulation of Ras-MAPK signaling in the vasculature: implications for the treatment of EPHB4- and RASA1-related vascular anomalies in humans. Pharmaceuticals (Basel). 2023;16:165. https://doi.org/10.3390/ph16020165.
17. Revencu N, Fastre E, Ravoet M, Helaers R, Brouillard P, Bisdorff-Bresson A, et al. RASA1 mosaic mutations in patients with capillary malformation-arteriovenous malformation. J Med Genet. 2020;57:48–52. https://doi.org/10.1136/jmedgenet-2019-106024.
18. Hammill AM, Boscolo E. Capillary malformations. J Clin Invest. 2024;134:e172842. https://doi.org/10.1172/jci172842.
19. Hirose K, Hori Y, Ozeki M, Motooka D, Hata K, Tahara S, et al. Comprehensive phenotypic and genomic characterization of venous malformations. Hum Pathol. 2024;145:48–55. https://doi.org/10.1016/j.humpath.2024.02.004.
20. Andreoti TA, Maiolo M, Tuleja A, Döring Y, Schaller A, Vassella E, et al. Non-hotspot PIK3CA variants have higher variant allele frequency and are more common in syndromic vascular malformations. Am J Med Genet A. 2025;197:e63883. https://doi.org/10.1002/ajmg.a.63883.
21. Kapp FG, Bazgir F, Mahammadzade N, Mehrabipour M, Vassella E, Bernhard SM, et al. Somatic RIT1 delins in arteriovenous malformations hyperactivate RAS-MAPK signaling amenable to MEK inhibition. Angiogenesis. 2024;27:739–52. https://doi.org/10.1007/s10456-024-09934-8.
22. Schmidt VF, Kapp FG, Goldann C, Huthmann L, Cucuruz B, Brill R, et al. Extracranial vascular anomalies driven by RAS/MAPK variants: spectrum and genotype-phenotype correlations. J Am Heart Assoc. 2024;13:e033287. https://doi.org/10.1161/jaha.123.033287.
23. Bernhard SMTA, Döring Y, Vassella E, Amstutz U, Zweier C, Rössler J, Boon LM, Vikkula M, Haupt F, Hamvas G, Schindewolf M, Kammer R, Baumgartner I. Oncogene targeted next-generation-sequencing in extracranial arterio-venous malformation. Zenodo EU Open Res Repo. 2025. https://doi.org/10.5281/zenodo.14643334.
24. Latif MA, Sobreira NLD, Guthrie KS, Motaghi M, Robinson GM, Shafaat O, et al. Clinical and molecular characterization of patients with hereditary hemorrhagic telangiectasia: experience from an HHT center of excellence. Am J Med Genet A. 2021;185:1981–90. https://doi.org/10.1002/ajmg.a.62193.
25. Al Tabosh T, Al Tarrass M, Tourvieilhe L, Guilhem A, Dupuis-Girod S, Bailly S. Hereditary hemorrhagic telangiectasia: from signaling insights to therapeutic advances. J Clin Invest. 2024;134:e176379. https://doi.org/10.1172/jci176379.
26. Diociaiuti A, Paolantonio G, Zama M, Alaggio R, Carnevale C, Conforti A, et al. Vascular birthmarks as a clue for complex and syndromic vascular anomalies. Front Pediatr. 2021;9:730393. https://doi.org/10.3389/fped.2021.730393.
27. Van Trigt WK, Kelly KM, Hughes CCW. GNAQ mutations drive port wine birthmark-associated Sturge-weber syndrome: a review of pathobiology, therapies, and current models. Front Hum Neurosci. 2022;16:1006027. https://doi.org/10.3389/fnhum.2022.1006027.

28. Ramirez EL, Jülich K. Sturge-weber syndrome: an overview of history, genetics, clinical manifestations, and management. Semin Pediatr Neurol. 2024;51:101151. https://doi.org/10.1016/j.spen.2024.101151.
29. Rodríguez Bandera AI, Sebaratnam DF, Wargon O, Wong LF. Infantile hemangioma. Part 1: epidemiology, pathogenesis, clinical presentation and assessment. J Am Acad Dermatol. 2021;85:1379–92. https://doi.org/10.1016/j.jaad.2021.08.019.
30. Haefliger S, Adams S, Nandakumar A, Nguyen L, Wargon O. CM-AVM syndrome - a prospective observational study of unrelated paediatric cases. Australas J Dermatol. 2021;62:347–53. https://doi.org/10.1111/ajd.13651.
31. Kanji A, Cobben J, Laguda B. CLOVES Syndrome. JAMA Dermatol. 2023;159:659–60. https://doi.org/10.1001/jamadermatol.2022.6180.
32. Markovic JN, Shortell CK. Venous malformations. J Cardiovasc Surg. 2021;62:456–66. https://doi.org/10.23736/s0021-9509.21.11911-1.
33. Mir-Bonafé JF, Mir-Bonafé M, Piquero-Casals J, Rozas-Muñoz E. Familial cutaneomucosal venous malformations. Dermatol Pract Concept. 2020;10:e2020082. https://doi.org/10.5826/dpc.1004a82.
34. Kozai L, Nishimura Y. Clinical characteristics of blue rubber bleb nevus syndrome in adults: systematic scoping review. Scand J Gastroenterol. 2023;58:1108–14. https://doi.org/10.1080/00365521.2023.2214263.
35. Asghar F, Aqeel R, Farooque U, Haq A, Taimur M. Presentation and management of Klippel-Trenaunay syndrome: a review of available data. Cureus. 2020;12:e8023. https://doi.org/10.7759/cureus.8023.
36. Andreoti TA, Berg S, Holm A, Angerer M, Oberlin M, Foeldi E, et al. Complex lymphatic anomalies: report on a patient registry using the latest diagnostic guidelines. Lymphat Res Biol. 2023;21:230–43. https://doi.org/10.1089/lrb.2022.0041.
37. Reynolds G, Cardaropoli S, Carli D, Luca M, Gazzin A, Coppo P, et al. Epidemiology of the disorders of the Pik3ca-related overgrowth spectrum (Pros). Eur J Hum Genet. 2023;31:1333–6. https://doi.org/10.1038/s41431-023-01414-9.
38. Klimeczek-Chrapusta MK, Kachnic M, Chrapusta A. Proteus syndrome: case report and updated literature review. Arch Plast Surg. 2024;51:423–31. https://doi.org/10.1055/a-2300-7002.
39. Wang YP, Di WJ, Qin SL, Yang S, Wang Z, Xu YF, et al. A rare presentation of Maffucci syndrome: a case report and literature review. Exp Ther Med. 2023;26:435. https://doi.org/10.3892/etm.2023.12134.
40. Shovlin CL, Buscarini E, Sabbà C, Mager HJ, Kjeldsen AD, Pagella F, et al. The European rare disease network for HHT frameworks for management of hereditary haemorrhagic telangiectasia in general and speciality care. Eur J Med Genet. 2022;65:104370. https://doi.org/10.1016/j.ejmg.2021.104370.
41. Pilz RA, Skowronek D, Ehresmann T, Felbor U, Rath M. Novel postzygotic RASA1 mutation in a patient with Parkes Weber syndrome: a case report and literature review. Clin Case Rep. 2024;12:e9543. https://doi.org/10.1002/ccr3.9543.
42. Takaya K, Sakamoto Y, Miwa T, Yoshida K, Kishi K. Gorham-Stout disease with parietal bone osteolysis: a case series and review of literature. Br J Neurosurg. 2021;35:27–31. https://doi.org/10.1080/02688697.2020.1744524.
43. Zenker M, Edouard T, Blair JC, Cappa M. Noonan syndrome: improving recognition and diagnosis. Arch Dis Child. 2022;107:1073–8. https://doi.org/10.1136/archdischild-2021-322858.
44. Cogan G, Bourgon N, Borghese R, Julien E, Jaquette A, Stos B, et al. Diagnosis of Menke-Hennekam syndrome by prenatal whole exome sequencing and review of prenatal signs. Mol Genet Genomic Med. 2023;11:e2219. https://doi.org/10.1002/mgg3.2219.
45. Fahrni JO, Cho EY, Engelberger RP, Baumgartner I, von Känel R. Quality of life in patients with congenital vascular malformations. J Vasc Surg Venous Lymphat Disord. 2014;2:46–51. https://doi.org/10.1016/j.jvsv.2013.09.001.

46. Muir T, Wohlgemuth WA, Cemazar M, Bertino G, Groselj A, Ratnam LA, et al. Current operating procedure (COP) for bleomycin ElectroScleroTherapy (BEST) of low-flow vascular malformations. Radiol Oncol. 2024;58:469–79. https://doi.org/10.2478/raon-2024-0061.
47. Lee BB, Baumgartner I, Berlien HP, Bianchini G, Burrows P, Do YS, et al. Consensus document of the International Union of Angiology (IUA)-2013. Current concept on the management of arterio-venous management. Int Angiol. 2013;32:9–36.
48. Gu Y, Sebaratnam DF. Adjuvant topical sirolimus for pulsed dye laser in pediatric capillary malformation. Dermatologic Surg. 2024;50:300–1. https://doi.org/10.1097/dss.0000000000004047.
49. Giovanni C, Marina PB, Tiziano Z. A retrospective 10 years- experience overview of dye laser treatments for vascular pathologies. Skin Res Technol. 2023;29:e13427. https://doi.org/10.1111/srt.13427.
50. Sodha P, Wang JV, Aboul-Fettouh N, Martin K, Geronemus RG, Friedman PM. Largest comparative analysis: novel large spot size 595 nm, high-energy, pulsed dye laser reduces number of treatments for improvement of adult and pediatric port wine birthmarks. Lasers Surg Med. 2023;55:741–7. https://doi.org/10.1002/lsm.23693.
51. Patil UA. Application of lasers in vascular anomalies. Indian J Plast Surg. 2023;56:395–404. https://doi.org/10.1055/s-0043-1775871.
52. Kim H, Joh J, Labropoulos N. Characteristics, clinical presentation, and treatment outcomes of venous malformation in the extremities. J Vasc Surg Venous Lymphat Disord. 2022;10:152–8. https://doi.org/10.1016/j.jvsv.2021.05.011.
53. Kim KR. Percutaneous sclerotherapy of venous malformations. Tech Vasc Interv Radiol. 2024;27:100960. https://doi.org/10.1016/j.tvir.2024.100960.
54. Swerdlin RF, Briones MA, Gill AE, Hawkins CM. Coagulopathy and related complications following sclerotherapy of congenital venous malformations. Pediatr Blood Cancer. 2022;69:e29610. https://doi.org/10.1002/pbc.29610.
55. Steiner F, FitzJohn T, Tan ST. Ethanol sclerotherapy for venous malformation. ANZ J Surg. 2016;86:790–5. https://doi.org/10.1111/ans.12833.
56. Li HB, Zhang J, Li XM, Zhou SY, Niu CQ, Liu ZY, et al. Clinical efficacy of absolute ethanol combined with n-butyl cyanoacrylate sclerotherapy in the treatment of Puig's classified advanced venous malformation in children. Exp Ther Med. 2019;17:1276–81. https://doi.org/10.3892/etm.2018.7051.
57. Polites SF, Watanabe M, Scorletti F, Patel MN, Ricci KW, Hammill AM, et al. Single-stage embolization with n-butyl cyanoacrylate and surgical resection of venous malformations. Pediatr Blood Cancer. 2020;67:e28029. https://doi.org/10.1002/pbc.28029.
58. Han YY, Sun LM, Yuan SM. Localized intravascular coagulation in venous malformations: a system review. Phlebology. 2021;36:38–42. https://doi.org/10.1177/0268355520946211.
59. Dompmartin A, Acher A, Thibon P, Tourbach S, Hermans C, Deneys V, et al. Association of localized intravascular coagulopathy with venous malformations. Arch Dermatol. 2008;144:873–7. https://doi.org/10.1001/archderm.144.7.873.
60. Ghahremani JS, Chapek MA, Singh Rana SS, Lee J, Safran BA, Lau DL, et al. Endovascular embolization of aneurysmal renal arteriovenous malformation. Vasc Endovasc Surg. 2025;59:198–203. https://doi.org/10.1177/15385744241286675.
61. Botsford A, Tradi F, Loubet A, Tantawi S, Soulez G, Giroux MF, et al. Transarterial embolization of simple pulmonary arteriovenous malformations: long-term outcomes of 0.018-inch coils versus vascular plugs. J Vasc Interv Radiol. 2024;35:349–60. https://doi.org/10.1016/j.jvir.2023.11.018.
62. Kohlbrenner R, Fidelman N, Kohi MP, Kumar V, Kolli KP. Onyx embolization of an enlarging arterioportal pancreatic AVM using a balloon-occlusion microcatheter. Diagn Interv Radiol. 2021;27:458–9. https://doi.org/10.5152/dir.2020.20416.
63. Chen CJ, Norat P, Ding D, Mendes GAC, Tvrdik P, Park MS, et al. Transvenous embolization of brain arteriovenous malformations: a review of techniques, indications, and outcomes. Neurosurg Focus. 2018;45:E13. https://doi.org/10.3171/2018.3.Focus18113.

64. Dabhi N, Sokolowski J, Zanaty M, Kellogg RT, Park MS, Mastorakos P. Primary embolization of cerebral arteriovenous malformations with intention to cure: a systematic review of literature and meta-analysis. Neurosurgery. 2024;95:1232–44. https://doi.org/10.1227/neu.0000000000003001.
65. Li XY, Wang DM, Wen MZ, Zheng LZ, Wang ZF, Ren C, et al. Ethanol embolization of chest wall arteriovenous malformations: four-year findings. J Endovasc Ther. 2024;31:919–26. https://doi.org/10.1177/15266028221149908.
66. Soulez G, Gilbert MFP, Giroux MFMF, Racicot MFJN, Dubois J. Interventional management of arteriovenous malformations. Tech Vasc Interv Radiol. 2019;22:100633. https://doi.org/10.1016/j.tvir.2019.100633.
67. Seront E, Van Damme A, Legrand C, Bisdorff-Bresson A, Orcel P, Funck-Brentano T, et al. Preliminary results of the European multicentric phase III trial regarding sirolimus in slow-flow vascular malformations. JCI Insight. 2023;8:e173095. https://doi.org/10.1172/jci.insight.173095.
68. Al-Samkari H, Kasthuri RS, Parambil JG, Albitar HA, Almodallal YA, Vázquez C, et al. An international, multicenter study of intravenous bevacizumab for bleeding in hereditary hemorrhagic telangiectasia: the InHIBIT-bleed study. Haematologica. 2021;106:2161–9. https://doi.org/10.3324/haematol.2020.261859.
69. Dupuis-Girod S, Shovlin CL, Kjeldsen AD, Mager HJ, Sabba C, Droege F, et al. European reference network for rare vascular diseases (VASCERN): when and how to use intravenous bevacizumab in hereditary haemorrhagic telangiectasia (HHT)? Eur J Med Genet. 2022;65:104575. https://doi.org/10.1016/j.ejmg.2022.104575.
70. Seebauer CT, Wiens B, Hintschich CA, Platz Batista da Silva N, Evert K, Haubner F, et al. Targeting the microenvironment in the treatment of arteriovenous malformations. Angiogenesis. 2024;27:91–103. https://doi.org/10.1007/s10456-023-09896-3.
71. Muster R, Ko N, Smith W, Su H, Dickey MA, Nelson J, et al. Proof-of-concept single-arm trial of bevacizumab therapy for brain arteriovenous malformation. BMJ Neurol Open. 2021;3:e000114. https://doi.org/10.1136/bmjno-2020-000114.
72. Dupuis-Girod S, Rivière S, Lavigne C, Fargeton AE, Gilbert-Dussardier B, Grobost V, et al. Efficacy and safety of intravenous bevacizumab on severe bleeding associated with hemorrhagic hereditary telangiectasia: a national, randomized multicenter trial. J Intern Med. 2023;294:761–74. https://doi.org/10.1111/joim.13714.
73. Venot Q, Blanc T, Rabia SH, Berteloot L, Ladraa S, Duong JP, et al. Targeted therapy in patients with PIK3CA-related overgrowth syndrome. Nature. 2018;558:540–6. https://doi.org/10.1038/s41586-018-0217-9.
74. Adams DM, Trenor CC 3rd, Hammill AM, Vinks AA, Patel MN, Chaudry G, et al. Efficacy and safety of sirolimus in the treatment of complicated vascular anomalies. Pediatrics. 2016;137:e20153257. https://doi.org/10.1542/peds.2015-3257.
75. Wiegand S, Dietz A, Wichmann G. Efficacy of sirolimus in children with lymphatic malformations of the head and neck. Eur Arch Otorrinolaringol. 2022;279:3801–10. https://doi.org/10.1007/s00405-022-07378-8.
76. Maruani A, Tavernier E, Boccara O, Mazereeuw-Hautier J, Leducq S, Bessis D, et al. Sirolimus (rapamycin) for slow-flow malformations in children: the observational-phase randomized clinical PERFORMUS trial. JAMA Dermatol. 2021;157:1289–98. https://doi.org/10.1001/jamadermatol.2021.3459.
77. Cavazos R, Patil MS, Gowda SH, Iacobas I, Rosenberg T, Fernandes CJ, et al. Sirolimus for vascular anomalies in the first year of life: a systematic review. J Perinatol. 2024;44:1087–97. https://doi.org/10.1038/s41372-024-01868-9.
78. Goldenberg DC, Carvas M, Adams D, Giannotti M, Gemperli R. Successful treatment of a complex vascular malformation with sirolimus and surgical resection. J Pediatr Hematol Oncol. 2017;39:e191–e5. https://doi.org/10.1097/mph.0000000000000702.

79. Liu H, Yang X, Jia H, Hu L, Xu Z, Chen H, et al. Recurrence and restart of sirolimus in vascular anomalies after withdrawal. J Dermatol. 2023;50:e119–20. https://doi.org/10.1111/1346-8138.16649.
80. Durán-Romero AJ, Hernández-Rodríguez JC, Ortiz-Álvarez J, Domínguez-Cruz JJ, Monserrat-García MT, Conejo-Mir Sánchez J, et al. Efficacy and safety of oral sirolimus for high-flow vascular malformations in real clinical practice. Clin Exp Dermatol. 2022;47:57–62. https://doi.org/10.1111/ced.14841.
81. Kalbfell R, Cohen-Cutler S, Grisham E, Bereitschaft C, Borst AJ, Green AM, et al. Infectious complications of vascular anomalies treated with sirolimus: a systematic review. Pediatr Blood Cancer. 2024;71:e30758. https://doi.org/10.1002/pbc.30758.
82. Bevacqua M, Baldo F, Pastore S, Valencic E, Tommasini A, Maestro A, et al. Off-label use of sirolimus and everolimus in a pediatric center: a case series and review of the literature. Paediatr Drugs. 2019;21:185–93. https://doi.org/10.1007/s40272-019-00337-7.
83. Rössler J, Baselga E, Davila V, Celis V, Diociaiuti A, El Hachem M, et al. Severe adverse events during sirolimus "off-label" therapy for vascular anomalies. Pediatr Blood Cancer. 2021;68:e28936. https://doi.org/10.1002/pbc.28936.
84. Smits PJ, Konczyk DJ, Sudduth CL, Goss JA, Greene AK. Endothelial MAP2K1 mutations in arteriovenous malformation activate the RAS/MAPK pathway. Biochem Biophys Res Commun. 2020;529:450–4. https://doi.org/10.1016/j.bbrc.2020.06.022.
85. Nguyen HL, Boon LM, Vikkula M. Trametinib as a promising therapeutic option in alleviating vascular defects in an endothelial KRAS-induced mouse model. Hum Mol Genet. 2023;32:276–89. https://doi.org/10.1093/hmg/ddac169.
86. Gordon K, Moore M, Van Zanten M, Pearce J, Itkin M, Madden B, et al. Case report: progressive central conducting lymphatic abnormalities in the RASopathies. Two case reports, including successful treatment by MEK inhibition. Front Genet. 2022;13:1001105. https://doi.org/10.3389/fgene.2022.1001105.
87. Lekwuttikarn R, Lim YH, Admani S, Choate KA, Teng JMC. Genotype-guided medical treatment of an arteriovenous malformation in a child. JAMA Dermatol. 2019;155:256–7. https://doi.org/10.1001/jamadermatol.2018.4653.
88. Nicholson CL, Flanagan S, Murati M, Boull C, McGough E, Ameduri R, et al. Successful management of an arteriovenous malformation with trametinib in a patient with capillary-malformation arteriovenous malformation syndrome and cardiac compromise. Pediatr Dermatol. 2022;39:316–9. https://doi.org/10.1111/pde.14912.
89. Nakano TA, Rankin AW, Annam A, Kulungowski AM, McCallen LM, Hill LR, et al. Trametinib for refractory chylous effusions and systemic complications in children with Noonan syndrome. J Pediatr. 2022;248:81–8.e1. https://doi.org/10.1016/j.jpeds.2022.05.030.
90. Seront E, Froidure A, Revencu N, Dekeuleneer V, Clapuyt P, Dumitriu D, et al. Targeted treatment in complex lymphatic anomaly: a case of synergistic efficacy of trametinib and sirolimus. Orphanet J Rare Dis. 2024;19:199. https://doi.org/10.1186/s13023-024-03211-z.
91. Edwards EA, Phelps AS, Cooke D, Frieden IJ, Zapala MA, Fullerton HJ, et al. Monitoring arteriovenous malformation response to genotype-targeted therapy. Pediatrics. 2020;146:e20193206. https://doi.org/10.1542/peds.2019-3206.
92. Feng N, Chen H, Fu S, Bian Z, Lin X, Yang L, et al. HIF-1α and HIF-2α induced angiogenesis in gastrointestinal vascular malformation and reversed by thalidomide. Sci Rep. 2016;6:27280. https://doi.org/10.1038/srep27280.
93. Blatt J, Brondon JE, Nieman EL, Phillips K, Pandya A. Repurposing of antiangiogenic agents for treatment of vascular anomalies. Pharmacol Ther. 2023;250:108520. https://doi.org/10.1016/j.pharmthera.2023.108520.
94. Al-Samkari H. Systemic antiangiogenic therapies for bleeding in hereditary hemorrhagic telangiectasia: a practical, evidence-based guide for clinicians. Semin Thromb Hemost. 2022;48:514–28. https://doi.org/10.1055/s-0042-1743467.

95. Nip L, Evans N, Bali S, Hopper C, Papadopoulou A, Khalifa M, et al. Early experience of thalidomide therapy for high-grade peripheral and facial arteriovenous malformations. Int Angiol. 2023;42:448–56. https://doi.org/10.23736/s0392-9590.23.05111-8.
96. Bongetta D, Zoia C, Lafe E, Gaetani P. Could thalidomide be a treatment option for arteriovenous malformations? World Neurosurg. 2017;99:802. https://doi.org/10.1016/j.wneu.2016.10.068.
97. Seront E, Hermans C, Boon LM, Vikkula M. Targeted treatments for vascular malformations: current state of the art. J Thromb Haemost. 2024;22:2961–75. https://doi.org/10.1016/j.jtha.2024.07.013.
98. Gopishetty A, Amarnath K, Uma Magesh DP, Saichand G. Successful treatment of low-flow vascular malformation in the lip using intralesional bleomycin: a case report. Cureus. 2024;16:e74119. https://doi.org/10.7759/cureus.74119.
99. Viglione M, Discalzi A, Mistretta F, Mancini A, Nardelli F, Bergui M. Bilateral congenital pelvic arteriovenous malformation: a case report and review of literature. J Endovasc Ther. 2024;33(2):543–54. https://doi.org/10.1177/15266028241267747.

Chapter 10
Lymphoedema

Kristiana Gordon

SN Flashcards
Test your learning and check your understanding of this book's contents: use the "Springer Nature Flashcards" app to access questions using ▶ https://sn.pub/wppvze. To use the app, please follow the instructions in Chap. 1.

Key Learning Points

- The lymphatic system has several functions, including maintenance of fluid balance and maintaining immune function with the help of lymphoid organs, and nutrition (fat absorption via the intestinal lymphatics). The lymphatic system also plays a role in disease, such as inflammatory disorders and cancer metastasis.
- Unlike the larger collecting vessels, initial lymphatic capillaries have a discontinuous basement membrane. The gaps permit entry of interstitial fluid, macromolecules and leucocytes.
- Lymphatic vessels are essentially of three types: (1) initial non-contractile lymphatic vessels that absorb capillary filtrate, leucocytes and macrophages, (2) pre-collectors that are sparsely covered by smooth muscle cells and (3) the larger collecting lymphatic vessels that actively pump lymph to the regional lymph nodes.
- Lymphoedema occurs when the rate of microvascular filtration overwhelms lymphatic drainage capacity. This can occur because either the microvascular filtra-

K. Gordon (✉)
Department of Dermatology and Lymphovascular Medicine, St George's University Hospitals NHS Foundation Trust, London, UK
e-mail: Kristiana.Gordon@stgeorges.nhs.uk

R. Fitridge et al. (eds.), *Pathophysiology of Vascular Disease*,
https://doi.org/10.1007/978-3-032-31459-8_10

tion rate is increased (e.g. in the case of venous insufficiency), or the rate of lymphatic flow has decreased, or a combination of the two. Failure of the lymphatic system leads to the accumulation of protein-rich lymph fluid within interstitial spaces, manifesting as lymphoedema.
- Primary lymphoedema arises as a result of a genetic predisposition. The lymphatic system fails to develop normally or to be maintained adequately, causing impaired drainage of lymph and swelling of the affected region. Primary lymphoedema is an umbrella term, and there are many subtypes that can be divided into five different categories. A diagnostic pathway has been developed that describes the specific primary lymphoedema phenotypes and guides clinicians on relevant gene testing that may be available.
- Secondary lymphoedema develops from an acquired disruption to lymph drainage routes, e.g. damage to the lymphatic vessels and/or lymph nodes. Causes of secondary lymphoedema include infection (e.g. recurrent cellulitis or Filariasis), malignancy, surgery, inflammatory conditions, trauma, venous disease and immobility.
- The management of lymphoedema is aimed at reducing swelling through physical treatments designed to stimulate flow through existing or collateral drainage routes. This physical therapy management approach is the same for patients with primary and secondary lymphoedema.
- Patients with primary or secondary lymphoedema are susceptible to a number of complications, including infections, almost certainly due to reduced immune surveillance secondary to lymphatic dysfunction. Recurrent cellulitis is a particular problem. The use of prophylactic penicillin has been shown to reduce the rate of infection.

10.1 Introduction

The lymphatic system forms part of the human circulatory and immune systems. It has several functions, including (1) maintenance of fluid balance by returning lymphatic fluid from interstitial spaces to the blood circulation, (2) maintaining immune function with the help of lymphoid organs and (3) nutritional, as fat is absorbed via the intestinal lymphatics. The lymphatic system also plays a role in disease, e.g. inflammatory disorders and cancer metastasis.

Lymphoedema occurs when the rate of microvascular filtration overwhelms lymphatic drainage capacity. This can occur because either the microvascular filtration rate is increased (e.g. in the case of venous insufficiency), or the rate of lymphatic flow has decreased, or a combination of the two. Failure of the lymphatic system leads to the accumulation of protein-rich lymph fluid within interstitial spaces, manifesting as lymphoedema, a debilitating swelling with associated changes of the skin.

Primary lymphoedema refers to *chronic swelling due to an intrinsic anomaly affecting the lymphatic system*, which is often genetic in origin. It arises as a result of the lymphatic system failing to develop normally or to be maintained adequately, causing impaired drainage of lymph resulting in swelling of the affected region. Primary lymphoedema may occur as a non-syndromic Mendelian condition, or less commonly as part of a complex syndromic disorder. A diagnostic algorithm has been developed in order to facilitate diagnosis [1].

Secondary lymphoedema develops from an acquired disruption to lymphatic drainage routes, e.g. damage to the lymphatic vessels and/or lymph nodes. Causes of secondary lymphoedema include infection (e.g. recurrent cellulitis or filariasis), malignancy, surgery, inflammatory conditions, trauma, venous disease and immobility [2–4].

Patients with primary or secondary lymphoedema are susceptible to a number of complications. These include infections due to reduced immune surveillance secondary to lymphatic dysfunction. Recurrent cellulitis is a particular problem. Constitutional symptoms such as fever, vomiting or headaches may develop suddenly without typical heralding skin signs of cellulitis. Repeated episodes of infection will exacerbate lymphoedema and predispose to further infections, thus creating a vicious cycle of events. The use of prophylactic penicillin has been shown to reduce the rate of infection [5].

Unfortunately, there is no proven curative treatment for lymphoedema. Management is aimed at reducing the swelling through physical treatments designed to stimulate flow through existing or collateral drainage routes. This physical therapy management approach is the same for those patients with primary and secondary lymphoedema. Several surgical techniques have been implemented in an attempt to improve lymphatic drainage or achieve limb volume reduction via liposuction. However, in the absence of robust data to support most surgical techniques, we must rely on physical therapies for the majority of patients until new and improved therapeutic options are available.

10.2 Lymphangiogenesis

Lymphangiogenesis is the term used to describe the growth of new lymphatic vessels. Developmental lymphangiogenesis occurs in the foetus when the lymphatic system is developing. However, lymphangiogenesis may also occur postnatally in association with inflammatory disease and malignancy. Research has identified several lymphatic endothelial cell-specific molecular markers and genes involved in lymphatic development and lymphangiogenesis, but there is still much to learn about the process. Expression of these endothelial markers can occur in both lymphatic and blood vessels, which may explain the high rate of coexistent venous abnormalities in patients with primary lymphoedema and genetically determined lymphatic vessel abnormalities.

10.2.1 Origin and Differentiation of Lymphatic Endothelial Cells

There is still much that is not known about the development of the lymphatic system. It is a challenging system to study thanks to its fragile and transparent ('see through') nature. The most widely accepted model of the origin of lymphatic endothelium was proposed by Florence Sabin in 1902 [6]. Other models have been proposed but are less widely accepted and not supported by mammalian animal models. Current literature reports that lymph sacs develop in the human embryo at 6–7 weeks of gestation, nearly 1 month after the blood vascular system has started to develop [7]. Research in animal models demonstrates that a subpopulation of blood endothelial cells, arising from cardinal and peripheral veins, differentiates into lymphatic endothelial cells (LECs) [8]. These LECs then bud off as strings of cells to form primitive lymphatic structures called 'lymph sacs' [9]. Differentiation of LECs is thought to be governed by the action of transcription factors, including Prox1, Sox18 and COUP-TFII [10]. Prox1-expressing LECs up-regulate Vascular Endothelial Growth Factor Receptor 3 (VEGFR3), lymphatic vessel endothelial hyaluronan receptor 1 (LYVE1) and other lymphatic endothelial-specific molecules [11]. Sox18 is expressed in the cardinal vein and is responsible for regulating Prox1 expression [12]. COUP-TFII has been shown to establish venous endothelial cell identity and LEC specification by suppressing Notch signalling [13].

10.2.2 Sprouting of Lymphatic Endothelial Cells

These individual lymphatic endothelial cells connect to other LECs by adherens junctions and start 'sprouting' into primitive lymphatic structures (lymph sacs) [14]. A direct connection is created between the primordial thoracic duct and the cardinal vein to permit eventual return of lymphatic fluid back into the cardiovascular system. Valves develop at the connection site in order to prevent retrograde flow of blood into the newly formed lymphatic system [15]. The LECs produce podoplanin (a mucin-type protein) that interacts with C-type lectin domain family 1 member B (Clec-2) in platelets to induce platelet aggregation and induce a 'sealing' process and subsequent separation of the two vascular systems [16]. Animal studies suggest that the VEGFC/VEGFR3 and CCBE1 (collagen and calcium-binding EGF domain-1) signalling pathways regulate sprouting. Venous sprouting is inhibited by the absence of VEGFC or CCBE1, resulting in the complete absence of lymphatic vessels in animal models [15].

The ligands VEGFC and VEGFD bind and activate the tyrosine kinase receptors VEGFR2 and VEGFR3 on LECs. VEGFR3 is considered the main VEGFC receptor for lymphangiogenesis [17]. Both VEGFC and VEGFD promote migration and proliferation of LECs in vitro, and lymphatic vessel hyperplasia in vivo. However, it appears that only VEGFC is required for embryonic lymphatic development [18, 19]. CCBE1 does not appear to have lymphangiogenic activity on its own but enhances the lymphangiogenic effects of VEGFC in vivo [20]. CCBE1 up-regulates levels of mature VEGFC. CCBE1 also promotes in vitro proteolytic cleavage of the otherwise poorly active 29/31-kDa form of VEGFC by the A disintegrin and metalloprotease with thrombospondin motifs-3 protease (ADAMTS3), resulting in the mature form of VEGFC, which subsequently induces increased VEGFC receptor signalling [21].

Whilst we do not yet fully understand all mechanisms involved in lymphangiogenesis, the identification of mutations in *SOX18*, *VEGFR3*, *VEGFC*, *CCBE1* and

ADAMTS3 in humans with primary lymphoedema and lymphatic insufficiency supports the critical role these genes play. Gene therapy may one day be available to treat patients with these mutations to cure their disease.

10.2.3 Remodelling of the Lymphatic Vascular System

Further development of the lymphatic system occurs by lymphatic vessel sprouting from the primitive lymph sacs mentioned above. The primitive lymphatic vessels must now mature into a functional network with vessel-type features that serve their critical functions. Remodelling processes lead to the formation of flap valves in lymphatic capillaries, the establishment of pre-collecting and collecting vessels via smooth muscle cell recruitment and luminal valve development.

Flap-like openings called 'primary valves' form between the LECs of lymphatic capillaries to create button-like intercellular junctions. These facilitate the entry of interstitial fluid and leucocytes into the initial lymphatic vessels [22]. Prox1 and FOXC2 transcription factors are expressed by clusters of cells within developing collecting vessels to form intraluminal valves [23]. FOXC2 (forkhead box C2) is a significant regulator of lymphatic valve formation. FOXC2 deficiency in humans results in lymphatic vessel valve aplasia, manifesting with lymphatic reflux and lymphoedema in patients with Lymphoedema Distichiasis Syndrome due to *FOXC2* mutations [24].

The lymphatic pre-collectors and collecting lymphatic vessels are covered by smooth muscle cells (SMCs), except in the luminal valve areas, to assist with proximal propulsion of lymph [25]. SMCs play a significant role in lymphatic remodelling and function. Unlike the larger collecting vessels, initial lymphatic capillaries have a discontinuous basement membrane. The gaps permit entry of interstitial fluid, macromolecules and leucocytes [26]. Initial lymphatic capillary LECs remain attached to the interstitial matrix by anchoring filaments [27].

It is clear how some primary lymphoedema subtypes are caused by abnormal gene function (e.g. *VEGFR3* mutations and Milroy disease; *CCBE1* and Hennekam Syndrome; *FOXC2* and Lymphoedema Distichiasis Syndrome), as the causal genes play a significant role in the lymphangiogenic pathway. However, some genes implicated in other forms of primary lymphoedema are not known to play a role in lymphangiogenesis. There is clearly more to learn about lymphangiogenesis and the genes that regulate it.

10.3 Structure and Function of the Lymphatic System

The lymphatic system is comprised of an extensive network of lymphatic vessels and lymph nodes found in almost all of the tissues in the human body. The primary function of the lymphatic system is to drain fluid and materials from tissue spaces that cannot directly return to the bloodstream. These include capillary filtrate, proteins, macrophages, lymphocytes and malignant cells [28]. The lymphatic system ensures that capillary filtrate (known as lymph/lymphatic fluid once it has entered the lymphatic capillaries) is returned to the blood circulation via the thoracic duct.

The lymphatic system is not a circular system, unlike the blood vascular system. Lymphatic vessels are essentially of three types: (1) initial non-contractile lymphatic vessels that absorb capillary filtrate, leucocytes and macrophages, (2) pre-collectors that are sparsely covered by smooth muscle cells and (3) the larger collecting lymphatic vessels that actively pump lymph to the regional lymph nodes.

10.3.1 Formation of Lymphatic Fluid and Maintenance of Fluid Balance

Lymphatic fluid is derived from the interstitial fluid found in the extracellular spaces in our tissues. This fluid passes into the initial lymphatic capillaries as a result of a pressure gradient via the LEC cell junctions. These junctions act as a form of primary valves, as once interstitial fluid is permitted to enter the initial lymphatics, it cannot easily escape. Once interstitial fluid has entered the lymphatic capillaries, it is called 'lymph'. Alongside this fluid, other cells enter the lymphatic capillaries, including macromolecules, leucocytes and pathogens [26].

The source of interstitial fluid, and therefore lymph, is the transcapillary filtrate from the blood plasma. The rate of capillary filtration is governed by the Starling principle of fluid exchange. Microvascular filtration of fluid from the capillary into the interstitium is driven by the hydraulic pressure gradient across the blood vessel wall and is opposed by the osmotic pressure gradient, which is the suction force retaining fluid within the vessel. The recently revised Starling model proves it is lymphatic drainage that prevents accumulation of transcapillary plasma filtrate in the interstitial spaces, and not via reabsorption in the venous system as originally thought [29]. The subsequent transport of lymph through the lymphatic capillaries is dependent on cyclical changes in hydrostatic and osmotic pressures largely generated by skeletal muscle contractions, arterial pulsation, breathing, intestinal peristalsis and external body compression [30].

Lymphoedema occurs when microvascular (capillary and venular) filtration exceeds the drainage capacity/function of the lymphatic drainage system. This can occur because (1) the microvascular filtration rate is increased, or (2) the rate of lymphatic flow has decreased, or a combination of the two. If lymphatic drainage fails to cope with excessive microvascular filtration caused by an increase in capillary pressure (e.g. heart failure), or a reduction in plasma colloid osmotic pressure (e.g. malnutrition, liver disease), or increased endothelial conductance (e.g. in inflammatory conditions), then lymphoedema will develop. If the lymphatic system fails to adequately drain the capillary filtrate due to (1) damage to a previously healthy lymphatic system (as in a secondary lymphoedema scenario), or (2) an abnormal development of the lymphatic system (as in primary lymphoedema), then the clinical signs of lymphoedema will develop.

We have much still to learn about the transport of lymph, but we are realising that mechanisms of disease vary between different types of lymphoedema. For example, in primary lymphoedema due to Milroy disease, there is a paucity of the initial lymphatic vessels and a failure of them to absorb the interstitial fluid, which accumulates within the lower limb peripheries. In contrast, patients with Lymphoedema Distichiasis Syndrome have normal absorption of interstitial fluid into the lymphatic capillaries but develop lymphoedema as a result of abnormal lymphatic valves. Their mutation in the *FOXC2* gene results in abnormal valvular structure, which causes lymphatic fluid to reflux and accumulate in the lower limbs [1].

10.3.2 Immunity and Infection

The lymphatic system plays a vital role in immune function by mediating the transport of soluble antigens, macrophages, lymphocytes and dendritic cells to draining lymph nodes via afferent lymphatic vessels. It also assists with the trafficking of leucocytes to and from lymph nodes [31]. This transport system allows for an adaptive immune response to be generated to pathogens trying to invade the body.

Local infections (e.g. warts, cellulitis or athlete's foot) are a frequent concern for patients with lymphoedema of any aetiology. Lymphoedema has been reported to convey a relative risk of 71 times the normal for the development of cellulitis [32]. The underlying mechanism is likely to be a disturbance in immune cell trafficking that compromises local tissue immune surveillance.

10.3.3 Lymphatics, Fat and Inflammation

The intestinal lymphatics (lacteals) are responsible for the majority of fat absorption. They absorb dietary fats in the villi of the small intestine in the form of a milky substance called chyle. The lacteals merge to form larger lymphatic vessels and the chyle is transported to the thoracic duct and later to the subclavian vein [33]. The relationship between fat and lymphatics may extend beyond the gut. Clinicians are realising that fat deposition may be a defining clinical characteristic of lymphoedema. Management of lymphoedema by liposuction has confirmed that the swelling is not just fluid but includes large volumes of fat [34]. Evidence is also emerging that the lymphatic system is involved in the regulation of lipids, adipocytes and inflammatory cells. Lymphatic impairment (i.e. lymphoedema) leads to disorders of inflammation and fat homeostasis and deposition and would explain the increased adipose deposition seen in chronic lymphoedema [35].

10.4 Lymphoedema

10.4.1 Introduction

Failure of the lymphatic system leads to the accumulation of protein-rich fluid within interstitial spaces, manifesting as lymphoedema. This may present as debilitating swelling, usually of a limb or limbs, with associated brawny changes of the skin. Primary lymphoedema arises due to an intrinsic abnormality involving a genetically determined aplasia, hypoplasia, malformation or dysfunction of lymphatic vessels. Secondary lymphoedema results from lymphatic damage due to extrinsic factors such as surgical lymphadenectomy, radiotherapy or chronic venous disease. Recurrent lower limb cellulitis can also lead to lymphoedema. Interestingly, a significant number of the latter group will have an intrinsic lymphatic abnormality predisposing them to cellulitis, indicating that this can be both a cause of lymphoedema and occur secondary to a primary lymphoedema [36].

10.4.2 Epidemiology

Estimates of prevalence have been difficult to calculate, as it is presumed that many affected individuals do not come to medical attention. However, it is acknowledged that lymphoedema/chronic oedema is an underestimated health problem that remains widely unrecognised despite affecting an estimated 250 million individuals worldwide, of which 400,000 are in the UK, and ten million in the United States [37, 38].

10.4.3 Clinical Features

The clinical signs of lymphoedema can range from mild swelling to massive enlargement in chronic cases that have not received adequate treatment. The severity of lymphoedema may be classified according to the clinical features (Table 10.1), and this may be useful in monitoring response to therapy over a prolonged period.

Protein-rich materials, lipids and debris accumulate in addition to the fluid. This results in 'solid' and 'fluid' components to the swelling, giving rise to the brawny nature of chronic oedema that resists pitting [40]. Skin changes may be present, including thickened fibrotic skin and the presence of the Kaposi-Stemmer sign (the failure to pinch/pick up a fold of skin at the base of the second toe as a result of its thickness) that is pathognomonic of lymphoedema [41]. Papillomatosis (small flesh-coloured papules) occurs as a result of dilatation within the upper dermal lymphatics and subsequent fibrosis of the dermis. Lymphangiectasia appears as small blisters on the skin surface as a result of engorgement of lymphatic vessels. Lymphatic fluid frequently leaks as a result of minimal trauma and is termed lymphorrhoea (Fig. 10.1).

Table 10.1 Stages of lymphoedema, adapted from the International Society of Lymphology Consensus Documents [39]

Stage	Clinical signs
Stage 0	A latent/subclinical state where swelling is not evident despite impaired lymphatic transport. This stage may exist for many months or years before oedema becomes evident
Stage I	Early onset of lymphoedema, where there is accumulation of tissue fluid that reduces with limb elevation; pitting may be present
Stage II	Accumulation of fluid that does not reduce on elevation; at later stages may be non-pitting
Stage III	Fibrotic tissue and absent pitting; elephantiasis skin changes develop, e.g. acanthosis, fatty and fibrous tissue changes and warty overgrowths

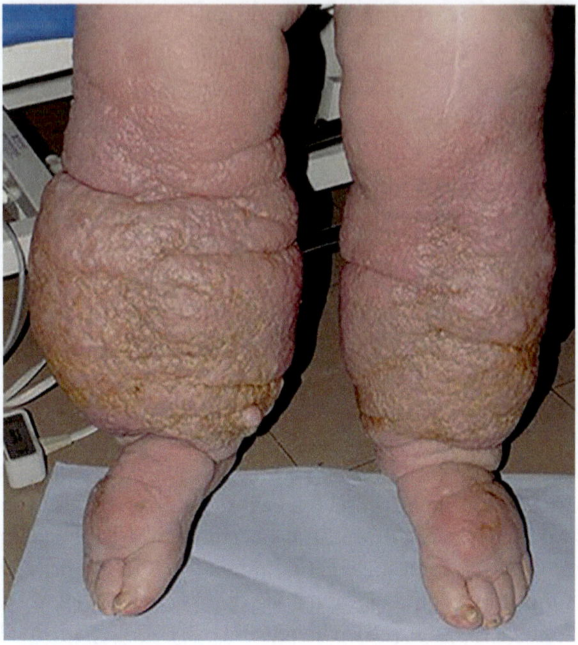

Fig. 10.1 Bilateral lower limb lymphoedema due to lymphovenous disease and immobility (note the left knee replacement) with signs of lipodermatosclerosis, papillomatosis and lymphorrhoea (the yellow encrusted areas)

10.4.4 Complications of Lymphoedema

Patients with primary or secondary lymphoedema are susceptible to a number of complications. These include infections with bacteria and fungi, almost certainly due to reduced immune surveillance secondary to lymphatic dysfunction. Recurrent cellulitis is a particular problem. Constitutional symptoms such as fever, vomiting or headaches may develop suddenly without heralding skin signs of cellulitis. Repeated episodes of infection will exacerbate lymphoedema and predispose to further infections, thus creating a vicious cycle of events. The use of prophylactic penicillin has been shown to reduce the rate of infection [5].

Rarely, lymphoedema may be complicated by the development of cutaneous malignancy. The most frequently reported malignancy is lymphangiosarcoma [42]. Stewart-Treves syndrome refers to the development of lymphangiosarcoma in patients with chronic post-mastectomy lymphoedema. However, it is now accepted that lymphangiosarcoma may occur in longstanding lymphoedema of any primary or secondary cause [43, 44]. Patients with longstanding lymphoedema are also at increased risk of local skin tumours, e.g. Kaposi's sarcoma, basal cell carcinoma, squamous cell carcinoma and malignant melanoma, presumably as a result of impaired immune surveillance within the lymphoedematous region [45, 46].

10.5 Secondary Lymphoedema

Secondary lymphoedema develops from any acquired disruption of lymph drainage routes, e.g. damage to the lymphatic vessels and/or lymph nodes. Lymphatic filariasis is the most common cause of lymphoedema worldwide, affecting an estimated 40 million people [47]. Mosquitoes are the vectors that transmit larvae to the lymphatics, where they hatch into adult worms, causing progressive disruption to lymphatic function. Filarial infection is concentrated in the tropics and does not account for the majority of lymphoedema seen in temperate zones. The World Health Organisation (WHO) has undertaken a Global Programme to Eliminate Lymphatic Filariasis (GPELF) with large-scale preventative chemotherapy treatment.

Other causes of secondary lymphoedema include infection (e.g. recurrent cellulitis), malignancy, surgery, inflammatory conditions, trauma, venous disease and immobility [2–4] (Table 10.2).

Perhaps the most recognised form of secondary lymphoedema in the developed world is that of breast cancer-related lymphoedema (BCRL). Despite recent advances in breast cancer treatment, including the introduction of minimal surgery guided by sentinel lymph node biopsy, the prevalence of BCRL remains stubbornly high at 15–20% [48]. The reasons why some patients develop BCRL and others do not, despite similar treatment plans, remain a mystery. Other unanswered questions include 'why is there a delay of years before lymphoedema manifests in some patients', and 'why can the distribution of swelling within the limb vary', e.g. the arm may be swollen, but the hand spared. The detection of Connexin47/*GJC2* gene mutations in a number of women with BCRL suggests that underlying gene mutations lead to an increased susceptibility for developing lymphoedema following cancer treatment [49].

Table 10.2 Causes of the swollen limb

Cause of impaired lymphatic function	Examples
Malignancy and cancer treatment	Lymph node biopsy/clearance Radiotherapy Active/recurrent cancer
Infection	Filariasis Recurrent cellulitis
Elevated venous pressures	Varicose veins, deep vein thrombosis Heart failure Obstructive sleep apnoea
Dependency	Immobility (e.g. post-CVA)
Obesity	
Medications	Calcium channel blockers Corticosteroids Non-steroidal anti-inflammatory drugs Taxanes
Trauma to lymphatic pathways	Accidental trauma to the lymphatic system Surgical 'trauma' (e.g. 'thighplasty' procedure)
Chronic cutaneous inflammatory disease	Acne, rosacea Hidradenitis suppurativa Cutaneous Crohn's disease
Low protein states	Protein-losing enteropathy Liver disease Nephrotic syndrome
Primary lymphoedema	Meige disease (pubertal onset lower limb lymphoedema)

10.5.1 Venous Lymphoedema

Venous lymphoedema results from venous valve failure and subsequent venous hypertension, creating excessive microvascular filtration into the interstitial spaces. Varicose veins or post-thrombotic syndrome are the commonest causes. If the lymph drainage is able to compensate, then the patient will not develop lymphoedema. Therefore, oedema in the presence of venous disease indicates lymphatic failure, and treatment should address improvements in lymph drainage as well as control of the venous disease. Surgical treatment of varicose veins will often not resolve 'venous' oedema because lymph drainage is already compromised and surgery will not improve it. Therefore, compression is the treatment of choice for venous oedema because compression garments (hosiery) have the advantage of reducing microvascular filtration (from the venous hypertension) and at the same time improve lymphatic drainage.

10.6 Primary Lymphoedema

Primary lymphoedema occurs as a result of a genetic predisposition causing the lymphatic system to fail to develop normally, or to be maintained adequately, causing abnormal drainage of lymph which results in swelling of the affected region. Primary lymphoedema may occur as an inherited condition, or less commonly as part of a complex syndromic disorder [50]. A patient with primary lymphoedema may only have problems with swelling, but some forms of primary lymphoedema occur in association with other health problems, e.g. congenital heart disease, systemic/internal lymphatic abnormalities (pleural and/or pericardial effusions, ascites), or very rarely haematological malignancy (leukaemia). The various subtypes of primary lymphoedema are discussed below, together with a classification pathway that has been developed in order to facilitate diagnosis for clinicians involved in the care of patients with primary lymphoedema [1].

Specific phenotyping facilitates the identification of subgroups of patients with the same type of primary lymphoedema. This leads to a better understanding of the natural history and management of the specific conditions and more accurate recurrence risks for future offspring/generations. Primary lymphoedema is not one disease, but the presenting feature of several distinct clinical entities. Historically, primary lymphoedema was categorised into three groups depending on the patient's age at onset of swelling: congenita (presenting at birth, Fig. 10.2), praecox (pubertal onset) or tarda (onset after 35 years of age). However, this classification system should no longer be used as it is out of date and fails to take into account associated health issues that need to be screened for.

Mutations in several genes are known to cause primary lymphoedema. Some, but not all, of these genes have been shown to play a role in lymphangiogenesis (the process of developing and maintaining a healthy lymphatic system). The discovery of these gene mutations has changed our diagnostic approach in the clinic, which is now based on clinical phenotyping (the process of associating a patient's lymphoedema with other health problems) and genotyping (DNA tests looking for the underlying causal gene mutation) in addition to the age of onset of swelling. Experience and research by the National Lymphoedema Service in the UK has led to the realisation that primary lymphoedema can be broadly divided into five different categories (see Table 10.3). Causal gene mutations have been identified for a number of disease subtypes within the five categories. A colour-coded diagnostic pathway (Fig. 10.3) has been developed that describes specific primary lymphoedema phenotypes and guides the clinician on gene tests that may be available for their patient (annotated in red within the pathway boxes).

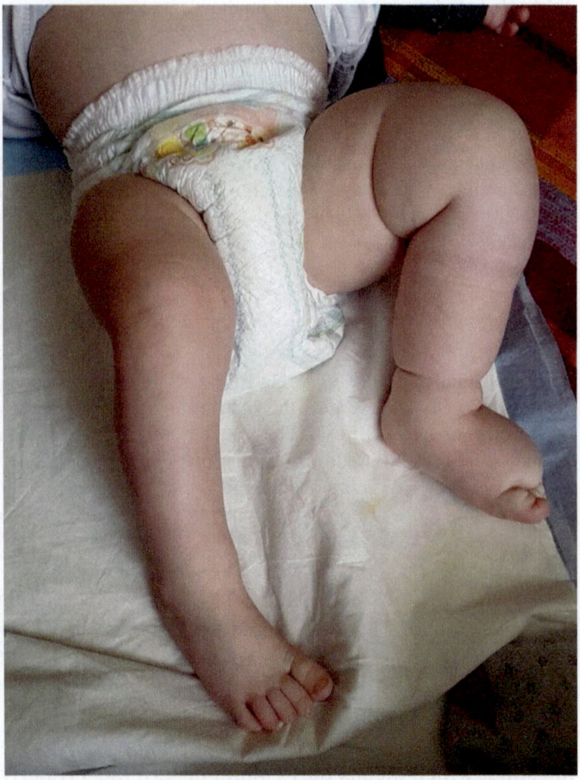

Fig. 10.2 Primary lymphoedema of one limb in a baby

10.6.1 Genetic Syndromes Associated with Lymphoedema (Blue Section of the Pathway)

The swelling is not the predominant feature of the child's health problems, but simply part of their overall condition. Examples include Turner syndrome, where girls are born with swollen feet ± hands because they are missing one X chromosome. Some children with Noonan syndrome also develop lymphoedema of their legs ± genitalia in childhood.

10.6.2 Lymphoedema with Systemic (Internal) Lymphatic Abnormalities (Pink Section of the Pathway)

This rare form of primary lymphoedema does not affect many children. These children may be swollen at birth (usually affecting several limbs/body parts) and have internal lymphatic problems. These internal problems may include fluid around the heart and/or lungs. They may also have abnormal lymphatic drainage of the small

Table 10.3 Subtypes of primary lymphoedema

Subtype	Examples	Comment
Genetic syndromes associated with lymphoedema	Turner syndrome, Noonan syndrome	The swelling is not the predominant feature of the child's health problems, but simply part of their overall condition
Lymphoedema with systemic (internal) lymphatic abnormalities	Hennekam syndrome (e.g. due to a mutation in the *CCBE1* gene)	A rare form of primary lymphoedema. These children may be swollen at birth (usually affecting several limbs/body parts) and have internal lymphatic problems, e.g. fluid around the heart and/or lungs. They may also have abnormal lymphatic drainage of the small intestine, causing them to have diarrhoea when they eat fatty foods
Lymphoedema in association with overgrowth of tissues	PIK3CA-related overgrowth syndrome (PROS). There are several conditions within this group, including Klippel-Trenaunay syndrome	Lymphoedema may develop in association with overgrowth of tissues within the swollen limb, e.g. the muscle, bone or fatty tissues are increased in size. These conditions are mosaic, with mutations confirmed on tissue biopsy of affected sites
Congenital lymphoedema	Milroy disease (*VEGFR3*)	Lower limb lymphoedema present at birth (or develops within the first few months of life)
Late-onset primary lymphoedema	Lymphoedema distichiasis syndrome (*FOXC2*), Meige disease	Swelling of lower limbs (+/− upper limbs) develops after the first year of the patient's life. The majority present after puberty

intestine, which means they cannot absorb fats properly, causing them to have diarrhoea when they eat fatty foods. One example of this rare problem is Hennekam syndrome due to a mutation in the *CCBE1* or *FAT4* genes [1].

10.6.3 Lymphoedema in Association with Overgrowth of Tissues (Yellow Section)

Lymphoedema may develop in patients who have overgrowth of tissues within the swollen limb—e.g. the muscle, bone or fatty tissues are increased in size. There are several conditions within this group, including Klippel-Trenaunay syndrome, where the child may have lymphoedema, varicose veins, red birthmarks of the skin and a longer limb. We are realising that many of these conditions develop because of a genetic mutation in the *PIK3CA/AKT1* overgrowth pathway just within the swollen limb (i.e. a mosaic/somatic mutation), and a skin biopsy of affected tissue is needed to confirm the gene mutation, as it will not be found in their blood. In patients with progressive overgrowth of tissues, it may be possible to treat them with Sirolimus, a repurposed medication that can inhibit the overgrowth pathway [51].

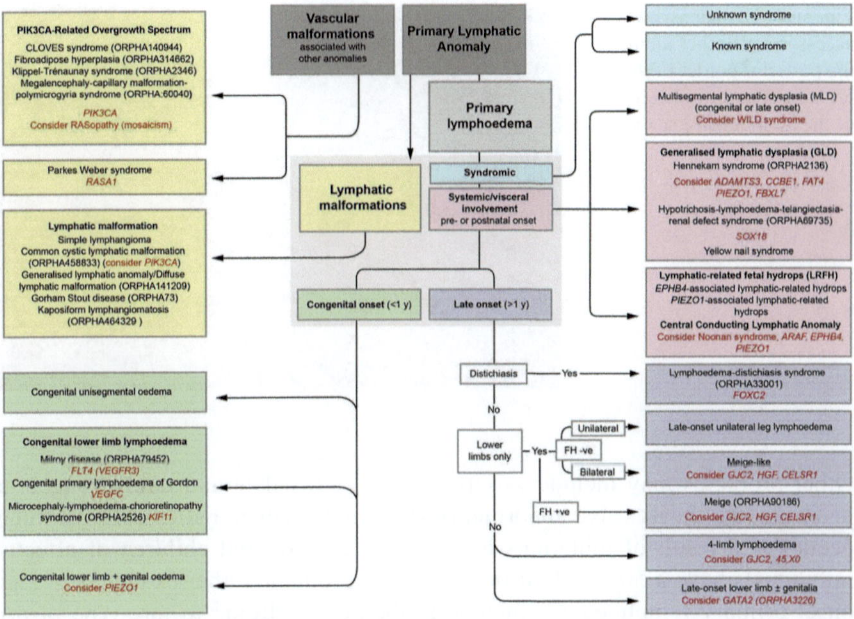

Fig. 10.3 St George's classification algorithm for primary lymphatic anomalies. The five main groupings (colour-coded) with their various clinical subtypes of disease. Primary lymphoedema is the major clinical feature in the green, pink and purple sections. Text in red indicates the suggested genetic test and/or differential diagnosis for the subgroup

10.6.4 Congenital Lymphoedema (Green Section)

Congenital lymphoedema describes children with lymphoedema that is present at birth (or develops within the first few months of life). There are several different causes, but the most recognised is Milroy's disease. This condition causes swelling of the feet and ankles at birth, varicose veins after puberty and one-third of boys will develop a build-up of lymphatic fluid in the scrotum (hydroceles). Milroy disease is due to a mutation in the *VEGFR3* gene. Children of affected individuals have a 50% risk of inheriting the problem.

10.6.5 Late-Onset Primary Lymphoedema (Purple Section)

The term 'late-onset lymphoedema' is used to describe a primary lymphoedema that develops after the first year of the patient's life (i.e. non-congenital lymphoedema). Lymphoedema distichiasis syndrome is one example. It presents with pubertal onset of bilateral lower limb lymphoedema. Distichiasis (extra eyelashes) is present from early childhood and may cause eye irritation (Fig. 10.4).

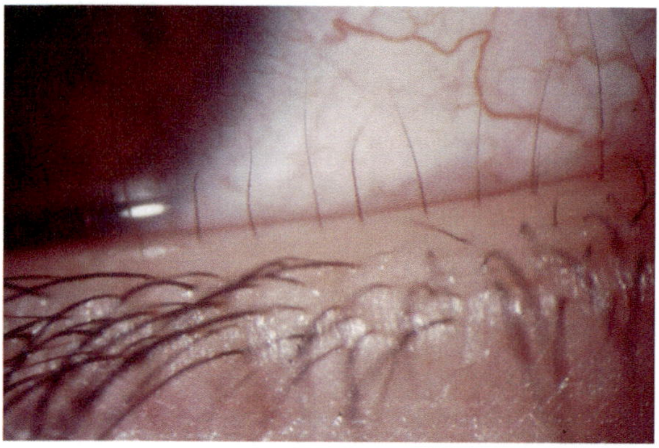

Fig. 10.4 Distichiasis with accessory eyelashes along the posterior border of the lid margin in the position of the Meibomian glands

Other problems may include varicose veins, cleft palate and rarely congenital heart disease (heart valve abnormalities). Lymphoedema distichiasis syndrome occurs as a result of mutations in the *FOXC2* gene, and children of affected individuals have a 50% risk of inheriting the problem. Other examples of late-onset primary lymphoedema include Emberger syndrome (a rare type of primary lymphoedema associated with a risk of developing leukaemia) and Meige disease (the commonest form of primary lymphoedema that is not associated with other health problems).

The diagnostic pathway helps the clinician to offer appropriate genetic testing (assuming the underlying gene mutation is known), and screen and treat for associated health problems. Testing for the primary lymphoedema gene panel is now widely available. Patients and families benefit hugely from receiving a formal genetic diagnosis of their primary lymphoedema as it allows the clinician to confidently predict the clinical prognosis and offer screening for family members.

Unfortunately, there is no curative treatment for primary lymphoedema. Hopefully, gene therapy will be available to treat some forms of primary lymphoedema in the future. In the meantime, a number of repurposed medications have been successfully used in the management of complex cases of primary lymphoedema with progressive, and often internal, lymphatic problems [51–53].

Routine management of primary lymphoedema is aimed at controlling swelling through physical treatments designed to stimulate flow through existing or collateral drainage routes. This physical therapy management approach is the same for those patients with secondary lymphoedema. Several reconstructive surgical techniques have been implemented in recent years in a bid to improve lymphatic drainage in patients with secondary lymphoedema. These are unlikely to benefit patients with primary lymphoedema as the fault with lymphatic drainage is not an 'obstruction', rather a molecular/genetic abnormality that cannot simply be bypassed.

10.7 Investigating Lymphoedema

Most patients with lymphoedema are diagnosed based on the history and clinical findings. The use and value of imaging techniques are highly dependent on availability and expertise. Techniques used to investigate the lymphatic system are discussed below, but some patients will benefit from additional imaging in order to fully understand the cause of their swelling. For example, magnetic resonance imaging (MRI) and computerised tomography (CT) scanning may be indicated to assess for the presence of intra-abdominal or pelvic pathology/masses obstructing lymphatic drainage. MRI may also be requested to assess for tissue hypertrophy or signs of overgrowth (e.g. in Klippel-Trenaunay syndrome). Venous duplex imaging may be requested to investigate the possibility that a patient's lymphoedema is associated with venous incompetence. Table 10.4 compares the different techniques available for imaging the lymphatic system.

10.7.1 Lymphography and Lymphoscintigraphy

Imaging with X-ray contrast lymphography (lymphangiography) was previously the best investigation tool for demonstrating lymphatic collectors and lymph nodes. However, it is now rarely used as the technique requires the invasive procedure of direct cannulation of the lymphatics.

Lymphoscintigraphy (isotope lymphography) is the current gold standard investigation for determining whether chronic oedema may be due to lymphatic failure. It involves a simple intradermal/subcutaneous injection of a radio-labelled tracer protein, exclusively cleared by lymphatics. Measurement of tracer uptake and transit through the lymphatics permits the qualitative and quantitative analyses of lymph drainage and may discriminate lymphoedema from lipoedema [54, 55]. Lymphoscintigraphy has the potential to distinguish between different types of primary lymphoedema and their mechanisms of lymphatic failure, i.e. initial lymphatic dysfunction in Milroy disease, versus lymph collector reflux in lymphoedema-distichiasis syndrome (Fig. 10.5). However, lymphoscintigraphy is a relatively crude test as it suffers from poor spatial resolution and cannot provide functional measurements of flow [56].

10.7.2 Near Infra-Red Lymphangiography

Near infra-red lymphangiography (NIRL) using indocyanine green (ICG) is a recently introduced and potentially useful technique used to demonstrate superficial lymphatic vessels [57]. NIR imaging techniques use tracers that fluoresce under the excitation of near infra-red waves and external fluorescent detectors. ICG is a dye with properties of NIR absorption and fluorescence emission. ICG-solution is injected intradermally or subcutaneously and enables real-time detection of the lymphatic vessels. NIRL has been used to assess lymphatic vessel structure and

Table 10.4 A comparison of the different techniques available for imaging the lymphatic system

Imaging technique	Contrast agent	Depth of imaging	Invasiveness	Availability
Lymphography/ lymphangiography	Intralymphatic injection of a radio-opaque oil (e.g. lipiodol)	Anatomical imaging of lymphatic collectors and lymph nodes	Very invasive: Requires the identification of a lymphatic collecting vessel by exploratory surgery	Rarely performed anymore
Lymphoscintigraphy	Simple intradermal/subcutaneous injection of a radio-labelled tracer protein (e.g. ^{99}Technetium-labelled dextran)	Lymphatic collectors and lymph nodes Poor resolution compared to the lymphography technique Limited functional data acquired Not anatomical	Minimally	Readily available in hospitals
Fluorescence microlymph-angiography	Simple intradermal injection of fluorescent contrast agent (FITC-dextran)	Superficial dermal lymphatic vessels	Minimally	Research tool
Near infra-red lymphangiography	Simple intradermal/subcutaneous injection of indocyanine green	Superficial dermal lymphatic vessels and superficial lymph nodes. Peristalsis can be visualised but not quantified	Minimally	Increasing availability in departments offering lymphatic microsurgery
MR lymphangiography	Simple intradermal/subcutaneous injection of a gadolinium-based contrast agent	Lymphatic collectors and lymph nodes. Subcutaneous fat and oedema also visualised	Minimally	Research tool in the UK. Offered in a few centres in the USA & Europe

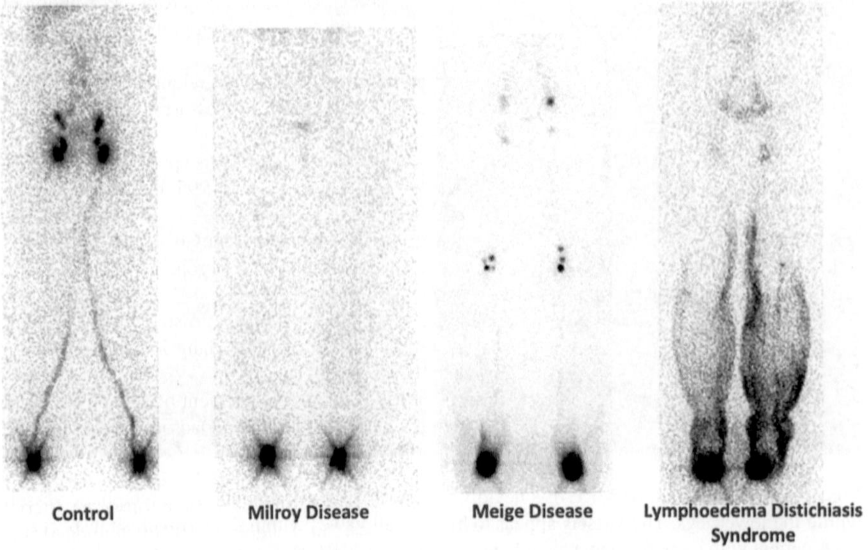

Fig. 10.5 Comparison of lymphoscintigraphy results in primary lymphoedema. (1) A healthy control demonstrating uptake of tracer from the injection sites in the feet to the inguinal lymph nodes via the main lymphatic tracts. These images were taken 2 h after the tracer was injected into the subjects' feet. (2) A patient with Milroy disease is unable to transport tracer from the injection sites in the feet because the initial lymphatic vessels are unable to function adequately. After 2 h, there is no uptake of tracer within the lymphatic vessels or lymph nodes due to a 'functional aplasia' of the lymphatic system. (3) A patient with Meige disease is able to transport tracer from the injection site in the feet up to the inguinal lymph nodes. However, tracer is re-routed via the deep lymphatic system, as demonstrated by uptake of tracer within the popliteal lymph nodes. (4) Patients with lymphoedema distichiasis syndrome have abnormal lymphatic function due to valve defects within the vessels. This is demonstrated on lymphoscintigraphy imaging: the tracer is absorbed by the initial lymphatic vessels and begins to be transported up the limb, but then refluxes back down, creating an outline of the limb in the process

function [58]. NIRL is now used to assess lymphatic vessel patency before lymphaticovenous or lymphatico-lymphatic anastomosis surgery [59].

10.7.3 Magnetic Resonance Lymphangiography

The use of contrast-enhanced magnetic resonance lymphangiography (MRL) has been used in the investigation of patients with lymphoedema [60]. MRL has been used to demonstrate the presence of abnormally enlarged and tortuous lymphatic vessels in patients with unspecified limb lymphoedema [61] (Fig. 10.6). However, it has yet to prove helpful in refining the subtype of primary lymphoedema as a clear correlation between the phenotype of primary lymphoedema and the MRL findings is lacking [62]. A developing area is the use of MRL to visualise central lymphatic

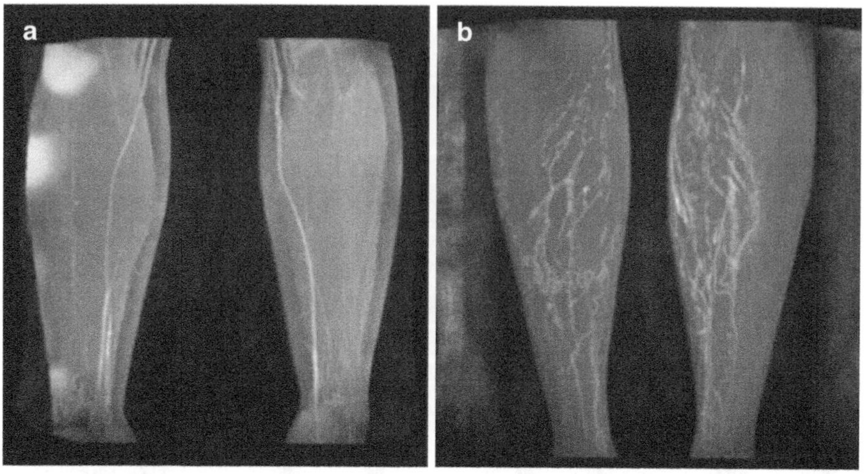

Fig. 10.6 (**a**) Post-contrast MRL of a healthy volunteer demonstrating multiple lymphatic vessels within the lower legs. The vessels appear to have small valves within them (on close inspection). (**b**) A patient with Lymphoedema distichiasis syndrome's MRL images (post-contrast) demonstrating multiple dilated, tortuous lymphatic vessels are seen in the below-knee regions

abnormalities and assist with interventional treatment, e.g. in patients with chylous effusions of the heart/lungs/ascites [63].

10.8 Management of Lymphoedema

Unfortunately, there is no curative treatment for lymphoedema. Management is aimed at controlling swelling through physical treatments designed to stimulate flow through existing or collateral drainage routes. Several surgical techniques have been implemented in recent years in a bid to improve lymphatic drainage or achieve limb volume reduction via liposuction. However, in the absence of robust data to support most surgical techniques, we must rely on so-called 'conservative' physical therapies for the majority of patients. Hopefully, gene/medical therapy will be available as an additional treatment for some forms of primary lymphoedema in the future.

10.8.1 Physical Therapies

Compression is the most important component of lymphoedema treatment and cannot be replaced by any other modality. The International Society of Lymphology has developed guidelines regarding the management of lymphoedema [39]. The physical treatment of lymphoedema, often called 'Decongestive

Lymphatic Therapy' (DLT), should occur in two distinct stages. The goal of the intensive first stage (Reduction Phase) is to 'disorganise' the fibrosis within the lymphoedema, reduce the volume and discomfort. In order to do so, a combination of techniques are used: manual lymph drainage, multi-layered bandages, exercise and skin care. The use of intermittent pneumatic compression has also been suggested. The goal of the second stage of treatment (Maintenance Phase) is to maintain the results achieved in the reduction phase. The techniques used in this phase are: compression with low-stretch elastic hosiery garments, specific exercises and skin care.

10.8.1.1 Reduction Phase Treatment

The intensive reduction phase of lymphoedema treatment is usually offered to patients with significant swelling (of any body site) in order to achieve considerable volume reduction (with inelastic bandages or Velcro strapping systems) before fitting them with compression hosiery with a view to maintaining the smaller (limb) volumes. The majority of patients with mild lymphoedema, typically of a limb, do not require intensive bandaging therapy and can be directly measured for appropriate compression hosiery.

The duration of reduction phase therapy varies across the globe but typically involves daily bandaging and exercises once daily for an approximate duration of 2–4 weeks. Manual lymphatic drainage (MLD) massage may be offered depending on local protocols and availability. Treatment duration will be determined by the assessing physician or lymphoedema therapist, but should be continued until pitting oedema has resolved and long-term compression hosiery has been commenced. A small number of patients require a prolonged course of treatment if they have significant limb distortion or severe, neglected chronic lymphoedema.

10.8.1.2 Maintenance Phase Treatment

Compression hosiery limits the amount of fluid accumulation within the tissues affected by lymphoedema. It acts as a counterforce to muscle contractions to improve lymphatic drainage. Compression garments have a graduated compression profile (more strength at the foot/hand than at the top of the garment), ensuring lymphatic fluid is directed towards the root of the limb (groin/axilla). Effects are enhanced when a patient wears their compression hosiery during exercise. Compression hosiery is available in many different styles (below-knee or full-length stockings, half or full tights and sleeves) and degrees of asserted pressure. Complex limb lymphoedema may require the use of high compression and/or double layers of garments. Most garments last no more than 6 months. A minimum of two sets of garments should be provided (one to wear whilst the other is washed). The patient's technique for the application, removal and care of garments is crucial for a successful outcome. Compression garments are beneficial in the management of lymphoedema, and it is possible to achieve volume reduction with compression hosiery and exercise alone.

Compression can also be achieved with the use of Velcro strapping systems applied to swollen limbs (Fig. 10.7). These adjustable garments are utilised in the 'maintenance' phase of lymphoedema treatment, often for patients with significant comorbidities who are unable to comply with standard compression hosiery. These Velcro garments can be applied by the patient and/or carers after minimal training. One advantage over bandaging is the option to adjust them (i.e. apply more pressure to the limb) during the day to overcome issues with 'slippage' during periods of limb volume reduction. There is a recent realisation that these Velcro strapping systems can also be utilised in the intensive reduction phase of treatment. A recent randomised controlled trial demonstrated significantly more leg volume reduction from the use of the Velcro system when compared to conventional inelastic bandages [64].

10.8.1.3 Manual Lymphatic Drainage

Manual lymphatic drainage (MLD) is a massage technique performed by lymphoedema therapists. The aim is to re-route the accumulation of lymph from the swollen region via collateral lymphatic pathways to lymphatic basins that are able to drain normally. The initial step in MLD is to decongest the central/proximal areas before

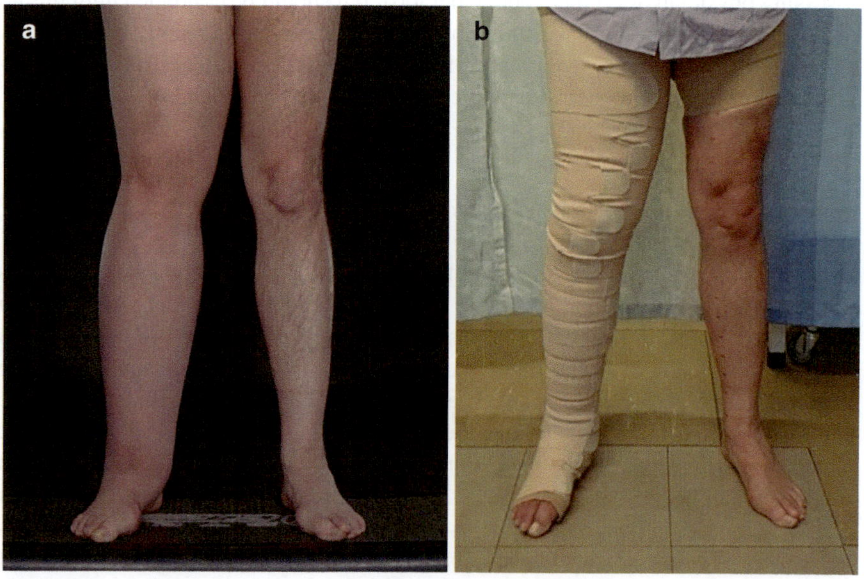

Fig. 10.7 (**a**) Patient with right lower limb secondary lymphoedema. (**b**) Same patient as above (**a**) receiving compression treatment with Velcro strapping system

massaging the oedematous region. This facilitates the drainage of lymph via lymphatic vessels and pathways that have been stimulated by the massage technique. Tissue movement must be gentle if it is to stimulate lymph flow without increasing blood flow [65]. There is little evidence in the literature to support its use, and it is offered less frequently in many lymphoedema clinics [66–68]. However, MLD is still widely practised, and many patients, therapists and physicians advocate the benefits.

The recent development of lymphofluoroscopy (Indocyanine Green Lymphography) as a tool to map patients' superficial lymphatic drainage pathways is proving of interest to patients and lymphoedema therapists alike. Lymphatic drainage pathways differ between patients as a result of differences in normal anatomy and damage from external factors (e.g. cancer treatment or infection). Lymphofluoroscopy mapping involves the intradermal injection of indocyanine green tracer that is taken up by the initial lymphatic vessels, and the superficial lymphatic pathways can be mapped out on the skin and documented for future MLD treatments. This imaging technique could facilitate the development of a bespoke treatment protocol, maximising the benefits of MLD for each patient, but efficacy must be demonstrated before it becomes an established treatment option.

10.8.1.4 Intermittent Pneumatic Compression

Pneumatic compression therapy (intermittent sequential pneumatic compression) should not be used in preference to compression garments and exercise, but can be a useful adjunct in the treatment of some cases of lymphoedema [69]. An inflatable boot or sleeve is connected to a motor-driven pump, and lymph is displaced proximally towards the root of the limb. If hosiery is not fitted immediately following the use of pneumatic compression, the lymphoedema will rapidly recur. Few studies support the beneficial use of pneumatic compression in lymphoedema [70]. Pneumatic compression may soften the tissues and reduce limb volume during treatment, but it is doubtful that any long-term benefit is gained over the use of compression hosiery and exercise.

10.8.2 Pharmacological Therapies

There is little use for drug therapy in the management of lymphoedema. Diuretics alone demonstrate minimal improvement in lymphoedema, as their mode of action is to reduce capillary filtration by a reduction in circulating blood volume. Paroven (an oxerutin) and Coumarin (a benzopyrone) have been trialled in lymphoedema and may create a small reduction in limb volume by reducing vascular permeability and thus the amount of fluid forming in the subcutaneous tissues. However, this has been shown to be of little clinical benefit to the patient [71].

The link between lymphatic function and inflammation has recently been explored from a therapeutic perspective. Research in animal models has demonstrated the efficacy of specific topical immunomodulatory therapies in treating secondary lymphoedema [72]. This exciting development has led to human trials with specific anti-inflammatory agents, with the results eagerly awaited by patients and clinicians alike [73].

10.8.3 Surgical Options

10.8.3.1 Excisional Methods

Excisional surgical procedures for the management of lymphoedema, regardless of the underlying cause, have been employed for more than a century. They are now rarely employed as the post-operative complications can be disastrous (e.g. with exacerbation of swelling and/or recurrent infections). An example of a recognised lymphatic surgical technique includes the 'Charles procedure', where the patient undergoes complete resection of the skin and subcutaneous tissue of the lymphoedematous region and receives a full-thickness skin graft to restore the tissue defect [74]. It has largely been abandoned because of problems with massive skin transplant necrosis, poor cosmetic results and worsening lymphoedema distal to the surgical site. None of the excisional procedures has curative potential as all chances of restoring effective lymphatic transport have been surgically removed. Volume reduction may be achieved through tissue reduction, but not through lymphatic drainage improvement. The indications for this type of surgery must be restricted to rare cases lacking alternative conservative or surgical treatment options.

10.8.3.2 Lymphaticovenous Anastomosis Surgery

As traditional excisional procedures have fallen out of favour, there has been much interest in a surgical procedure called lymphaticovenous anastomosis surgery (LVA). LVA is a type of lymphovenous bypass, utilising a supermicrosurgical technique to anastomose distal subdermal lymphatic vessels with adjacent venules less than 0.8 mm in diameter in an attempt to improve regional lymph drainage and potentially remove the need for using hosiery (a scenario that many patients are desperate to achieve). It is popular amongst surgeons as it is performed under local anaesthetic, and the surgical incisions are small. Post-operative complications are rare but include lymphatic vessel occlusion, possibly due to thrombus formation within the lumen [75]. Before LVA surgery, the patients undergo indocyanine green fluorescent imaging to locate functional patent lymphatic vessels within the affected limb. A review of the literature suggests that the efficacy of LVA surgery is variable, with studies reporting mean post-operative volume reduction ranging from just 4% to 67% [76, 77]. Lymphoscintigraphy failed to demonstrate patency of any bypass procedures, with the authors suggesting the evidence for LVA success is limited [76]. However, subjective symptom relief was found in the majority of patients, as well as a reduction in the number of cellulitis episodes [78].

In summary, there is a lack of long-term data as the technique is relatively new. However, some surgeons favour its use because of the low risk of complications. There is currently no method of determining its effect on lymphatic function. The development of better imaging techniques could provide a tool to answer the question of its place in lymphatic treatment strategies.

10.8.3.3 Lymph Node Transfer Surgery

Autologous transplantation of normal lymphatic tissue within a local or free flap to a region that is deficient in lymph nodes and vessels has been performed by surgeons. The aim is to transplant normal lymph nodes to encourage and improve lymphatic drainage in a previously oedematous region. Fewer centres perform this type of surgery than LVA, but the reported results appear encouraging in patients with secondary lymphoedema. For example, Becker et al. reported a series of 24 patients receiving Deep/Superficial Inferior Epigastric Perforator flap (DIEP/SIEP) transposition, and ten patients were reportedly cured of their lymphoedema (41.6%), an additional six patients experienced >50% volume reduction, six patients achieved <50% reduction and two patients had no improvement [79]. This surgery relies on the transfer of normal lymph nodes in order to improve lymphatic drainage. This may be possible in a patient with secondary lymphoedema, but concerns exist over its use in patients with primary lymphoedema who may not have 'normal' lymph nodes, or 'normal' lymphatic vasculature, even at unaffected sites.

10.8.3.4 Liposuction

Chronic lymphoedema may be associated with the development of fibrosis and excess fatty tissue deposition within the swollen region in some patients. The mechanism is thought to be due to abnormal adipogenesis secondary to inflammatory changes within lymphoedematous tissue [80].

Excess adipose tissue will not respond to decongestive lymphoedema treatments, anastomosis surgery or lymph node transfer procedures, and can only be removed surgically. Liposuction creates significant volume reduction in therapy-resistant lymphoedema of the extremities, when combined with lifelong compression therapy [81]. This adjunctive therapy is only offered to compliant patients willing to wear lifelong compression garments 24-h a day. Warren reports that if patients disregard regular use of their garments, a relapse or worsening of lymphoedema is observed, as liposuction may cause injury to remaining subcutaneous lymphatics within lymphoedematous extremities [81]. Brorson reports a long-term volume reduction of more than 100% in compliant patients who were followed for up to 17 years [34]. Liposuction techniques, although not curative, offer an effective symptomatic treatment [82].

10.9 Summary

This chapter aims to provide the clinician with a greater understanding of the aetiology of lymphoedema and increased knowledge for managing this condition. Lymphoedema is a chronic, debilitating condition that may lead to significant physical and psychological morbidity. Swelling results in discomfort, reduced mobility and impaired function. Recurrent infections further complicate the management of this challenging condition. Many patients currently receive inadequate care as lymphoedema fails to receive appropriate recognition by the medical community. Surgical management will only benefit select individuals, but daily compression therapy is proven to be effective in the majority. Emerging evidence of the relationship between the lymphatic system and chronic inflammation should lead to the development of adjunctive oral therapies. The future of lymphoedema care will undoubtedly improve thanks to research, but clinicians must still endeavour to diagnose and treat lymphoedema in a timely manner in order to avoid complications.

Key References

- Gordon K, Varney R, Keeley V, Riches K, Jeffery S, Van Zanten M, et al. Update and audit of the St George's classification algorithm of primary lymphatic anomalies: a clinical and molecular approach to diagnosis. J Med Genet. 2020;57:653–9. https://doi.org/10.1136/jmedgenet-2019-106084
- Executive Committee of the International Society of Lymphology. The diagnosis and treatment of peripheral lymphedema: 2023 Consensus Document of The International Society of Lymphology. Lymphology. 2023;56:133–51.

Acknowledgements I would like to thank and acknowledge the contributions of Mr. Matt Waltham to previous versions of this chapter.

Multiple Choice Questions

1. Failure of the lymphatic system leads to lymphoedema, characterised by the accumulation of a specific type of fluid within interstitial spaces. What are the key characteristics of this accumulated fluid that contributes to the non-pitting nature of chronic oedema?

   (a) It is protein-poor and high in glucose
   (b) It is clear water, easily reduced by diuretics
   (c) It is primarily chyle, high in dietary fats
   (d) It is protein-rich lymph fluid, leading to fibrosis and lipid accumulation
   (e) It is primarily plasma filtrate, retained by osmotic pressure

   Answer: (d) It is protein-rich lymph fluid, leading to fibrosis and lipid accumulation

2. Which subtype of primary lymphoedema is defined by swelling that develops after the first year of life, with the majority presenting after puberty, and includes examples such as lymphoedema distichiasis syndrome and Meige disease?
   (a) Genetic syndromes associated with lymphoedema
   (b) Congenital lymphoedema
   (c) Lymphoedema in association with overgrowth of tissue
   (d) Lymphoedema with systemic (internal) lymphatic abnormalities
   (e) Late-onset primary lymphoedema

   Answer: (e) Late-onset primary lymphoedema

References

1. Gordon K, Varney R, Keeley V, Riches K, Jeffery S, Van Zanten M, et al. Update and audit of the St George's classification algorithm of primary lymphatic anomalies: a clinical and molecular approach to diagnosis. J Med Genet. 2020;57:653–9. https://doi.org/10.1136/jmedgenet-2019-106084.
2. Stöberl C, Partsch H. Erysipelas and lymphedema–egg or hen? Z Hautkr. 1987;62:56–62.
3. Sakorafas GH, Peros G, Cataliotti L, Vlastos G. Lymphedema following axillary lymph node dissection for breast cancer. Surg Oncol. 2006;15:153–65. https://doi.org/10.1016/j.suronc.2006.11.003.
4. Nagai Y, Aoyama K, Endo Y, Ishikawa O. Lymphedema of the extremities developed as the initial manifestation of rheumatoid arthritis. Eur J Dermatol. 2007;17:175–6. https://doi.org/10.1684/ejd.2007.0144.
5. Thomas KS, Crook AM, Nunn AJ, Foster KA, Mason JM, Chalmers JR, et al. Penicillin to prevent recurrent leg cellulitis. N Engl J Med. 2013;368:1695–703. https://doi.org/10.1056/NEJMoa1206300.
6. Sabin F. On the origin of the lymphatic system from the veins and the development of the lymph hearts and thoracic duct in the pig. Am J Anat. 1902;1:367–89.
7. Oliver G, Alitalo K. The lymphatic vasculature: recent progress and paradigms. Annu Rev Cell Dev Biol. 2005;21:457–83. https://doi.org/10.1146/annurev.cellbio.21.012704.132338.
8. Okuda KS, Astin JW, Misa JP, Flores MV, Crosier KE, Crosier PS. lyve1 expression reveals novel lymphatic vessels and new mechanisms for lymphatic vessel development in zebrafish. Development. 2012;139:2381–91. https://doi.org/10.1242/dev.077701.
9. Schulte-Merker S, Sabine A, Petrova TV. Lymphatic vascular morphogenesis in development, physiology, and disease. J Cell Biol. 2011;193:607–18. https://doi.org/10.1083/jcb.201012094.
10. Wigle JT, Harvey N, Detmar M, Lagutina I, Grosveld G, Gunn MD, et al. An essential role for Prox1 in the induction of the lymphatic endothelial cell phenotype. EMBO J. 2002;21:1505–13. https://doi.org/10.1093/emboj/21.7.1505.
11. Tammela T, Petrova TV, Alitalo K. Molecular lymphangiogenesis: new players. Trends Cell Biol. 2005;15:434–41. https://doi.org/10.1016/j.tcb.2005.06.004.
12. François M, Caprini A, Hosking B, Orsenigo F, Wilhelm D, Browne C, et al. Sox18 induces development of the lymphatic vasculature in mice. Nature. 2008;456:643–7. https://doi.org/10.1038/nature07391.
13. You LR, Lin FJ, Lee CT, DeMayo FJ, Tsai MJ, Tsai SY. Suppression of notch signalling by the COUP-TFII transcription factor regulates vein identity. Nature. 2005;435:98–104. https://doi.org/10.1038/nature03511.

14. Yang Y, García-Verdugo JM, Soriano-Navarro M, Srinivasan RS, Scallan JP, Singh MK, et al. Lymphatic endothelial progenitors bud from the cardinal vein and intersomitic vessels in mammalian embryos. Blood. 2012;120:2340–8. https://doi.org/10.1182/blood-2012-05-428607.
15. Hägerling R, Pollmann C, Andreas M, Schmidt C, Nurmi H, Adams RH, et al. A novel multistep mechanism for initial lymphangiogenesis in mouse embryos based on ultramicroscopy. EMBO J. 2013;32:629–44. https://doi.org/10.1038/emboj.2012.340.
16. Bertozzi CC, Hess PR, Kahn ML. Platelets: covert regulators of lymphatic development. Arterioscler Thromb Vasc Biol. 2010;30:2368–71. https://doi.org/10.1161/atvbaha.110.217281.
17. Martinez-Corral I, Makinen T. Regulation of lymphatic vascular morphogenesis: implications for pathological (tumor) lymphangiogenesis. Exp Cell Res. 2013;319:1618–25. https://doi.org/10.1016/j.yexcr.2013.01.016.
18. Karkkainen MJ, Haiko P, Sainio K, Partanen J, Taipale J, Petrova TV, et al. Vascular endothelial growth factor C is required for sprouting of the first lymphatic vessels from embryonic veins. Nat Immunol. 2004;5:74–80. https://doi.org/10.1038/ni1013.
19. Veikkola T, Jussila L, Makinen T, Karpanen T, Jeltsch M, Petrova TV, et al. Signalling via vascular endothelial growth factor receptor-3 is sufficient for lymphangiogenesis in transgenic mice. EMBO J. 2001;20:1223–31. https://doi.org/10.1093/emboj/20.6.1223.
20. Bos FL, Caunt M, Peterson-Maduro J, Planas-Paz L, Kowalski J, Karpanen T, et al. CCBE1 is essential for mammalian lymphatic vascular development and enhances the lymphangiogenic effect of vascular endothelial growth factor-C in vivo. Circ Res. 2011;109:486–91. https://doi.org/10.1161/circresaha.111.250738.
21. Jeltsch M, Jha SK, Tvorogov D, Anisimov A, Leppänen VM, Holopainen T, et al. CCBE1 enhances lymphangiogenesis via a disintegrin and metalloprotease with thrombospondin motifs-3-mediated vascular endothelial growth factor-C activation. Circulation. 2014;129:1962–71. https://doi.org/10.1161/circulationaha.113.002779.
22. Baluk P, Fuxe J, Hashizume H, Romano T, Lashnits E, Butz S, et al. Functionally specialized junctions between endothelial cells of lymphatic vessels. J Exp Med. 2007;204:2349–62. https://doi.org/10.1084/jem.20062596.
23. Sabine A, Agalarov Y, Maby-El Hajjami H, Jaquet M, Hägerling R, Pollmann C, et al. Mechanotransduction, PROX1, and FOXC2 cooperate to control connexin37 and calcineurin during lymphatic-valve formation. Dev Cell. 2012;22:430–45. https://doi.org/10.1016/j.devcel.2011.12.020.
24. Petrova TV, Karpanen T, Norrmén C, Mellor R, Tamakoshi T, Finegold D, et al. Defective valves and abnormal mural cell recruitment underlie lymphatic vascular failure in lymphedema distichiasis. Nat Med. 2004;10:974–81. https://doi.org/10.1038/nm1094.
25. Bridenbaugh EA, Gashev AA, Zawieja DC. Lymphatic muscle: a review of contractile function. Lymphat Res Biol. 2003;1:147–58. https://doi.org/10.1089/153968503321642633.
26. Pflicke H, Sixt M. Preformed portals facilitate dendritic cell entry into afferent lymphatic vessels. J Exp Med. 2009;206:2925–35. https://doi.org/10.1084/jem.20091739.
27. Danussi C, Spessotto P, Petrucco A, Wassermann B, Sabatelli P, Montesi M, et al. Emilin1 deficiency causes structural and functional defects of lymphatic vasculature. Mol Cell Biol. 2008;28:4026–39. https://doi.org/10.1128/mcb.02062-07.
28. Oliver G, Srinivasan RS. Lymphatic vasculature development: current concepts. Ann N Y Acad Sci. 2008;1131:75–81. https://doi.org/10.1196/annals.1413.006.
29. Levick JR, Michel CC. Microvascular fluid exchange and the revised Starling principle. Cardiovasc Res. 2010;87:198–210. https://doi.org/10.1093/cvr/cvq062.
30. Martin-Almedina S, Mortimer PS, Ostergaard P. Development and physiological functions of the lymphatic system: insights from human genetic studies of primary lymphedema. Physiol Rev. 2021;101:1809–71. https://doi.org/10.1152/physrev.00006.2020.
31. Teijeira A, Russo E, Halin C. Taking the lymphatic route: dendritic cell migration to draining lymph nodes. Semin Immunopathol. 2014;36:261–74. https://doi.org/10.1007/s00281-013-0410-8.

32. Dupuy A, Benchikhi H, Roujeau JC, Bernard P, Vaillant L, Chosidow O, et al. Risk factors for erysipelas of the leg (cellulitis): case-control study. BMJ. 1999;318:1591–4. https://doi.org/10.1136/bmj.318.7198.1591.
33. Martin IC, Marinho LH, Brown AE, McRobbie D. Medium chain triglycerides in the management of chylous fistulae following neck dissection. Br J Oral Maxillofac Surg. 1993;31:236–8. https://doi.org/10.1016/0266-4356(93)90146-n.
34. Brorson H. From lymph to fat: complete reduction of lymphoedema. Phlebology. 2010;25(Suppl 1):52–63. https://doi.org/10.1258/phleb.2010.010s08.
35. Ly CL, Kataru RP, Mehrara BJ. Inflammatory manifestations of lymphedema. Int J Mol Sci. 2017;18:171. https://doi.org/10.3390/ijms18010171.
36. Soo JK, Bicanic TA, Heenan S, Mortimer PS. Lymphatic abnormalities demonstrated by lymphoscintigraphy after lower limb cellulitis. Br J Dermatol. 2008;158:1350–3. https://doi.org/10.1111/j.1365-2133.2007.08423.x.
37. Greene AK. Epidemiology and morbidity of lymphedema. In: Greene A, Slavin S, Brorson H, editors. Lymphedema. Cham: Springer; 2015. p. 33–44.
38. Thomas MJ, Morgan K. The development of lymphoedema network Wales to improve care. Br J Nurs. 2017;26:740–50. https://doi.org/10.12968/bjon.2017.26.13.740.
39. Executive Committee of the International Society of Lymphology. The Diagnosis and Treatment of Peripheral Lymphedema: 2023 Consensus document of the International Society of Lymphology. Lymphology. 2023;56:133–51.
40. Mortimer PS. Managing lymphoedema. Clin Exp Dermatol. 1995;20:98–106. https://doi.org/10.1111/j.1365-2230.1995.tb02665.x.
41. Stemmer R. A clinical symptom for the early and differential diagnosis of lymphedema. Vasa. 1976;5:261–2.
42. Stewart FW, Treves N. Lymphangiosarcoma in postmastectomy lymphedema; a report of six cases in elephantiasis chirurgica. Cancer. 1948;1:64–81. https://doi.org/10.1002/1097-0142(194805)1:1<64::aid-cncr2820010105>3.0.co;2-w.
43. Offori TW, Platt CC, Stephens M, Hopkinson GB. Angiosarcoma in congenital hereditary lymphoedema (Milroy's disease)—diagnostic beacons and a review of the literature. Clin Exp Dermatol. 1993;18:174–7. https://doi.org/10.1111/j.1365-2230.1993.tb01008.x.
44. Dürr HR, Pellengahr C, Nerlich A, Baur A, Maier M, Jansson V. Stewart-Treves syndrome as a rare complication of a hereditary lymphedema. Vasa. 2004;33:42–5. https://doi.org/10.1024/0301-1526.33.1.42.
45. Peyron N, Dandurand M, Guillot B. Malignant tumors as complications of lymphedema. J Mal Vasc. 1993;18:293–8.
46. Schreiber H, Barry FM, Russell WC, Macon WL, Ponsky JL, Pories WJ. Stewart-Treves syndrome. A lethal complication of postmastectomy lymphedema and regional immune deficiency. Arch Surg. 1979;114:82–5. https://doi.org/10.1001/archsurg.1979.01370250084018.
47. de Almeida AB, Freedman DO. Epidemiology and immunopathology of bancroftian filariasis. Microbes Infect. 1999;1:1015–22. https://doi.org/10.1016/s1286-4579(99)80519-x.
48. Lin Y, Xu Y, Wang C, Song Y, Huang X, Zhang X, et al. Loco-regional therapy and the risk of breast cancer-related lymphedema: a systematic review and meta-analysis. Breast Cancer. 2021;28:1261–72. https://doi.org/10.1007/s12282-021-01263-8.
49. Finegold DN, Baty CJ, Knickelbein KZ, Perschke S, Noon SE, Campbell D, et al. Connexin 47 mutations increase risk for secondary lymphedema following breast cancer treatment. Clin Cancer Res. 2012;18:2382–90. https://doi.org/10.1158/1078-0432.Ccr-11-2303.
50. Connell F, Brice G, Jeffery S, Keeley V, Mortimer P, Mansour S. A new classification system for primary lymphatic dysplasias based on phenotype. Clin Genet. 2010;77:438–52. https://doi.org/10.1111/j.1399-0004.2010.01394.x.
51. Ricci KW, Hammill AM, Mobberley-Schuman P, Nelson SC, Blatt J, Bender JLG, et al. Efficacy of systemic sirolimus in the treatment of generalized lymphatic anomaly and Gorham-stout disease. Pediatr Blood Cancer. 2019;66:e27614. https://doi.org/10.1002/pbc.27614.

52. Gordon K, Moore M, Van Zanten M, Pearce J, Itkin M, Madden B, et al. Case report: progressive central conducting lymphatic abnormalities in the RASopathies. Two case reports, including successful treatment by MEK inhibition. Front Genet. 2022;13:1001105. https://doi.org/10.3389/fgene.2022.1001105.
53. Garlisi Torales LD, Sempowski BA, Krikorian GL, Woodis KM, Paulissen SM, Smith CL, et al. Central conducting lymphatic anomaly: from bench to bedside. J Clin Invest. 2024;134:e172839. https://doi.org/10.1172/jci172839.
54. Stewart G, Gaunt JI, Croft DN, Browse NL. Isotope lymphography: a new method of investigating the role of the lymphatics in chronic limb oedema. Br J Surg. 1985;72:906–9. https://doi.org/10.1002/bjs.1800721120.
55. Proby CM, Gane JN, Joseph AE, Mortimer PS. Investigation of the swollen limb with isotope lymphography. Br J Dermatol. 1990;123:29–37. https://doi.org/10.1111/j.1365-2133.1990.tb01821.x.
56. Modi S, Stanton AW, Mortimer PS, Levick JR. Clinical assessment of human lymph flow using removal rate constants of interstitial macromolecules: a critical review of lymphoscintigraphy. Lymphat Res Biol. 2007;5:183–202. https://doi.org/10.1089/lrb.2007.5306.
57. Xiong L, Engel H, Gazyakan E, Rahimi M, Hünerbein M, Sun J, et al. Current techniques for lymphatic imaging: state of the art and future perspectives. Eur J Surg Oncol. 2014;40:270–6. https://doi.org/10.1016/j.ejso.2013.11.027.
58. Unno N, Inuzuka K, Suzuki M, Yamamoto N, Sagara D, Nishiyama M, et al. Preliminary experience with a novel fluorescence lymphography using indocyanine green in patients with secondary lymphedema. J Vasc Surg. 2007;45:1016–21. https://doi.org/10.1016/j.jvs.2007.01.023.
59. Yamamoto T, Yamamoto N, Azuma S, Yoshimatsu H, Seki Y, Narushima M, et al. Near-infrared illumination system-integrated microscope for supermicrosurgical lymphaticovenular anastomosis. Microsurgery. 2014;34:23–7. https://doi.org/10.1002/micr.22115.
60. Lohrmann C, Pache G, Felmerer G, Foeldi E, Schaefer O, Langer M. Posttraumatic edema of the lower extremities: evaluation of the lymphatic vessels with magnetic resonance lymphangiography. J Vasc Surg. 2009;49:417–23. https://doi.org/10.1016/j.jvs.2008.08.069.
61. Lohrmann C, Foeldi E, Bartholomä JP, Langer M. Interstitial MR lymphangiography—a diagnostic imaging method for the evaluation of patients with clinically advanced stages of lymphedema. Acta Trop. 2007;104:8–15. https://doi.org/10.1016/j.actatropica.2007.07.001.
62. Liu NF, Yan ZX, Wu XF. Classification of lymphatic-system malformations in primary lymphoedema based on MR lymphangiography. Eur J Vasc Endovasc Surg. 2012;44:345–9. https://doi.org/10.1016/j.ejvs.2012.06.019.
63. Chavhan GB, Amaral JG, Temple M, Itkin M. MR lymphangiography in children: technique and potential applications. Radiographics. 2017;37:1775–90. https://doi.org/10.1148/rg.2017170014.
64. Damstra RJ, Partsch H. Prospective, randomized, controlled trial comparing the effectiveness of adjustable compression Velcro wraps versus inelastic multicomponent compression bandages in the initial treatment of leg lymphedema. J Vasc Surg Venous Lymphat Disord. 2013;1:13–9. https://doi.org/10.1016/j.jvsv.2012.05.001.
65. Mortimer PS, Simmonds R, Rezvani M, Robbins M, Hopewell JW, Ryan TJ. The measurement of skin lymph flow by isotope clearance–reliability, reproducibility, injection dynamics, and the effect of massage. J Invest Dermatol. 1990;95:677–82. https://doi.org/10.1111/1523-1747.ep12514347.
66. Williams AF, Vadgama A, Franks PJ, Mortimer PS. A randomized controlled crossover study of manual lymphatic drainage therapy in women with breast cancer-related lymph-

oedema. Eur J Cancer Care. 2002;11:254–61. https://doi.org/10.1046/j.1365-2354.2002.00312.x.
67. Woods M. The experience of manual lymph drainage as an aspect of treatment for lymphoedema. Int J Palliat Nurs. 2003;9:336–42; discussion 42. https://doi.org/10.12968/ijpn.2003.9.8.11524.
68. McNeely ML, Magee DJ, Lees AW, Bagnall KM, Haykowsky M, Hanson J. The addition of manual lymph drainage to compression therapy for breast cancer related lymphedema: a randomized controlled trial. Breast Cancer Res Treat. 2004;86:95–106. https://doi.org/10.1023/B:BREA.0000032978.67677.9f.
69. Compression for lymphoedema (editorial). Lancet. 1986;1:896.
70. Devoogdt N, Van Kampen M, Geraerts I, Coremans T, Christiaens MR. Different physical treatment modalities for lymphoedema developing after axillary lymph node dissection for breast cancer: a review. Eur J Obstet Gynecol Reprod Biol. 2010;149:3–9. https://doi.org/10.1016/j.ejogrb.2009.11.016.
71. Loprinzi CL, Kugler JW, Sloan JA, Rooke TW, Quella SK, Novotny P, et al. Lack of effect of coumarin in women with lymphedema after treatment for breast cancer. N Engl J Med. 1999;340:346–50. https://doi.org/10.1056/nejm199902043400503.
72. Gardenier JC, Kataru RP, Hespe GE, Savetsky IL, Torrisi JS, Nores GD, et al. Topical tacrolimus for the treatment of secondary lymphedema. Nat Commun. 2017;8:14345. https://doi.org/10.1038/ncomms14345.
73. Rockson SG, Tian W, Jiang X, Kuznetsova T, Haddad F, Zampell J, et al. Pilot studies demonstrate the potential benefits of antiinflammatory therapy in human lymphedema. JCI Insight. 2018;3:e123775. https://doi.org/10.1172/jci.insight.123775.
74. Dumanian GA, Futrell JW. The Charles procedure: misquoted and misunderstood since 1950. Plast Reconstr Surg. 1996;98:1258–63. https://doi.org/10.1097/00006534-199612000-00022.
75. Nielubowicz J, Olszewski W. Surgical lymphaticovenous shunts in patients with secondary lymphoedema. Br J Surg. 1968;55:440–2. https://doi.org/10.1002/bjs.1800550609.
76. Damstra RJ, Voesten HG, van Schelven WD, van der Lei B. Lymphatic venous anastomosis (LVA) for treatment of secondary arm lymphedema. A prospective study of 11 LVA procedures in 10 patients with breast cancer-related lymphedema and a critical review of the literature. Breast Cancer Res Treat. 2009;113:199–206. https://doi.org/10.1007/s10549-008-9932-5.
77. Campisi C, Bellini C, Campisi C, Accogli S, Bonioli E, Boccardo F. Microsurgery for lymphedema: clinical research and long-term results. Microsurgery. 2010;30:256–60. https://doi.org/10.1002/micr.20737.
78. Forte AJ, Khan N, Huayllani MT, Boczar D, Saleem HY, Lu X, et al. Lymphaticovenous anastomosis for lower extremity lymphedema: a systematic review. Indian J Plast Surg. 2020;53:17–24. https://doi.org/10.1055/s-0040-1709372.
79. Becker C, Assouad J, Riquet M, Hidden G. Postmastectomy lymphedema: long-term results following microsurgical lymph node transplantation. Ann Surg. 2006;243:313–5. https://doi.org/10.1097/01.sla.0000201258.10304.16.
80. Zampell JC, Aschen S, Weitman ES, Yan A, Elhadad S, De Brot Andrade M, et al. Regulation of adipogenesis by lymphatic fluid stasis: part I. Adipogenesis, fibrosis, and inflammation. Plast Reconstr Surg. 2012;129:825–34. https://doi.org/10.1097/PRS.0b013e3182450b2d.
81. Warren AG, Brorson H, Borud LJ, Slavin SA. Lymphedema: a comprehensive review. Ann Plast Surg. 2007;59:464–72. https://doi.org/10.1097/01.sap.0000257149.42922.7e.
82. Schaverien MV, Munnoch DA, Brorson H. Liposuction treatment of lymphedema. Semin Plast Surg. 2018;32:42–7. https://doi.org/10.1055/s-0038-1635116.

Key References

Gordon K, Varney R, Keeley V, Riches K, Jeffery S, Van Zanten M, et al. Update and audit of the St George's classification algorithm of primary lymphatic anomalies: a clinical and molecular approach to diagnosis. J Med Genet. 2020;57:653–9. https://doi.org/10.1136/jmedgenet-2019-106084.

Executive Committee of the International Society of Lymphology. The diagnosis and treatment of peripheral lymphedema: 2023 Consensus Document of The International Society of Lymphology. Lymphology. 2023;56:133–51.

Chapter 11
Graft Materials: Present and Future

Mital Desai and George Hamilton

SN Flashcards
Test your learning and check your understanding of this book's contents: use the "Springer Nature Flashcards" app to access questions using ▶ https://sn.pub/wppvze. To use the app, please follow the instructions in Chap. 1.

Key Learning Points

- Synthetic materials such as polyethylene terephthalate (Dacron) and expanded polytetrafluoroethylene (ePTFE) have been successfully used in large diameter vascular grafts, but their results are consistently poor when the diameter decreases below 6 mm.
- Thrombosis, lack of endothelial coverage, compliance mismatch and haemodynamic imbalance are the main factors responsible for early and late graft failure.
- Both Dacron and ePTFE have undergone several modifications to address their limitations, including heparin bonding, electrospinning, gelatin/polymer coatings and modification with sulphonated silk fibroin, without any significant success.

M. Desai
St George's Vascular Institute and St George's University Hospitals, London, UK
e-mail: mdesai@nhs.net

G. Hamilton (✉)
Department of Vascular Surgery, Royal Free London NHS Foundation Trust, and University College London, London, UK
e-mail: g.hamilton@ucl.ac.uk

R. Fitridge et al. (eds.), *Pathophysiology of Vascular Disease*,
https://doi.org/10.1007/978-3-032-31459-8_11

- Polyurethane grafts have been investigated with studies showing superior-thrombo-resistance, rapid ingrowth of living tissue and reduced anastomotic hyperplasia. However, the major problems have been relative thrombogenicity and aneurysmal degeneration.
- Biografts, which are vascular grafts made from biological sources such as bacterial cellulose, allogeneic grafts and biotubes, have been used but have not yet gained widespread clinical acceptance.
- Over the last decade, we have seen significant progress in cardiovascular tissue engineering. The three essential components of tissue engineering consist of (i) the cells that are seeded onto the graft, (ii) the scaffold onto which the extracellular matrix (ECM) forms and (iii) the humoral and mechanical signals that regulate neotissue formation and maintenance.
- The current climate of vascular tissue engineering is very promising. Significant progress has been made in the development of recent technologies in scaffold engineering and cell engineering, including gene delivery and improvement of endothelial progenitor cells.
- With ongoing development to match as closely as possible both the mechanical characteristics and biological functions of normal human arteries, there is real potential for new graft development within the next decade.
- Challenges in the clinical translation of decellularised extracellular matrix (dECM)-based vascular grafts, such as thrombosis, intimal hyperplasia and ensuring long-term patency, are areas of active research. Strategies to address these challenges include facilitating early endothelialisation and avoiding intravascular thrombosis through scaffold design and surface modifications.

11.1 Introduction

Vascular graft materials serve as critical components in the repair, bypass, or replacement of diseased blood vessels. The selection of an appropriate graft material is often a pivotal decision in the success of vascular interventions, as it directly influences both the short- and long-term outcomes for the patient.

Vascular grafts can be broadly classified into biological, synthetic and biosynthetic (Fig. 11.1). Biological grafts, such as autologous veins or arteries, offer superior biocompatibility and patency rates but may be limited by availability or the condition of the patient's own vessels. Synthetic grafts, on the other hand, provide an alternative when biological options are not feasible, and advances in material science have significantly improved their performance over the years. Synthetic materials such as polyethylene terephthalate (Dacron) and expanded polytetrafluoroethylene (ePTFE) have been used in vascular surgery for several decades. These materials are much stiffer compared to normal arteries. Compliance mismatch and haemodynamic imbalance are factors leading to intimal hyperplasia (IH), one of the fundamental causes of graft failure. Both Dacron and ePTFE have been very successful in replacing medium- and large-diameter

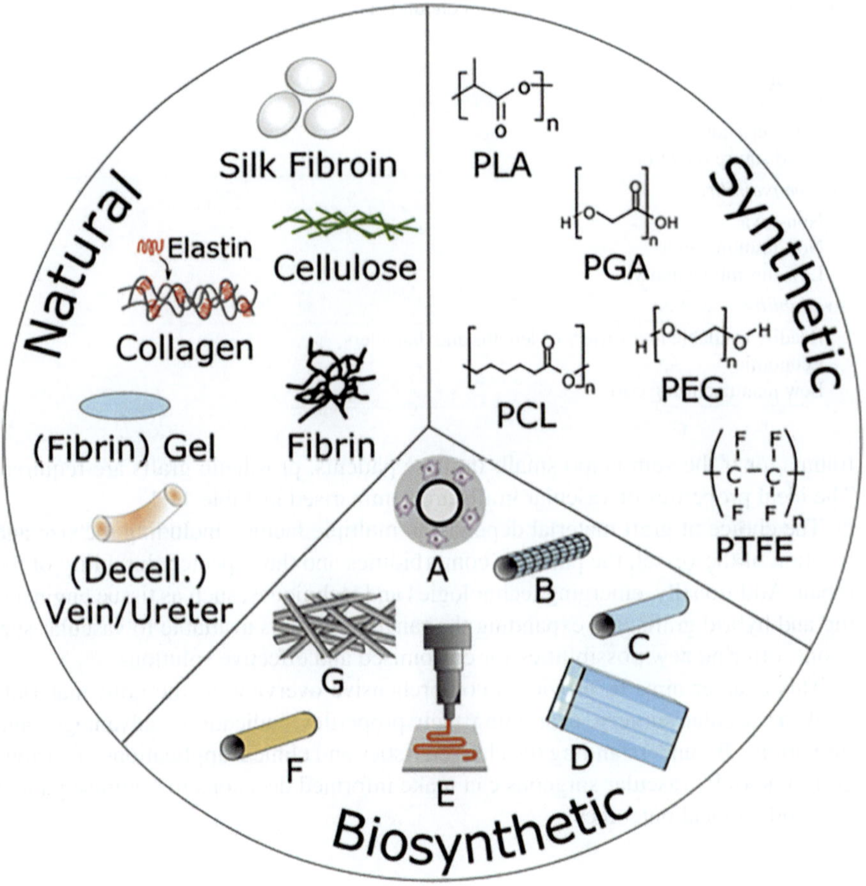

Fig. 11.1 This schematic categorises vascular graft materials into natural, synthetic and biosynthetic types, providing a clear overview of the materials utilised in vascular tissue engineering [89]. Natural materials used for vascular grafts contain decellularised ECM such as collagen, silk fibroin or fibrin. Furthermore, decellularised vein allografts display satisfactory mechanical stability, minimal evidence of antigenicity and a recolonisation with smooth muscle cells. Besides natural, synthetic materials are an attractive alternative due to their flexibility, mechanical strength and stiffness. Combining natural and synthetic materials (biosynthetic) opens more possibilities for tailoring the graft's properties to suit the needs of a particular application. Possible materials are collagen layers containing cells and an acellular support sleeve (A), fibrin-based scaffolds (B), nanostructured polyurethane blended with gelatin (C), microchannels in methacrylated gelatin (D), 3D printed scaffolds (E), hybrid meshes (F) or heparin functionalised polymers (G)

vessels. However, as diameters decrease below 6 mm, their performance has been consistently poor.

Autologous vein remains the conduit of choice for infrageniculate bypasses. However, almost a third of patients do not have a suitable available vein [1] due to the patient having varicose veins, previous removal, bypass or phlebitis, fibrosis or

Table 11.1 Properties of an ideal vascular conduit [91]

Mechanical features
Strong
Compliant
Kink resistant
Good suture retention
Biocompatibility
Non-toxic
Non-immunogenic
Low thrombogenicity
Availability
Readily available in a variety of lengths and diameters
Economic
Low manufacturing cost

trauma, or if the vein is too small. In these patients, prosthetic grafts are required. The ideal properties of vascular grafts are summarised in Table 11.1.

The choice of graft material depends on multiple factors, including the size and location of the vessel, the patient's comorbidities and the expected durability of the repair. Additionally, emerging technologies and techniques, such as tissue engineering and hybrid grafts, are expanding the range of options available to vascular surgeons, offering new possibilities for customised and effective solutions.

This chapter aims to provide a comprehensive overview of the graft materials used in vascular surgery, examining their properties, indications, advantages and limitations. By understanding the characteristics and clinical applications of various graft materials, vascular surgeons can make informed decisions to optimise patient care and surgical outcomes.

11.2 Historical Perspective

The development of peripheral vascular grafts has evolved from basic biological conduits to advanced synthetic and bioengineered constructs designed to overcome limitations in long-term patency and functionality. The saphenous vein has been a cornerstone for peripheral arterial bypass since the early twentieth century. Vein availability, variable quality and susceptibility to intimal hyperplasia were key issues. Early experiments used cadaveric arterial segments for bypass, but outcomes were limited by rapid degeneration and immune response [2]. The limitations of biological grafts spurred the development of synthetic alternatives. Introduced in the 1950s, these synthetic materials provided durability and consistency for arterial bypass [3]. Dacron was particularly effective for larger arteries but showed reduced success in small-diameter vessels (<6 mm) due to thrombosis and lack of endothelialisation. Knitted Dacron offered greater flexibility, while woven variants provided higher strength. Improvements in pore size facilitated tissue ingrowth and healing.

ePTFE grafts gained popularity for peripheral applications due to their low thrombogenicity and mechanical stability. The addition of external ridges helped resist kinking and compression in challenging anatomical locations. The evolution of peripheral vascular grafts highlights the interplay between biological and synthetic solutions to address clinical challenges.

11.3 Pathophysiology of Graft Healing

The tissue response to implantation of a prosthetic graft is complex, with many variable factors involved, such as the material used, its construction, its porosity and its length. Further important factors relate to the interaction between the graft and the host artery at the anastomotic areas. A major stimulus for the study of this area is the still unresolved puzzle of man's inability to endothelialise a prosthetic graft beyond the immediate 2 cm or so from the anastomosis.

Recent evidence on the pathophysiology of vascular graft healing reveals several key mechanisms that influence graft integration, remodelling and long-term performance. Vascular graft healing is a multifaceted process involving several key mechanisms.

11.3.1 Endothelialisation

Prosthetic grafting involves injury to the artery from the direct trauma of implantation, and subsequent exposure of the anastomotic areas to haemodynamic stress (compliance mismatch, turbulent flow and altered shear stress). Following implantation, in arteries or veins and especially in the peri-anastomotic area, there is fibroblast and smooth muscle cell (SMC) accumulation in the intima with extracellular matrix (ECM) deposition. The end result of this excessive cellular deposition is expansion of the intimal layer, termed as 'neointima', which is associated with loss of peri-anastomotic luminal area. The formation of a new endothelial layer over the graft's inner surface is crucial for reducing thrombosis and enhancing long-term graft performance. This endothelial coverage can originate from the migration of endothelial cells from the adjacent native vessel or through capillary ingrowth from the graft's exterior.

11.3.2 Capillary Ingrowth

Healing of prosthetic grafts occurs through capillary ingrowth into the graft wall and the proliferation of endothelial cells along the graft's luminal surface from each anastomosis [4]. Studies have shown that short grafts can develop a complete endothelial lining, highlighting the importance of capillary ingrowth in graft healing. Capillary ingrowth helps anchor the graft to the host tissue by promoting the formation of a new vascular network within the graft wall. Ingrowing capillaries supply the graft with essential nutrients and oxygen, which are critical for cellular survival and proliferation during the healing process. By enhancing vascularisation, capillary ingrowth reduces the likelihood of ischaemia and necrosis in the graft tissue, particularly in bioengineered or tissue-derived grafts.

The primary process driving capillary ingrowth is angiogenesis, where new capillaries sprout from pre-existing blood vessels near the graft site. This process is mediated by:

- Pro-Angiogenic Growth Factors: Vascular endothelial growth factor (VEGF) and basic fibroblast growth factor (bFGF) are key drivers of angiogenesis.
- Endothelial Cell Activity: Endothelial cells proliferate, migrate and align to form new capillary structures. As capillaries grow into the graft wall, fibroblasts and other stromal cells contribute to the deposition of ECM, providing structural support for the newly formed vessels. Porous grafts allow better infiltration of capillaries compared to non-porous ones. Biodegradable scaffolds are designed to degrade as capillary networks develop, leaving behind native tissue. Incorporating pro-angiogenic agents like VEGF or platelet-derived growth factor (PDGF) into the graft material accelerates capillary formation. Capillary ingrowth is a cornerstone of vascular graft healing, enabling vascularisation and long-term graft functionality.

11.3.3 Intimal Hyperplasia

This refers to the thickening of the tunica intima due to the proliferation and migration of vascular smooth muscle cells (VSMCs) to the intima, leading to extracellular matrix deposition. Intimal hyperplasia is a common cause of late graft failure, particularly in veins and synthetic grafts. The three phases of intimal hyperplasia develop quite rapidly, with the first being proliferation of medial smooth muscle cells as soon as 24 hours after injury and lasting up to 4 weeks. The second phase of SMC migration into the intima starts as early as 4 days after injury and continues for about a month. The final phase is of intimal expansion due to the dual action of SMC migration and intimal proliferation by deposition of matrix proteins such as collagen, elastin and proteoglycans. This phase is complex and is mostly self-limiting but may continue unabated if certain factors are present.

11.3.4 *Haemodynamic Factors*

Abnormal blood flow within the graft can impair healing and overall patency. Disturbed flow patterns can promote adverse remodelling, contributing to graft failure. The tangential force exerted by blood flow on the endothelial surface is vital for maintaining vascular homeostasis and promoting endothelial cell alignment and function. Circumferential stress from pulsatile blood flow impacts the mechanical integrity and adaptation of the graft wall. Laminar (smooth) flow supports healthy endothelialisation, while disturbed or turbulent flow predisposes to thrombosis, intimal hyperplasia (IH) and graft failure.

Optimising shear stress, reducing turbulence and ensuring mechanical compatibility between the graft and native vessels can significantly enhance healing and long-term graft patency. Advances in graft design, bioactive materials and surgical techniques continue to improve outcomes by addressing haemodynamic challenges. Understanding these mechanisms is essential for developing strategies to enhance graft healing and longevity.

11.4 Natural Materials

11.4.1 *Autologous Veins*

Multiple large-scale trials and meta-analyses show superior patency of autologous veins compared to synthetic materials (e.g. ePTFE, Dacron) in femoropopliteal and tibial bypasses [5]. Vein grafts have a five-year primary patency rate of up to 70% for below-knee bypass, compared to approximately 30%–50% for prosthetic grafts in the same setting. The biological and mechanical advantages and disadvantages of autologous bypass conduit are summarised in Table 11.2, and approaches to enhance the performance of autologous vein grafts are shown in Table 11.3.

Table 11.2 Biological and mechanical advantages and disadvantages of autologous bypass conduit

Endothelial lining	Autologous veins retain a native endothelial layer that inhibits thrombosis and promotes healing
Elasticity and compliance	Veins can adapt to arterial pressure conditions better than rigid synthetic alternatives
Resistance to infection	The biological nature of vein grafts offers superior resistance to infection, critical in contaminated or high-risk fields
Availability	Suitable veins may be unavailable due to prior harvest, varicosities, or systemic disease
Harvest-related morbidity	Complications include wound infection, seroma and nerve injury
Degeneration and intimal hyperplasia	Late graft failure is often due to remodelling and intimal thickening at anastomotic sites

Table 11.3 Approaches to enhance the performance of autologous vein grafts

Preconditioning	External supports, flow preconditioning, or pharmacological agents are being explored to enhance adaptation
Bioengineering	Decellularised autologous vein scaffolds seeded with stem cells show potential to rejuvenate compromised veins
Hybrid grafting	Combining short autologous segments with synthetic materials to reduce synthetic graft length and associated risks

Professional societies, including the Society for Vascular Surgery (SVS) and European Society for Vascular Surgery (ESVS), endorse autologous vein grafts as the first-line conduit for infrainguinal bypass surgery and complex revascularisation procedures.

11.4.2 Allografts

Allografts, derived from human donors, have historically served as alternative conduits in vascular surgery, particularly when autologous veins are unavailable or unsuitable. These grafts include cryopreserved veins and arteries, as well as decellularised vessels, offering biological compatibility and potential for integration with host tissue [6].

Cryopreserved allografts, such as saphenous veins and femoral arteries, are utilised in various vascular procedures, including infrainguinal bypasses and haemodialysis access, especially in infected fields where synthetic grafts pose higher risks [7]. Their advantages include resistance to infection and availability for urgent interventions. However, challenges such as limited long-term patency and potential for immunogenic responses persist.

The future of allografts in vascular surgery is poised to benefit from advancements in regenerative medicine and bioengineering. Efforts are underway to enhance the mechanical properties and longevity of allografts, including the incorporation of stem cells and growth factors to promote endothelialisation and integration. Additionally, the development of off-the-shelf, universally compatible grafts aims to address the limitations of donor availability and immunogenicity [8].

11.5 Prosthetic Grafts

11.5.1 Polyethylene Terephthalate (Dacron)

Dacron (polyethylene terephthalate) has been one of the most widely used materials for vascular grafts since its introduction in the 1960s. It is known for its durability, biocompatibility and resistance to degradation.

Dacron is a synthetic polyester fibre that offers a balance of strength, flexibility and resistance to infection. Its ability to withstand physiological pressures without significant deformation makes it particularly useful for large-calibre arterial bypass procedures. However, despite its physical properties, Dacron lacks inherent endothelialisation, which predisposes to thrombosis, IH and long-term occlusion [9].

Long-term follow-up studies suggest that Dacron grafts maintain high patency rates, especially in large-calibre applications like aorto-femoral bypass procedures. Patency rates of over 70% at 5 years have been reported for Dacron grafts used in these procedures [10]. In contrast, when Dacron is used for small-calibre grafts (e.g. femoro-popliteal bypass), the patency rate significantly drops due to the aforementioned compliance mismatch, flow disturbances and heightened risk of thrombosis.

Studies have shown that the lack of endothelialisation of Dacron grafts increases the likelihood of platelet aggregation and thrombus formation, particularly in the early post-operative period. Infections, although less frequent than thrombosis, can lead to graft loss and require revascularisation or graft removal [11].

Grafts that combine Dacron with endothelial cells or coated with biologic substances have shown promise in improving endothelialisation and reducing the risk of thrombosis [12]. Further research is needed to develop Dacron grafts that better mimic the dynamic compliance of native vessels and integrate more effectively with the surrounding tissue. The role of drug-eluting coatings and biodegradable scaffolds in reducing graft failure through improved healing and prevention of intimal hyperplasia (IH) is another area of active investigation [13].

11.5.1.1 Heparin Bonding

Increased thrombogenicity arises due to the lack of endothelial cells on the surface of the graft, leading to platelet aggregation and thrombus formation [9]. Heparin, an anticoagulant that naturally binds to antithrombin III to inhibit clotting factors, has been used to modify the surface of Dacron grafts in an effort to enhance the graft's thromboresistance.

Heparin bonding to Dacron is typically achieved by covalent attachment or electrostatic interactions between heparin molecules and the surface of the graft material. Heparin are immobilised onto the Dacron surface through chemical modifications such as glutaraldehyde crosslinking or silanisation (coating surface with silicon molecules) [14]. These modifications enable the heparin to remain stably bound to the graft while still retaining its anticoagulant activity. When bound to the graft surface, heparin promotes the binding of antithrombin III, which in turn inhibits thrombin and other clotting factors, thus reducing thrombogenicity [15].

Studies examining heparin-coated Dacron grafts have demonstrated promising results in terms of reduced thrombosis and improved patency rates, particularly in the first year after surgery, when the risk of thrombosis is highest. Despite these promising outcomes, the long-term effectiveness of heparin bonding remains a subject of ongoing research. Some studies have indicated that while heparin bonding offers substantial initial benefits in reducing thrombogenicity, the effect may diminish over time. Degradation of heparin due to hydrolysis or shear forces from blood flow can limit the long-term efficacy of heparin-coated grafts [16]. Consequently, strategies are being developed to enhance the stability and durability of heparin coatings, such as the use of biodegradable polymers or hydrogel-based matrices to create a more stable anticoagulant interface [17]. Growth factors such as vascular endothelial growth factor (VEGF) and endothelial cell adhesion peptides have been explored as adjuncts to heparin coatings to improve graft integration and further reduce the risk of thrombosis [18].

11.5.1.2 Electrospinning

The process of electrospinning offers a promising solution by creating nanofibrous mats that mimic the natural ECM, which can support cell attachment, proliferation and endothelialisation. Electrospinning involves the application of a high-voltage electric field to a polymer solution, causing the polymer to form fine nanofibres. These fibres are deposited onto a collector, creating a non-woven fibrous mat. The size, alignment and porosity of the electrospun fibres can be precisely controlled by adjusting parameters such as the polymer concentration, voltage and collection distance. In the context of vascular grafts, electrospinning can be applied to Dacron to create a fibrous scaffold that provides a more suitable environment for cellular growth and infiltration.

Electrospinning can address thrombogenicity by creating a nanofibrous surface that promotes cell adhesion and proliferation, mimicking the natural ECM. This allows for the improved growth of endothelial cells, which can line the surface of the graft and create a more biocompatible interface between the graft and native vessel [19].

Recent studies have shown that Dacron grafts modified with electrospun nanofibres improve endothelial cell attachment and reduce thrombus formation compared to non-modified Dacron grafts. Wang et al. demonstrated that Dacron grafts electrospun with a blend of polycaprolactone (PCL) and gelatin significantly enhanced endothelial cell attachment and proliferation [20].

In addition to enhancing endothelialisation, electrospinning can also modify the mechanical properties of Dacron grafts. Electrospun nanofibres can be tailored to produce grafts with improved flexibility and compliance. By incorporating biodegradable polymers or elastomeric materials into the electrospun fibres, researchers have been able to produce Dacron grafts that exhibit enhanced elasticity and dynamic response to blood pressure fluctuations. This compliance improvement can reduce mechanical stresses at the graft-vessel interface and promote better long-term graft function [21].

The modification of Dacron grafts through electrospinning has been shown to reduce the risk of thrombosis and IH. The nanofibrous structure of electrospun scaffolds mimics the structure of the native vascular wall, promoting the infiltration of cells that are crucial for graft healing. In particular, SMCs and fibroblasts can migrate into the electrospun scaffold, leading to the development of a more natural tissue-like structure within the graft. Moreover, the electrospun nanofibres can be functionalised with bioactive molecules such as heparin, VEGF, or PDGF, which further enhance endothelialisation and SMC migration [22].

The clinical use of electrospun Dacron grafts is still in the early stages, but several studies have shown promising results in improving graft outcomes. Challenges remain in terms of scalability, cost-effectiveness and the long-term stability of the electrospun coatings. The durability of electrospun fibres and their ability to maintain their beneficial properties in the physiological environment for extended periods remain critical areas for improvement. Future research focusing on advanced biofunctionalisation techniques, composite materials and long-term clinical trials will be essential to realising the full potential of electrospun Dacron grafts in clinical practice.

11.5.1.3 Gelatin Coatings

Gelatin coatings have emerged as a widely used surface modification to enhance the biocompatibility and healing potential of Dacron grafts.

Gelatin is a natural, biodegradable and biocompatible polymer derived from collagen, the primary structural protein in the ECM. It possesses numerous arginine–glycine–aspartic acid (RGD) motifs that facilitate cell adhesion and proliferation [23]. These properties make it an ideal candidate for coating synthetic vascular grafts.

The gelatin coating serves multiple functions:

- Improved Haemostasis: The porous structure of woven or knitted Dacron can allow blood leakage post-implantation. Gelatin coatings reduce permeability and promote rapid sealing of the graft, with the potential to minimise intraoperative and post-operative blood loss.
- Enhanced Endothelialisation: By mimicking components of the native ECM, gelatin-coated grafts better support endothelial cell adhesion and migration [24].
- Reduced Thrombogenicity: Gelatin acts as a carrier for bioactive agents such as heparin, VEGF, or growth factors, which can be embedded in the coating to provide local, controlled release. This functionalisation further reduces thrombotic events and supports neointimal regeneration.
- Biodegradability: Gelatin coatings are designed to degrade over time, typically within a few weeks after implantation. This temporary presence provides early protection without interfering with long-term integration of the graft.

Gelatin is typically applied to Dacron grafts via dip-coating or spray-coating, followed by crosslinking using agents like glutaraldehyde or genipin (see Glossary) to improve mechanical stability and control degradation kinetics. The degree of crosslinking influences the release profile of embedded agents, mechanical properties and biodegradation rate. Modern coatings may be further enhanced by the addition of nanoparticles, growth factors, or antimicrobial agents. Table 11.4 discusses the limitations of gelatin coating of grafts.

Table 11.4 Limitations of gelatin coating of grafts

Batch variability	Due to gelatin's natural origin, can impact reproducibility
Immunogenicity	May arise in sensitive patients, particularly with animal-derived gelatin
Temporary nature of gelatin	May not suffice for long-term benefits unless combined with other modifications or drug delivery systems
Crosslinking agents	May introduce cytotoxicity if not thoroughly neutralised (particularly glutaraldehyde)

Recent developments have focused on functionalising gelatin coatings to impart additional bioactivities. For example, gelatin-heparin conjugates have been shown to maintain antithrombotic effects while supporting endothelialisation [25]. Electrospun gelatin coatings, often in combination with other polymers like PCL, provide structural support and enhance compliance matching [26].

Additionally, gelatin coatings are being explored as a delivery vehicle for stem cells or endothelial progenitor cells to accelerate vascular tissue regeneration, further enhancing the biological integration of Dacron grafts [27]. Advances in crosslinking chemistry, drug incorporation and surface engineering are necessary to fully realise the long-term potential of this approach.

11.5.2 Expanded Polytetrafluoroethylene (ePTFE)

ePTFE has been a cornerstone in the field of vascular surgery for decades. Its biocompatibility, durability and ease of handling have made it a preferred material for creating vascular grafts.

ePTFE is a synthetic polymer derived from polytetrafluoroethylene (PTFE), commonly known as Teflon. The expansion process creates a microporous structure characterised by nodes and interconnecting fibrils. This unique structure imparts several advantageous properties:

- Biocompatibility: ePTFE is chemically inert and hydrophobic, minimising its interaction with blood components and reducing the risk of thrombosis and inflammation [28].
- Durability and Mechanical Strength: ePTFE grafts exhibit good tensile strength and resistance to degradation, allowing them to withstand physiological blood pressure and mechanical stress [6].
- Porosity: The microporous structure allows for tissue ingrowth, which can promote graft integration and long-term patency. The internodal distance is a critical parameter that determines the porosity and influences tissue ingrowth [28].

Despite their widespread use, ePTFE grafts have several limitations, particularly in small-diameter applications (Table 11.5).

Table 11.5 Limitations of ePTFE grafts

Thrombosis	The most significant limitation is the risk of thrombosis, especially in low-flow conditions or small-diameter grafts (<6 mm) due to its hydrophobic nature
Intimal hyperplasia	This is a common complication leading to stenosis and graft failure at the graft-host anastomosis
Infection	ePTFE grafts are susceptible to bacterial infection, which can lead to graft failure, sepsis and significant morbidity [92]
Compliance mismatch	The difference in mechanical properties between the relatively stiff ePTFE graft and the more compliant native artery can lead to haemodynamic disturbances and contribute to failure

11.5.2.1 Heparin-Bonded ePTFE Grafts

ePTFE, while biocompatible, lacks the natural antithrombotic properties of the endothelium, resulting in activation of platelets and clotting factors leading to thrombus formation. To mitigate this, various modifications have been explored, with heparin bonding being a prominent strategy.

Several techniques have been developed to attach heparin to ePTFE graft surfaces. These methods can be broadly classified into:

- Physical Adsorption: This involves simple coating of heparin onto the graft surface. However, this method results in poor stability and rapid release of heparin, limiting its long-term effectiveness.
- Ionic Bonding: Heparin, being negatively charged, can be attached to positively charged sites on the ePTFE surface. While this method offers improved stability compared to physical adsorption, the bonding is still relatively weak.
- Covalent Bonding: Provides the most durable and effective means of heparin immobilisation, minimising heparin release and maximising its antithrombotic activity. A commonly used technique involves the use of a linker molecule to covalently bind heparin to the ePTFE surface.
- End-Point Covalent Bonding: This advanced technique, employed in grafts like the GORE PROPATEN Vascular Graft, involves a proprietary method (Carmeda BioActive Surface or CBAS) to anchor heparin molecules to the luminal surface while maintaining heparin's intrinsic bioactive properties. This method has shown promising results in enhancing thromboresistance and patency [29].

Despite the advantages, there are some limitations to heparin-bonded ePTFE grafts:

- Cost: Heparin-bonded grafts are generally more expensive than standard ePTFE grafts.
- Long-Term Efficacy: While studies have shown improved short- to mid-term patency, more research is needed to fully evaluate the long-term efficacy and durability of heparin-bonded grafts in all clinical settings.

- Variability in Performance: The clinical performance of heparin-bonded grafts can vary depending on the specific bonding technique, the patient population and the anatomical location of the graft.

Future research should focus on:

- Novel Antithrombotic Agents: Exploring the use of other antithrombotic agents, such as tissue plasminogen activator (tPA) or antiplatelet drugs, in combination with heparin or as alternatives.
- Improved Bonding Techniques: Developing even more stable and durable methods for attaching heparin or other agents to ePTFE surfaces.
- Tissue Engineering: Combining heparin bonding with tissue engineering approaches to create grafts that not only resist thrombosis but also promote endothelialisation and graft remodelling.
- Personalised Medicine: Identifying patient-specific factors that influence graft patency to optimise the selection of graft type and antithrombotic therapy.

11.5.2.2 Sulphonated Silk Fibroin-Modified ePTFE Grafts

Silk fibroin (SF) is a natural protein derived from Bombyx mori silkworm silk. It has garnered significant attention in tissue engineering due to its:

- Biocompatibility: SF exhibits minimal immunogenicity and supports cell adhesion and proliferation [30].
- Biodegradability: SF can be enzymatically degraded, allowing for tissue remodelling and regeneration [31].
- Mechanical Properties: SF can be processed into various forms, including films, scaffolds and nanofibres, with tunable mechanical properties [32].

Sulphonation is a chemical modification that introduces sulphonic acid groups ($-SO_3H$) onto the SF molecule. This modification enhances several properties of SF [33]:

- Anticoagulant Activity: Sulphonated SF exhibits anticoagulant properties by mimicking the structure and function of glycosaminoglycans, such as heparin.
- Improved Cell Adhesion: The negatively charged sulphonic acid groups can enhance the adsorption of positively charged growth factors and promote cell adhesion.
- Increased Hydrophilicity: Sulphonation increases the hydrophilicity of SF, which can improve its biocompatibility and reduce protein adsorption.

The modification of ePTFE grafts with sulphonated SF aims to overcome the limitations of ePTFE and improve graft patency. Several studies have demonstrated the benefits of this approach:

- Enhanced Haemocompatibility: Sulphonated SF coatings on ePTFE grafts have been shown to reduce platelet adhesion and activation, leading to improved haemocompatibility and reduced thrombosis [34].
- Promoted Endothelialisation: Sulphonated SF surfaces can enhance endothelial cell adhesion, proliferation and migration, facilitating the formation of a functional endothelium [35].
- Improved Patency Rates: In vivo studies have demonstrated that sulphonated SF-modified ePTFE grafts exhibit higher patency rates compared to unmodified grafts, particularly in small-diameter applications [34].

Future research directions may include:

- Long-term in vivo studies to evaluate the durability and remodelling potential of sulphonated SF-modified ePTFE grafts.
- The development of tissue-engineered vascular grafts using sulphonated SF in combination with other biomaterials and cell-seeding techniques.
- Clinical trials to assess the safety and efficacy of sulphonated SF-modified ePTFE grafts in humans.

Sulphonated SF modification of ePTFE grafts represents a promising strategy. The enhanced haemocompatibility, improved endothelialisation and improved patency rates associated with this modification offer significant advantages. Continued research and development in this area may lead to the development of more effective and durable vascular grafts for the treatment of vascular diseases.

11.5.2.3 Polymer-Coated ePTFE Grafts

Polymer and heparin coatings have been employed to impart antithrombogenic properties to ePTFE grafts. Táborská et al. developed a fibrin/heparin coating enriched with VEGF and FGF, which promoted endothelialisation and exhibited excellent antithrombogenic properties in vitro [36].

To enhance endothelial cell adhesion and proliferation, biofunctional coatings have been explored. A study by Ding et al. introduced a differentiated inner and outer surface modification of ePTFE grafts using heparin and epigallocatechin gallate (see Glossary) on the luminal side, and polyethyleneimine (see Glossary) and rapamycin on the outer surface. This dual modification promoted endothelialisation while inhibiting smooth muscle cell proliferation and inflammation [37].

Poly(diol-co-citrate-co-ascorbate) (POCA) elastomers have been applied as coatings to reduce neointimal hyperplasia. These coatings demonstrated antioxidant properties, supported endothelial cell growth and inhibited SMC proliferation, indicating their potential in improving graft patency [38].

Fluorosurfactant polymers (FSPs) have been utilised to modify the luminal surface of ePTFE grafts, enhancing endothelial cell adhesion and reducing thrombogenicity. In a porcine carotid artery bypass model, FSP-coated ePTFE grafts exhibited improved endothelialisation and reduced platelet adhesion compared to uncoated grafts [39].

The conjugation of Substance P (SP) (see Glossary) and heparin onto poly(L-lactide-co-caprolactone) (PLCL) coatings has been investigated to promote endothelial and smooth muscle cell recruitment. This approach facilitated vascular regeneration and reduced thrombosis in small-diameter ePTFE grafts [40].

Future research should focus on long-term clinical studies to evaluate the efficacy and safety of these coatings in human subjects. Additionally, the development of multifunctional coatings that combine antithrombogenic, anti-inflammatory and pro-endothelialisation properties could further improve graft outcomes.

11.6 Polyurethane Grafts

Polyurethane (PU)-based vascular grafts have emerged as a promising alternative due to their tunable mechanical properties, haemocompatibility and ability to mimic the compliance of native vessels. Polyurethanes are segmented block copolymers composed of alternating soft and hard segments, which allow for fine-tuning of elasticity, tensile strength and degradation rates. Early generations of PU grafts were limited by biodegradation and loss of mechanical integrity; however, advances in polymer chemistry and fabrication technologies have led to the development of new PU formulations with improved biostability and biofunctionality.

Recent research has focused on modifying the surface properties of PU grafts to promote endothelialisation, reduce thrombogenicity and minimise the inflammatory response. Strategies such as surface coating with bioactive molecules, incorporation of heparin and fabrication of nanofibrous structures through electrospinning have been employed to enhance graft performance. Furthermore, biodegradable polyurethane scaffolds offer the potential for vascular regeneration by serving as a temporary matrix that is gradually replaced by native tissue.

11.6.1 Polycarbonate Polyurethane (PCU)

A study by Eilenberg et al. evaluated electrospun, bioabsorbable PCU grafts in a rat model over 12 months. The grafts demonstrated excellent patency rates (92.9%) and promoted neo-vessel formation with minimal inflammatory response, indicating their potential for in situ vascular tissue engineering [41].

In another investigation, Jalaie et al. compared two variants of PCU patches with Dacron in sheep carotid arteries. Both PCU variants showed nearly complete endothelialisation and thinner neointimal layers compared to Dacron [42]. Additionally, a review highlighted the development of composite materials combining PCU with polyhedral oligomeric silsesquioxane (POSS) (see Glossary). These composites exhibited enhanced mechanical strength and resistance to degradation, making them suitable candidates for small-diameter vascular grafts [28].

11.6.2 Composite Polyurethane Grafts

Recent research has focused on enhancing PU grafts through composite strategies, incorporating other polymers, bioactive agents and structural modifications to improve performance.

A study developed electrospun composite grafts combining PU and PCL, integrated with growth factors and coated with heparin and iloprost. These grafts exhibited a micro/nanofibrous structure with interconnected pores, promoting endothelialisation and reducing thrombogenicity. Mechanical properties such as tensile strength and compliance were comparable to native vessels, suggesting potential for improved patency in preclinical models [43].

Das and team fabricated trilayered electrospun grafts using PU layers infused with gallic acid and a middle layer of poly(glycolic acid)-poly(caprolactone) blend. These grafts demonstrated high burst pressure and suture retention strength. In vivo studies in rat femoral arteries showed maintained patency and promoted endothelialisation, indicating the grafts' efficacy in reducing oxidative stress and supporting tissue integration [44].

Another approach involved creating bilayered PU grafts with a macroporous outer layer and a nanofibrous inner layer, surface-modified with methacrylated sulphated alginate. This modification enhanced anticoagulant properties and protein adsorption, facilitating endothelial cell attachment. Implantation in rat abdominal aortas demonstrated the grafts' functionality and biocompatibility over a five-month period [45].

Using the roto-evaporation technique, a three-layer PU graft was engineered to mimic the architecture of native coronary arteries. The graft exhibited superior mechanical properties, including high burst pressure and compliance. Cytocompatibility tests showed high cell viability, although fibroblast adhesion varied among the different PU layers [46].

These studies underscore the potential of composite PU-based grafts in addressing the limitations of traditional small-diameter vascular prostheses. By integrating bioactive compounds, optimising structural design and enhancing mechanical properties, composite PU grafts are advancing towards clinical applicability.

11.6.3 Endothelial Progenitor Cell (EPC) Homing

The integration of endothelial progenitor cells (EPCs) into vascular grafts has emerged as a promising strategy. EPCs, originating from the bone marrow and circulating in peripheral blood, have the capacity to differentiate into mature endothelial cells, contributing to vascular repair and neovascularisation. Their recruitment and homing to sites of vascular injury are regulated by various chemokines and adhesion molecules, notably the stromal cell-derived factor-1 (SDF-1)/CXCR4 axis [47].

Recent advancements have focused on biofunctionalising vascular graft surfaces to enhance EPC capture. For instance, immobilising EPC-specific capture molecules on graft surfaces can mimic natural homing signals, facilitating in vivo endothelialisation. Additionally, modifying graft materials, such as incorporating gold nanoparticles into polyurethane matrices, has been shown to promote EPC differentiation and maturation, leading to improved antithrombotic properties [48]. Furthermore, the use of electrospun scaffolds coated with ECM proteins like fibronectin has demonstrated enhanced EPC adhesion and proliferation, supporting the formation of a functional endothelial layer. These strategies aim to create a conducive microenvironment for EPC homing, ultimately improving the performance of small-diameter vascular grafts [49].

In conclusion, leveraging EPC homing mechanisms through graft surface modifications holds significant potential. Continued research into optimising these approaches is essential for translating these findings into clinical applications.

Despite encouraging preclinical data, the clinical translation of polyurethane small-diameter grafts remains limited. Critical challenges include achieving long-term patency, preventing early thrombosis and ensuring mechanical durability under physiological conditions. There may be degradation of PU materials during long-term implantation in vivo, resulting in a decline in the physical properties of artificial blood vessels, such as weakened strength and cracks, affecting normal use [50].

Continued research into polyurethane chemistry, surface biofunctionalisation and scaffold design holds promise for the development of next-generation vascular grafts capable of meeting the complex demands of small-calibre vessel replacement.

11.7 Biological Vascular Grafts

Biological small-diameter grafts are typically derived from natural tissues, including autologous, allogeneic, or xenogeneic sources, or are engineered from biomaterials designed to support cell integration and tissue regeneration. Strategies include decellularised vascular scaffolds, tissue-engineered blood vessels (TEBVs) and

ECM-based constructs. These biological approaches aim to create grafts with appropriate mechanical strength, haemocompatibility and the ability to remodel and integrate into the host vasculature.

Recent advances in decellularisation techniques, stem cell seeding and scaffold functionalisation have significantly improved the mechanical integrity and biological performance of these grafts. Nevertheless, challenges such as immunogenicity, risk of infection and achieving consistent endothelialisation remain key barriers to clinical translation. Ongoing research focuses on optimising scaffold design, enhancing cell recruitment and promoting long-term graft patency.

11.7.1 Bacterial Cellulose

Bacterial cellulose (BC), a biopolymer synthesised by certain bacterial species, has garnered significant attention as a material due to its remarkable mechanical strength, biocompatibility and structural similarity to the native extracellular matrix. One innovative approach involves the in situ compaction and heparin immobilisation of BC to create vascular patches with improved mechanical properties and anticoagulant activity. This method enhances the tensile and burst strength of the grafts while promoting endothelial cell proliferation and reducing platelet adhesion, thereby facilitating endothelialisation [51].

Another study developed hierarchical-structured BC/potato starch composite tubes, which exhibited favourable physicochemical properties and biocompatibility. These grafts demonstrated a 75% patency rate in rabbit models, with complete endothelialisation and organised SMC formation, indicating their potential for in situ blood vessel regeneration [52].

Furthermore, the incorporation of magnetic properties into BC scaffolds has been investigated to improve cell retention. Magnetic bacterial cellulose was shown to effectively capture and retain magnetically labelled smooth muscle cells under dynamic flow conditions in vitro, suggesting a novel strategy to enhance cell homing and integration in vascular grafts [53].

In vivo studies have also demonstrated the feasibility of using BC-based grafts in large animal models. For instance, small-diameter BC grafts reinforced with a cobalt-chromium mesh were successfully implanted as aortocoronary bypasses in pigs, showing complete patency and evidence of functional remodelling after 4 weeks [54].

Collectively, these advancements underscore the potential of bacterial cellulose as a versatile and effective material for small-diameter vascular grafts. Ongoing research focusing on optimising its mechanical properties, biocompatibility and functionalisation strategies will be crucial for its translation into clinical applications.

11.7.2 Allogeneic Grafts

Allogeneic vascular grafts—derived from human donors—have emerged as a promising alternative to synthetic and autologous grafts, particularly in scenarios where autologous vessels are unavailable or unsuitable. These grafts offer the potential for improved biocompatibility and integration, aiming to reduce complications such as thrombosis and intimal hyperplasia.

Recent advancements have focused on the development of tissue-engineered allogeneic grafts. For instance, a study reported the first clinical use of a completely biological, allogeneic, non-living, human tissue-engineered vascular graft. These grafts, constructed from human fibroblasts, were implanted as arteriovenous shunts in haemodialysis patients. The grafts demonstrated mechanical strength comparable to native vessels and showed no signs of degradation or dilation up to 11 months post-implantation, with no evidence of immune responses, indicating their potential for clinical application [55].

Another innovative approach involves the use of double allogeneic human-engineered tissue grafts. In preclinical studies, these grafts have shown promising results in promoting tissue revascularisation, reducing infarct size, preventing adverse remodelling and fibrosis and ultimately enhancing cardiac function [56]. Furthermore, research into small-diameter artery grafts engineered from pluripotent stem cells has demonstrated the feasibility of creating 3 mm-diameter artery grafts by using arterial endothelial cells derived from pluripotent stem cells. These grafts were evaluated in a rhesus arterial interposition grafting model, showing potential [57]. Despite these advancements, challenges remain in the widespread clinical adoption of allogeneic vascular grafts. Issues such as immunogenicity, long-term patency and the risk of infection require ongoing research and development.

11.7.3 Biotubes

Biotubes are autologous, tissue-engineered vascular grafts created through in-body tissue architecture (iBTA), wherein a biocompatible mould is implanted subcutaneously, allowing the host's tissue to encapsulate it over time. Upon retrieval, the mould is removed, leaving behind a collagen-rich tubular structure suitable for vascular grafting [58].

Recent studies have demonstrated the potential of biotubes in both preclinical and clinical settings. In a goat model, 4-mm diameter biotubes implanted as carotid artery bypass grafts remained patent over a six-month period. Histological analyses revealed neointima formation, endothelialisation and minimal inflammation, although instances of stenosis and dilatation were observed, indicating areas for further optimisation [59].

Innovations in biotube fabrication have focused on enhancing mechanical properties and surgical handling. For instance, the development of wing-attached moulds has accelerated tissue formation, while the incorporation of reinforcement cuffs at anastomosis sites has improved graft stability [60]. Despite promising results, challenges such as preventing graft stenosis and aneurysm formation remain. Ongoing research aims to address these issues to improve the long-term efficacy and safety of biotubes as viable options.

11.8 Vascular Tissue Engineering

Vascular tissue engineering (VTE) has emerged as a transformative approach in the development of vascular grafts, aiming to overcome the limitations of traditional synthetic and autologous grafts. This process involves scaffold fabrication followed by cell seeding and maturation. The scaffold involves the use of a dense and cohesive sheet of cells to create a tubular structure. The sheet is rolled around and matured to develop vessel-like properties. Cells are accurately positioned into a mould using a microtissue aggregation approach. The production of ECM allows the merging of the aggregates into a complex structure. Finally, bioprinting is used to extrude supporting material to increase the flexibility of the fabrication.

VTE seeks to address these challenges by creating bioengineered vascular conduits that mimic the structural, mechanical and biological properties of native blood vessels. Recent advancements in scaffold fabrication techniques, including electrospinning, 3D bioprinting and multi-part microfluidic channel systems, have enabled the production of intricate and customised tubular scaffolds with improved functional and biomechanical properties. These scaffolds can be seeded with various cell types, such as endothelial cells, smooth muscle cells, or stem cells, to promote in vivo integration and functionality [61].

11.8.1 Decellularised Extracellular Matrix (dECM)

Decellularised extracellular matrix (dECM) has emerged as a promising material for vascular graft development. By removing cellular components from native tissues while preserving the structural and biochemical cues of the ECM, dECM scaffolds aim to promote host cell integration and functional tissue regeneration.

Recent studies have explored various sources and modifications of dECM for vascular graft applications. For instance, decellularised human umbilical arteries have been investigated as potential small-diameter vascular grafts, demonstrating preserved ECM, support for endothelialisation and maintained function in vivo for up to 8 weeks [62]. Similarly, decellularised pericardial extracellular matrix combined with poly(propylene fumarate) has been developed to create biohybrid scaffolds [63]. Innovative approaches have also considered non-traditional sources for dECM. Decellularised plant scaffolds, such as spinach leaves, have been evaluated, leveraging their inherent vascular networks and mechanical properties conducive to recellularisation [64].

To enhance the performance of dECM-based grafts, hybrid materials have been developed. Combining dECM with synthetic polymers like PU has shown positive effects on the inflammatory and pro-thrombotic state of aged endothelial cells, suggesting improved biocompatibility and functionality of the grafts [65]. Additionally, blending dECM with silk fibroin has been explored to synergistically combine the mechanical strength of silk with the bioactivity of dECM, aiming to create scaffolds that support tissue regeneration while maintaining structural integrity [66].

Despite these advances, challenges remain in the clinical translation of dECM-based vascular grafts. Issues such as thrombosis, intimal hyperplasia and ensuring long-term patency continue to be areas of active research. Strategies to address these challenges include facilitating early endothelialisation and avoiding intravascular thrombosis through scaffold design and surface modifications [67].

11.8.2 Synthetic Scaffolds

Synthetic scaffolds play a pivotal role in VTE, offering customisable platforms designed to mimic the mechanical and biological properties of native blood vessels, promoting integration and functionality.

Common synthetic polymers used in scaffold fabrication include polycaprolactone (PCL), polylactic acid (PLA) and PU. These materials are favoured for their tunable degradation rates, mechanical strength and ease of processing. Advanced fabrication techniques such as electrospinning and 3D bioprinting have been employed to create scaffolds with micro- and nanoscale architectures that facilitate cell adhesion and proliferation.

To address the thrombogenic nature of synthetic materials, various strategies have been adopted to enhance scaffold bioactivity. Surface modification with heparin and the incorporation of bioactive molecules such as VEGF have significantly improved endothelialisation and reduced platelet adhesion [68]. These functionalised scaffolds provide a more favourable microenvironment for endothelial cell attachment and survival.

Blending synthetic polymers with natural biomaterials, such as collagen or silk fibroin, has led to the development of hybrid scaffolds that combine mechanical robustness with biological activity [69]. For instance, silk fibroin–PCL composite scaffolds have demonstrated enhanced endothelial cell attachment and mechanical properties, offering a synergistic approach to scaffold design.

Despite significant progress, major challenges persist, including achieving long-term patency, preventing intimal hyperplasia and matching the compliance of native vessels. New trends involve the development of 'smart' scaffolds that can release growth factors in response to physiological cues and the use of patient-derived cells to engineer personalised vascular grafts [68, 70]. Furthermore, the integration of bioprinting technologies with synthetic scaffolds holds promise for fabricating complex, multilayered vascular structures tailored to specific clinical needs. Another concept showing promise recently is the use of an acellular graft, composed of ECM proteins found in human arteries and with similar mechanical strength [71]. In clinical studies, it provides benefits in terms of limb salvage, patency and infection resistance in trauma scenarios.

Despite significant progress, several challenges remain in the clinical translation of tissue-engineered vascular grafts (TEVGs) in general. Adverse host responses, such as inflammation and immune rejection, can lead to graft failure. Moreover, achieving functional maturity of induced pluripotent stem cell (iPSC)-derived vascular cells, ensuring adequate elastogenesis, and improving the efficiency of obtaining iPSC-derived seed cells are ongoing areas of research. Additionally, the development of TEVGs that can withstand physiological pressures and exhibit long-term patency remains a critical objective. Innovative strategies are being explored to enhance the performance of TEVGs. For instance, the incorporation of controlled release systems within biodegradable scaffolds has shown promise in improving the mechanical properties and biocompatibility of vascular grafts. Furthermore, the use of natural materials, such as dECM, is gaining attention for their potential to provide bioactive cues that facilitate tissue regeneration.

In conclusion, vascular tissue engineering represents a promising frontier in the development of small-diameter vascular grafts. While significant advancements have been made in scaffold design, cell sourcing and bioreactor technologies, further research is needed to address the remaining challenges and translate these innovations into clinically viable solutions.

11.9 Biodegradable Polymers

Unlike permanent synthetic grafts, biodegradable polymers are designed to provide temporary mechanical support while gradually degrading and being replaced by native tissue, thus promoting natural vessel regeneration and reducing long-term complications such as chronic inflammation, thrombosis and infection.

Commonly used biodegradable polymers include poly(lactic acid) (PLA), poly(glycolic acid) (PGA), poly(lactic-co-glycolic acid) (PLGA) and polycaprolactone (PCL), each offering tunable degradation rates and mechanical properties suited for VTE. Recent advances have also incorporated copolymers and functionalised materials to optimise endothelialisation, mechanical compliance and bioactivity.

The dynamic interplay between scaffold degradation and tissue remodelling remains a critical focus in the design of next-generation biodegradable vascular grafts. Achieving a balance between maintaining structural integrity during healing and ensuring timely resorption is essential for successful long-term outcomes. As research continues to refine material formulations and scaffold architectures, biodegradable polymers are poised to play a pivotal role in advancing vascular graft technologies.

11.9.1 Polylactic Acid (PLA)

PLA is a biodegradable, biocompatible polyester derived from renewable resources. Its mechanical strength, tunable degradation and safe metabolic byproducts make it a promising material. PLA scaffolds aim to provide temporary support while encouraging native tissue regeneration, addressing the limitations of non-degradable synthetic grafts.

PLA's properties can be tailored by adjusting its molecular weight and blending with other polymers. Techniques like electrospinning and 3D printing enable the fabrication of porous, nanofibrous scaffolds that promote vascular cell adhesion and proliferation [70]. These structures aim to replicate the extracellular matrix and maintain mechanical compliance with host vessels. In vitro, PLA scaffolds support endothelial and smooth muscle cell growth. In vivo studies in animal models have shown encouraging results, though challenges such as incomplete endothelialisation and graft stenosis persist. Surface modification with bioactive molecules like VEGF is being explored to enhance endothelialisation and haemocompatibility.

Despite its potential, PLA-based grafts face hurdles related to long-term patency and immune responses. Emerging strategies include smart, bio-responsive scaffolds and patient-specific cell seeding to improve outcomes. Continued advances in fabrication and functionalisation technologies are critical for clinical translation.

11.9.2 Polyglycolic Acid (PGA)

PGA is a biodegradable, thermoplastic polymer with favourable mechanical properties and a rapid degradation profile. Recent studies have explored the fabrication of trilayered electrospun small-diameter vascular grafts incorporating a blend of PGA and PCL as the middle layer, with antioxidant polyurethane layers containing gallic acid on the inner and outer surfaces. These grafts demonstrated commendable mechanical properties, including an elastic modulus of 6 MPa, suture retention strength of 4 Newton and burst pressure of 2500 mm Hg. In vivo evaluations in rodent femoral arteries showed satisfactory patency over 35 days, with ultrasound imaging confirming adequate blood flow and histological analyses revealing significant endothelial and smooth muscle cell infiltration, as well as matrix deposition [44].

Another approach involved the development of tissue-engineered vascular grafts using a core/shell fibrous structure, where the core comprised a faster-degrading poly(lactic-co-glycolic acid) (PLGA) and the shell consisted of poly(ε-caprolactone) (PCL). These grafts were surface heparinised to enhance haemocompatibility. After implantation in rat abdominal aortas for 12 months, the grafts exhibited good endothelialisation, low inflammation and no calcification. The neointimal layer showed organised elastin and collagen deposition, indicating successful vascular remodelling [72].

Additionally, braided PGA fibres coated with poly(glycerol sebacate) (PGS) have been utilised. This design promotes in vivo tissue engineering, allowing neo-tissue formation within the body post-implantation. Adjustments in scaffold braid design and coating have been shown to influence neo-tissue formation, highlighting the importance of scaffold architecture in vascular graft development [73].

In summary, PGA-based scaffolds, particularly when combined with other polymers and bioactive coatings, offer promising avenues for the development of small-diameter vascular grafts. Ongoing research focuses on optimising scaffold designs to enhance mechanical properties, promote endothelialisation and ensure long-term patency.

11.10 Hybrid Materials

Hybrid materials are increasingly pivotal in vascular graft development, combining the mechanical robustness of synthetic polymers with the bioactivity of natural tissues to enhance graft performance and integration. Recent studies have demonstrated the efficacy of hybrid materials in promoting cellular repopulation and improving blood compatibility. For instance, a study evaluated hybrid scaffolds composed of decellularised bovine pericardium coupled with synthetic polymers like Chronoflex AR and Chronoflex ARLT. These materials exhibited favourable physicochemical, structural, mechanical and biological properties, confirming their potential for vascular graft applications [74].

Another approach involved the fabrication of hybrid electrospun fibrous materials that mimic the crimped microstructure of natural collagen. This biomimetic design, achieved through electrospinning techniques, allows for precise control over the scaffold's mechanical properties, closely resembling those of native vascular tissue [75]. Furthermore, the development of biohybrid TEVGs has shown promise in adapting to host needs over time. These grafts, monitored using advanced imaging techniques, demonstrate the potential for long-term durability and functionality in vivo [76].

In summary, the integration of synthetic and natural components in hybrid materials offers a synergistic approach to vascular graft design, aiming to replicate the complex structure and function of native blood vessels while ensuring mechanical strength and biocompatibility.

11.11 Real-Time Haemodynamic Monitoring

Real-time haemodynamic monitoring is crucial for assessing the performance and longevity of vascular grafts. Traditional surveillance methods, such as Doppler ultrasound and angiography, provide intermittent data and may not detect early signs of graft dysfunction. To address this limitation, recent advancements have focused on integrating sensors directly into vascular graft materials, enabling continuous monitoring of haemodynamic parameters.

One innovative approach involves the development of smart vascular grafts equipped with flexible flow biosensors. These biosensors, constructed by encapsulating patterned porous graphene within biocompatible polymers, allow for seamless integration into the graft structure. Such integration facilitates real-time monitoring of blood flow dynamics, aiding in the early detection of potential complications and improving patient outcomes.

Another notable development is the creation of self-monitoring prosthetic bypass grafts. These grafts incorporate microsensors and microelectronics on their extraluminal surface, enabling wireless transmission of haemodynamic data. In vitro studies have demonstrated the system's ability to detect changes in flow parameters under various conditions, including simulated stenosis. Subsequent in vivo experiments in an ovine model confirmed the feasibility of this technology, showing successful signal acquisition through biological tissues and a favourable healing response over a 30-day period [77].

The integration of real-time haemodynamic monitoring into vascular grafts represents a significant advancement in vascular surgery. By providing continuous data on graft performance, these smart materials have the potential to enhance patient management, reduce the incidence of graft failure and pave the way for more personalised therapeutic strategies.

11.12 Graft Materials for Aortic Stent-Grafts

Endovascular aortic repair (EVAR) and thoracic endovascular aortic repair (TEVAR) have become standard treatments for aortic aneurysms and dissections. The success of these procedures heavily relies on the properties of the stent-graft materials used.

The primary materials used in aortic stent-grafts are PTFE and Dacron. PTFE is known for its chemical inertness and low thrombogenicity, while Dacron offers high tensile strength and durability. Despite their widespread use, there is a lack of direct comparative studies evaluating the long-term outcomes associated with each material. Both materials have demonstrated satisfactory performance, but differences in flexibility and compliance may influence clinical decisions [78].

Material fatigue remains a concern in stent-graft longevity. Studies have reported instances of stent fractures, suture disruptions and graft fabric wear, leading to complications such as endoleaks and device failure, especially in the early generation devices. These issues underscore the importance of material selection and device design in stent-graft durability [79].

Advancements in material science have led to the exploration of bioresorbable materials, such as magnesium-based alloys and polymeric scaffolds. These materials aim to provide temporary support, reducing long-term complications associated with permanent implants. However, challenges related to mechanical strength and controlled degradation rates need to be addressed before widespread clinical adoption [80].

The stiffness of stent-graft materials can alter native aortic haemodynamics, potentially leading to increased cardiac workload and adverse cardiovascular events. Efforts are ongoing to develop materials and designs that better mimic the compliance of the native aorta, aiming to minimise these haemodynamic disturbances [78].

The development of hybrid materials combining synthetic and natural components, as well as the integration of smart technologies for real-time monitoring, represents promising avenues for improving stent-graft performance. Further research and clinical trials are necessary to evaluate the long-term benefits and potential risks associated with these innovations.

11.13 Vascular Graft Failure

11.13.1 Early Failure

Vascular graft failure remains a significant clinical concern, particularly in the early post-operative period. Early graft failure, typically defined as occurring within 30 days of implantation, is primarily attributed to thrombosis, technical errors during surgery and poor run-off due to distal vessel disease [10].

Thrombosis is the most common cause of early graft failure and results from a complex interplay between the graft material, blood elements and haemodynamic forces. Grafts with poor haemocompatibility, such as early-generation synthetic polymers (e.g. Dacron and ePTFE), tend to activate coagulation cascades and platelet adhesion, leading to acute thrombus formation [13]. Native endothelium possesses antithrombotic properties that are lacking in synthetic grafts, making them particularly vulnerable to clot formation in the immediate post-implantation period.

Technical factors such as anastomotic misalignment, kinking, or torsion of the graft can severely compromise blood flow, contributing to turbulent flow patterns and stasis—conditions conducive to thrombus formation. These mechanical issues are especially critical in small-diameter grafts (<6 mm), where even slight perturbations in geometry can dramatically alter flow dynamics.

Poor distal runoff refers to the presence of distal arterial disease or small-calibre outflow vessels, which can increase resistance to blood flow and predispose the graft to occlusion. This is particularly relevant in infrainguinal bypass grafts in patients with peripheral arterial disease (PAD) [81].

Infection and inflammation, although less common as causes of early failure, can compromise graft integrity. Infections may induce localised thrombosis or lead to systemic pro-coagulant states [11]. Moreover, the absence of endothelialisation on synthetic grafts may prolong the inflammatory response and delay healing, further predisposing to occlusion.

In conclusion, early vascular graft failure is predominantly due to thrombosis triggered by poor hemocompatibility of materials, suboptimal surgical technique and unfavourable patient anatomy. A deep understanding of these mechanisms is essential to improve graft design and surgical outcomes.

11.13.2 Late Failure

Late vascular graft failure, occurring beyond 30 days post-implantation, is primarily associated with intimal hyperplasia, graft atherosclerosis, infection and mechanical degeneration of the graft material. While early failures are often due to thrombosis or technical issues, late failures reflect longer-term biological and biomechanical interactions between the graft and host tissue.

Intimal hyperplasia (IH) is the predominant cause of late graft failure, especially in synthetic grafts. IH involves the proliferation and migration of VSMCs and accumulation of extracellular matrix at the graft anastomoses, leading to progressive luminal narrowing [82]. This response is typically stimulated by endothelial injury and altered shear stress, especially at regions of flow turbulence and compliance mismatch between the graft and native vessel [83]. Synthetic grafts like ePTFE and Dacron do not fully endothelialise over time, especially in low-flow regions, exacerbating the risk for hyperplasia and failure.

Neoatherosclerosis, a phenomenon characterised by lipid-laden macrophage infiltration and fibroatheroma formation within the neointima, can develop in autologous vein grafts and, to a lesser extent, in synthetic conduits. It mirrors traditional atherosclerosis but progresses more rapidly due to the pro-inflammatory and haemodynamic environment within grafts.

Late graft infections may present months or even years after implantation, often manifesting with pseudoaneurysm, sepsis, or graft-enteric fistulae. These are commonly caused by low-grade organisms such as *Staphylococcus epidermidis* and can be difficult to detect in early stages. The long-term consequences of graft infection often necessitate complete graft excision and alternative revascularisation.

Mechanical degeneration or structural fatigue of grafts over time—especially in locations subject to flexion or compression, such as the femoropopliteal segment—can lead to material fatigue, graft kinking, or fracture. Dacron grafts, in particular, may develop aneurysmal dilatation, especially when implanted in high-pressure arterial systems [84].

Late vascular graft failure reflects a combination of biological responses—most notably intimal hyperplasia and neoatherosclerosis—and mechanical wear of the implanted material. Understanding these long-term interactions is essential for improving graft longevity and for guiding both surveillance and secondary intervention strategies.

11.13.3 Tubular Compliance Mismatch

One of the critical but often underappreciated factors contributing to vascular graft failure—especially at the anastomotic sites—is tubular compliance mismatch between the graft material and the native vessel. Compliance refers to the ability of a blood vessel to expand and contract with pulsatile blood flow. Native arteries are highly compliant, particularly in younger or healthy individuals, whereas most synthetic grafts are significantly stiffer and less distensible [85, 86].

The stiffness of synthetic materials creates a rigid transition zone that disrupts the normal pulse wave transmission and increases pulsatile energy reflection, leading to oscillatory shear stress and flow disturbances [87]. These altered biomechanical conditions are known triggers for IH, which is the primary mechanism behind late graft stenosis and occlusion.

A notable study by Post et al. [88] utilised an ex vivo organ culture model to investigate the effects of graft compliance mismatch on vascular remodelling. They found that low-compliance grafts led to reduced wall shear stress at the distal anastomosis, which correlated with increased smooth muscle cell proliferation and extracellular matrix deposition—key indicators of IH. This study underscores the mechanobiological link between compliance mismatch and vascular remodelling [88]. Furthermore, the resulting disturbed flow contributes to endothelial dysfunction, further amplifying the risk of thrombosis and chronic inflammation in the peri-anastomotic region.

Clinically, compliance mismatch is especially problematic in small-diameter grafts (<6 mm), where haemodynamic sensitivity is more pronounced. It also plays a role in the long-term failure of grafts placed in the femoropopliteal or coronary circulations, where vessel dynamics are more complex due to movement, bending and smaller calibres [13].

To mitigate these effects, recent research has focused on biomimetic materials and tissue-engineered vascular grafts (TEVGs) that better replicate the mechanical properties of native vessels. These newer materials, including decellularised scaffolds and polymer blends, aim to restore compliance continuity and reduce the biomechanical triggers of neointimal formation [12].

11.13.4 Anastomotic Compliance Mismatch

Anastomotic compliance mismatch between vascular grafts and native vessels is a major contributor to graft failure, especially in the long term. The anastomotic site, where the graft is sutured to the native vessel, is particularly vulnerable to mechanical stresses, given the significant differences in compliance between the two structures.

Haemodynamic consequences at the anastomosis are critical in the development of graft failure. Native vessels are highly compliant and can adapt to the pulsatile forces generated by the heart, whereas synthetic grafts are less compliant and do not respond to pressure changes in the same way. This difference in mechanical properties results in altered blood flow patterns, with disturbed and non-laminar flow often occurring at the graft-vessel junction [9]. The irregular flow and shear stress at the anastomosis can trigger endothelial injury, inflammatory responses and the development of IH.

The disruption of normal endothelial function leads to the proliferation of SMCs and ECM deposition, narrowing the graft lumen and impairing blood flow [82]. This process is exacerbated in small-calibre grafts, where the mechanical forces are more pronounced, and even minor mismatches in compliance can lead to significant complications.

One strategy to address anastomotic compliance mismatch is the use of compliant graft materials or biologically engineered grafts that better mimic the properties of native vessels. For example, grafts made from polyurethane or biological materials such as decellularised veins show improved compliance characteristics, reducing the risk of hyperplasia and improving graft patency [12]. Figure 11.2 illustrates various fabrication methods.

However, despite these advancements, synthetic grafts remain prone to compliance mismatch in long-term clinical use, particularly when they are used in high-stress areas or in patients with complex vascular anatomy [13]. Furthermore, surgical technique plays a crucial role in mitigating the effects of compliance mismatch. The precise alignment of grafts with native vessels during the anastomotic procedure is essential to minimise turbulence and optimise blood flow across the junction. Poor surgical technique or failure to adequately match the diameters of the graft and the vessel can exacerbate the effects of compliance mismatch, leading to an increased risk of failure.

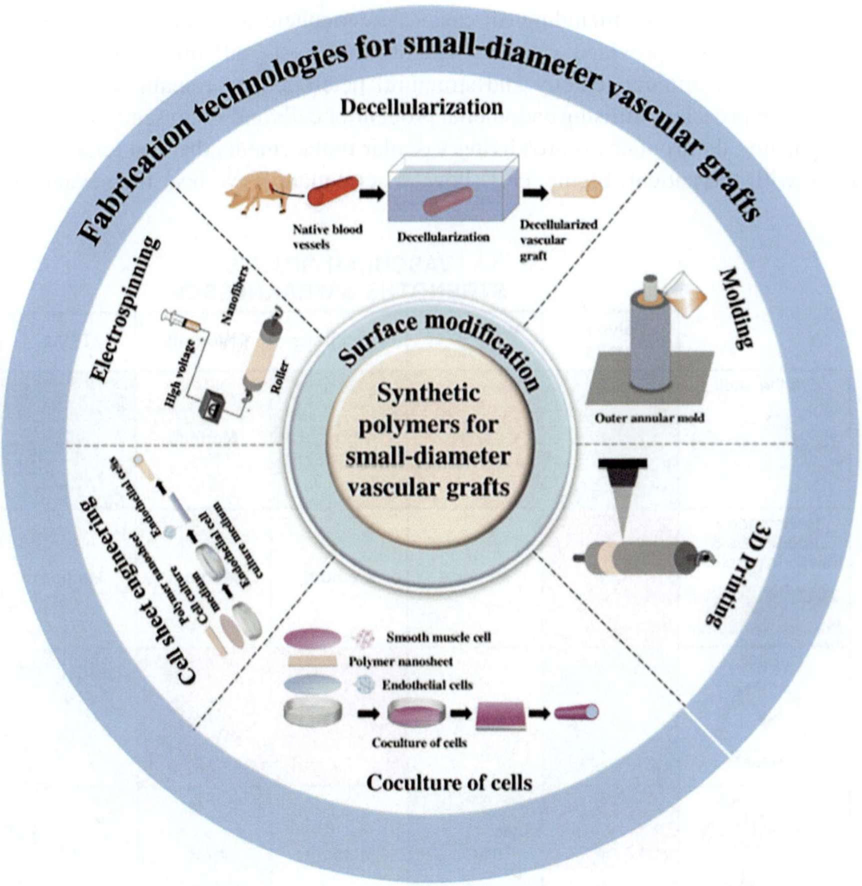

Fig. 11.2 This diagram illustrates various fabrication methods for small-diameter vascular grafts, including decellularisation, electrospinning and cell sheet engineering, highlighting the complexity and diversity of current approaches. (Source: Biomaterials Research (2023) [90])

11.14 Conclusions and Future Directions

Vascular graft materials have evolved significantly over the past decades, transitioning from inert synthetic polymers to sophisticated biomimetic and bioactive scaffolds. Conventional materials such as ePTFE and Dacron have demonstrated clinical durability in large-diameter applications but consistently underperform in small-diameter (<6 mm) grafts due to thrombosis, intimal hyperplasia and compliance mismatch. Biodegradable polymers such as PLA and PGA have emerged as promising alternatives, offering temporary mechanical support and promoting endogenous tissue regeneration.

Biological grafts—including allogeneic, xenogeneic and decellularised ECM constructs—have provided valuable insights into host-graft interactions, though challenges in immunogenicity and structural heterogeneity remain. Tissue engineering approaches, utilising endothelial progenitor cells and smart scaffold designs, are pushing the frontier towards living vascular replacements that can remodel and grow with the patient. Figure 11.3 shows a semiquantitative heat map evaluating

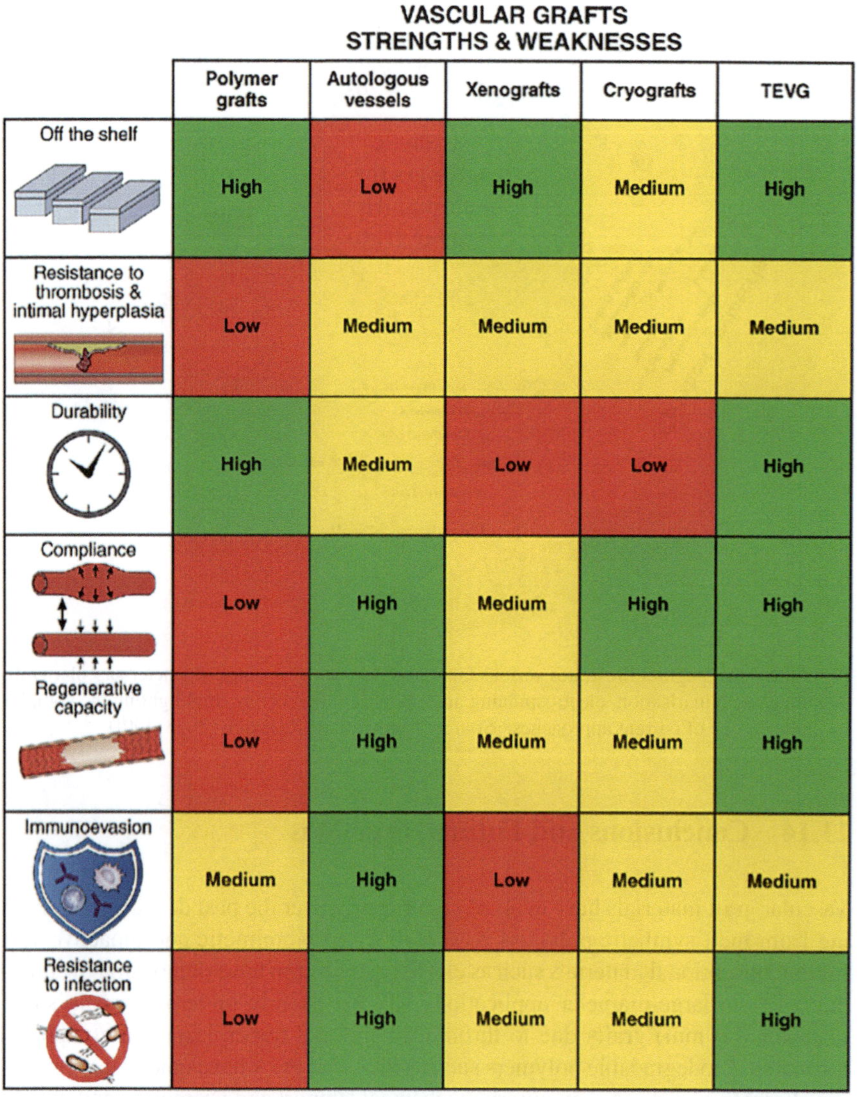

Fig. 11.3 This semiquantitative heat map evaluates various vascular graft materials based on criteria such as durability, compliance and immunoresistance, aiding in material selection decisions. (Source: 'Strengths and weaknesses of different vascular graft materials' [6])

various vascular graft materials based on criteria such as durability, compliance and immunoresistance, aiding in material selection decisions. Innovations in hybrid materials, integrating synthetic strength with biological functionality and real-time haemodynamic monitoring systems embedded within grafts represent critical steps towards more personalised, dynamic therapeutic options.

The future of vascular graft development lies at the intersection of biomaterials science, tissue engineering and regenerative medicine. Several key avenues demand focused research:

1. *Biomimetic Scaffold Design*
   Replicating the hierarchical structure, mechanical compliance and bioactivity of native vessels remains a central goal. Next-generation scaffolds should incorporate gradients of stiffness, biochemical cues and anisotropic (see Glossary) microstructures to guide cellular organisation and function.
2. *Dynamic and Bioresponsive Materials*
   The integration of stimuli-responsive polymers capable of adapting to physiological changes, such as inflammation, mechanical stress, or hypoxia, could improve graft performance and long-term patency.
3. *Advanced Cell Sources and Conditioning*
   The use of patient-specific induced pluripotent stem cells (iPSCs) combined with dynamic bioreactor conditioning (e.g. pulsatile flow, cyclic strain) can enhance endothelialisation and smooth muscle cell maturation, yielding truly autologous tissue-engineered grafts.
4. *Real-Time Monitoring and Smart Grafts*
   The incorporation of flexible biosensors and wireless communication technologies into graft materials will enable continuous monitoring of blood flow, pressure and biochemical markers, facilitating early detection of complications such as thrombosis, infection or structural failure.
5. *Immunomodulatory Strategies*
   Future grafts must not only avoid immune rejection but also actively modulate the host immune response to promote constructive remodelling. Surface modifications, controlled release of immunoregulatory factors and engineered 'immune-privileged' materials are critical research areas.
6. *Clinical Translation and Regulatory Frameworks*
   As complexity in graft design increases, robust preclinical models and standardised evaluation protocols must be developed. A major bottleneck lies in the choice and relevance of animal models. Most preclinical evaluations rely on young, healthy animals—often rodents—with rapid healing responses and juvenile vascular cells, which do not accurately reflect the aged, diseased vasculature of typical human patients. Additionally, small animal models fail to replicate the haemodynamic and immunologic environment of the human vasculature. While large animal models (e.g. sheep, pigs, primates) provide better physiological analogues, they are expensive, ethically complex and less frequently used.

Moreover, many clinical grafts that initially show promise exhibit disappointing long-term outcomes due to chronic inflammation, compliance mismatch, calcification, or thrombosis—issues often underrepresented in short-duration animal studies. To bridge the gap between bench and bedside, the field must prioritise the development of standardised, clinically relevant animal models, longer-term studies and robust translational frameworks. Without these, the transition from experimental grafts to durable, functional clinical implants will remain a persistent challenge. Close collaboration between material scientists, bioengineers, clinicians and regulatory agencies will be essential to streamline the path from bench to bedside.

The development of next-generation vascular grafts demands a multidisciplinary effort, combining the rigour of engineering design with the nuances of biological systems. Although significant challenges remain, the convergence of advanced biomaterials, regenerative strategies and real-time monitoring technologies offers unprecedented opportunities to revolutionise vascular surgery and improve patient outcomes in the years ahead.

Multiple Choice Questions

1. For small-diameter vascular grafts, synthetic materials such as Dacron and ePTFE consistently show poor long-term results. Which pathological process is the predominant cause of late graft failure in these conduits?

   (a) Technical error
   (b) Thrombosis
   (c) Aneurysm dilatation
   (d) Graft infection
   (e) Intimal hyperplasia

   Answer: (e) Intimal hyperplasia

2. Which specific modification of Dacron grafts involves coating the surface with a natural biodegradable polymer derived from collagen to promote rapid graft sealing, cell adhesion, and acts as a carrier for bioactive agents?

   (a) Gelatin coatings
   (b) Heparin bonding
   (c) Electrospinning
   (d) Sulphonation with silk fibroin
   (e) PGA coating

   Answer: (a) Gelatin coatings

References

1. Sayers RD, Raptis S, Berce M, Miller JH. Long-term results of femorotibial bypass with vein or polytetrafluoroethylene. Br J Surg. 1998;85:934–8. https://doi.org/10.1046/j.1365-2168.1998.00765.x.
2. Cooley DA, Crawford ES, Creech O Jr, De Bakey ME. Arterial homografts for peripheral arteriosclerotic occlusive disease. Circulation. 1957;15:21–30. https://doi.org/10.1161/01.cir.15.1.21.
3. Blakemore AH, Voorhees AB. The use of tubes constructed from Vinyon N-cloth in bridging arterial defects - experimental and clinical. Ann Surg. 1954;140:324–34. https://doi.org/10.1097/00000658-195409000-00008.
4. Shi Q, Wu MH, Hayashida N, Wechezak AR, Clowes AW, Sauvage LR. Proof of fallout endothelialization of impervious Dacron grafts in the aorta and inferior vena cava of the dog. J Vasc Surg. 1994;20:546–56. https://doi.org/10.1016/0741-5214(94)90279-8.
5. Vossen RJ, Fokkema TM, Vahl AC, Balm R. Systematic review and meta-analysis comparing the autogenous vein bypass versus a prosthetic graft for above-the-knee femoropopliteal bypass surgery in patients with intermittent claudication. Vascular. 2024;32:91–101. https://doi.org/10.1177/17085381221124701.
6. Naegeli KM, Kural MH, Li Y, Wang J, Hugentobler EA, Niklason LE. Bioengineering human tissues and the future of vascular replacement. Circ Res. 2022;131:109–26. https://doi.org/10.1161/circresaha.121.319984.
7. Quint C, Arief M, Muto A, Dardik A, Niklason LE. Allogeneic human tissue-engineered blood vessel. J Vasc Surg. 2012;55:790–8. https://doi.org/10.1016/j.jvs.2011.07.098.
8. Lawson JH, Glickman MH, Ilzecki M, Jakimowicz T, Jaroszynski A, Peden EK, et al. Bioengineered human acellular vessels for dialysis access in patients with end-stage renal disease: two phase 2 single-arm trials. Lancet. 2016;387:2026–34. https://doi.org/10.1016/s0140-6736(16)00557-2.
9. Salacinski HJ, Goldner S, Giudiceandrea A, Hamilton G, Seifalian AM, Edwards A, et al. The mechanical behavior of vascular grafts: a review. J Biomater Appl. 2001;15:241–78. https://doi.org/10.1106/na5t-j57a-jtdd-fd04.
10. Veith FJ, Gupta SK, Ascer E, White-Flores S, Samson RH, Scher LA, et al. Six-year prospective multicenter randomized comparison of autologous saphenous vein and expanded polytetrafluoroethylene grafts in infrainguinal arterial reconstructions. J Vasc Surg. 1986;3:104–14. https://doi.org/10.1067/mva.1986.avs0030104.
11. Kieffer E, Gomes D, Chiche L, Fléron MH, Koskas F, Bahnini A. Allograft replacement for infrarenal aortic graft infection: early and late results in 179 patients. J Vasc Surg. 2004;39:1009–17. https://doi.org/10.1016/j.jvs.2003.12.040.
12. Konig G, McAllister TN, Dusserre N, Garrido SA, Iyican C, Marini A, et al. Mechanical properties of completely autologous human tissue engineered blood vessels compared to human saphenous vein and mammary artery. Biomaterials. 2009;30:1542–50. https://doi.org/10.1016/j.biomaterials.2008.11.011.
13. Zilla P, Bezuidenhout D, Human P. Prosthetic vascular grafts: wrong models, wrong questions and no healing. Biomaterials. 2007;28:5009–27. https://doi.org/10.1016/j.biomaterials.2007.07.017.
14. Murugesan S, Xie J, Linhardt RJ. Immobilization of heparin: approaches and applications. Curr Top Med Chem. 2008;8:80–100. https://doi.org/10.2174/156802608783378891.
15. Kodama K, Pasche B, Olsson P, Swedenborg J, Adolfsson L, Larm O, et al. Antithrombin III binding to surface immobilized heparin and its relation to F Xa inhibition. Thromb Haemost. 1987;58:1064–7.
16. Radke D, Jia W, Sharma D, Fena K, Wang G, Goldman J, et al. Tissue engineering at the blood-contacting surface: a review of challenges and strategies in vascular graft development. Adv Healthc Mater. 2018;7:e1701461. https://doi.org/10.1002/adhm.201701461.

17. Gupta S, Puttaiahgowda YM, Deiglmayr L. Recent advances in the design and immobilization of heparin for biomedical application: a review. Int J Biol Macromol. 2024;264:130743. https://doi.org/10.1016/j.ijbiomac.2024.130743.
18. Arkonac BM, Foster LC, Sibinga NE, Patterson C, Lai K, Tsai JC, et al. Vascular endothelial growth factor induces heparin-binding epidermal growth factor-like growth factor in vascular endothelial cells. J Biol Chem. 1998;273:4400–5. https://doi.org/10.1074/jbc.273.8.4400.
19. Li D, Xia Y. Electrospinning of nanofibers: reinventing the wheel? Adv Mater. 2004;16:1151–70. https://doi.org/10.1002/adma.200400719.
20. Wang Z, Sun B, Zhang M, Ou L, Che Y, Zhang J, et al. Functionalization of electrospun poly(ε-caprolactone) scaffold with heparin and vascular endothelial growth factors for potential application as vascular grafts. J Bioact Compat Polym. 2012;28:154–66. https://doi.org/10.1177/0883911512469707.
21. Zulkifli MZA, Nordin D, Shaari N, Kamarudin SK. Overview of electrospinning for tissue engineering applications. Polymers (Basel). 2023;15:2418. https://doi.org/10.3390/polym15112418.
22. Hengqing C JZ, Lishuai S, Wenjum Z, Haiyan C. Smart carriers in scar therapy: bridging mechanisms to innovative treatments. Available at SSRN: https://ssrn.com/abstract=5185607.
23. D'Souza SE, Ginsberg MH, Plow EF. Arginyl-glycyl-aspartic acid (RGD): a cell adhesion motif. Trends Biochem Sci. 1991;16:246–50. https://doi.org/10.1016/0968-0004(91)90096-e.
24. Ikada Y, Tabata Y. Protein release from gelatin matrices. Adv Drug Deliv Rev. 1998;31:287–301. https://doi.org/10.1016/s0169-409x(97)00125-7.
25. Claaßen C, Southan A, Grübel J, Tovar GEM, Borchers K. Interactions of methacryloylated gelatin and heparin modulate physico-chemical properties of hydrogels and release of vascular endothelial growth factor. Biomed Mater. 2018;13:055008. https://doi.org/10.1088/1748-605X/aacdb2.
26. Fu W, Liu Z, Feng B, Hu R, He X, Wang H, et al. Electrospun gelatin/PCL and collagen/PLCL scaffolds for vascular tissue engineering. Int J Nanomedicine. 2014;9:2335–44. https://doi.org/10.2147/ijn.S61375.
27. Heng JW, Yazid MD, Abdul Rahman MR, Sulaiman N. Coatings in decellularized vascular scaffolds for the establishment of a functional endothelium: a scoping review of vascular graft refinement. Front Cardiovasc Med. 2021;8:677588. https://doi.org/10.3389/fcvm.2021.677588.
28. Zizhou R, Wang X, Houshyar S. Review of polymeric biomimetic small-diameter vascular grafts to tackle intimal hyperplasia. ACS Omega. 2022;7:22125–48. https://doi.org/10.1021/acsomega.2c01740.
29. Fujimura N, Obara H, Matsubara K, Toya N, Isogai N, Ogino H, et al. Long-term outcomes of a Japanese prospective multicenter registry using a heparin-bonded expanded polytetrafluoroethylene graft for above-the-knee femoropopliteal bypasses. Circ J. 2024;88:1656–63. https://doi.org/10.1253/circj.CJ-24-0135.
30. Fan H, Liu H, Toh SL, Goh JC. Enhanced differentiation of mesenchymal stem cells co-cultured with ligament fibroblasts on gelatin/silk fibroin hybrid scaffold. Biomaterials. 2008;29:1017–27. https://doi.org/10.1016/j.biomaterials.2007.10.048.
31. Kundu B, Rajkhowa R, Kundu SC, Wang X. Silk fibroin biomaterials for tissue regenerations. Adv Drug Deliv Rev. 2013;65:457–70. https://doi.org/10.1016/j.addr.2012.09.043.
32. Koh L-D, Cheng Y, Teng C-P, Khin Y-W, Loh X-J, Tee S-Y, et al. Structures, mechanical properties and applications of silk fibroin materials. Prog Polym Sci. 2015;46:86–110. https://doi.org/10.1016/j.progpolymsci.2015.02.001.
33. Shi P, Zhang L, Tian W, Li H, Wang Q, Yi H, et al. Preparation and anticoagulant activity of functionalised silk fibroin. Chem Eng Sci. 2019;199:240–8. https://doi.org/10.1016/j.ces.2019.01.022.
34. Zhang J, Huang H, Ju R, Chen K, Li S, Wang W, et al. In vivo biocompatibility and hemocompatibility of a polytetrafluoroethylene small diameter vascular graft modified with sulfonated silk fibroin. Am J Surg. 2017;213:87–93. https://doi.org/10.1016/j.amjsurg.2016.04.005.

35. Liu H, Li X, Niu X, Zhou G, Li P, Fan Y. Improved hemocompatibility and endothelialization of vascular grafts by covalent immobilization of sulfated silk fibroin on poly(lactic-co-glycolic acid) scaffolds. Biomacromolecules. 2011;12:2914–24. https://doi.org/10.1021/bm200479f.
36. Táborská J, Riedelová Z, Brynda E, Májek P, Riedel T. Endothelialization of an ePTFE vessel prosthesis modified with an antithrombogenic fibrin/heparin coating enriched with bound growth factors. RSC Adv. 2021;11:5903–13. https://doi.org/10.1039/d1ra00053e.
37. Ding K, Yu X, Wang D, Wang X, Li Q. Small diameter expanded polytetrafluoroethylene vascular graft with differentiated inner and outer biomacromolecules for collaborative endothelialization, anti-thrombogenicity and anti-inflammation. Colloids Surf B Biointerfaces. 2023;229:113449. https://doi.org/10.1016/j.colsurfb.2023.113449.
38. Yu L, Newton ER, Gillis DC, Sun K, Cooley BC, Keith AN, et al. Coating small-diameter ePTFE vascular grafts with tunable poly (diol-co-citrate-co-ascorbate) elastomers to reduce neointimal hyperplasia. Biomater Sci. 2021;9:5160–74. https://doi.org/10.1039/d1bm00101a.
39. Bastijanic JM, Marchant RE, Kligman F, Allemang MT, Lakin RO, Kendrick D, et al. In vivo evaluation of biomimetic fluorosurfactant polymer-coated expanded polytetrafluoroethylene vascular grafts in a porcine carotid artery bypass model. J Vasc Surg. 2016;63:1620–30 e4. https://doi.org/10.1016/j.jvs.2015.01.060.
40. Kim D, Chung JJ, Jung Y, Kim SH. The effect of substance P/heparin conjugated PLCL polymer coating of bioinert ePTFE vascular grafts on the recruitment of both ECs and SMCs for accelerated regeneration. Sci Rep. 2019;9:17083. https://doi.org/10.1038/s41598-019-53514-6.
41. Eilenberg M, Enayati M, Ehebruster D, Grasl C, Walter I, Messner B, et al. Long-term evaluation of nanofibrous, bioabsorbable polycarbonate urethane grafts for small diameter vessel replacement in rodents. Eur J Vasc Endovasc Surg. 2020;59:643–52. https://doi.org/10.1016/j.ejvs.2019.11.004.
42. Jalaie H, Steitz J, Afify M, Barbati ME, Hoeft K, Assar MAM, et al. In vivo endothelialization and neointimal hyperplasia assessment after angioplasty of sheep carotid artery with a novel polycarbonate polyurethane patch. J Biomater Appl. 2019;34:208–18. https://doi.org/10.1177/0885328219849368.
43. Senokosova EA, Prokudina ES, Krivkina ES, Glushkova TV, Velikanova EA, Khanova MY, et al. Composite tissue-engineered small-diameter vascular grafts based on polycaprolactone and polyurethane with growth factors and atrombogenic drug coatings: surface ultrastructure, physical and mechanical properties. Sovrem Tekhnol Med. 2024;16:18–25. https://doi.org/10.17691/stm2024.16.5.02.
44. Das A, Nikhil A, Kumar A. Antioxidant and trilayered electrospun small-diameter vascular grafts maintain patency and promote endothelialisation in rat femoral artery. ACS Biomater Sci Eng. 2024;10:1697–711. https://doi.org/10.1021/acsbiomaterials.4c00006.
45. Amiri Heydari H, Kazemi Ashtiani M, Mostafaei F, Alipour Choshali M, Shiravandi A, Rajabi S, et al. Functional efficacy of tissue-engineered small-diameter nanofibrous polyurethane vascular grafts surface-modified by methacrylated sulfated alginate in the rat abdominal aorta. ACS Appl Mater Interfaces. 2024;16:67255–74. https://doi.org/10.1021/acsami.4c13925.
46. Zumbardo-Bacelis GA, Peponi L, Vargas-Coronado RF, Rodríguez-Velázquez E, Alatorre-Meda M, Chevallier P, et al. A comparison of three-layer and single-layer small vascular grafts manufactured via the roto-evaporation method. Polymers (Basel). 2024;16:1314. https://doi.org/10.3390/polym16101314.
47. Miller-Kasprzak E, Jagodziński PP. Endothelial progenitor cells as a new agent contributing to vascular repair. Arch Immunol Ther Exp. 2007;55:247–59. https://doi.org/10.1007/s00005-007-0027-5.
48. Hung HS, Yang YC, Lin YC, Lin SZ, Kao WC, Hsieh HH, et al. Regulation of human endothelial progenitor cell maturation by polyurethane nanocomposites. Biomaterials. 2014;35:6810–21. https://doi.org/10.1016/j.biomaterials.2014.04.076.
49. Daum R, Visser D, Wild C, Kutuzova L, Schneider M, Lorenz G, et al. Fibronectin adsorption on electrospun synthetic vascular grafts attracts endothelial progenitor cells and promotes

endothelialization in dynamic in vitro culture. Cells. 2020;9:778. https://doi.org/10.3390/cells9030778.
50. Ji H, Shi X, Yang H. Recent advances in polyurethane for artificial vascular application. Polymers (Basel). 2024;16:3528. https://doi.org/10.3390/polym16243528.
51. Yang Z, Zhang Y, Chen Y, Fu L, Sun Y, Yang Z, et al. In situ densification and heparin immobilization of bacterial cellulose vascular patch for potential vascular applications. Int J Biol Macromol. 2024;270:132181. https://doi.org/10.1016/j.ijbiomac.2024.132181.
52. Liu L, Ji X, Mao L, Wang L, Chen K, Shi Z, et al. Hierarchical-structured bacterial cellulose/potato starch tubes as potential small-diameter vascular grafts. Carbohydr Polym. 2022;281:119034. https://doi.org/10.1016/j.carbpol.2021.119034.
53. Arias SL, Shetty A, Devorkin J, Allain JP. Magnetic targeting of smooth muscle cells in vitro using a magnetic bacterial cellulose to improve cell retention in tissue-engineering vascular grafts. Acta Biomater. 2018;77:172–81. https://doi.org/10.1016/j.actbio.2018.07.013.
54. Fusco D, Meissner F, Podesser BK, Marsano A, Grapow M, Eckstein F, et al. Small-diameter bacterial cellulose-based vascular grafts for coronary artery bypass grafting in a pig model. Front Cardiovasc Med. 2022;9:881557. https://doi.org/10.3389/fcvm.2022.881557.
55. Wystrychowski W, McAllister TN, Zagalski K, Dusserre N, Cierpka L, L'Heureux N. First human use of an allogeneic tissue-engineered vascular graft for hemodialysis access. J Vasc Surg. 2014;60:1353–7. https://doi.org/10.1016/j.jvs.2013.08.018.
56. Bayes-Genis A, Gastelurrutia P, Monguió-Tortajada M, Cámara ML, Prat-Vidal C, Cediel G, et al. Implantation of a double allogeneic human engineered tissue graft on damaged heart: insights from the PERISCOPE phase I clinical trial. EBioMedicine. 2024;102:105060. https://doi.org/10.1016/j.ebiom.2024.105060.
57. Zhang J, Tabima DM, Vereide D, Zeng W, Albano NJ, Lyon S, et al. Small-diameter artery grafts engineered from pluripotent stem cells maintain 100% patency in an allogeneic rhesus macaque model. Cell Rep Med. 2025;6:102002. https://doi.org/10.1016/j.xcrm.2025.102002.
58. Higashita R, Miyazaki M, Oi M, Ishikawa N. First-in-human results of an in-body tissue architecture-induced tissue-engineered vascular graft "Biotube" for application in distal bypass for chronic limb-threatening ischemia. J Vasc Surg Cases Innov Tech. 2022;8:488–93. https://doi.org/10.1016/j.jvscit.2022.07.007.
59. Mori K, Umeno T, Kawashima T, Shuto T, Iwai R, Teng L, et al. Six-month patency of long carotid bypass grafts constructed with in-body tissue architecture-induced small-diameter biotubes in a goat model. Bioengineering (Basel). 2025;12:260. https://doi.org/10.3390/bioengineering12030260.
60. Sakai O, Kanda K, Ishibashi-Ueda H, Takamizawa K, Ametani A, Yaku H, et al. c. J Biomed Mater Res B Appl Biomater. 2007;83:240–7. https://doi.org/10.1002/jbm.b.30789.
61. West-Livingston L, Lim JW, Lee SJ. Translational tissue-engineered vascular grafts: from bench to bedside. Biomaterials. 2023;302:122322. https://doi.org/10.1016/j.biomaterials.2023.122322.
62. Gui L, Muto A, Chan SA, Breuer CK, Niklason LE. Development of decellularized human umbilical arteries as small-diameter vascular grafts. Tissue Eng Part A. 2009;15:2665–76. https://doi.org/10.1089/ten.tea.2008.0526.
63. Kimicata M, Allbritton-King JD, Navarro J, Santoro M, Inoue T, Hibino N, et al. Assessment of decellularized pericardial extracellular matrix and poly(propylene fumarate) biohybrid for small-diameter vascular graft applications. Acta Biomater. 2020;110:68–81. https://doi.org/10.1016/j.actbio.2020.04.013.
64. Gorbenko N, Rinaldi G, Sanchez A, Merna N. Small-caliber vascular grafts engineered from decellularized leaves and cross-linked gelatin. Tissue Eng Part A. 2023;29:397–409. https://doi.org/10.1089/ten.TEA.2022.0223.
65. Specht SJ, Rohringer S, Hager P, Grasl C, Schmitt AM, Pach VJC, et al. Decellularized extracellular matrix and polyurethane vascular grafts have positive effects on the inflammatory and pro-thrombotic state of aged endothelial cells. J Biomed Mater Res A. 2025;113:e37830. https://doi.org/10.1002/jbm.a.37830.

66. Ghosh S, Pati F. Decellularized extracellular matrix and silk fibroin-based hybrid biomaterials: a comprehensive review on fabrication techniques and tissue-specific applications. Int J Biol Macromol. 2023;253:127410. https://doi.org/10.1016/j.ijbiomac.2023.127410.
67. Li Y, Zhou Y, Qiao W, Shi J, Qiu X, Dong N. Application of decellularized vascular matrix in small-diameter vascular grafts. Front Bioeng Biotechnol. 2022;10:1081233. https://doi.org/10.3389/fbioe.2022.1081233.
68. Jia W, Liu L, Li M, Zhou Y, Zhou H, Weng H, et al. Construction of enzyme-laden vascular scaffolds based on hyaluronic acid oligosaccharides-modified collagen nanofibers for anti-thrombosis and in-situ endothelialization of tissue-engineered blood vessels. Acta Biomater. 2022;153:287–98. https://doi.org/10.1016/j.actbio.2022.09.041.
69. Valsecchi E, Biagiotti M, Alessandrino A, Gastaldi D, Vena P, Freddi G. Silk vascular grafts with optimized mechanical properties for the repair and regeneration of small caliber blood vessels. Materials (Basel). 2022;15:3735. https://doi.org/10.3390/ma15103735.
70. Weekes A, Bartnikowski N, Pinto N, Jenkins J, Meinert C, Klein TJ. Biofabrication of small diameter tissue-engineered vascular grafts. Acta Biomater. 2022;138:92–111. https://doi.org/10.1016/j.actbio.2021.11.012.
71. Moore EE, Curi M, Namias N, Kundi R, Lum YW, Fox CJ, et al. Bioengineered Human arteries for the repair of vascular injuries. JAMA Surg. 2025;160:181–8. https://doi.org/10.1001/jamasurg.2024.4893.
72. Xiao Y, Cai Z, Xing Y, Fang Z, Ye L, Geng X, et al. Fabrication of small-diameter in situ tissue engineered vascular grafts with core/shell fibrous structure and a one-year evaluation via rat abdominal vessel replacement model. Biomater Adv. 2024;165:214018. https://doi.org/10.1016/j.bioadv.2024.214018.
73. Zbinden JC, Blum KM, Berman AG, Ramachandra AB, Szafron JM, Kerr KE, et al. Effects of braiding parameters on tissue engineered vascular graft development. Adv Healthc Mater. 2020;9:e2001093. https://doi.org/10.1002/adhm.202001093.
74. Todesco M, Casarin M, Sandrin D, Astolfi L, Romanato F, Giuggioli G, et al. Hybrid materials for vascular applications: a preliminary in vitro assessment. Bioengineering (Basel). 2024;11:436. https://doi.org/10.3390/bioengineering11050436.
75. Beachley V, Kuo J, Kasyanov V, Mironov V, Wen X. Biomimetic crimped/aligned microstructure to optimize the mechanics of fibrous hybrid materials for compliant vascular grafts. J Mech Behav Biomed Mater. 2024;150:106301. https://doi.org/10.1016/j.jmbbm.2023.106301.
76. Rama E, Mohapatra SR, Sugimura Y, Suzuki T, Siebert S, Barmin R, et al. In vitro and in vivo evaluation of biohybrid tissue-engineered vascular grafts with transformative (1)H/(19)F MRI traceable scaffolds. Biomaterials. 2024;311:122669. https://doi.org/10.1016/j.biomaterials.2024.122669.
77. Neville RF, Gupta SK, Kuraguntla DJ. Initial in vitro and in vivo evaluation of a self-monitoring prosthetic bypass graft. J Vasc Surg. 2017;65:1793–801. https://doi.org/10.1016/j.jvs.2016.06.114.
78. Sultan S, Acharya Y, Soliman O, Parodi JC, Hynes N. TEVAR and EVAR, the unknown knowns of the cardiovascular hemodynamics; and the immediate and long-term consequences of fabric material on major adverse clinical outcome. Front Surg. 2022;9:940304. https://doi.org/10.3389/fsurg.2022.940304.
79. Jacobs TS, Won J, Gravereaux EC, Faries PL, Morrissey N, Teodorescu VJ, et al. Mechanical failure of prosthetic human implants: a 10-year experience with aortic stent graft devices. J Vasc Surg. 2003;37:16–26. https://doi.org/10.1067/mva.2003.58.
80. Vahabli E, Mann J, Heidari BS, Lawrence-Brown M, Norman P, Jansen S, et al. The technological advancement to engineer next-generation stent-grafts: design, material, and fabrication techniques. Adv Healthc Mater. 2022;11:e2200271. https://doi.org/10.1002/adhm.202200271.
81. Abbott WM, Green RM, Matsumoto T, Wheeler JR, Miller N, Veith FJ, Above-Knee Femoropopliteal Study Group, et al. Prosthetic above-knee femoropopliteal bypass grafting: results of a multicenter randomized prospective trial. J Vasc Surg. 1997;25:19–28. https://doi.org/10.1016/s0741-5214(97)70317-3.

82. Owens GK, Kumar MS, Wamhoff BR. Molecular regulation of vascular smooth muscle cell differentiation in development and disease. Physiol Rev. 2004;84:767–801. https://doi.org/10.1152/physrev.00041.2003.
83. Szafron JM, Heng EE, Boyd J, Humphrey JD, Marsden AL. Hemodynamics and wall mechanics of vascular graft failure. Arterioscler Thromb Vasc Biol. 2024;44:1065–85. https://doi.org/10.1161/atvbaha.123.318239.
84. Sottiurai VS, Yao JS, Flinn WR, Batson RC. Intimal hyperplasia and neointima: an ultrastructural analysis of thrombosed grafts in humans. Surgery. 1983;93:809–17.
85. L'Heureux N, Pâquet S, Labbé R, Germain L, Auger FA. A completely biological tissue-engineered human blood vessel. FASEB J. 1998;12:47–56. https://doi.org/10.1096/fasebj.12.1.47.
86. Berger K, Sauvage LR, Rao AM, Wood SJ. Healing of arterial prostheses in man: its incompleteness. Ann Surg. 1972;175:118–27. https://doi.org/10.1097/00000658-197201000-00018.
87. Day T. Role of arterial pressure, wall stiffness, pulse pressure and waveform in Arterial Wall stress/strain and its clinical implications. In: Risk factors for cardiovascular disease. IntechOpen; 2022. p. 1–19. https://doi.org/10.5772/intechopen.100048.
88. Post A, Diaz-Rodriguez P, Balouch B, Paulsen S, Wu S, Miller J, et al. Elucidating the role of graft compliance mismatch on intimal hyperplasia using an ex vivo organ culture model. Acta Biomater. 2019;89:84–94. https://doi.org/10.1016/j.actbio.2019.03.025.
89. Hielscher D, Kaebisch C, Braun BJV, Gray K, Tobiasch E. Stem cell sources and graft material for vascular tissue engineering. Stem Cell Rev. 2018;14:642–67. https://doi.org/10.1007/s12015-018-9825-x.
90. Li MX, Wei QQ, Mo HL, Ren Y, Zhang W, Lu HJ, et al. Challenges and advances in materials and fabrication technologies of small-diameter vascular grafts. Biomater Res. 2023;27:58. https://doi.org/10.1186/s40824-023-00399-2.
91. Baguneid M, de Mel A, Yildirimer L, Fuller BJ, Hamilton G, Seifalian AM. In vivo study of a model tissue-engineered small-diameter vascular bypass graft. Biotechnol Appl Biochem. 2011;58:14–24. https://doi.org/10.1002/bab.8.
92. Kirkton RD, Prichard HL, Santiago-Maysonet M, Niklason LE, Lawson JH, Dahl SLM. Susceptibility of ePTFE vascular grafts and bioengineered human acellular vessels to infection. J Surg Res. 2018;221:143–51. https://doi.org/10.1016/j.jss.2017.08.035.

Chapter 12
Vascular Graft Infections

Mauro Vicaretti

SN Flashcards
Test your learning and check your understanding of this book's contents: use the "Springer Nature Flashcards" app to access questions using ▶ https://sn.pub/wppvze. To use the app, please follow the instructions in Chap. 1.

Key Learning Points

- Vascular graft infection is associated with significant mortality and morbidity (including limb loss).
- Bacteriology of graft infections varies with the affected site of the body.
- Early graft infections (within the first 4 months of graft implantation) are uncommon (approx. 1%) and are caused by virulent microorganisms.
- Graft infections are more common following emergency surgery and surgery in the groin.
- Late graft infections tend to be caused by less virulent organisms such as *Staphylococcus epidermidis*.
- Late graft infections often present insidiously with sinus tracts, perigraft fluid collections, graft occlusion and development of pseudo-aneurysms.
- Many bacteria can produce biofilms, which form a capsule of extracellular polymer substances protecting the bacteria from conventional antibiotics.
- Small colony variants often form biofilms and are difficult to isolate. They are likely to be a common cause of recurrent and relapsing infection.

M. Vicaretti (✉)
Department of Vascular Surgery, Westmead Hospital, Westmead, NSW, Australia
e-mail: mauro.vicaretti@sydney.edu.au

R. Fitridge et al. (eds.), *Pathophysiology of Vascular Disease*,
https://doi.org/10.1007/978-3-032-31459-8_12

- The management of vascular graft infection is complex, and a multi-disciplinary approach is required to optimise outcomes. The "gold standard" approach is total graft excision and extra-anatomical revascularisation. More conservative approaches may be required in individual cases. Treatment is not infrequently individualised.
- The management of stent graft infection is challenging, and best outcomes are obtained with explantation and revascularisation. Conservative management is associated with significantly inferior outcomes.

12.1 Introduction

The introduction of prosthetic grafts has revolutionised the management of vascular disease, but graft infection, although uncommon, remains a dreaded complication with significant morbidity and mortality. Mortality occurs in approximately one-third of all graft infections [1], with mortality highest when an aortic prosthesis is involved [2, 3]. As many as 75% of survivors of an infected aortic prosthesis require amputation of a limb [3], with the incidence of amputation highest when the infection involves more distal prosthetic grafts [4]. The incidence of graft infections is difficult to quantify as infection may be manifested many years after implantation [1], with many reports being isolated or as part of case series. Nevertheless, the reported incidence is in the order of 5%, varying according to the site of operation (Table 12.1), being higher when a groin incision is used, or if the procedure is an emergency or a redo procedure. However, to date, there continues to be a paucity of randomised controlled trial literature with respect to the optimal management of graft infection. This is understandable considering the complexity of such a medical and surgical problem. As such, treatment strategies are generally based on individual surgical experience and generalised recommendations for treatment [12].

Table 12.1 Incidence of prosthetic graft infection according to location

Author	Location of graft	Incidence (%)
Berger et al. [5]	Abdominal aorta	4.5
O'Sullivan et al. [6]	Thoracic aorta	1–3
Lorentzan et al. [7]	Aortofemoral	3.0
Lorentzan et al. [7]	Femoropopliteal	3.5
Exton and Galland [8]	Femoropopliteal	2.8
Eiberg et al. [9]	Femoro-femoro	2.5
Criado [10]	Carotid-subclavian	1.5
Argyriou [11]	Aortic endograft	0.6

12.2 Natural History of Prosthetic Vascular Graft Infections

Early prosthetic vascular graft infections typically occurring in the first 4 months following placement are relatively uncommon (1%) and are usually caused by the more virulent microorganisms, such as *S. aureus*, *E. coli*, *Pseudomonas*, *Klebsiella*, *Proteus* and *Enterobacter* [1]. Late prosthetic vascular graft infections are the result of two possible mechanisms. Firstly, by haematogenous seeding from a septic focus elsewhere or by the prosthetic graft becoming infected with enteric contents following a graft-enteric erosion [13]. In both the haematogenous and graft-enteric erosion situations, the usual causative organisms are those with high virulence and clinical manifestations are signs and symptoms of sepsis. The second mode of presentation is insidious, caused by the less virulent coagulase-negative staphylococci such as *S. epidermidis* with contamination likely occurring at the time of implantation [1]. Clinically, the mode of presentation of these late appearing infections are as sinus tracts, perigraft fluid collection and anastomotic pseudo-aneurysm formation [2]. This is illustrated in Fig. 12.1, which shows an extensive perigraft fluid collection around a prosthetic femoro-femoral cross-over graft. Figure 12.2 demonstrates an unincorporated graft with perigraft fluid collection.

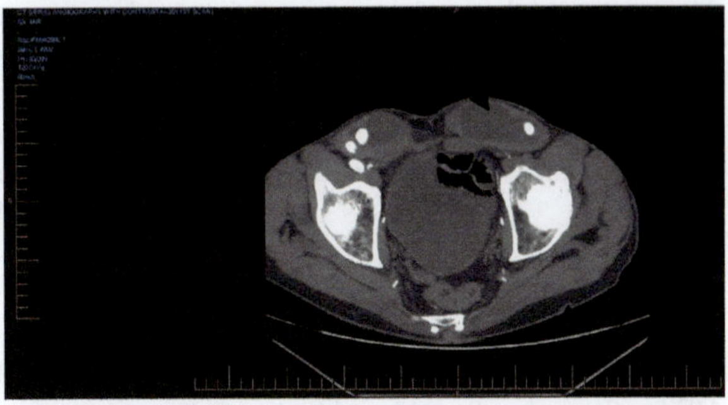

Fig. 12.1 Collections in both groins around prosthetic graft

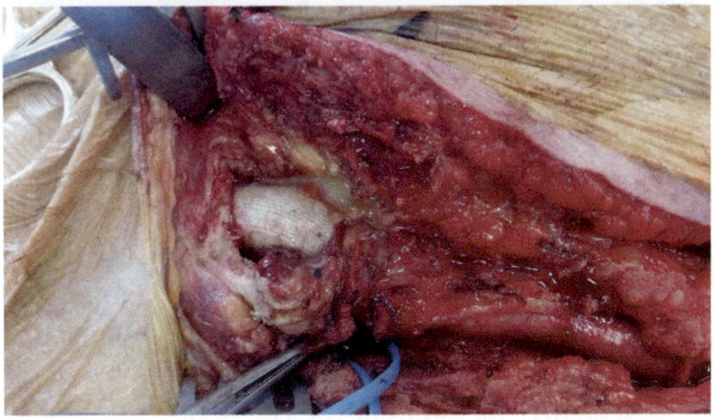

Fig. 12.2 Unincorporated Dacron graft with biofilm infection

12.3 Mechanisms of Graft Contamination at Operation

There is general agreement that the most common mechanism by which grafts become infected is at the time of implantation either by contamination from the surgical team or by colonised microorganisms on the patient. It has been demonstrated that the majority of patients undergoing arterial revascularisation are colonised with coagulase-negative staphylococci [14] and colonisation of patients with nosocomial bacteria is enhanced when the preoperative hospitalisation is lengthy [15].

The incidence of graft infection following emergency aneurysmorrhaphy has been reported to be as high as 7.5% [16]. The evidence of other potential mechanisms such as division of lymph nodes [17], infected transudated fluid during aortic surgery [18] and infected laminated thrombus [4, 18, 19] is conflicting. In addition, patients who develop superficial and/or deep surgical infections are 7.1 times more likely to develop graft infections [20].

12.4 Pathogenesis of Graft Infections

The exact aetiology of vascular graft infections is not completely understood but likely to be multi-factorial. According to Bandyk and Esses [21], the risk of vascular graft infection, as demonstrated by animal models, can be predicted by the formula:

$$\text{Risk of biomaterial infection} = \text{Dose of bacterial contamination} \times \text{virulence} / \text{Host resistance}$$

The dose of bacterial contamination is dependent on the infecting microorganism. Experimentation in a canine aortic model has demonstrated that the infective threshold for bacteria to cause graft infection in over 50% of grafts was 10^7, 10^9 and 10^2 for *S. aureus, S. epidermidis and P. Aeruginosa*, respectively [22]. Virulence of microorganisms is often associated with the production of secreted toxins and enzymes with a resultant decline in structural integrity of the artery wall [21, 22]. Many bacterial strains, including *S. epidermidis*, *S. aureus*, *P. aeruginosa*, *Klebsiella pneumoniae* and *Escherichia coli* are known to produce extracellular polymer substances (EPS) (slime), forming a capsule incorporating the bacteria. This is referred to as a biofilm and protects the microorganism against host defences and antibiotic therapy and allows greater adherence of the microorganism to the biomaterial [23, 24]. Biofilms protect the invading bacteria by increasing their resistance against conventional antibiotics, and in a sense the biofilm constitutes a protected mode of growth that allows survival in a hostile environment, allowing bacteria to resist biocides [25].

Essentially, the steps involved in the development of biomaterial-associated infection include the following: (a) bacterial adherence; (b) microcolony formation

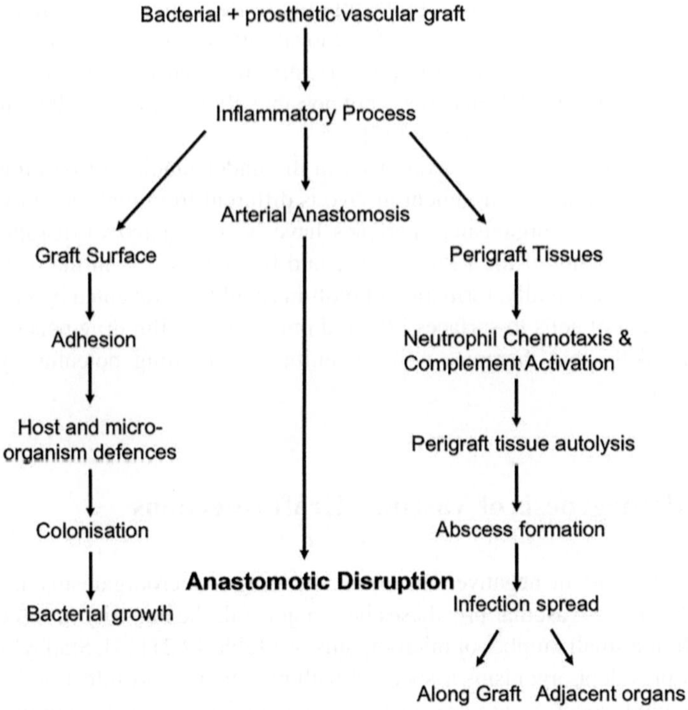

Fig. 12.3 Pathogenesis of vascular biomaterial-associated infections

within a biofilm; (c) activation of host defences; and (d) the inflammatory response involving perigraft tissues and the graft/artery anastomoses (Fig. 12.3) [2].

Bacterial adherence is initiated when planktonic (see Glossary) bacteria adhere to a surface and become irreversibly attached within a few minutes [26]. Adherence is influenced by microorganism characteristics, graft properties including graft electronegativity, hydroporosity and smoothness of the graft [23]. Microcolony formation within the biofilm ensues as the microorganisms secrete a protective layer of exopolysaccharides giving the biofilm the so-called slimy appearance. It is the interaction between the graft and the host that produces inflammatory stimuli activating the host's humoral and cellular immune system with the release of cytokines and polymorphonuclear granulocytes [2]. In addition, the acidic, ischaemic microenvironment produced by the immune foreign body reaction to the synthetic vascular grafts promotes bacterial biofilm formation and proliferation. The isolation of the graft and the microenvironment produced prevents antibiotics and immune complexes exerting their maximal effect, which contributes to the ultimate manifestations of graft infection, including tissue autolysis, arterial vessel wall or anastomotic disruption and haemorrhage [2]. The dynamic communities within the biofilm continually shed new planktonic cells [26].

It is the nature of the biofilm protecting the resident microorganisms which not infrequently mandates prosthetic graft removal, often followed by antibiotic treatment to prevent regrowth and to target bacteria released into the bloodstream or surrounding tissues [27]. When this is not possible, then aggressive alternate antimicrobial strategies are implemented [25].

Significant advances have been made in the understanding of biofilms, yet the dynamics of the microenvironment in vivo is different from that seen in vitro [25]. To act on the microorganisms, therapies have been targeted to disrupt the EPS matrix. Components of the EPS matrix could be vital targets in the disruption of biofilm structure. Equally, formation of biofilms could be prevented by inhibition of the attachment of cells to surfaces [25] and improved biofilm drug penetration [25, 28]. It is likely that therapies will be multiple, exploiting potential synergistic effects [28].

12.5 Pathogenesis of Vascular Graft Infections

Gram positive, gram negative, anaerobic and fungal microorganisms all have the potential to infect vascular prostheses but, in general, the majority of infections are the result of a small number of microorganisms (Table 12.2) [29]. Staphylococci are the most prevalent organisms associated with prosthetic graft infection [2, 30, 31]. Of the staphylococci, *S. aureus* is generally regarded as the most common causative bacterium [2, 30], particularly MRSA [31]. *S. epidermidis* is now being recognised as the leading cause of vascular graft infection, particularly chronic and late-onset infections [19].

The gram-negative organisms, *E. coli*, *Pseudomonas*, *Klebsiella*, *Enterobacter* and *Proteus*, although relatively uncommon causative organisms for graft infections, are of particular interest and concern because of their high virulence and their tendency to destroy the vessel wall [23, 32, 33]. Virulent microorganisms are significantly associated with an increased risk of re-infection [34].

Candida, *Mycobacteria* and *Aspergillus* infections are uncommon but pose a significant risk especially to patients who are immunocompromised [2]. Although uncommon, they are all expected to increase in frequency because of their increasing resistance to standard prophylactic antibiotics [33]. A major risk factor for fungal infection is the presence of graft-enteric fistula [35].

There is an association between the type of infecting organism, the type of vascular complication and the arteries that are involved in the anastomosis to the prosthetic graft. Bandyk and Bergamini [2], in a collective survey of 1258 patients who had a vascular graft infection, found that the majority of aortoenteric fistulas were the result of either *Streptococci or E. coli* and, if the anastomosis involved the femoral artery, the thoracic aorta, the subclavian, carotid or innominate arteries, *S. epidermidis or S aureus* was the likely causative organism. *E. coli*, *Enterococci* and

Table 12.2 Bacteriology of prosthetic vascular graft infections from collected series (location and incidence (%))

Microorganism	Thoracic aorta (% of total)	Graft enteric erosion/ graft enteric fistula	Aortofemoral	Femoro-popliteal-tibial
S. aureus	22	4	27	28
S. epidermidis	25	2	26	11
Strep sp.	2	9	10	11
Pseudomonas sp.	14	3	6	16
Coliforms and gram negative	10	49	28	29
Other species	11	15	1	3
No growth/no culture	16	18	2	2

Modified from Back [29]

Enterobacter were the more likely organisms to be involved in aortoiliac anastomoses.

Significant interest has developed in the role of small colony variants (SCVs) [34]. Many clinical studies and observations have been published associating recurrent, persistent staphylococcal infections, including device-associated infections to this special phenotype. It has been shown that SCV were strong biofilm (slime) formers, indicating that biofilm formation is a special feature of the pathogenesis of SCVs [36]. As with biofilm producing microorganisms, SCVs are associated with alterations in metabolism and host-pathogen interplay, resulting in chronic and relapsing, often therapy-refractory infections. SCV are difficult to identify by conventional methods with identification mostly performed by 16S rRNA gene sequencing [34].

12.6 Investigations for Detection of Prosthetic Graft Infections

The diagnosis of vascular prosthetic infections can be difficult as the presentation may be subtle especially if it is a late-onset infection, the prosthesis is intra-abdominal and the microorganism is one of low virulence. The presentation of vascular graft infection is thus very dependent on the location of infection and the causative microorganism(s). The diagnosis is aided by multiple available microbiological and imaging testing, but in general is directed more at proving the absence of infection rather than its presence. It is infrequent that single modality imaging is sufficient in establishing the presence of vascular graft infection [37].

In response to the challenges in diagnosing vascular graft infection, the multidisciplinary Management of Aortic Graft Infection Collaboration (MAGIC) has proposed a comprehensive set of criteria, which have been validated and endorsed by the European Society of Vascular Surgery. The MAGIC criteria encompass major

Table 12.3 MAGIC criteria for vascular graft infection

Criterion	Clinical/surgical	Radiological	Laboratory
Major	Pus (confirmed by microscopy) around graft or in aneurysm sac at surgery Open wound with exposed graft or communicating sinus Fistula development, e.g. aorto-enteric or aortobronchial Graft insertion in an infected site, e.g. fistula, mycotic aneurysm, or infected pseudo-aneurysm	Perigraft fluid on CT scan ≥ 3 months after insertion Perigraft gas on CT scan ≥ 7 weeks after insertion Increase in perigraft gas volume demonstrated on serial imaging	Organisms recovered from an explanted graft Organisms recovered from an intraoperative specimen Organisms recovered from a percutaneous, radiologically guided aspirate of perigraft fluid
Minor	Localised clinical features of graft infection, e.g. erythema, warmth, swelling, purulent discharge, pain Fever ≥38 °C with graft infection as most likely cause	Other, e.g. suspicious perigraft gas/fluid soft tissue inflammation; aneurysm expansion; pseudo-aneurysm formation: focal bowel wall thickening; discitis/ osteomyelitis; suspicious metabolic activity on FDGPET/CT; radiolabelled leukocyte uptake	Blood culture(s) positive and no apparent source except graft infection Abnormally elevated inflammatory markers with graft infection as most likely cause, e.g. erythrocyte sedimentation rate, C-reactive protein, white cell count

Adapted from Lyons et al. [38]

and minor criteria across four key categories: clinical, surgical, radiological and laboratory findings [38, 39]. Suspicion of graft infection is raised when a single *major* criterion or two or more *minor* criteria from different categories are present. However, a diagnosis of graft infection requires the presence of at least one major criterion along with at least one criterion (either major or minor) from a different category [38] (Table 12.3).

12.6.1 History and Physical Examination

Clinical signs and symptoms are typically non-diagnostic for the presence of vascular graft infections. The clinical clues suggesting graft infection especially those placed superficially include an inflammatory perigraft mass, overlying cellulitus, presence of exposed prosthetic graft, a sinus tract with persistent purulent drainage and/or bleeding and/or a palpable anastomotic pseudo-aneurysm, graft thrombosis and distal septic embolisation [2–4, 40]. The presence of intra-abdominal prosthetic graft infection may be non-specific, such as fever of unknown origin, septicaemia, or abdominal pain [3]. Upper or lower gastrointestinal haemorrhage of either an acute or chronic nature may indicate a graft-enteric fistula [19, 40]. Occasionally, indirect evidence, such as the presence of hydronephrosis or osteomyelitis of the spine, may be indicative of perigraft inflammation.

12.6.2 Laboratory Investigations

Routine laboratory studies such as white cell count and differential, erythrocyte sedimentation rate (ESR), C-reactive protein (CRP) and blood cultures are obtained. However, the results may be non-specific and even normal if the organism is *S. epidermidis* [2]. Wherever possible, pus, exudates, tissue specimens, blood and wound cultures should be analysed microbiologically to aid in microorganism identification and to allow the use of appropriate and specific treatment. Ideally, samples should be harvested before the start of antimicrobial therapy. To increase the chances of recovering biofilm-forming microorganisms, such as *S. epidermidis*, various specimen processing techniques can be employed. These techniques include serial dilution techniques, sonicating a harvested graft, or vortex mixing tissue samples. These methods aim to dislodge microorganisms from the biofilm and improve their availability for subsequent culture and analysis [41–43].

12.6.3 Diagnostic Imaging

Various diagnostic modalities (computerised tomography (CT), ultrasonography, magnetic resonance imaging, leucocyte or immunoglobulin-labelled scanning, transoesophageal ultrasound, Positron Emission Tomography (PET) scanning ± CT, angiography and/or endoscopy) may assist the vascular surgeon in determining the presence and extent of prosthetic graft infection. Not infrequently, a combination of diagnostic modalities to improve sensitivity and specificity is utilised to confirm the presence or absence of a vascular prosthetic graft infection. These modalities are also helpful in planning definitive surgery. The utility of CT angiography with the capability of vascular three-dimensional reconstruction has largely replaced digital subtraction angiography as the method of diagnosis and therapeutic planning. In general, the features suggestive of graft infection include perigraft fluid and/or gas (Fig. 12.4), graft disruption, absence of graft incorporation and pseudo-aneurysm formation. The presence of periprosthetic gas more than 7 weeks following graft implantation is an abnormal finding and should alert the physician to the possibility of a graft infection. Oesophagogastroduodenoscopy (Fig. 12.5) and/or colonoscopy is of value to exclude other gastrointestinal causes of bleeding in patients with aortic prosthesis and gastrointestinal bleeding [40].

While CTA provides excellent spatial resolution for visualising vascular anatomy and related pathology, its ability to definitively diagnose graft infection is

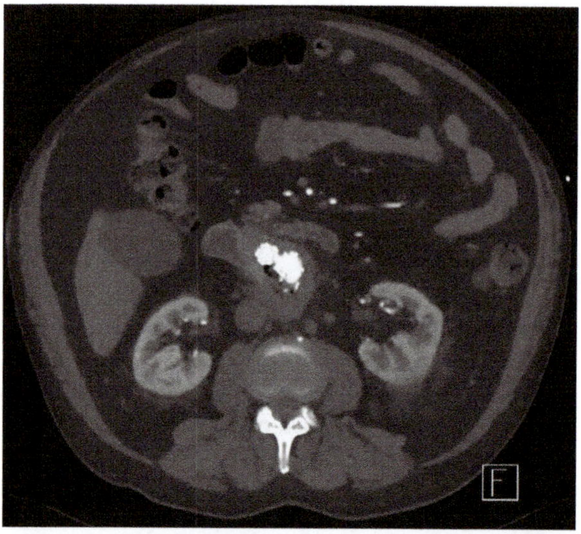

Fig. 12.4 CT scan demonstrating perigraft inflammatory mass and gas around stent graft

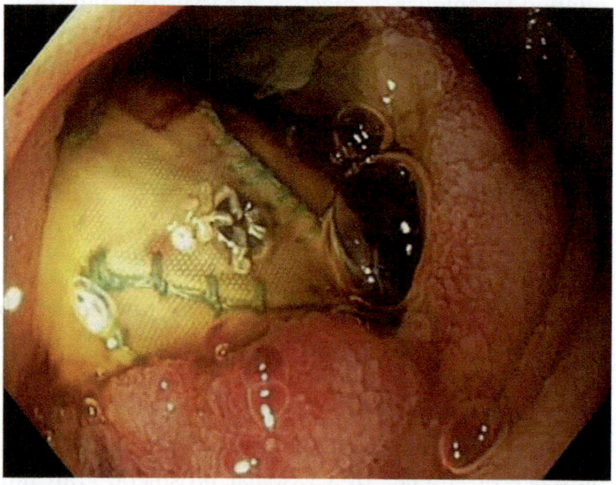

Fig. 12.5 Duodenoscopy demonstrating graft enteric fistula with graft on view in duodenum

limited. Nuclear medicine techniques offer a valuable tool to confirm or exclude infection, particularly when CTA findings are inconclusive. PET/CT using [18F] FDG has high sensitivity and is particularly useful for ruling out infection. However, to minimise false positive from post-surgical inflammation, it is ideally performed at least 4 months after the procedure. Analysing PET/CT images involves several criteria, including visual assessment, semiquantitative measures like maximum standardised uptake value (SUVmax) and comparing target-to-background ratios. Among several qualitative and semiquantitative parameters measured for interpretation for PET/CT, focal uptake seems to be a reliable tool to diagnose infection as demonstrated by high positive predictive and negative predictive values reported [12, 44, 45].

Radiolabelled white blood cell (WBC) scintigraphy, especially when combined with single-photon emission computed tomography co-registered with CT (SPECT/CT), provides a compelling alternative, particularly soon after surgery, where PET/CT may be unreliable. SPECT/CT enhances the precision of WBC scintigraphy by providing better localisation and assessment of suspected infection sites [12, 45].

Despite their strengths, both PET/CT and WBC scintigraphy have limitations. PET/CT, while sensitive, suffers from lower specificity and a high false positive rate within 4 months of surgery due to non-specific uptake in inflammatory tissue. Furthermore, the lack of standardised interpretation criteria can affect its diagnostic accuracy. WBC scintigraphy, though highly accurate in differentiating infection from inflammation, has limited availability and involves blood manipulation. It often requires late acquisitions and specialised facilities, with trained personnel [12, 45]. Ultimately, a comprehensive approach combining clinical findings with appropriate imaging modalities is essential for accurate diagnosis and timely management of vascular graft or endograft infections.

12.7 Management of Prosthetic Graft Infections

In general, the management of prosthetic graft infections is dependent on patient comorbidities, clinical presentation, extent of graft involvement, site of the prosthetic graft (intra-cavitary vs. extra-cavitary), initial indication for the prosthesis, revascularisation options and microbiology of infecting organisms. Procedures may be undertaken as single-staged or multi-staged accounting for these variables.

Preventive measures such as the routine use of skin preparations [46], the use of a depilatory agent [47], limiting the length of preoperative hospitalisation [15], operating time and intensive care stay all contribute to the reduction in wound infection, and more importantly, the chance of developing resistant multiple nosocomial infections [46]. Antimicrobial prophylaxis has been shown to reduce wound infections in vascular surgery and ideally should be given as close as possible prior to incision and repeated in the event of haemorrhage and lengthy operations every 4 h [48].

As a preventive measure, host resistance may be enhanced by the antimicrobial impregnation of grafts. A number of novel combinations of grafts and antibiotic with or without various forms of treatment have been trialled at both the in vitro and in vivo levels (Table 12.4) [49–63] Rifampicin, a known anti-staphylococcal agent, particularly for treatment of methicillin resistant (MRSA), is a hydrophobic semi-synthetic substance with a high affinity for gelatin [64]. It inhibits DNA-dependent RNA polymerase activity in bacterial cells without affecting mammalian cells [65] and has been passively incorporated into gelatin-sealed Dacron grafts as a mode of staphylococcal protection at the time of implantation. It has been shown to be resistant to experimental bacterial contamination [66–69], with in vivo bioactivity to 22 days [70], and in vitro bioactivity to 4 days [71–73]. It is these qualities plus its excellent tissue and intracellular penetration [64] that make rifampicin an

Table 12.4 Antimicrobial impregnation of vascular grafts

Antibiotics used in experimental models	Vehicles, agents
Silver allantoin-heparin [49]	Silver [49–52]
Norflaxacin [50], penicillin [53], oxacillin [51, 54–56]	Triododecylmethylammonium chloride (cationic surfactant) [50, 53]
Amikacin [57]	Benzalkonium chloride [53, 55]
Cephazolin [53], cefoxitin [58], ciprofloxacin [52, 59, 60], ofloxacin [54]	Luminal coated glycosaminoglycan-keratin fibrin glue (cryoprecipitate, bovine thrombin, aminocaproic acid) [58, 61]
Tobramycin [61, 62]	N-butyl-2 cyanoacrylate [62]
Gentamicin [63]	PTFE threads [54]

ideal antibiotic to be bonded to prosthetic grafts in order to prevent subsequent graft infection.

It has been shown in an ovine model [31], in which a segment of carotid artery was replaced with a rifampicin-soaked Gelsoft graft (1.2 or 10 mg/mL) and then directly inoculated with 10^8 colony forming units of either methicillin resistant staphylococcal aureus or methicillin resistant staphylococcal epidermidis, that the rifampicin-soaked grafts offered significant protection against the development of graft infection compared to non-rifampicin soaked grafts [74–76]. Although there is ample in vitro evidence supporting antibiotic impregnation of prosthetic grafts, there continues to be no clinical evidence that prophylactic rifampicin bonding to Dacron grafts reduced graft infection at either 1 month (RR 0.63, 95% CI 0.27–1.49) or 2 years (RR 1.05, 95% CI 0.46–2.40) [48].

12.8 Established Infection

12.8.1 Antibiotic Therapy

Once the diagnosis or suspicion of prosthetic vascular graft infection is made, then broad-spectrum antimicrobial therapy is initiated and subsequently converted to organism-specific antibiotics [3]. The duration of antimicrobial treatment for vascular graft infection is highly variable, ranging from weeks to lifelong, and depends on several factors. In cases of complete graft explanation, where the infected graft is entirely removed, meticulous debridement performed and vascular continuity is restored via an extra-anatomical bypass or using an autologous vein graft, a shorter course of antibiotics is generally sufficient. This typically involves a minimum of 2 weeks of intravenous antibiotics followed by a variable duration of oral antibiotics. However, when in situ reconstruction is performed, a longer duration on intravenous therapy (typically 6 weeks) is recommended. The total duration of antibiotics depends on the causative organism and its susceptibility, patient immune status, presence of metastatic infection (such as infective endocarditis) and the graft material used for reconstruction. For patients deemed unsuitable for surgical intervention, lifelong antimicrobial suppression may be warranted. Throughout treatment, close monitoring of clinical signs and symptoms, along with inflammatory markers, helps guide therapy [12, 77, 78].

12.8.2 Operative Approaches to Vascular Graft Infection

The operative technique largely depends on the vascular graft location and patient clinical status. Historically, the "gold standard" management of vascular graft infection was total removal of the infected graft, debridement of infected tissue and extra-anatomical revascularisation [12, 79]. The main advantages of this approach are that arterial reconstruction is performed outside the infected field and the procedure can be performed in one or two stages. The disadvantages of extra-anatomical reconstruction include concerns with long-term patency and limb loss and risk of stump rupture with life-threatening bleeding. Techniques to prevent stump rupture include double suture layers and reinforcement with venous or felt pledges. Most authors recommend covering the stump with healthy vascularised tissue such as omentum [12].

A number of alternative approaches, including in situ repair or partial graft removal, have been advocated depending on the site of the infection and the micro-organism involved. Extracavitary as compared to intracavitary grafts are more amenable to the more conservative approaches. The most conservative of treatments is aggressive local wound care with graft preservation providing the graft and anastomoses are intact, and the patient has no systemic features of sepsis [80]. A series of patients who had graft preservation concluded that, with the exception of *Pseudomonas and Staphylococcus aureus*, infra-inguinal vascular graft infections could be managed selectively with debridement, antibiotic therapy and wound closure [32]. The skeletonised prosthetic graft can be covered using viable regional rotational flaps [81]. The risk of such treatment is fatal graft disruption and persistent graft infection [82]. Graft excision without revascularisation may be considered in well collateralised distal arterial beds and/or grafts that are thrombosed with no symptoms of distal ischaemia. Some groups have advocated aggressive wound debridement with vacuum-assisted closure without rotational muscle flap coverage even with exposed grafts with minimal morbidity and mortality [81]. Others have proposed graft excision and replacement with cadaveric arterial allografts [83], venous autografts [84], cryopreserved saphenous vein homografts [85], autogenous arteries and/or veins [86] or prosthesis [87].

In situ reconstruction (ISR) is increasingly favoured for abdominal graft infections, utilising autologous veins, cryopreserved allografts, or antibiotic-impregnated grafts (silver-coated or rifampicin-bonded). This approach may offer lower long-term mortality rates compared to extra-anatomical bypass, according to some meta-analyses [88–90]. However, recent data from a nationwide Swedish study found no significant difference in survival or re-infection rates between the two strategies [91].

Despite the lack of definitive evidence, the 2020 European Society for Vascular Surgery Clinical Practice Guidelines on the Management of Vascular Graft and Endograft Infections recommends ISR, particularly with autologous vein grafts, as first-line treatment for abdominal aortic graft infection, especially in younger patients with good health and longer life expectancy. However, deep vein harvesting adds complexity and operative time, making it less suitable for elderly patients with comorbidities [12]. A critical technical aspect of ISR is ensuring adequate coverage of the new graft with biological material, such as a pedicled omentum flap, muscle, fascia, or retroperitoneal tissue. In cases involving multi-drug-resistant microorganisms, extra-anatomical reconstruction may be the preferred option [12].

The major concern with in situ reconstruction is recurrent and/or ongoing sepsis. Experimental evidence for in situ prosthetic replacement [23] was provided in an in vitro model which compared the bacterial adherence of four strains of bacteria (*S. aureus*, "mucin" and "non-mucin" producing *S. epidermidis* and *E. coli*) to ePTFE, woven Dacron and velour knitted Dacron. The study demonstrated that bacterial adherence was greatest to velour knitted Dacron and least with ePTFE. In addition, "mucin" producing *S. epidermidis* adhered to Dacron in 10- to 100-fold greater numbers compared to PTFE [23]. Two meta-analyses demonstrated relatively low re-infection rates with ISR techniques. Furthermore, there was no statistically significant difference in re-infection rates between different graft types (veins 2%; cryopreserved allografts 9%, rifampicin-bonded or silver-coated prosthesis 11%). Importantly, all these options showed significantly improved outcomes compared to standard ePTFE and Dacron grafts [88, 92].

To date, a number of groups [83, 93, 94] have successfully managed prosthetic graft infections with rifampicin-impregnated grafts with zero mortality, no requirement for limb amputation and to date, no recurrence of infection. Interestingly, a prospective United Kingdom trial defining the role of extra-anatomical bypass with rifampicin-bonded grafts, found no evidence to support their use when compared to non-treated collagen-impregnated grafts, with respect to graft infection and mortality [84]. The same group reported fewer amputations, conduit failures and early mortalities with the use of rifampicin-bonded grafts than other treatment modalities for aortic graft infection, but reinfection was the worst for rifampicin-bonded prostheses and lowest for autogenous veins. When considering all revascularisation options and outcomes, the in situ reconstruction for aortic graft infections was the preferred option over extra-anatomic bypass [84].

Stent grafts have become a viable alternative in the management of not only infected prosthetic grafts but also in infective native aortic aneurysms (previously known as mycotic aneurysms) in patients presenting with pseudo-anastomotic active bleeding, acute fistulisation or rupture/impending rupture [85, 95]. In patients with an aortic-enteric fistula, a stent graft can be a valuable tool in emergency settings. It provides rapid haemorrhage control and temporary physiologic stabilisation, allowing time for later definitive repair. While this may be considered definitive management for patients with limited life expectancy (less than 6 months), those with longer predicted lifespan should be considered for graft removal and definitive surgical repair following the initial endovascular procedure [85]. For native aortic aneurysm infections, multiple reports support endovascular aneurysm repair (EVAR) as a potentially acceptable long-term alternative to open surgical repair [96, 97].

12.9 Stent Graft Infection

Stent grafts are increasingly being utilised for the management of arterial occlusive and/or aneurysmal disease. Although stent graft infection is uncommon, with widespread aortic endograft placement for the treatment of aortic pathology, complications of endografts are increasingly being reported. Infection of an endograft placed during an abdominal endovascular aortic repair (EVAR) or thoracic endovascular aortic repair (TEVAR) is reported to have an incidence in small series of 0.2–5% [86, 87]. There are, to date, no large multi-institutional studies.

The management of stent graft infection can be complicated and associated with significant morbidity and mortality. A recent meta-analysis [98] demonstrated superior results with conventional surgical therapies, namely explantation of the endoprosthesis and revascularisation independent of means of revascularisation and conduit type compared to conservative management. Patients in the surgical group had a higher survival rate compared with conservative group (58% vs 33%, $P = 0.002$). Outcomes were worse with infected thoracic aortic endografts compared to abdominal aortic endo-grafts with survival rates of 27% versus 58%, respectively ($P = 0.000$) [98].

12.10 Conclusion

The future management of vascular graft infections will be reliant on a better understanding of the interaction between the microorganism, the prosthesis and the immune system. This will allow a more directed approach towards prevention and treatment. Possibilities would include more powerful antibiotics either administered parenterally or incorporated into the prosthesis, acting as a local delivery system for prolonged periods of time. The role of the biofilm in the pathogenesis of graft infection needs further understanding from both a molecular and an immune level.

Multiple Choice Questions

1. Early prosthetic vascular graft infections, typically occurring within the first 4 months of implantation are relatively uncommon. Which group of microorganisms is generally responsible for these early infections?
   (a) Coagulase-negative staphylococci such as *S. epidermidis*
   (b) Fungal microorganisms such as *Candida* and *Aspergillus*
   (c) Small colony variants
   (d) More virulent microorganisms, such as *S. aureus*, *E. coli* and *Pseudomonas*
   (e) *Streptococci and Enterococci*

   Answer: (d) More virulent microorganisms, such as S. aureus, E. coli and Pseudomonas
2. The management of aortic graft infection collaboration (MAGIC) criteria require the presence of at least one major criterion along with at least one criterion (either major or minor) from a different category to establish a diagnosis of graft infection. Which of the following is listed as a major criterion?
   (a) Abnormally elevated inflammatory markers, such as C-reactive protein
   (b) Perigraft gas on CT scan < 7 weeks after graft insertion
   (c) Focal bowel thickening
   (d) Blood culture(s) positive with no apparent source except the graft
   (e) Perigraft fluid on CT scan ≥ 3 months after insertion

   Answer: (e) Perigraft fluid on CT scan ≥ 3 months after insertion

References

1. Back MR. Infections and antibiotics in vascular surgery. In: White RA, Hollier LH, editors. Vascular surgery: basic science and clinical correlations. Philadelphia: J. B. Lippincott Company; 1994. p. 613–24.
2. Bandyk DF, Bergamini TM. Infection in prosthetic vascular grafts. In: Rutherford RB, editor. Vascular surgery. 4th ed. Philadelphia: W. B. Saunders Company; 1995. p. 588–604.
3. Moore WS, Deaton WH. Infection in prosthetic vascular grafts. In: Moore WS, editor. Vascular surgery: a comprehensive review. 4th ed. Philadelphia: W. B. Saunders; 1993. p. 694–706.
4. Buckels JA, Wilson SE. Prevention and management of prosthetic graft infection. In: Veith FJ, Hobson II RW, Williams RA, Wilson SE, editors. Vascular surgery: principles and practice. 2nd ed. New York: McGraw-Hill Inc; 1994. p. 1081–9.
5. Berger P, De Borst GJ, Moll FL. Current opinions about diagnosis and treatment strategy for aortic graft infections in The Netherlands. J Cardiovasc Surg. 2015;56:867–76.
6. O'Sullivan KE, Casey L, Sidhu P, Graham A, Austin C, Hunter M. Exploring thoracic aortic graft infection: a comprehensive review of diagnosis and treatment options with a management strategy algorithm. J Cardiac Surg. 2024;2024:2821237. https://doi.org/10.1155/2024/2821237.
7. Lorentzen JE, Nielsen OM, Arendrup H, Kimose HH, Bille S, Andersen J, et al. Vascular graft infection: an analysis of sixty-two graft infections in 2411 consecutively implanted synthetic vascular grafts. Surgery. 1985;98:81–6.

8. Exton RJ, Galland RB. Major groin complications following the use of synthetic grafts. Eur J Vasc Endovasc Surg. 2007;34:188–90. https://doi.org/10.1016/j.ejvs.2007.03.012.
9. Eiberg JP, Røder O, Stahl-Madsen M, Eldrup N, Qvarfordt P, Laursen A, et al. Fluoropolymer-coated dacron versus PTFE grafts for femorofemoral crossover bypass: randomised trial. Eur J Vasc Endovasc Surg. 2006;32:431–8. https://doi.org/10.1016/j.ejvs.2006.04.018.
10. Criado FJ. Extrathoracic management of aortic arch syndrome. Br J Surg. 1982;69(Suppl):S45–51. https://doi.org/10.1002/bjs.1800691316.
11. Argyriou C, Georgiadis GS, Lazarides MK, Georgakarakos E, Antoniou GA. Endograft infection after endovascular abdominal aortic aneurysm repair: a systematic review and meta-analysis. J Endovasc Ther. 2017;24:688–97. https://doi.org/10.1177/1526602817722018.
12. Chakfé N, Diener H, Lejay A, Assadian O, Berard X, Caillon J, et al. Editor's choice – European Society for Vascular Surgery (ESVS) 2020 clinical practice guidelines on the management of vascular graft and endograft infections. Eur J Vasc Endovasc Surg. 2020;59:339–84. https://doi.org/10.1016/j.ejvs.2019.10.016.
13. Armstrong PA, Back MR, Wilson JS, Shames ML, Johnson BL, Bandyk DF. Improved outcomes in the recent management of secondary aortoenteric fistula. J Vasc Surg. 2005;42:660–6. https://doi.org/10.1016/j.jvs.2005.06.020.
14. Levy MF, Schmitt DD, Edmiston CE, Bandyk DF, Krepel CJ, Seabrook GR, et al. Sequential analysis of staphylococcal colonization of body surfaces of patients undergoing vascular surgery. J Clin Microbiol. 1990;28:664–9. https://doi.org/10.1128/jcm.28.4.664-669.1990.
15. Perry M. Infection in vascular surgery. In: Davis JM, Shires GT, editors. Principles and management of surgical infections. Philadelphia: JB Lippincott; 1991. p. 371–82.
16. Jamieson GG, DeWeese JA, Rob CG. Infected arterial grafts. Ann Surg. 1975;181:850–2. https://doi.org/10.1097/00000658-197506000-00016.
17. Rubin JR, Malone JM, Goldstone J. The role of the lymphatic system in acute arterial prosthetic graft infections. J Vasc Surg. 1985;2:92–8.
18. Russell HE, Barnes RW, Baker WH. Sterility of intestinal transudate during aortic reconstructive procedures. Arch Surg. 1975;110:402–4. https://doi.org/10.1001/archsurg.1975.01360100044009.
19. O'Brien T, Collin J. Prosthetic vascular graft infection. Br J Surg. 1992;79:1262–7. https://doi.org/10.1002/bjs.1800791205.
20. Langenberg JCM, Kluytmans J, de Groot HGW, Ho GH, Veen EJ, Buimer MG, et al. Surgical site and graft infections in endovascular and open abdominal aortic aneurysm surgery. Surg Infect. 2018;19:424–9. https://doi.org/10.1089/sur.2017.302.
21. Bandyk DF, Esses GE. Prosthetic graft infection. Surg Clin North Am. 1994;74:571–90.
22. White JV, Nessel CC, Whang K. Differential effect of type of bacteria on peripheral graft infections. In: Calligaro KD, Veith FJ, editors. Management of infected arterial grafts. St Louis: Quality Medical Publishing Incorporated; 1994. p. 25–42.
23. Schmitt DD, Bandyk DF, Pequet AJ, Malangoni MA, Towne JB. Mucin production by Staphylococcus epidermidis. A virulence factor promoting adherence to vascular grafts. Arch Surg. 1986;121:89–95. https://doi.org/10.1001/archsurg.1986.01400010103013.
24. Malangoni MA, Livingston DH, Peyton JC. The effect of protein binding on the adherence of staphylococci to prosthetic vascular grafts. J Surg Res. 1993;54:168–72. https://doi.org/10.1006/jsre.1993.1027.
25. Rabin N, Zheng Y, Opoku-Temeng C, Du Y, Bonsu E, Sintim HO. Biofilm formation mechanisms and targets for developing antibiofilm agents. Future Med Chem. 2015;7:493–512. https://doi.org/10.4155/fmc.15.6.
26. Hall-Stoodley L, Costerton JW, Stoodley P. Bacterial biofilms: from the natural environment to infectious diseases. Nat Rev Microbiol. 2004;2:95–108. https://doi.org/10.1038/nrmicro821.
27. Davies DG, Geesey GG. Regulation of the alginate biosynthesis gene algC in Pseudomonas aeruginosa during biofilm development in continuous culture. Appl Environ Microbiol. 1995;61:860–7. https://doi.org/10.1128/aem.61.3.860-867.1995.

28. Wolfmeier H, Pletzer D, Mansour SC, Hancock REW. New perspectives in biofilm eradication. ACS Infect Dis. 2018;4:93–106. https://doi.org/10.1021/acsinfecdis.7b00170.
29. Back MR. Infections and antibiotics in vascular surgery. In: White RA, Hollier LH, editors. Vascular surgery: basic science and clinical correlations. 2nd ed. Hoboken: Blackwell; 2005. p. 477–92.
30. Golan JF. Vascular graft infection. Infect Dis Clin N Am. 1989;3:247–58.
31. Fletcher JP, Dryden M, Munro R, Xu JH, Hehir MD. Establishment of a vascular graft infection model in the sheep carotid artery. Aust N Z J Surg. 1990;60:801–3. https://doi.org/10.1111/j.1445-2197.1990.tb07477.x.
32. Calligaro KD, Westcott CJ, Buckley RM, Savarese RP, DeLaurentis DA. Infrainguinal anastomotic arterial graft infections treated by selective graft preservation. Ann Surg. 1992;216:74–9. https://doi.org/10.1097/00000658-199207000-00011.
33. Treiman GS. Bacteriology of aortic graft infections. In: Gewartz BL, Schwartz LB, editors. Surgery of the aorta and its branches. Philadelphia: W. B. Saunders Company; 2000. p. 375–83.
34. Kahl BC, Becker K, Löffler B. Clinical significance and pathogenesis of staphylococcal small colony variants in persistent infections. Clin Microbiol Rev. 2016;29:401–27. https://doi.org/10.1128/cmr.00069-15.
35. Monnier B, Couture T, Dechartres A, Sitruk S, Gaillard J, Bleibtreu A, et al. Fungal versus non-fungal supra-inguinal prosthetic vascular graft infections: a cohort study. Infect Dis Now. 2024;54:104792. https://doi.org/10.1016/j.idnow.2023.104792.
36. Baddour LM, Barker LP, Christensen GD, Parisi JT, Simpson WA. Phenotypic variation of Staphylococcus epidermidis in infection of transvenous endocardial pacemaker electrodes. J Clin Microbiol. 1990;28:676–9. https://doi.org/10.1128/jcm.28.4.676-679.1990.
37. Reinders Folmer EI, Von Meijenfeldt GCI, Van der Laan MJ, Glaudemans A, Slart R, Saleem BR, et al. Diagnostic imaging in vascular graft infection: a systematic review and meta-analysis. Eur J Vasc Endovasc Surg. 2018;56:719–29. https://doi.org/10.1016/j.ejvs.2018.07.010.
38. Lyons O, Baguneid M, Barwick T, Bell R, Foster N, Homer-Vanniasinkam S, et al. Diagnosis of aortic graft infection: a case definition by the Management of Aortic Graft Infection Collaboration (MAGIC). Eur J Vasc Endovasc Surg. 2016;52:758–63. https://doi.org/10.1016/j.ejvs.2016.09.007.
39. Anagnostopoulos A, Mayer F, Ledergerber B, Bergadà-Pijuan J, Husmann L, Mestres CA, et al. Editor's choice – Validation of the Management of Aortic Graft Infection Collaboration (MAGIC) criteria for the diagnosis of vascular graft/endograft infection: results from the prospective Vascular Graft Cohort study. Eur J Vasc Endovasc Surg. 2021;62:251–7. https://doi.org/10.1016/j.ejvs.2021.05.010.
40. Murray SP, Goldstone J. Diagnostic advances. In: Calligaro KD, Veith FJ, editors. Management of infected arterial grafts. St Louis: Quality Medical Publishing Incorporated; 1994. p. 43–53.
41. Bergamini TM, Bandyk DF, Govostis D, Kaebnick HW, Towne JB. Infection of vascular prostheses caused by bacterial biofilms. J Vasc Surg. 1988;7:21–30.
42. Bergamini TM, Bandyk DF, Govostis D, Vetsch R, Towne JB. Identification of Staphylococcus epidermidis vascular graft infections: a comparison of culture techniques. J Vasc Surg. 1989;9:665–70. https://doi.org/10.1067/mva.1989.vs0090665.
43. Wengrovitz M, Spangler S, Martin LF. Sonication provides maximal recovery of staphylococcus epidermidis from slime-coated vascular prosthetics. Am Surg. 1991;57:161–4.
44. Rojoa D, Kontopodis N, Antoniou SA, Ioannou CV, Antoniou GA. 18F-FDG PET in the diagnosis of vascular prosthetic graft infection: a diagnostic test accuracy meta-analysis. Eur J Vasc Endovasc Surg. 2019;57:292–301. https://doi.org/10.1016/j.ejvs.2018.08.040.
45. Lauri C, Signore A, Glaudemans AW, Treglia G, Gheysens O, Slart RH, et al. Evidence-based guideline of the European Association of Nuclear Medicine (EANM) on imaging infection in vascular grafts. Eur J Nucl Med Mol Imaging. 2022;49:3430–51. https://doi.org/10.1007/s00259-022-05769-x.
46. Cruse PJ, Foord R. A five-year prospective study of 23,649 surgical wounds. Arch Surg. 1973;107:206–10. https://doi.org/10.1001/archsurg.1973.01350200078018.

47. Seropian R, Reynolds BM. Wound infections after preoperative depilatory versus razor preparation. Am J Surg. 1971;121:251–4. https://doi.org/10.1016/0002-9610(71)90199-1.
48. Stewart AH, Eyers PS, Earnshaw JJ. Prevention of infection in peripheral arterial reconstruction: a systematic review and meta-analysis. J Vasc Surg. 2007;46:148–55. https://doi.org/10.1016/j.jvs.2007.02.065.
49. Clark RE, Margraf HW. Antibacterial vascular grafts with improved thromboresistance. Arch Surg. 1974;109:159–62. https://doi.org/10.1001/archsurg.1974.01360020021005.
50. Shah PM, Modak S, Fox CL, Babu SC, Sampath L, Clauss RH, et al. PTFE graft treated with silver norfloxacin (AgNF): drug retention and resistance to bacterial challenge. J Surg Res. 1987;42:298–303. https://doi.org/10.1016/0022-4804(87)90147-8.
51. Benvenisty AI, Tannenbaum G, Ahlborn TN, Fox CL, Modak S, Sampath L, et al. Control of prosthetic bacterial infection: evaluation of an easily incorporated, tightly bound, silver antibiotic PTFE graft. J Surg Res. 1988;44:1–7. https://doi.org/10.1016/0022-4804(88)90116-3.
52. Kinney EV, Bandyk DF, Seabrook GA, Kelly HM, Towne JB. Antibiotic-bonded PTFE vascular grafts: the effect of silver antibiotic on bioactivity following implantation. J Surg Res. 1991;50:430–5. https://doi.org/10.1016/0022-4804(91)90020-m.
53. Harvey RA, Greco RS. The noncovalent bonding of antibiotics to a polytetrafluoroethylene-benzalkonium graft. Ann Surg. 1981;194:642–7. https://doi.org/10.1097/00000658-198111000-00015.
54. Okahara K, Kambayashi J, Shibuya T, Kawasaki T, Sakon M, Dohi Y, et al. An infection-resistant PTFE vascular graft; spiral coiling of the graft with ofloxacin-bonded PTFE thread. Eur J Vasc Endovasc Surg. 1995;9:408–14. https://doi.org/10.1016/s1078-5884(05)80008-5.
55. Webb LX, Myers RT, Cordell AR, Hobgood CD, Costerton JW, Gristina AG. Inhibition of bacterial adhesion by antibacterial surface pretreatment of vascular prostheses. J Vasc Surg. 1986;4:16–21.
56. Shue WB, Worosilo SC, Donetz AP, Trooskin SZ, Harvey RA, Greco RS. Prevention of vascular prosthetic infection with an antibiotic-bonded Dacron graft. J Vasc Surg. 1988;8:600–5.
57. Moore WS, Chvapil M, Seiffert G, Keown K. Development of an infection-resistant vascular prosthesis. Arch Surg. 1981;116:1403–7. https://doi.org/10.1001/archsurg.1981.01380230027004.
58. Sobinsky KR, Flanigan DP. Antibiotic binding to polytetrafluoroethylene via glucosaminoglycan-keratin luminal coating. Surgery. 1986;100:629–34.
59. Phaneuf MD, Ozaki CK, Bide MJ, Quist WC, Alessi JM, Tannenbaum GA, et al. Application of the quinolone antibiotic ciprofloxacin to Dacron utilizing textile dyeing technology. J Biomed Mater Res. 1993;27:233–7. https://doi.org/10.1002/jbm.820270213.
60. Ozaki CK, Phaneuf MD, Bide MJ, Quist WC, Alessi JM, LoGerfo FW. In vivo testing of an infection-resistant vascular graft material. J Surg Res. 1993;55:543–7. https://doi.org/10.1006/jsre.1993.1181.
61. Ney AL, Kelly PH, Tsukayama DT, Bubrick MP. Fibrin glue-antibiotic suspension in the prevention of prosthetic graft infection. J Trauma. 1990;30:1000–5; discussion 5–6. https://doi.org/10.1097/00005373-199008000-00009.
62. Shenk JS, Ney AL, Tsukayama DT, Olson ME, Bubrick MP. Tobramycin-adhesive in preventing and treating PTFE vascular graft infections. J Surg Res. 1989;47:487–92. https://doi.org/10.1016/0022-4804(89)90125-x.
63. Haverich A, Hirt S, Karck M, Siclari F, Wahlig H. Prevention of graft infection by bonding of gentamycin to Dacron prostheses. J Vasc Surg. 1992;15:187–93. https://doi.org/10.1067/mva.1992.30301.
64. Turnidge J, Grayson ML. Optimum treatment of staphylococcal infections. Drugs. 1993;45:353–66. https://doi.org/10.2165/00003495-199345030-00004.
65. Farr B, Mandell GL. Rifampin. Med Clin North Am. 1982;66:157–68. https://doi.org/10.1016/s0025-7125(16)31449-3.
66. Powell TW, Burnham SJ, Johnson G Jr. A passive system using rifampin to create an infection-resistant vascular prosthesis. Surgery. 1983;94:765–9.

67. McDougal EG, Burnham SJ, Johnson G Jr. Rifampin protection against experimental graft sepsis. J Vasc Surg. 1986;4:5–7. https://doi.org/10.1067/mva.1986.avs0040005.
68. Avramovic JR, Fletcher JP. Rifampicin impregnation of a protein-sealed Dacron graft: an infection-resistant prosthetic vascular graft. Aust N Z J Surg. 1991;61:436–40. https://doi.org/10.1111/j.1445-2197.1991.tb00258.x.
69. Chervu A, Moore WS, Gelabert HA, Colburn MD, Chvapil M. Prevention of graft infection by use of prostheses bonded with a rifampin/collagen release system. J Vasc Surg. 1991;14:521–4; discussion 4–5.
70. Chervu A, Moore WS, Chvapil M, Henderson T. Efficacy and duration of antistaphylococcal activity comparing three antibiotics bonded to Dacron vascular grafts with a collagen release system. J Vasc Surg. 1991;13:897–901. https://doi.org/10.1067/mva.1991.27349.
71. Goëau-Brissonnière O, Leport C, Bacourt F, Lebrault C, Comte R, Pechère JC. Prevention of vascular graft infection by rifampin bonding to a gelatin-sealed Dacron graft. Ann Vasc Surg. 1991;5:408–12. https://doi.org/10.1007/bf02133043.
72. Lachapelle K, Graham AM, Symes JF. Antibacterial activity, antibiotic retention, and infection resistance of a rifampin-impregnated gelatin-sealed Dacron graft. J Vasc Surg. 1994;19:675–82. https://doi.org/10.1016/s0741-5214(94)70041-9.
73. Gahtan V, Esses GE, Bandyk DF, Nelson RT, Dupont E, Mills JL. Antistaphylococcal activity of rifampin-bonded gelatin-impregnated Dacron grafts. J Surg Res. 1995;58:105–10. https://doi.org/10.1006/jsre.1995.1017.
74. Sardelic F, Ao PY, Taylor DA, Fletcher JP. Prophylaxis against Staphylococcus epidermidis vascular graft infection with rifampicin-soaked, gelatin-sealed Dacron. Cardiovasc Surg. 1996;4:389–92. https://doi.org/10.1016/0967-2109(95)00075-5.
75. Fletcher JP, Avramovic JR, Kenny J, Sardelic F. Increased resistance to staphylococcal graft infection by rifampicin impregnation of gelatin sealed Dacron. In: Chang JB, editor. Modern vascular surgery, vol. 6. New York: Springer; 1994. p. 483–7.
76. Vicaretti M, Hawthorne W, Ao PY, Fletcher JP. Does in situ replacement of a staphylococcal infected vascular graft with a rifampicin impregnated gelatin sealed Dacron graft reduce the incidence of subsequent infection? Int Angiol. 2000;19:158–65.
77. Tabaja H, Chesdachai S, Shah AS, Stevens RW, DeMartino RR, Erben YM, et al. Fostering collaborative teamwork—a comprehensive approach to vascular graft infection following arterial reconstructive surgery. Clin Infect Dis. 2024;78:e69–80. https://doi.org/10.1093/cid/ciae150.
78. Halim RA, Challita C, Omeirat N, Kanafani ZA. Vascular graft infections: updates on a challenging problem. Infect Dis Clin N Am. 2024;38:657–71. https://doi.org/10.1016/j.idc.2024.07.003.
79. Curl GR, Ricotta JJ. Total prosthetic graft excision and extra-anatomic bypass. In: Calligaro KD, Veith FJ, editors. Management of infected arterial grafts. St Louis: Quality Medical Publishing Incorporated; 1994. p. 82–94.
80. Calligaro KD, Veith FJ, Schwartz ML, Savarese RP, Goldsmith J, Westcott CJ, et al. Management of infected lower extremity autologous vein grafts by selective graft preservation. Am J Surg. 1992;164:291–4. https://doi.org/10.1016/s0002-9610(05)81090-6.
81. Dosluoglu HH, Loghmanee C, Lall P, Cherr GS, Harris LM, Dryjski ML. Management of early (<30 day) vascular groin infections using vacuum-assisted closure alone without muscle flap coverage in a consecutive patient series. J Vasc Surg. 2010;51:1160–6. https://doi.org/10.1016/j.jvs.2009.11.053.
82. Fletcher JP, Dryden M, Sorrell TC. Infection of vascular prostheses. Aust N Z J Surg. 1991;61:432–5. https://doi.org/10.1111/j.1445-2197.1991.tb00257.x.
83. Oderich GS, Bower TC, Hofer J, Kalra M, Duncan AA, Wilson JW, et al. In situ rifampin-soaked grafts with omental coverage and antibiotic suppression are durable with low reinfection rates in patients with aortic graft enteric erosion or fistula. J Vasc Surg. 2011;53:99–106. https://doi.org/10.1016/j.jvs.2010.08.018.
84. Braithwaite BD, Davies B, Heather BP, Earnshaw JJ. Early results of a randomized trial of rifampicin-bonded Dacron grafts for extra-anatomic vascular reconstruction. Joint Vascular

Research Group. Br J Surg. 1998;85:1378–81. https://doi.org/10.1046/j.1365-2168.1998.00878.x.
85. Haidar GM, Hicks TD, Strosberg DS, El-Sayed HF, Davies MG. "In situ" endografting in the treatment of arterial and graft infections. J Vasc Surg. 2017;65:1824–9. https://doi.org/10.1016/j.jvs.2016.12.134.
86. Capoccia L, Mestres G, Riambau V. Current technology for the treatment of infection following abdominal aortic aneurysm (AAA) fixation by endovascular repair (EVAR). J Cardiovasc Surg. 2014;55:381–9.
87. Heyer KS, Modi P, Morasch MD, Matsumura JS, Kibbe MR, Pearce WH, et al. Secondary infections of thoracic and abdominal aortic endografts. J Vasc Interv Radiol. 2009;20:173–9. https://doi.org/10.1016/j.jvir.2008.10.032.
88. O'Connor S, Andrew P, Batt M, Becquemin JP. A systematic review and meta-analysis of treatments for aortic graft infection. J Vasc Surg. 2006;44:38–45.e8. https://doi.org/10.1016/j.jvs.2006.02.053.
89. Antonopoulos CN, Papakonstantinou NA, Hardy D, Lyden SP. Editor's choice – Cryopreserved allografts for arterial reconstruction after aorto-iliac infection: a systematic review and meta-analysis. Eur J Vasc Endovasc Surg. 2019;58:120–8. https://doi.org/10.1016/j.ejvs.2019.03.003.
90. Post IC, Vos CG. Systematic review and meta analysis on the management of open abdominal aortic graft infections. Eur J Vasc Endovasc Surg. 2019;58:258–81. https://doi.org/10.1016/j.ejvs.2019.03.013.
91. Gavali H, Mani K, Furebring M, Olsson KW, Lindström D, Sörelius K, et al. Editor's choice – Outcome of radical surgical treatment of abdominal aortic graft and endograft infections comparing extra-anatomic bypass with in situ reconstruction: a nationwide multicentre study. Eur J Vasc Endovasc Surg. 2021;62:918–26. https://doi.org/10.1016/j.ejvs.2021.09.033.
92. Batt M, Feugier P, Camou F, Coffy A, Senneville E, Caillon J, et al. A meta-analysis of outcomes after in situ reconstructions for aortic graft infection. Angiology. 2018;69:370–9. https://doi.org/10.1177/0003319717710114.
93. Torsello G, Sandmann W, Gehrt A, Jungblut RM. In situ replacement of infected vascular prostheses with rifampin-soaked vascular grafts: early results. J Vasc Surg. 1993;17:768–73. https://doi.org/10.1067/mva.1993.40229.
94. Naylor AR, Clark S, London NJ, Sayers RD, Macpherson DS, Barrie WW. Treatment of major aortic graft infection: preliminary experience with total graft excision and in situ replacement with a rifampicin bonded prosthesis. Eur J Vasc Endovasc Surg. 1995;9:252–6. https://doi.org/10.1016/s1078-5884(05)80101-7.
95. Wyss TR, Giardini M, Sörelius K. Infective native aortic aneurysm: a Delphi consensus document on treatment, follow up, and definition of cure. Eur J Vasc Endovasc Surg. 2024;67:654–61. https://doi.org/10.1016/j.ejvs.2023.12.008.
96. Sörelius K, Wanhainen A, Furebring M, Björck M, Gillgren P, Mani K. Nationwide study of the treatment of mycotic abdominal aortic aneurysms comparing open and endovascular repair. Circulation. 2016;134:1822–32. https://doi.org/10.1161/CIRCULATIONAHA.116.024021.
97. Wanhainen A, Van Herzeele I, Goncalves FB, Montoya SB, Berard X, Boyle JR, et al. Editor's choice – European Society for Vascular Surgery (ESVS) 2024 clinical practice guidelines on the management of abdominal aorto-iliac artery aneurysms. Eur J Vasc Endovasc Surg. 2024;67:192–331. https://doi.org/10.1016/j.ejvs.2023.11.002.
98. Li HL, Chan YC, Cheng SW. Current evidence on management of aortic stent-graft infection: a systematic review and meta-analysis. Ann Vasc Surg. 2018;51:306–13. https://doi.org/10.1016/j.avsg.2018.02.038.

Key References

Anagnostopoulos A, Mayer F, Ledergerber B, Bergadà-Pijuan J, Husmann L, Mestres CA, et al. Editor's choice – Validation of the Management of Aortic Graft Infection Collaboration (MAGIC) criteria for the diagnosis of vascular graft/endograft infection: results from the prospective Vascular Graft Cohort study. Eur J Vasc Endovasc Surg. 2021;62:251–7. https://doi.org/10.1016/j.ejvs.2021.05.010.

Chakfé N, Diener H, Lejay A, Assadian O, Berard X, Caillon J, et al. Editor's choice – European Society for Vascular Surgery (ESVS) 2020 clinical practice guidelines on the management of vascular graft and endograft infections. Eur J Vasc Endovasc Surg. 2020;59:339–84. https://doi.org/10.1016/j.ejvs.2019.10.016.

Haidar GM, Hicks TD, Strosberg DS, El-Sayed HF, Davies MG. "In situ" endografting in the treatment of arterial and graft infections. J Vasc Surg. 2017;65:1824–9. https://doi.org/10.1016/j.jvs.2016.12.134.

Kahl BC, Becker K, Löfflerb B. Clinical significance and pathogenesis of staphylococcal small colony variants in persistent infections. Clin Microbiol Rev. 2016;29:401–27. https://doi.org/10.1128/cmr.00069-15.

Langenberg CM, Kluytmans JA, De Groot HG, Ho GW, Veen EJ, Buimer MG, et al. Surgical site and graft infections in endovascular and open abdominal aortic aneurysm surgery. Surg Infect (Larchmt). 2018;19:424–9. https://doi.org/10.1089/sur.2017.302.

Li HL, Chan YC, Cheng SW. Current evidence on management of aortic stent-graft infection: a systematic review and meta-analysis. Ann Vasc Surg. 2018;51:306–13. https://doi.org/10.1016/j.avsg.2018.02.038.

Lyons O, Baguneid M, Barwick T, Bell R, Foster N, Homer-Vanniasinkam S, et al. Diagnosis of aortic graft infection: a case definition by the Management of Aortic Graft Infection Collaboration (MAGIC). Eur J Vasc Endovasc Surg. 2016;52:758–63. https://doi.org/10.1016/j.ejvs.2016.09.007.

Rabin N, Zheng Y, Opoku-Temeng C, Du Y, Bonsu E, Sintim HO. Biofilm formation mechanisms and targets for developing antibiofilm agents. Future Med Chem. 2015;7:493–512. https://doi.org/10.4155/fmc.15.6.

Chapter 13
Radiation Physics and Biological Effects of Radiation in Vascular Surgery

Joseph Dawson and Stephan Haulon

SN Flashcards
Test your learning and check your understanding of this book's contents: use the "Springer Nature Flashcards" app to access questions using ▶ https://sn.pub/wppvze. To use the app, please follow the instructions in Chap. 1.

Key Learning Points

- X-Rays used in endovascular procedures are a form of electromagnetic radiation with high energy and short wavelength, enabling penetration of tissue but also carrying the risk of ionisation and cellular damage.
- The use of radiation in medicine has increased significantly, making it the largest man-made source of radiation exposure for the general population.
- Scatter radiation, generated by X-ray interaction with tissue, is the primary source of radiation exposure for the interventionalist and can be minimised by distance, shielding and technique.
- Radiation dose is measured in various ways, including absorbed dose (Gy), Integral dose (Gy), equivalent dose (Sv), effective dose (Sv), air kerma (Gy) and

J. Dawson (✉)
Vascular and Endovascular Service, Royal Adelaide Hospital, and Discipline of Surgery, Adelaide University, Adelaide, South Australia
e-mail: joseph.dawson@adelaide.edu.au

S. Haulon
Department of Vascular Surgery—Aortic Centre Hospital Marie Lannelongue, University Paris-Sud, Paris, France
e-mail: s.haulon@hml.fr

R. Fitridge et al. (eds.), *Pathophysiology of Vascular Disease*,
https://doi.org/10.1007/978-3-032-31459-8_13

dose area product (Gy-cm^2), each reflecting different aspects of radiation interaction and biological effect.

- Cumulative Air Kerma (CAK) is a practical measure of radiation exposure during fluoroscopy, closely related to Peak Skin Dose (PSD) and useful for estimating the risk of deterministic effects (e.g. Skin burns).
- Dose Area Product (DAP) reflects the total energy imparted to the patient, providing an estimate of stochastic risk and allowing comparison of radiation doses across different procedures.
- Deterministic effects of radiation, such as skin burns and cataracts, have a threshold dose and increase in severity with higher exposures.
- Stochastic effects, primarily cancer and genetic mutations, are considered to have no threshold, and their probability increases with radiation dose, following the linear no-threshold model.
- Obesity significantly increases radiation dose to both patients and operators due to increased tissue attenuation and the automatic brightness control (ABC) of the X-ray machine.
- Vascular Surgeons are at risk of occupational radiation exposure, particularly to the eyes (cataracts) and potentially to the brain, emphasising the importance of consistent use of protective measures.
- The ALARA principles (As Low As Reasonably Achievable) should guide all radiation-related practices in the interventional suite to minimise both patient and operator exposure.
- Individual genetic susceptibility to radiation injury varies, highlighting the need for consistent adherence to radiation safety protocols for all personnel.

13.1 A Brief History of Radiation Use in Vascular Surgery

13.1.1 The Discovery of Radiation

X-rays were first discovered by Wilhelm Conrad Roentgen in Germany in 1895 when he discovered the emission of a ray from a cathode-ray tube that passed through heavy black paper shielding [1]. One of the first images using this discovery was the now-famous picture of his wife's hand. The interest in uptake of this exciting new technology was unsurprising, and within 6 months, a direct medical utility was born with radiographs being used on the battlefield to help locate bullets in wounded soldiers [1].

Concurrently, Henri Becquerel discovered another form of penetrating rays produced by uranium, which was radioactivity. His work was complemented and expanded by Marie Curie, and together they won the Nobel Prize for Physics in 1903 [1]. The concurrent discoveries of X-rays and radioactivity led to a new aspect of health care. There was initially no concern regarding any potential harmful effects due to the apparent similarity of these X-rays to harmless light and the delayed onset of symptoms [1]. However, as early as 2 years after radiation was discovered, some of these early pioneers reported what we now know were radiation-induced injuries due to overexposure: skin burns, pigmentations, eye irritations, ulceration, hair loss, limb loss and even death [2], most noticeably Marie Curie dying from aplastic anaemia [3]. Further realisation that X-rays and gamma rays, whilst similar to light in that they are electromagnetic waves, have much shorter wavelengths, which led to the understanding that, with much higher inherent energy, they could penetrate material that light cannot. The disadvantage of this additional energy was the propensity to alter and break chemical bonds in tissues and cells, leading to radiation-induced injury [1].

13.1.2 Endovascular Pioneers

A handful of events occurred in the early and mid-twentieth century that contributed to the inception of endovascular surgery, with the true revolution occurring in the latter two decades of the century. In 1920, Dos Santos performed the first angiogram, and in 1953, the Seldinger technique was developed, allowing safe percutaneous access to vessels [4, 5]. Towards the end of the 1950s, Thomas Fogarty invented the first minimally invasive endovascular device, the embolectomy catheter, which gained popularity during the 1960s. In 1964, Dotter performed the first percutaneous transluminal angioplasty [6], but this was not widely accepted by surgeons and remained limited to use by radiologists. In 1978, Andreas Grüntzig, a Swiss cardiologist, published his first series of cases of percutaneous transluminal angioplasty (PTA) of the coronary vessels using a balloon he had developed. In 1985, Julio Palmaz, an Argentinian radiologist, introduced stenting to complement PTA, which really 'lit the fuse' for the endovascular revolution [5]. One of his large Palmaz stents was used as the proximal segment in the first widely publicised endovascular repair of an abdominal aortic aneurysm (EVAR), performed in 1990 by fellow Argentinian vascular surgeon, Juan Parodi [7]. However, behind the Iron Curtain, similar innovations had been occurring, with the Ukrainian cardiovascular surgeon Nicolai Volodos using his stent delivery system in the common iliacs in 1985, leading to the first ever EVAR in 1987 [8]. New technology followed thereafter to advance these concepts, and by the late 1990s, all of the elements were in place for the endovascular explosion [5].

13.1.3 Exposure to Medical Radiation

13.1.3.1 General Population

With at least two-thirds of all medical imaging involving ionising radiation [9], it now represents the greatest man-made source of ionising radiation to the general population [10]. In 1980, medical radiation only contributed 15% all-cause radiation exposure per capita, but by 2006, this had risen to 48% [9]. In 1987, the estimated total annual medical radiation exposure per person was 0.6 milliSieverts (mSv), but by 2006, this had risen to 3.2 mSv, representing a fivefold increase [11] and overtaking the natural background dose per person of 3.0 mSv per year [11]. This is the equivalent of 150 chest X-rays for every member of the population [11].

The causes for this pattern are multifactorial:

1. Modern medicine has a growing reliance on imaging technology [2].
2. Higher radiation doses usually accompany advances in medical imaging, for example, abdominal CT delivers 500 times the radiation of a routine CXR and multiphase scans routinely double that [2].
3. Radiation doses for the same scan can vary considerably among institutions, and even within the same institution [12].
4. Many investigations are not medically justified, with 30% of CT examinations thought to be unnecessary [2].
5. Medical personnel seriously underestimate the radiation dose attributable to CT scans, and their association with increased lifetime risk of cancer [13].

This poses a real risk to individual patients, with an estimated 1.5–2.0% of all cancers in the USA potentially being attributable to the radiation from CT scans [13]. It also increases the risk to occupationally exposed medical workers [11], who now have a similar radiation hazard to those working in the nuclear industry [14].

13.1.3.2 Vascular Patients

Vascular patients, and particularly those undergoing endovascular aortic repairs, demand particular mention. These patients often undergo multiple and repeated studies [2] comprising pre-operative diagnostic investigations including CT scans, nuclear stress tests and coronary interventions [2, 15, 16], complex prolonged procedures [17], multiple reinterventions [17] and often prolonged CT follow-up [15–17]. All of these modalities can help establish accurate diagnosis, stratify operative risk, reduce the risk of vascular interventions and evaluate post-operative success [2]. However, the benefits of these medical procedures must outweigh any potential risk from the attendant radiation [2]. Cumulative radiation dose needs to be seriously considered in such patients, as their cancer risk is not insignificant [16], cancer being the second most common cause of death in EVAR patients [10]. The challenge remains to definitively link medical radiation exposure to cancer risk in these patients, as everyone is exposed to not insignificant background radiation, and radiation-induced illnesses have a long lead time [11].

The considerable radiation dose delivered at the time of endovascular aortic repair pales in significance compared to that received during routine follow-up with CT [18]. Surveillance scans in the first year exceed the radiation dose during EVAR (15 mSv vs. 12.6 mSv) [19]. One study calculated the contribution of follow-up CT after TEVAR to the patient's total radiation exposure associated with the procedure over a 5-year period (pre-op work-up, the procedure itself and post-op surveillance)

[20]. They found that the follow-up CT surveillance alone contributed to 87% of the total radiation exposure after 1 year, 92% at 5 years and 96% in a lifetime [20]. These calculations suggest that a 2-year radiation exposure of >100 mSv with a life expectancy of >15 years leads to a lifetime risk of radiation-induced leukaemia and solid tumour malignancy of greater than 2.7% [20]. The lifetime cancer risk for a 70-year-old undergoing EVAR followed by conventional CT surveillance is 0.6%, and for a 50-year old, this rises to 1.0% [21]. When considering a young patient for open repair versus EVAR, it has been suggested that the patient's lifetime attributable risk of cancer associated with lifelong surveillance and reinterventions should contribute the same weight to the decision-making and consent process as do anatomy and durability [15, 22]. Once the need to perform endovascular repair has been duly justified, the true need for follow-up with CT needs to be justified [18], with consideration of other options such as a minimised-dose 'light' protocol, or use of plain or contrast-enhanced ultrasound [22].

These risks could be better managed if the cumulative radiation dose of patients was routinely monitored [2]. An electronic national registry documenting and recording radiation doses for every medical procedure using ionising radiation has been suggested [10]. Dose information tracking systems have been developed to incorporate into institutions' IT systems, performing statistical analysis and sending alerts to medical staff [23].

13.2 Radiation Physics, Measurements, Dosimetry and Units

13.2.1 X-Rays

X-rays are a form of electromagnetic radiation (EMR) lying on a spectrum with light, radio waves and microwaves. What characterises these various forms of radiation are their wavelength and frequency; the shorter the wavelength, the greater the frequency and also the greater amount of energy they carry [24]. X-rays have a short wavelength and therefore carry a high amount of energy, which is why they can penetrate material, including tissue.

X-rays are produced by a cathode-ray tube when high-speed electrons strike a solid target and rapidly decelerate, releasing energy [25]. Energy is carried through space in a bundle of energy, or a packet, called a photon [24]. Photons travel at the speed of light and carry no mass or charge [11]. Their electromagnetic energy can range from a few electron volts (eV) to millions of eV and is set by the voltage applied across the X-ray tube. The ranges typically found in fluoroscopy have a photon energy spectrum of 30–140 keV, the higher the keV, the higher the X-ray energy [11].

What differentiates X-rays (ionising radiation) from other forms of EMR (non-ionising radiation) is their ability to displace an outer electron from an atom when they collide with it (ionisation). Non-ionising radiation, such as light and microwaves, only has enough energy to move electrons to a higher energy state without actually displacing them [24].

The other type of radiation is particulate, a non-EMR form in which small particles, such as electrons, carry both mass and energy. This is the form of radiation produced by radioactive materials and linear accelerators and doesn't have a role in diagnostic imaging, as commonly used forms have limited ability to penetrate matter [24].

13.2.2 Interaction with the Body

When X-rays interact with the body, they are absorbed, either completely or partially. This degree of energy transfer to the tissues, or absorption, not only accounts for the difference in transparency of the subsequent shadow image obtained from various tissue densities, but also the radiation 'dose' delivered to the patient [23]. This dose is related to the photons that enter but do not leave the body [25]. If the energy transferred is large enough, or cumulative, it can cause DNA and tissue damage.

The energy exchange in this process is due to the loss of energy from the photon and increased motion in the ejected electron. If the photon is not extinguished from this interaction, it can continue to travel, but at a lower energy. This weakened photon is known as scatter radiation and may collide with further tissue, potentially ionising them as well, until either all of its energy is used up or it escapes into the environment.

13.2.3 Scatter Radiation and the Inverse Square Law

X-rays that enter a patient from the primary beam can either be fully absorbed by the body, pass straight through the patient, or be partially absorbed by the tissues and change direction. These X-rays that exit the patient after changing direction are known as 'scatter' radiation, with the highest level occurring at the entry point of the patient's skin. Although scatter causes blurring of the image, of far greater consequence is that it comprises the main source of radiation to the operator and staff, and controlling patient dose generally reduces scatter and subsequent operator doses [23, 26]. Scatter is affected by many variables, including beam size, large distances between the X-ray source and the image intensifier, patient BMI, gantry angulation, fluoroscopy and acquisition settings [26]. Most of these factors, and therefore scatter radiation production, are controllable by the interventionalist, and their effect on reducing radiation exposure will be explained in Chap. 14.

Scatter is the reason why fluoroscopy machines are set up with the primary source positioned under the patient (posteroanterior imaging) [27]. This results in scatter being deflected towards the legs of the operator, an area that is less susceptible to radiation than the torso, head and neck, and easier to protect with lead drapes

[28]. With an anteroposterior set-up, the head, neck and upper body exposure would be approximately four times greater where shielding is less effective [27].

As these scattered X-rays leave the body, they travel in straight, but divergent directions. With an increase in distance, there is an exponential decrease in the number of photons per unit area and hence energy; doubling the distance from the X-ray source decreases exposure by a factor of 4, tripling the distance results in a reduction by a factor of 9. This 'inverse square law' ($X = 1/d^2$, X = exposure, d = distance) has a simple yet profound impact on radiation safety and is a cornerstone in reducing radiation exposure, namely increasing the distance between yourself and the X-ray source [3, 24]. It is important to stress that maximising distance between operator and source is a fundamental principle of radiation safety behaviour, but it must also be appreciated that the inverse square law pertains to radiation in a vacuum. The interaction of the radiation beam on solid structures within a working vascular suite has a profound effect on this otherwise formulaic scatter pattern, producing an eccentric 'scatter cloud' which is less easy to predict [29].

13.2.4 Measuring Radiation Dose

Radiation dose is the quantity of radiation that an exposed tissue absorbs. Therefore, understanding how radiation dose is measured is fundamental to good Radiation Stewardship. Unfortunately, there are many factors that make radiation dosimetry difficult to comprehend. These include (i) two different nomenclature systems (conventional and International System of Units (IS)); (ii) no direct way to measure radiation absorption in the body; (iii) several surrogate methods for estimating dose; (iv) terms such as exposure and dose are often used interchangeably in the literature without specific meanings; (v) different units used to describe the radiation exposure for the same procedure making comparisons between studies challenging [10, 11]. The following section aims to clarify radiation dose calculations.

13.2.4.1 Conceptual, Direct and Indirect Measurements

Radiation dose terminology can be best understood by categorising it in the following manner:

1. Conceptual Measurements: Those that are impossible or difficult to measure (Absorbed dose, Integral dose, Equivalent dose, Effective Dose).
2. Direct Measurements: Possible to measure but labour-intensive and not real-time (Peak Skin Dose).
3. Indirect Measurements: Used in daily practice but are surrogates of the above and therefore have limitations (Cumulative Air Kerma, Dose Area Product and Fluoroscopy Time).

Patient radiation dose is most accurately evaluated by the direct measurement of radiation exposure. For deterministic risks (e.g. skin burns), this is best estimated by Peak Skin Dose (PSD), and for stochastic risks (e.g. cancer), this is best estimated by Effective Dose (ED). However, these conceptual or direct measurements are either impossible or impractical for everyday practice, labour-intensive and not real-time [23]. Therefore, a range of indirect measurements (e.g. Cumulative Air Kerma (CAK) and Dose Area Product (DAP)) have been developed as surrogates to measure radiation exposure and estimate these risks. PSD and ED can then be calculated from these indirect measurements using equations [30]. The advantage of indirect measurements is the provision of real-time data allowing pragmatic monitoring during a procedure [23], but due to their indirect nature, they have potential for considerable error [18]. In a study comparing direct and indirect measures during complex aortic repairs, the authors found that even though indirect measures (CAK and DAP) correlated reasonably with direct measures (PSD), they were higher than direct measurements, giving rise to three sentinel threshold events of >15 Gy, which were well below this threshold on direct measurement [18].

13.2.4.2 Medical Radiation Units

Gray (Gy)
SI unit for radiation absorbed by a mass of tissue
1 Gy = 1 J/kg = 1 joule of energy deposited in 1 kg of irradiated tissue

Radiation Absorbed Dose (rad)
Legacy unit for radiation absorbed dose—now superseded by SI unit Gy
1 rad = 0.01 Gy = 0.01 J/kg

Sievert (Sv)
SI unit for biological risk of absorbed dose according to specific radiation type (Equivalent Dose) and tissue susceptibility (Effective Dose)
1 Sv = 1 Gy (for medical radiation)

Roentgen Equivalent in Man (rem)
Legacy unit for biological risk of absorbed dose—now superseded by SI unit Sv
1 rem = 0.01 Sv

13.2.4.3 Conceptual Measurements

Absorbed Dose (Gray (Gy))

This is the concentration of energy deposited by radiation into the absorbing tissue and gives an index of the potential biological risk [25]. Only a fraction of the radiation energy that reaches the body is absorbed, depending on the tissue's mass, composition, type of radiation and exposure time [31]. Whilst 1 Gy represents a relatively small dose in terms of energy deposition (it would only raise the temperature of water by 0.00024 °C), the effects of this energy transfer on biological functions are complex and can be deleterious [23]. It is the concentration of energy deposited, not the total amount deposited. Not all the radiation that tissues are exposed to is absorbed; some will pass through without imparting any energy (thus producing an X-ray image) whilst some is deflected, thus imparting smaller amounts of energy [11]. In this way, absorbed dose differs from exposure in that the radiation present at a given location will not deposit all of its energy there [11]. This is dependent on the energy of the radiation, the tissue type and depth from the skin [11].

Integral Dose (Gray (Gy))

The 'Integral Dose' is the cumulative dose absorbed by all the tissues corresponding to the amount of potential tissue damage. It is extrapolated from exposure because there is no way to measure radiation absorption in the body [24].

Equivalent Dose (Sievert (Sv))

Different forms of radiation have different tissue-injuring potential, some causing more biological damage than others [24]. The Equivalent Dose concept allows the biological effects of different forms of radiation to be compared with each other. Equivalent Dose is calculated by multiplying the Absorbed Dose (in Gy) by a weighting factor (W_R) specific to each form of radiation. Fortunately, X-rays have a W_R of 1, so from the point of view of medical radiation (X-rays and gamma rays), the Equivalent Dose and the Absorbed Dose are equal, with 1 Sievert being equivalent to 1 Gray [11, 24, 25]. The Equivalent Dose is more useful when assessing for potential tissue injury due to highly ionising particles such as alpha particles, protons and neutrons, rather than X-rays, gamma radiation and electrons.

Effective Dose (Sievert (Sv))

In the same way that various forms of radiation have different capacities for biological damage, different tissues and organs have different sensitivities to radiation damage. In addition, radiation exposure is not uniform. Some organs and tissues receive more than others [11]. The Effective Dose (ED) for a particular organ is calculated by taking the Equivalent Dose and multiplying it by a specific tissue weighting factor (W_T) for that organ [24]. The W_T relates to the organ's specific susceptibility to cancer and genetic defects as a result of radiation exposure. For example, the W_T for the breast (0.12) is 10 times higher than that for the brain (0.01) [23]. The potential stochastic (see Sect. 13.3.3) risk contributions from all the various exposed organs are then added to calculate a whole-body risk, expressed as the Effective Dose [11]. In this way, the effective dose is a measure of the estimated potential for a biological effect on the whole body caused by a particular absorbed radiation dose [11]. It is a hypothetical uniform whole-body dose that confers the same stochastic risk as the non-uniform regional dose actually delivered and estimates the radiation dose's contribution to stochastic risk [11, 18]. In this way, it reflects the overall biological risk from radiation to an average person from a specific radiation exposure scenario [11]. The effective dose provides the same whole-person stochastic risk as an absorbed dose for a limited portion of the body; it allows comparison of the risk among several individuals regardless of the body areas irradiated [25].

Advantages of Effective Dose [18, 30]:

- Accounts for the portion of the body exposed
- Accurate reflection of stochastic risk

Disadvantages of Effective Dose [18, 30]:

- Impossible to measure or calculate; can only be estimated
- No real-time assessment
- Cannot predict radiation risk for an individual due to the nature of stochastic risk

13.2.4.4 Direct Measurements

Peak Skin Dose (Gray (Gy))

The 'Peak Skin Dose' (PSD) refers to the maximally irradiated area (including both primary beam and scatter) in a defined skin area [23]. PSD is measured using thermoluminescent dosimeters (TLDs), radiochromic film (Gafchromic™) or optically stimulated luminescence dosimeters (OSLDs) [23].

Advantages of Peak Skin Dose

- A reliable direct measurement of specific points of interest at the most irradiated area [18]
- Directly attributable to deterministic effects [10, 30]

Disadvantages of Peak Skin Dose

- Expensive and labour-intensive to measure using radiochromic film [10, 18, 30]
- Not real-time, therefore usually used only for research purposes [18, 32]

13.2.4.5 Indirect Measurements

Cumulative Air Kerma at the Interventional Reference Point (CAK) (Gray (Gy))

Also known as:

- *Cumulative Air Kerma*
- *Cumulative Dose*

Air Kerma at the Reference Point (Gray (Gy))

Also known as:

- *Reference Air Kerma (RAK)*
- *Reference Point Air Kerma (RPAK)*
- *Entrance Surface Dose*
- *Entrance Skin Dose*

CAK is used to assess the quantity of external radiation at a constant distance from the patient [11]. 'Kerma' describes 'Kinetic Energy Released in MAtter' [25]; i.e. the amount of energy released by the interaction of radiation with a unit mass of absorbing material. 'Air Kerma' refers to the amount of energy released if the absorbing material is 1 kg of air [11]. The 'Interventional Reference Point' (IRP) is where in space 'Air Kerma' is measured in relation to the patient, and it approximates the point where the X-rays reach the patient's skin. The IRP is a constant position fixed along the central ray of the X-ray beam at a distance of 15 cm towards the X-ray tube side of the isocentre of the C-arm [25]. Therefore, the 'Air Kerma at the IRP' provides an index of the dose reaching the skin and the risk of skin injury. In this way, the 'Air Kerma at the IRP' is also known as the 'Entrance Surface Dose', or more commonly the 'Entrance Skin Dose' [25]. The Air Kerma accumulates at a specific point (the reference point) in space relative to the fluoroscopy gantry. As the gantry rotates, the reference point will change over the full surface of a 15 cm radius sphere representing a 30 cm diameter patient. The Cumulative Air Kerma (CAK) is the sum of all the energy liberated in air at the IRP during the whole procedure. It can be appreciated that during a procedure where the C-arm remains static (e.g. cardiac catheterisation), the beam 'Entrance Skin Dose' will approximate well to the area of skin to which the beam is directed. In these situations, the Entrance Skin Dose correlates accurately with the deterministic effects of radiation [32]. However, during procedures where the C-arm is frequently moved (e.g. EVAR), the Entrance Skin Dose may actually be spread over a larger area, so no one point receives the total dose. In order to correct for some of the shortfalls of CAK, manufacturers have developed more sophisticated tools to correct Air Kerma at the IRP to the actual position of the patient, taking into account patient size, system geometry, backscatter and table attenuation. Maps can be displayed of dose distribution in real time, giving a more accurate estimation of deterministic effects [23].

Advantages of Cumulative Air Kerma

- Easy to calculate.
- Easy to interpret.
- Accounts for high-dose acquisitions.
- Best estimation of Peak Skin Dose to monitor deterministic effects [10, 30, 33, 34].
- Provided by most fluoroscopy units.
- Recommended over fluoroscopy time or DAP for high-dose procedures by the National Council on Radiation Protection and Measurements (NCRP) [23].

- Since 2006, real-time display of CAK became mandatory in new systems in the USA [32].

Disadvantages of Cumulative Air Kerma

- Does not represent Entrance Skin Dose if the patient's size or table height results in the IRP being inside or outside of the patient, rather than on the surface.
- Does not account for the area exposed [10, 18].
- Does not account for the patient's location in relation to the C-arm or different beam projections [18].
- Does not account for backscatter from the patient which can increase skin dose by one-third.
- It tends to overestimate deterministic risk compared to direct measures of PSD [23, 34].

Dose Area Product (DAP) (Gray-Centimetre Squared ($Gy.cm^2$))

Also known as:

Kerma Area Product (KAP)

The Dose Area Product (DAP) is the Air Kerma multiplied by the beam cross-sectional area at the point of measurement [25]. One disadvantage of CAK is that it does not take into consideration the area exposed and therefore the volume. Whilst CAK is a good surrogate for dose at the surface, deeper structures receive smaller doses. For every 5 cm of tissue that X-rays pass through, they are attenuated by a factor of 2, thereby decreasing exponentially with depth from the entrance [11]. Therefore, to estimate the dose to a particular body part within the path of an X-ray beam, adjustments need to be made for the beam's absorbance; this is the DAP [11]. The DAP is the cumulative sum of the product of the air kerma and the X-ray cross-sectional beam area. It provides a good measure of the total energy output of the X-ray tube and therefore a good approximation of the total energy absorbed by the patient [25, 35]. In this way, it provides the basis of the estimated effective dose from a procedure [11].

Advantages of Dose Area Product (DAP)

- Modern machines have an integral DAP meter built in with a mandatory real-time display since 2006 [25, 32].
- Correlates to the amount of scatter during a procedure, and therefore the best measure of stochastic risk to staff [3, 25, 30, 34, 35].
- Surrogate measure for the entire amount of energy delivered to the patient and therefore relates to the stochastic risk to the patient [23].
- Widely used, allowing comparisons of doses between procedures and institutions [23].
- Best correlates with Effective Dose and can be used to estimate Effective Dose per organ or anatomical region using conversion factors [23, 30].
- Provides a measure of the efficacy of radiation protection practices within a unit [25].

Disadvantages of Dose Area Product

- Not as intuitive as CAK [30].
- Does not account for different projections [18].
- Estimation of absorbed skin dose can be inaccurate—a large dose delivered to a small area yields the same DAP as a small dose delivered to a large area [16].

Fluoroscopy Time (Minutes (min))

Fluoroscopy time (FT) is the total time the X-ray beam is activated [18, 30]. However, some machines record total pedal time and others total fluoroscopy time, which can differ if using pulsed fluoroscopy, and by variations in pulse rate.

Advantages of Fluoroscopy Time

- Provided by all fluoroscopy units
- Easy to measure and interpret
- Correlates with the complexity of a procedure [23]
- Can be used as a quality assurance tool for assessing the efficiency of an interventionalist at completing a procedure

Disadvantages of Fluoroscopy Time

- Poor correlation to dose, biological risk and clinical outcomes [23].
- Does not account for system settings, field size, dose contributions of various modes such as acquisitions, beam quality [18], output rate, differences in equipment, technique, patient BMI and angulation of gantry [16, 32].
- Ambiguous, as some machines measure total pedal time, others are limited to the sum of X-ray pulses [23, 34].
- Not recommended for routine use unless other parameters are unavailable, or as a correlation with procedural complexity [23].

13.2.4.6 Documenting Dose, Reporting Threshold Limits and Diagnostic Reference Levels

In daily practice, the CAK, DAP and FT should be recorded in the operative report, and this, in turn, should encourage interventionalists to become familiar with their procedural doses. Maximum dose limits have been determined for any single procedure as: CAK >5 Gy, PSD >3 Gy, DAP >500 Gy.cm^2 and FT > 60 min, irrespective of the complexity of intervention [23]. If any of these maximum dose limits are reached in a single case, this should stimulate documentation, prolonged patient follow-up to identify possible deterministic radiation injury, and a review of operator and institutional radiation safety behaviours and systems. Diagnostic Reference Levels (DRLs), on the other hand, differ in that they have been determined for specific diagnostic or interventional procedures and are indicative benchmark doses that are not expected to be exceeded in normal circumstances.

13.3 The Biological Effects of Radiation

13.3.1 Interaction of X-Rays with Tissue

When X-rays enter the body, they can either pass straight through with no interaction, transfer varying degrees of energy to the tissues with a resultant deviation in their path (scatter), or completely transfer all their energy to the tissues (photoelectric effect) [23]. This transfer of energy can form ions within tissues by ejecting electrons from the atoms that make up molecules, which is the basis for the term 'ionising' radiation, and is what differentiates X-rays from most other forms of Electromagnetic Radiation [11]. This process can subsequently modify the chemical, physical or biological effects of the tissues and cause radiation-induced injury in two ways:

1. Direct cellular damage due to molecular alterations, leading to a change in structure and function
2. Indirect cellular damage from hydrolysis of intra-cellular water leading to unstable and highly destructive free radicals which go on and interact with other molecules, proteins or nucleic acids, causing a cascade of injury [10, 11, 23]

The most susceptible cells to damage are immature or dividing cells. At low doses, the body's repair mechanisms can mitigate direct cellular damage and can bind proteins to free radicals, forming stable complexes. However, higher doses overwhelm these repair mechanisms, leading to apoptosis (see "Glossary"), and the resulting clinical manifestations of radiation injury, namely 'deterministic' and 'stochastic' effects [23, 24].

13.3.2 Deterministic Effects

Deterministic effects, also known as tissue reactions, are predictable injuries that will occur in every person subjected to a sufficient radiation dose [11, 25]. Once a threshold dose has been exceeded, cellular death will occur if the molecular damage exceeds the cell's own repair mechanisms. The severity of the injury typically correlates with the exposure in a dose-dependent manner [11, 23], in the same way that sunburn occurs as a result of a threshold of sun exposure, and worsens with increased exposure [34]. Although the corollary is that one is safe from such effects under threshold values, subclinical injury may occur if a sufficient proportion of cells are able to maintain function despite a certain number undergoing necrosis [11]. Another important point is that there may be a significant time lag between the damage occurring and the clinical manifestation of injury. Examples of deterministic injuries include skin burns, hair loss, bone injury, cataracts and infertility [24, 36].

13.3.2.1 Skin Injury

This is the most common deterministic injury and is estimated to occur between 1:10,000 and 1:100,000 examinations [23]. Skin injuries can present as mild skin erythema resembling sunburn and occur hours, days or even weeks after injury [36]. It is probably under-reported due to a combination of factors, including delays in presentation, commonly located on the back, a failure to link burns to previous radiation exposure both by patient and physician and failure to follow-up patients [23, 25]. Typically, radiation-induced skin burns resemble the rectangular shape of the X-ray beam and will be present at the site of beam entrance, usually the back. They present in a spectrum of forms ranging from erythema, hair loss, hyperpigmentation, telangiectasia, desquamation, dermal atrophy and ulceration [11].

Thresholds for skin injury are:

1. <2 Gy; no observed injury.
2. 2–5 Gy; transient temporary erythema.
3. 5–10 Gy; erythema and epilation with dermal atrophy towards 10 Gy.
4. 10–15 Gy; prolonged erythema, possible desquamation, permanent epilation and dermal atrophy.
5. >15 Gy; desquamation, dermal atrophy, ulceration and necrosis of subcutaneous tissues [37].

It must be remembered when treating vascular patients that these thresholds are for single first dose exposures, and repeated doses, especially those in close temporal proximity, may lead to injuries at lower doses than expected, due to inadequate time for DNA repair to occur [23]. The typical patient to suffer a skin injury is a smoking, obese, person with diabetes who has undergone 1 or more long-duration fluoroscopically guided procedures over a period of a few months [11]. Another group at risk of multiple interventions is dialysis patients, with increasing endovascular interventions for dialysis access maintenance [34].

Interestingly, in a study comparing direct versus indirect measures of skin dose during complex aortic repairs, investigators failed to identify any skin changes in half of their cohort that had a measured skin dose >2 Gy [18]. Whilst this is certainly not cause for complacency or lowering of the thresholds, this study does highlight the benefit of distributing the dose over relatively large and varying areas during aortic repairs, compared to coronary procedures, which tend to be more static, leading to a higher Peak Skin Dose in one area.

Additional risk factors for radiation-induced skin injury include obesity, extreme degrees of angulation of the C-arm, connective tissue disorders (scleroderma, systemic lupus erythematosus and ataxia telangiectasia), diabetes, hyperthyroidism and some chemotherapy agents [11, 16, 23, 25, 36]. Extraneous body parts within the radiation field of view, such as limbs, breasts, overlapping skin folds and obesity per se, will all lead to increased radiation dose due to the X-ray machine's Automatic Brightness Control (ABC), thus increasing skin injury risk [32, 36, 38].

The global obesity epidemic demands an appreciation of the profound effect obesity has on elevating both patient skin dose and operator scatter exposure [25, 39]. Due to overlapping skin folds and excess soft tissue, more energy is required to penetrate tissue. Radiation dose decreases by a factor of 2 for every 5 cm travelled in soft tissues; therefore, twice as much radiation is required to penetrate 10 cm of fat than 1 cm [3]. ABC settings force the dose up to obtain an adequate image [3, 15, 35, 40], with subsequent doses reaching 4–10 times higher in obese patients [3, 39]. For example, during EVAR, obese patients received up to 3× PSD [41] and 2× DAP [41, 42] than those with normal BMI, with BMI predicting radiation burden similarly to fluoroscopy time [43].

At the end of a procedure, the CAK should be recorded and used to estimate the patient's entrance skin dose to provide an index of the risk of deterministic effects [25]. Current recommendations suggest that patients receiving >5 Gy CAK should be counselled regarding the possibility of skin injury and followed up closely, in addition to involving institutional and local radiation regulatory authorities [11, 32].

13.3.2.2 Bone Injury

Whilst bone requires a higher dose than skin to undergo necrosis, the calcium content of bone leads to a greater capacity to absorb X-rays and thus a higher absorbed dose than the overlying skin [11]. Occasionally, this may manifest as osteonecrosis of superficial bones such as ribs at doses below those that cause skin necrosis [11].

13.3.2.3 Eye Injury

Unlike skin injuries, cataracts comprise a deterministic effect far more relevant to interventionists than patients. Cataracts describe a permanent clouding of the lens of the eye, which leads to loss of acuity and even sight. They are classified according to their location in the lens: (i) nuclear (centre), (ii) cortical (edge) and (iii) posterior subcapsular (back) [44].

Radiation exposure leads to direct protein and DNA damage, and indirect oxidative stress through free radical generation. The dividing epithelial cells are particularly susceptible and, when damaged, migrate to the posterior of the lens, resulting in opacities.

A higher incidence of cataracts was first noted in atomic bomb survivors, astronauts, radiation workers and radiotherapy patients but more recently has been identified in interventionalists [45]. For example, cardiologists were found to have three times the incidence of posterior subcapsular cataracts (PSC) than matched non-radiation-exposed doctors [45].

Already known to be one of the most radiosensitive tissues, emerging evidence suggests that the lens is much more radiosensitive than previously thought, and thresholds for the development of cataracts are far lower than previously assumed, and in fact may not exist at all [36, 45]. The International Commission on Radiation

Protection (ICRP) has stated that such a threshold is 4 Gy for fractionated exposure, but single-dose thresholds of 0.5 [46] to 1 Gy [36] may be enough to induce cataracts. The delay between exposure and onset of symptoms is many years, making it difficult to determine if they develop as a result of continued accumulation of small doses over time, but the latent period between exposure and formation seems to be inversely related to radiation dose [11].

PSC represents the most common type of radiation-induced cataract, followed by cortical cataract [36, 44]. This compounds the problem for interventionalists because in the general population, PSCs are uncommon, difficult to detect and treatment is suboptimal. Ophthalmologists may not even consider the possibility of radiation-induced cataracts. Routine eye chart testing is not sensitive for their detection, as they affect contrast prior to acuity, and most clinics won't have the sophisticated equipment required for their detection. Finally, even after diagnosis and treatment, 'successful' cataract surgery can still result in reduced visual acuity, 20/25 being considered an excellent surgical outcome [45]. Therefore, prevention should be every interventionalist's priority from the outset of their career and is highly achievable through the wearing of lead glasses and use of ceiling-mounted lead shields (see Chap. 14).

13.3.2.4 Impaired Fertility

Impaired fertility appears to be a deterministic effect of prolonged radiation exposure [3], although foetal abnormalities in offspring can represent stochastic effects [23].

13.3.3 Stochastic Effects

Stochastic effects describe genetic mutations and cancer that occur due to a cumulative radiation dose that overwhelms the individual's ability to repair DNA damage [43]. They are less predictable than deterministic effects, as any level of exposure can cause them, but not every exposure will, and as such there is no threshold dose [36]. Tissues that have a rapid cellular turnover such as bone marrow and breast tissue are more susceptible than more quiescent tissues [24].

13.3.3.1 DNA Damage

Stochastic effects are due to irreparable DNA damage and consequential genetic mutations. The type of damage, the body's repair mechanisms and the person's age will determine whether radiation-induced DNA damage leads to genetic mutations that cause cancer, the most feared stochastic effect, or go by unnoticed. Stochastic effects lead to the development of solid tumours and blood malignancies months or even years following exposure [23].

Sublethal damage to non-coding areas of DNA may be inconsequential and repaired successfully, avoiding a stochastic event [36]. However, damage to coding areas, regulatory regions, or double-stranded breaks that are harder to repair could affect genetic products or regulation, turning a normal gene into a cancer-inducing oncogene [11, 47]. Thereafter, the clinical development of cancer still depends on many other biological factors, including genetics and age. Children and young adults are at a greater risk of stochastic events simply due to a longer life expectancy in which a long latent cancer may develop, with those less than 30 years having the greatest dose sensitivity [11]. Solid organs that are most sensitive to radiation are those with a high mitotic activity, such as colon, thyroid, breast, lung and bladder. Haemopoietic tissues are highly sensitive for the induction of leukaemia [11].

13.3.3.2 The Linear No-Threshold Theory

Stochastic effects differ from deterministic effects in that they do not conform to a dose relationship. Whereas deterministic effects do not occur below a certain threshold and thereafter follow a dose-dependent severity, stochastic effects are not associated with a threshold, and there is no correlation with dose. They can occur at any dose, and there is no dose at which they will never occur. However, the likelihood of development is probabilistic, with increasing total doses, but the severity of the effect is not related to the dose that induced it [25].

This linear relationship of dose and stochastic risk has led to the concept of the so-called 'linear no-threshold theory'. Although stochastic risk increases with dose exposure, there is no threshold below which stochastic risk is zero [11]. This is because, in theory, a single X-ray photon could ionise a critical portion of DNA, creating an oncogene [11]. Therefore, even the lowest exposure to radiation increases stochastic risk [23]. This forms the foundation of the ALARA principle (As Low As Reasonably Achievable) [48], which maintains that radiation exposure should always be minimised as much as possible within the limits of clinical need [11].

13.3.3.3 Predicting Stochastic Risk

Despite the linear no-threshold theory, stochastic risk can still be estimated. At small doses, it is difficult to distinguish from zero [11], but the Biological Effects of Radiation VII Committee (BEIR VII) has suggested an estimate of lifetime attributable risk of cancer due to low-dose exposure based on mathematical models [23]. For example, the estimated risk of lifetime fatal malignancy in the US population is 21%, and this risk increases by 5% for each 1 Sv of Effective Dose radiation one is exposed to, assuming a normal life expectancy [34]. In this way, Effective Dose provides an index for stochastic risk [25].

This has implications for younger patients who may undergo multiple medical exposures in their lifetime, and career interventionalists regularly exposed to low-dose radiation.

13.3.4 *What Is the Risk for Interventionalists?*

Recent health issues in prominent interventionalists have highlighted the long-held concerns regarding the risk of occupational radiation exposure [49]. Most data on human stochastic effects are gleaned from epidemiological studies on survivors of atomic bombs in Nagasaki and Hiroshima, or nuclear power plant accidents such as Chernobyl [11]. However, these relate to large doses received over a short period of time, whereas occupational radiation workers are subject to small cumulative doses over longer periods. There are some observational data from nuclear plant operators and some longitudinal studies in healthcare workers suggesting that chronic exposure increases the risk of cancer compared to the general population [36]. However, one of the problems with developing any causal link between occupational radiation exposure and stochastic risk is the long latency of effects [10], coupled with the fact that radiation-induced malignancies are often indistinguishable from cancers developing de novo [2].

Nonetheless, since the first case report published in 1912 highlighting leukaemia in radiologists [45], and a case series in 1942 reporting a tenfold increase in the incidence of leukaemia in this specialty [50], there have been numerous studies reporting several-fold increases in the incidence of potential radiation injuries amongst angiography suite staff [51]. These include skin cancer [52], cataracts [53], solid organ and haematological cancers [54] and brain and neck cancers [55]. However, outside of cataract formation, it is currently impossible to draw definite conclusions from the existing evidence that these associations are due to occupational exposure [23, 56]. Whilst there is no conclusive evidence that radiation due to medical imaging can induce cancer, radiation remains one of the most extensively studied carcinogens [2].

13.3.4.1 Statistical Risk of Cancer in Interventionalists

The BEIR VII statistical models based on the linear no-threshold theory suggest a small but measurable risk for the development of cancer in medical radiation-exposed healthcare workers. In one scenario, a worker is exposed to the upper limit dose of 10 mGy/year from aged 18 years until retiring aged 66 years. This model suggests an additional risk of cancer incidence of 3.06% (male) or 4.29% (female) and cancer mortality of 1.7% (male) or 2.39% (female). This obviously needs to be put into the context of the background risk of developing cancer in the general population of 46% overall and 23% fatal [11].

13.3.4.2 Recommended Occupational Exposure Limits

Based on the BEIR VII models, the current ICRP recommended limits for occupationally exposed medical workers are [57, 58]:

- Total Body = 20 mSv/year (averaged over 5 years with no single annual exposure >50 mSv)
- Lens of Eye = 20 mSv/year (averaged over 5 years with no single annual exposure >50 mSv)
- Skin = 500 mSv/year
  Hands and Feet = 500 mSv/year (averaged over the most irradiated 1 cm^2 area of skin)

The total body dose is an Effective Dose relating to stochastic risk throughout the body, and the specific tissue doses are Equivalent Doses pertaining to deterministic risk in those tissues [26].

13.3.4.3 Occupational Limits in the Context of a Career in Vascular Surgery

A 3 mSv/year effective dose throughout a career translates to a less than 1:10,000 risk of radiation-induced cancer [59]. Based on the linear no-threshold theory, this risk increases with dose so that a lifetime cumulative exposure of 400 mSv correlates to an increased cancer risk of 1:250, with a cumulative dose of >100 mSv still being statistically relevant [60]. To put this into context, it has been estimated that an interventionalist performing 100 peripheral angiographic procedures a year will receive an annual dose of 30 mSv to the eyes and head, and 40 mSv to the hands [61]. Over a career of 40 years, this cumulative dose will approach the threshold for deterministic injury [36]. Although the Effective Dose under lead has been estimated to be 0.55 mSv for a vascular surgeon performing 50 elective non-complex EVARs over the course of a year, the equivalent dose to unprotected areas may exceed 10 mSv/year [62]. The consequences of receiving 10 mSv/year over a 30–40-year career are as yet unknown [11]. A similar estimation for a busy interventionalist adhering to ALARA principles is that their effective dose is unlikely to exceed 10 mSv/year, and more likely to be in the range of 1–4 mSv/year [26, 63]. However, the exposure in vascular surgery may be greater, with the endovascular case mix exposing the vascular surgeon to higher doses [47]. The per-case dose for EVAR was found to be almost sixfold higher than that of percutaneous coronary interventions, with peripheral endovascular interventions also being associated with higher operator exposure than coronary interventions [64]. This results in vascular surgeons being classified as Category A radiation-exposed workers (those likely to receive an Effective dose >6 mSv/year, equivalent dose of >15 mSv to the lens) [23].

13.3.4.4 Brain Cancer and Dementia

Studies have demonstrated significant doses to the unprotected left side of the head during endovascular procedures [65], and published case reports of brain tumours occurring in interventionalists have raised concerns. This has been compounded by the finding that, in one study of 31 interventionalists, a disproportionate number of brain and neck tumours were left-sided (85%), suggesting a causal relationship [55]. In addition, the majority of the malignant neoplasms reported have been associated with radiation exposure [56]. However, large epidemiological studies looking at the cause of death in workers exposed to fluoroscopically guided procedures, including interventionalists, failed to find any demonstrable increased radiogenic mortality in these groups [66]. The overall prevalence of malignant brain tumours is low, and in a group of 10,000 interventionalists, 25 may be expected to develop fatal brain tumours outside of any occupational risk, and four may develop fatal brain tumours from occupational exposure, giving a risk of 0.04% [67].

In addition to brain cancer, the question of radiation-induced dementia has been raised. Animal models have demonstrated that low-dose radiation downregulates the same neural pathways responsible for cognitive dysfunction seen in normal aging and Alzheimer's disease [68], but again a causal link has not been definitively identified.

13.3.4.5 Cataracts

Numerous studies have demonstrated an increased incidence of cataracts in radiation workers, particularly PLC, up to six times in some studies [45, 51]. The lens is one of the most radiosensitive tissues in the body, and cataracts can develop despite low-dose exposures [69]. As such, dose limits to the eye have been dropping since they were first evaluated by the ICRP; from 300 mSv/year in 1977, to 150 mSv in 1984, to 20 mSv/year in 2012, now identical to the whole-body effective dose limit [44]. Epidemiological evidence suggests an even lower threshold dose may be appropriate for radiation-induced cataracts, perhaps even a no-dose threshold [70].

Many endovascular procedures deliver considerable doses to the eye [71], with an estimated 23 h of fluoroscopy time resulting in the 20 mSv annual threshold [71]. Further studies highlighted EVAR, embolisation procedures, lower limb and renal interventions as delivering substantial doses to the eye [62, 63]. Again, extrapolating these doses to an annual workload exceeding the ICRP dose limit recommendations [72], with the completion of 50 EVARs over a year, results in eye exposure exceeding 30% of the ICRP limit, a threshold which, in the UK, would classify the surgeon as a radiation worker [62].

13.3.4.6 Genetic Susceptibility to Radiation Injury

When considering dose thresholds, one must bear in mind that they are based on average sensitivities to radiation injury from population data [45]. At an individual level, biological responses to injury vary, governed largely by genetically mediated mechanisms, resulting in natural variation with regard to one's individual sensitivity to radiation exposure [45]. Animal studies have demonstrated a genetic variation to radiation repair genes [73], and in a recent study measuring DNA damage markers in the circulating lymphocytes of vascular interventionalists exposed to radiation, it was found that significant individual variation existed regarding the induction of DNA repair markers to this exposure [47]. Certainly, there is growing awareness of personal radiation exposure amongst interventionalists; in a survey of over 600 European cardiac catheter laboratory workers, 11% had ceased working in the laboratory due to personal concerns regarding radiation exposure [74]. In the future, data regarding an individual's genetic susceptibility to radiation injury may help guide their career choice, but until that time, this uncertainty at an individual level highlights the importance of adherence to ALARA principles at all times.

13.4 Conclusion

A sound understanding of radiation physics and biology provides a solid foundation on which to apply the practical methods available to reduce exposure in daily practice. Although radiation dosimetry can be confusing, familiarity with the most common forms of dose measurement (CAK and DAP) will allow a deeper appreciation of the literature. In addition, auditing one's own dose reports in the context of DRLs will inevitably drive exposure down; after all, 'what gets measured gets managed'. Currently, there is no definitive evidence linking occupational radiation exposure to stochastic effects in interventionalists. However, a significant body of anecdotal evidence would suggest that keeping radiation doses to a minimum is, at the very least, highly prudent. Stronger evidence links deterministic cataract formation to occupational exposure, and adequate eye protection for interventionalists is essential, in addition to the other techniques available to minimise radiation exposure, as discussed further in Chap. 14.

Multiple Choice Questions

1. Which of the following measurements of radiation provides the best estimate of stochastic risk to operating staff?

   (a) Cumulative Air Kerma
   (b) Equivalent Dose
   (c) Fluoroscopy Time

(d) Air Kerma at the Reference Point
(e) Dose Area Product

Answer: (e) Dose Area Product

2. Which of the following statements is true?

(a) Radiation-induced cataracts are a stochastic effect
(b) Cancer is a deterministic effect of radiation exposure
(c) The lens is one of the most radiation-resistant tissues in the human body
(d) The Linear No-Threshold Theory describes the radiation risk of leukaemia in radiation workers
(e) Hands can safely enter the primary beam due to the low risk of skin cancer

Answer: (d) The Linear No-Threshold Theory describes the radiation risk of leukaemia in radiation workers

References

1. Reed AB. The history of radiation use in medicine. J Vasc Surg. 2011;53:3s–5s. https://doi.org/10.1016/j.jvs.2010.07.024.
2. Zhou W. Radiation exposure of vascular surgery patients beyond endovascular procedures. J Vasc Surg. 2011;53:39s–43s. https://doi.org/10.1016/j.jvs.2010.06.176.
3. Killewich LA, Falls G, Mastracci TM, Brown KR. Factors affecting radiation injury. J Vasc Surg. 2011;53:9s–14s. https://doi.org/10.1016/j.jvs.2010.07.025.
4. Seldinger SI. Catheter replacement of the needle in percutaneous arteriography; a new technique. Acta Radiol. 1953;39:368–76. https://doi.org/10.3109/00016925309136722.
5. The endovascular explosion: an interview with Dr Edward B Diethrich [Internet] Medscape [cited 2019 Jun 23]. Available from: https://www.medscapecom/viewarticle/549322.
6. Payne MM. Charles Theodore Dotter. The father of intervention. Tex Heart Inst J. 2001;28:28–38.
7. Parodi JC, Palmaz JC, Barone HD. Transfemoral intraluminal graft implantation for abdominal aortic aneurysms. Ann Vasc Surg. 1991;5:491–9. https://doi.org/10.1007/bf02015271.
8. Ivancev K, Vogelzang R. A 35 year history of stent grafting, and how EVAR conquered the world. Eur J Vasc Endovasc Surg. 2020;59:685–94. https://doi.org/10.1016/j.ejvs.2020.03.017.
9. Mastracci TM. Radiation safety: a call to arms. Eur J Vasc Endovasc Surg. 2015;50:1–2. https://doi.org/10.1016/j.ejvs.2015.02.001.
10. Monastiriotis S, Comito M, Labropoulos N. Radiation exposure in endovascular repair of abdominal and thoracic aortic aneurysms. J Vasc Surg. 2015;62:753–61. https://doi.org/10.1016/j.jvs.2015.05.033.
11. Hirshfeld JW Jr, Ferrari VA, Bengel FM, Bergersen L, Chambers CE, Einstein AJ, et al. 2018 ACC/HRS/NASCI/SCAI/SCCT expert consensus document on optimal use of ionizing radiation in cardiovascular imaging: best practices for safety and effectiveness: a report of the American College of Cardiology Task Force on expert consensus decision pathways. J Am Coll Cardiol. 2018;71:e283–351. https://doi.org/10.1016/j.jacc.2018.02.016.
12. Smith-Bindman R, Lipson J, Marcus R, Kim KP, Mahesh M, Gould R, et al. Radiation dose associated with common computed tomography examinations and the associated lifetime attributable risk of cancer. Arch Intern Med. 2009;169:2078–86. https://doi.org/10.1001/archinternmed.2009.427.

13. Brenner DJ, Hall EJ. Computed tomography—an increasing source of radiation exposure. N Engl J Med. 2007;357:2277–84. https://doi.org/10.1056/NEJMra072149.
14. Cole P, Hallard R, Broughton J, Coates R, Croft J, Davies K, et al. Developing the radiation protection safety culture in the UK. J Radiol Prot. 2014;34:469–84. https://doi.org/10.1088/0952-4746/34/2/469.
15. Machado R, Ferreira VM, Loureiro L, Gonçalves J, Oliveira P, Almeida R. Radiation exposure in endovascular infra-renal aortic aneurysm repair and factors that influence it. Braz J Cardiovasc Surg. 2016;31:415–21. https://doi.org/10.5935/1678-9741.20160084.
16. Ketteler ER, Brown KR. Radiation exposure in endovascular procedures. J Vasc Surg. 2011;53:35s–8s. https://doi.org/10.1016/j.jvs.2010.05.141.
17. Bannazadeh M, Altinel O, Kashyap VS, Sun Z, Clair D, Sarac TP. Patterns of procedure-specific radiation exposure in the endovascular era: impetus for further innovation. J Vasc Surg. 2009;49:1520–4. https://doi.org/10.1016/j.jvs.2009.02.015.
18. Panuccio G, Greenberg RK, Wunderle K, Mastracci TM, Eagleton MG, Davros W. Comparison of indirect radiation dose estimates with directly measured radiation dose for patients and operators during complex endovascular procedures. J Vasc Surg. 2011;53:885–94.e1; discussion 94. https://doi.org/10.1016/j.jvs.2010.10.106.
19. Walsh C, O'Callaghan A, Moore D, O'Neill S, Madhavan P, Colgan MP, et al. Measurement and optimization of patient radiation doses in endovascular aneurysm repair. Eur J Vasc Endovasc Surg. 2012;43:534–9. https://doi.org/10.1016/j.ejvs.2012.01.028.
20. Zoli S, Trabattoni P, Dainese L, Annoni A, Saccu C, Fumagalli M, et al. Cumulative radiation exposure during thoracic endovascular aneurysm repair and subsequent follow-up. Eur J Cardiothorac Surg. 2012;42:254–9; discussion 9–60. https://doi.org/10.1093/ejcts/ezr301.
21. White HA, Macdonald S. Estimating risk associated with radiation exposure during follow-up after endovascular aortic repair (EVAR). J Cardiovasc Surg. 2010;51:95–104.
22. Vallabhaneni R, Farber MA, Schneider F, Ricco JB. Debate: whether young, good-risk patients should be treated with endovascular abdominal aortic aneurysm repair. J Vasc Surg. 2013;58:1709–15. https://doi.org/10.1016/j.jvs.2013.09.017.
23. Hertault A, Maurel B, Midulla M, Bordier C, Desponds L, Saeed Kilani M, et al. Editor's choice—minimizing radiation exposure during endovascular procedures: basic knowledge, literature review, and reporting standards. Eur J Vasc Endovasc Surg. 2015;50:21–36. https://doi.org/10.1016/j.ejvs.2015.01.014.
24. Tonnessen BH, Pounds L. Radiation physics. J Vasc Surg. 2011;53:6s–8s. https://doi.org/10.1016/j.jvs.2010.05.138.
25. Walsh SR, Cousins C, Tang TY, Gaunt ME, Boyle JR. Ionizing radiation in endovascular interventions. J Endovasc Ther. 2008;15:680–7. https://doi.org/10.1583/08-2495.1.
26. Durán A, Hian SK, Miller DL, Le Heron J, Padovani R, Vano E. A summary of recommendations for occupational radiation protection in interventional cardiology. Catheter Cardiovasc Interv. 2013;81:562–7. https://doi.org/10.1002/ccd.24520.
27. Lipsitz EC, Veith FJ, Ohki T, Heller S, Wain RA, Suggs WD, et al. Does the endovascular repair of aortoiliac aneurysms pose a radiation safety hazard to vascular surgeons? J Vasc Surg. 2000;32:704–10. https://doi.org/10.1067/mva.2000.110053.
28. Boone JM, Levin DC. Radiation exposure to angiographers under different fluoroscopic imaging conditions. Radiology. 1991;180:861–5. https://doi.org/10.1148/radiology.180.3.1871307.
29. Haqqani OP, Agarwal PK, Halin NM, Iafrati MD. Defining the radiation "scatter cloud" in the interventional suite. J Vasc Surg. 2013;58:1339–45. https://doi.org/10.1016/j.jvs.2013.01.025.
30. Mohapatra A, Greenberg RK, Mastracci TM, Eagleton MJ, Thornsberry B. Radiation exposure to operating room personnel and patients during endovascular procedures. J Vasc Surg. 2013;58:702–9. https://doi.org/10.1016/j.jvs.2013.02.032.
31. Mehta K. Radiation: basic principles. J Vasc Surg. 2005;42:1237–8. https://doi.org/10.1016/j.jvs.2005.08.022.
32. Ahmed TAN, Taha S. Radiation exposure, the forgotten enemy: toward implementation of national safety program. Egypt Heart J. 2017;69:55–62. https://doi.org/10.1016/j.ehj.2016.10.001.

33. Kirkwood ML, Arbique GM, Guild JB, Timaran C, Chung J, Anderson JA, et al. Surgeon education decreases radiation dose in complex endovascular procedures and improves patient safety. J Vasc Surg. 2013;58:715–21. https://doi.org/10.1016/j.jvs.2013.04.004.
34. Beathard GA, Urbanes A, Litchfield T. Radiation dose associated with dialysis vascular access interventional procedures in the interventional nephrology facility. Semin Dial. 2013;26:503–10. https://doi.org/10.1111/sdi.12071.
35. Kirkwood ML, Guild JB, Arbique GM, Anderson JA, Valentine RJ, Timaran C. Surgeon radiation dose during complex endovascular procedures. J Vasc Surg. 2015;62:457–63. https://doi.org/10.1016/j.jvs.2015.02.050.
36. Brown KR, Rzucidlo E. Acute and chronic radiation injury. J Vasc Surg. 2011;53:15s–21s. https://doi.org/10.1016/j.jvs.2010.06.175.
37. Balter S, Hopewell JW, Miller DL, Wagner LK, Zelefsky MJ. Fluoroscopically guided interventional procedures: a review of radiation effects on patients' skin and hair. Radiology. 2010;254:326–41. https://doi.org/10.1148/radiol.2542082312.
38. Koenig TR, Wolff D, Mettler FA, Wagner LK. Skin injuries from fluoroscopically guided procedures: part 1, characteristics of radiation injury. Am J Roentgenol. 2001;177:3–11. https://doi.org/10.2214/ajr.177.1.1770003.
39. Connine T, Dukkipati S, Wolfe LG, Amendola MF. IP139. Is obesity associated with elevated radiation exposure during endovascular aortic aneurysm repair? J Vasc Surg. 2017;65:92S–3S. https://doi.org/10.1016/j.jvs.2017.03.173.
40. Bryk SG, Censullo ML, Wagner LK, Rossman LL, Cohen AM. Endovascular and interventional procedures in obese patients: a review of procedural technique modifications and radiation management. J Vasc Interv Radiol. 2006;17:27–33. https://doi.org/10.1097/01.Rvi.0000186953.44651.19.
41. Weiss DJ, Pipinos II, Longo GM, Lynch TG, Rutar FJ, Johanning JM. Direct and indirect measurement of patient radiation exposure during endovascular aortic aneurysm repair. Ann Vasc Surg. 2008;22:723–9. https://doi.org/10.1016/j.avsg.2008.06.008.
42. Maurel B, Sobocinski J, Perini P, Guillou M, Midulla M, Azzaoui R, et al. Evaluation of radiation during EVAR performed on a mobile C-arm. Eur J Vasc Endovasc Surg. 2012;43:16–21. https://doi.org/10.1016/j.ejvs.2011.09.017.
43. Kalef-Ezra JA, Karavasilis S, Ziogas D, Dristiliaris D, Michalis LK, Matsagas M. Radiation burden of patients undergoing endovascular abdominal aortic aneurysm repair. J Vasc Surg. 2009;49:283–7; discussion 7. https://doi.org/10.1016/j.jvs.2008.09.003.
44. Thome C, Chambers DB, Hooker AM, Thompson JW, Boreham DR. Deterministic effects to the lens of the eye following ionizing radiation exposure: is there evidence to support a reduction in threshold dose? Health Phys. 2018;114:328–43. https://doi.org/10.1097/hp.0000000000000810.
45. Machan L. The eyes have it. Tech Vasc Interv Radiol. 2018;21:21–5. https://doi.org/10.1053/j.tvir.2017.12.005.
46. Bouffler S, Ainsbury E, Gilvin P, Harrison J. Radiation-induced cataracts: the Health Protection Agency's response to the ICRP statement on tissue reactions and recommendation on the dose limit for the eye lens. J Radiol Prot. 2012;32:479–88. https://doi.org/10.1088/0952-4746/32/4/479.
47. El-Sayed T, Patel AS, Cho JS, Kelly JA, Ludwinski FE, Saha P, et al. Radiation-induced DNA damage in operators performing endovascular aortic repair. Circulation. 2017;136:2406–16. https://doi.org/10.1161/circulationaha.117.029550.
48. Report no. 107—implementation of the principle of As Low As Reasonably Achievable (ALARA) for Medical and Dental Personnel. National Council on Radiation Protection and Measurements [Internet]. 1990 [cited 2019 Feb 9];107 (ISBN 0-929600-15-0). Available from: https://ncrponline.org/shop/reports/report-no-107-implementation-of-the-principle-of-as-low-as-reasonably-achievable-alara-for-medical-and-dental-personnel-1990.
49. Marx MV. Live without regret. Tech Vasc Interv Radiol. 2018;21:1. https://doi.org/10.1053/j.tvir.2017.12.001.

50. March HC. Leukemia in radiologists/radiology. Radiology. 1944;43:275–8.
51. Andreassi MG, Piccaluga E, Guagliumi G, Del Greco M, Gaita F, Picano E. Occupational health risks in cardiac catheterization laboratory workers. Circ Cardiovasc Interv. 2016;9:e003273. https://doi.org/10.1161/circinterventions.115.003273.
52. Yoshinaga S, Hauptmann M, Sigurdson AJ, Doody MM, Freedman DM, Alexander BH, et al. Nonmelanoma skin cancer in relation to ionizing radiation exposure among U.S. radiologic technologists. Int J Cancer. 2005;115:828–34. https://doi.org/10.1002/ijc.20939.
53. Vano E, Kleiman NJ, Duran A, Romano-Miller M, Rehani MM. Radiation-associated lens opacities in catheterization personnel: results of a survey and direct assessments. J Vasc Interv Radiol. 2013;24:197–204. https://doi.org/10.1016/j.jvir.2012.10.016.
54. Rajaraman P, Doody MM, Yu CL, Preston DL, Miller JS, Sigurdson AJ, et al. Cancer risks in U.S. Radiologic Technologists working with fluoroscopically guided interventional procedures, 1994-2008. Am J Roentgenol. 2016;206:1101–8. https://doi.org/10.2214/ajr.15.15265.
55. Roguin A, Goldstein J, Bar O, Goldstein JA. Brain and neck tumors among physicians performing interventional procedures. Am J Cardiol. 2013;111:1368–72. https://doi.org/10.1016/j.amjcard.2012.12.060.
56. Kirkwood ML, Arbique GM, Guild JB, Zeng K, Xi Y, Rectenwald J, et al. Radiation brain dose to vascular surgeons during fluoroscopically guided interventions is not effectively reduced by wearing lead equivalent surgical caps. J Vasc Surg. 2018;68:567–71. https://doi.org/10.1016/j.jvs.2017.12.054.
57. Valentin J. The 2007 recommendations of the International Commission on Radiological Protection. ICRP publication 103. Ann ICRP. 2007;37:1–322. https://doi.org/10.1016/j.icrp.2007.10.003.
58. Stewart FA, Akleyev AV, Hauer-Jensen M, Hendry JH, Kleiman NJ, Macvittie TJ, et al. ICRP publication 118: ICRP statement on tissue reactions and early and late effects of radiation in normal tissues and organs—threshold doses for tissue reactions in a radiation protection context. Ann ICRP. 2012;41:1–322. https://doi.org/10.1016/j.icrp.2012.02.001.
59. Niklason LT, Marx MV, Chan HP. Interventional radiologists: occupational radiation doses and risks. Radiology. 1993;187:729–33. https://doi.org/10.1148/radiology.187.3.8497622.
60. Haqqani OP, Agarwal PK, Halin NM, Iafrati MD. Minimizing radiation exposure to the vascular surgeon. J Vasc Surg. 2012;55:799–805. https://doi.org/10.1016/j.jvs.2011.08.055.
61. Johnson DR, Kyriou J, Morton EJ, Clifton A, Fitzgerald M, Macsweeney E. Radiation protection in interventional radiology. Clin Radiol. 2001;56:99–106. https://doi.org/10.1053/crad.2000.0640.
62. Patel AP, Gallacher D, Dourado R, Lyons O, Smith A, Zayed H, et al. Occupational radiation exposure during endovascular aortic procedures. Eur J Vasc Endovasc Surg. 2013;46:424–30. https://doi.org/10.1016/j.ejvs.2013.05.023.
63. Miller DL. Make radiation protection a habit. Tech Vasc Interv Radiol. 2018;21:37–42. https://doi.org/10.1053/j.tvir.2017.12.008.
64. Ingwersen M, Drabik A, Kulka U, Oestreicher U, Fricke S, Krankenberg H, et al. Physicians' radiation exposure in the catheterization lab: does the type of procedure matter? JACC Cardiovasc Interv. 2013;6:1095–102. https://doi.org/10.1016/j.jcin.2013.05.012.
65. Albayati MA, Kelly S, Gallagher D, Dourado R, Patel AS, Saha P, et al. Editor's choice—angulation of the C-arm during complex endovascular aortic procedures increases radiation exposure to the head. Eur J Vasc Endovasc Surg. 2015;49:396–402. https://doi.org/10.1016/j.ejvs.2014.12.032.
66. Balter S. Always on my mind. Tech Vasc Interv Radiol. 2018;21:26–31. https://doi.org/10.1053/j.tvir.2017.12.006.
67. Fetterly K, Schueler B, Grams M, Sturchio G, Bell M, Gulati R. Head and neck radiation dose and radiation safety for interventional physicians. JACC Cardiovasc Interv. 2017;10:520–8. https://doi.org/10.1016/j.jcin.2016.11.026.
68. Lowe XR, Bhattacharya S, Marchetti F, Wyrobek AJ. Early brain response to low-dose radiation exposure involves molecular networks and pathways associated with cognitive func-

tions, advanced aging and Alzheimer's disease. Radiat Res. 2009;171:53–65. https://doi.org/10.1667/rr1389.1.
69. Rose A, Rae WID, Chikobvu P, Marais W. A multiple methods approach: radiation associated cataracts and occupational radiation safety practices in interventionalists in South Africa. J Radiol Prot. 2017;37:329–39. https://doi.org/10.1088/1361-6498/aa5eee.
70. Kim KP, Miller DL, Berrington de Gonzalez A, Balter S, Kleinerman RA, Ostroumova E, et al. Occupational radiation doses to operators performing fluoroscopically-guided procedures. Health Phys. 2012;103:80–99. https://doi.org/10.1097/HP.0b013e31824dae76.
71. Attigah N, Oikonomou K, Hinz U, Knoch T, Demirel S, Verhoeven E, et al. Radiation exposure to eye lens and operator hands during endovascular procedures in hybrid operating rooms. J Vasc Surg. 2016;63:198–203. https://doi.org/10.1016/j.jvs.2015.08.051.
72. Vanhavere F, Carinou E, Domienik J, Donadille L, Ginjaume M, Gualdrini G, et al. Measurements of eye lens doses in interventional radiology and cardiology: final results of the ORAMED project. Radiat Meas. 2011;46:1243–7. https://doi.org/10.1016/j.radmeas.2011.08.013.
73. Worgul BV, Smilenov L, Brenner DJ, Junk A, Zhou W, Hall EJ. Atm heterozygous mice are more sensitive to radiation-induced cataracts than are their wild-type counterparts. Proc Natl Acad Sci USA. 2002;99:9836–9. https://doi.org/10.1073/pnas.162349699.
74. Buchanan GL, Chieffo A, Mehilli J, Mikhail GW, Mauri F, Presbitero P, et al. The occupational effects of interventional cardiology: results from the WIN for safety survey. EuroIntervention. 2012;8:658–63. https://doi.org/10.4244/eijv8i6a103.

Key References

Hirshfeld JW, Ferrari VA, Bengel FM, Bergersen L, Chambers CE, Einstein AJ, et al. 2018 ACC/HRS/NASCI/SCAI/SCCT expert consensus document on optimal use of ionizing radiation in cardiovascular imaging: best practices for safety and effectiveness. J Am Coll Cardiol. 2018;71:e283–351. https://doi.org/10.1016/j.jacc.2018.02.016.

Hertault A, Maurel B, Midulla M, Bordier C, Desponds L, Saeed Kilani M, et al. Editor's Choice—Minimizing radiation exposure during endovascular procedures: basic knowledge, literature review, and reporting standards. Eur J Vasc Endovas Surg. 2015;50:21–36. https://doi.org/10.1016/j.ejvs.2015.01.014.

Tonnessen BH, Pounds L. Radiation physics. J Vasc Surg. 2011;53:6S–8S.

Report no. 107—Implementation of the Principle of As Low As Reasonably Achievable (ALARA) for Medical and Dental Personnel. National Council on Radiation Protection and Measurements [Internet]. 1990 [cited 2019 Feb 9];107 (ISBN 0-929600-15-0). Available from: https://ncrponline.org/shop/reports/report-no-107-implementation-of-the-principle-of-as-low-as-reasonably-achievable-alara-for-medical-and-dental-personnel-1990/.

Stewart FA, Akleyev AV, Hauer-Jensen M, Hendry JH, Kleiman NJ, MacVittie TJ, et al. ICRP PUBLICATION 118: ICRP Statement on tissue reactions and early and late effects of radiation in normal tissues and organs—threshold doses for tissue reactions in a radiation protection context. Ann ICRP. 2012;41:1–322.

Modarai B, Haulon S, Ainsbury E, Böckler D, Vano-Carruana E, Dawson J, et al. Editor's Choice—European Society for Vascular Surgery (ESVS) 2023 Clinical Practice Guidelines on Radiation Safety. Eur J Vasc Endovasc Surg. 2023;65:171–222. https://doi.org/10.1016/j.ejvs.2022.09.005.

Chapter 14
Radiation Stewardship: Radiation Exposure, Protection and Safety in Contemporary Endovascular Practice

Joseph Dawson and Stephan Haulon

> **SN Flashcards**
> Test your learning and check your understanding of this book's contents: use the "Springer Nature Flashcards" app to access questions using ▶ https://sn.pub/wppvze. To use the app, please follow the instructions in Chap. 1.

Key Learning Objectives

- Radiation stewardship mandates that surgeons understand machine control parameters and shielding efficacy to minimise occupational and patients' exposure during fluoroscopically guided intervention.
- EVAR, whilst a standard procedure, presents a possible scenario for exceeding 2 Gy estimated skin dose (ESD), emphasising the need for meticulous fluoroscopy time management and dose-reduction techniques.
- Complex endovascular aortic repairs, particularly involving thoracoabdominal procedures like FEVAR and challenging anatomies in infrarenal EVAR (high BMI, steep neck angulation), significantly increase radiation exposure for both patients and operators, necessitating careful pre-operative planning and intra-operative radiation minimisation strategies.

J. Dawson (✉)
Vascular and Endovascular Service, Royal Adelaide Hospital, and Discipline of Surgery, Adelaide University, Adelaide, SA, Australia
e-mail: joseph.dawson@adelaide.edu.au

S. Haulon
Department of Vascular Surgery – Aortic Centre Hospital Marie Lannelongue, University Paris-Sud, Paris, France
e-mail: s.haulon@hml.fr

R. Fitridge et al. (eds.), *Pathophysiology of Vascular Disease*,
https://doi.org/10.1007/978-3-032-31459-8_14

- Effective radiation safety culture requires standardised training curricula, regular dose audits and leadership endorsement of ALARA practices (as low as reasonably achievable), including consistent use of personal dosimeters.
- For female surgeons or trainees during childbearing years, especially during pregnancy, rigorous adherence to ALARA principles is paramount. Dedicated 1.0 mm lead equivalent (Pb LE) maternal gowns or equivalent multi-layered shielding, combined with foetal dosimeters for real-time monitoring and feedback, minimises foetal radiation exposure. Additionally, flexible rostering during critical gestational periods can further reduce radiation dose, respecting the 1 mSv/pregnancy International Commission on Radiation Protection (ICRP) limit.
- Application of inverse square law and judicious use of collimation are essential to minimise scatter radiation, particularly during high-dose digital subtraction angiography (DSA) runs and steep gantry angulations.
- Optimising fluoroscopy unit settings (automatic brightness control (ABC), pulse rate) and utilising advanced imaging software (3D-image fusion (3D-IF), preoperative planning, last image hold) reduces the dependency on high-dose DSA and minimises total radiation exposure.
- DSA delivers significantly higher radiation than fluoroscopy, and its use should be limited to critical diagnostic or documentation needs, with fluoroscopy loops and reduced DSA frame rate employed whenever possible to minimise patients' and operators' radiation exposure.
- Whilst magnification (reducing the field of view or FOV) improves image resolution, it significantly increases local patient radiation dose due to automatic brightness compensation, specifically increasing Cumulative Air Kerma (CAK) but decreasing dose area product (DAP); therefore, maximising FOV and utilising digital zoom on a large monitor for enhanced detail rather than optical magnification, is recommended to minimise radiation exposure.
- Imaging chain geometry (source-to-patient, patient-to detector distance) and C-arm positioning directly influence scatter radiation distribution, necessitating strategic table height and detector placement.
- Real-time dosimetry systems provide immediate feedback on operator exposure, enabling intra-procedural adjustments to minimise dose and reinforce ALARA compliance.
- Proper selection and consistent use of personal protective equipment (0.5 mmPb LE lead aprons, 0.75 mmPb LE leaded eyewear with side shielding) are paramount in mitigation scatter radiation exposure to radiosensitive organs.
- Innovative technologies, including robotic endovascular systems and advanced shielding designs, present promising solutions to significantly reduce or eliminate operator radiation exposure. These advancements aim to overcome the limitations of traditional lead-based protection, offering improved safety and reduced musculoskeletal strain for interventionalists.

14.1 Radiation Stewardship

Over the last 50 years, there has been a proliferation in fluoroscopically guided minimally invasive procedures, and endovascular interventions have frequently become the preferred choice with both patients and surgeons [1–3], due to a lower morbidity, mortality, reduced length of hospital stay [4] and favourable outcome data in almost every vascular territory [5].

This endovascular 'revolution' has now been superseded by 'evolution' where not only are the number of procedures increasing, but so is the complexity [1, 6]. The advent of the hybrid suite, combined with a pro-endovascular approach [4], has resulted in prolonged screening times with a substantial and significant increase in accompanying radiation dose [4, 6, 7]. To date, the majority of attention has been dedicated to developing and perfecting endovascular techniques to tackle increasingly complex pathology, with far less focus on the potential hazards that this cumulative radiation burden poses [8]. However, there has been a growing concern regarding this increasing radiation exposure, not only to the patient, but to the whole endovascular team [2, 9, 10]. With more patients being treated by more complex procedures, we will likely see this exposure continuing to rise dramatically in the future [11]. Whilst radiation exposure to patients has been studied in some detail, there is a relative paucity of data looking at occupational exposure for interventionalists [3, 4], although lessons learned from other specialties such as cardiology can be readily translated into the vascular field [12].

Whilst it is now accepted that ionising radiation is an inherent feature and accepted component of modern vascular practice [1, 13, 14] (the X-ray beam being described as the 'modern vascular surgeon's scalpel' [15]), the considerable clinical benefit of minimally invasive interventions must be tempered by the attendant disadvantage of a reliance on ionising radiation. Unfortunately, the risks of radiation exposure are not universally recognised by vascular operators [9] and perhaps underappreciated by those who learned their trade in the operating theatres of old [11]. As radiation is an entirely invisible threat, protection can be challenging for the surgeon to understand and enforce [16]. It is not as intuitive as, for example, blood-borne virus protection, a comparative safety issue of equal magnitude for the surgeon [16]. One of the hurdles identified in establishing an effective radiation protection culture is a lack of proper understanding of radiation risks by key players; knowledge and understanding of the real radiation risks relative to their benefits are critical [17].

With vascular surgeons now principal operators in the angiography suite, and no longer merely guests [15], their responsibilities must evolve beyond technical excellence. Whilst continuing to attend to the procedural and clinical needs of the patient, they must now also shoulder the responsibility of radiation protection for the patient, themselves, their trainees and team; we term this essential new leadership role 'radiation stewardship'.

The aim of this chapter is to aid in this task, to build on the concepts of Chap. 13 and to describe the numerous methods available to protect against radiation in practice. In this way, it is hoped that vascular surgeons feel empowered to implement radiation stewardship within their hospitals, to apply a heightened level of knowledge and responsibility regarding ionising radiation so they can protect themselves, their colleagues and their patients [18].

14.2 Radiation Exposure During Endovascular Interventions

The majority of the literature regarding radiation exposure and safety describes interventional procedures pertaining to cardiac interventions with an under-representation of peripheral vascular interventions [1, 19]. Meaningful comparisons of the data that do exist are hampered by significant methodological and outcome heterogeneity in small, non-randomised studies. Other limiting factors include significant differences regarding anatomical lesions, procedural complexity, technique, equipment, patient factors, operator experience, units of measurement and reporting [6, 20–22].

Some of these variables may explain the wide variations observed in the published literature. One reported a 1000-fold difference in minimum and maximum radiation doses for a range of cardiac interventions [23]. The same authors found operator dose varied up to three orders of magnitude for the same fluoroscopically guided intervention [22]. Similarly, in a study of 149 mixed endovascular procedures, it was found that the range of annual body effective dose was lower for vascular surgeons (0.13–0.27 mSv) compared to other published reports in cardiologists (1.9-37 mSv) and interventional radiologists (0.37–10.1 mSv) [6]. These low doses are in contrast to earlier reports of EVAR operators experiencing under-lead doses of 1.52 mSv, and over-lead doses of 13.7 mSv [19]. As increasing radiation awareness can lead to significant reductions in occupational dose, it has been suggested that large variations in operator dose could be substantially reduced with improved radiation safety practices [22].

14.2.1 Radiation Exposure During EVAR

EVAR remains the most common quintessential complex endovascular case, and as such, is the most investigated procedure regarding radiation dose in vascular surgery [8, 19, 20, 24–27]. In a systematic review reporting radiation during EVAR and other complex aortic repairs, the mean Dose Area Product (DAP) for standard infrarenal EVAR was 79 Gy/cm^2, but as expected increased proportionally with procedural complexity [20]. Although some studies report relatively low radiation doses for the majority of aortic repairs [28], others have found that one third of EVAR patients received an Entrance Skin Dose in excess of 2 Gy [27], the threshold for deterministic effects, with some patients receiving up to 6 Gy [27]. As previously discussed, these variations in dose are due, in part, to different operators and variations in technique, anatomical complexity, patient BMI and staff adherence to radiation safety principles [3]. Some investigators have gone on to investigate which part of the operator's body is most exposed during EVAR. By placing dosimeters near the eye, thyroid, chest, abdomen, hands and feet of interventionalists, investigators found that during EVAR 90% of the cases resulted in at least one body part receiving more than 1 mSv per procedure [29], usually in the lower body where scatter is known to be highest.

14.2.2 Procedural Complexity

Unsurprisingly, the more complex the procedure, the higher the associated radiation dose. Complex thoracoabdominal procedures such as FEVAR and TEVAR for aortic dissection [30] generate more radiation than EVAR and standard TEVAR [31], especially if associated with challenging renal or visceral artery stenting that requires steep C-arm angulation [32, 33]. In one study, one third of such repairs exceeded the 2 Gy skin dose deterministic threshold [28], and in another 21 patients, 70% of whom were undergoing FEVAR, the 6 Gy Cumulative Air Kerma (CAK) threshold for substantial radiation dose was exceeded [31]. Average operator doses associated with such repairs were reported at 0.17 mSv per procedure [32]. In addition to prolonged operative times, such procedures often require acute C-arm gantry angulations, further increasing the radiation dose [2].

Adverse features adding to the complexity of infrarenal EVAR associated with increased radiation doses include bilateral iliac aneurysms, AAA diameter >60 mm, neck diameter >28 mm, CIA diameter >20 mm and neck angulations >50° [13]. From this analysis, the authors determined that they could predict 40% of the case radiation pre-operatively from the BMI, neck angulation, AAA diameter and aneurysm type. Having more than two of these anatomical risk factors was related to increased radiation exposure, with BMI and neck angulation emerging as the two most predictive variables [13]. In another study, localisation of the proximal landing zone and main body deployment accounted for 24% of the total radiation dose during EVAR [34]. Significant contributors to radiation exposure during endovascular aortic repair include the number of acquisitions and acute C-arm angulation [9].

14.2.3 Other High-Dose Procedures

In addition to complex aortic repairs, other endovascular procedures have emerged as contributing high radiation doses. In 318 endovascular cases, atherectomy emerged as having the longest fluoroscopy time [35]. This may explain why, in another study of aortic, carotid and peripheral interventions, atherectomy had the highest estimated skin dose (ESD) of all endovascular procedures, approaching 1.5 Gy [16]. This finding has been corroborated in another study looking at 2103 mixed endovascular cases reporting an ESD of 1.26 mGy associated with atherectomy [14]. These findings are significant considering the threshold values for skin injury is 2 Gy. Other procedures associated with high peak skin doses include abdominal and pelvic procedures [35], particularly renal and visceral interventions [36] and embolisation [2, 30, 31, 35].

It is not only the total radiation dose that is important to consider but also the operator proximity to the source. For example, endovascular interventions for dialysis access often require the operator to be in close anatomical proximity to the area of interest, exposing them to potentially higher scatter, and inadvertent encroachment on the direct beam with their hands [2, 21]. As a result, fistulograms were found to have a twofold higher operator effective dose/DAP ratio, with cerebrovascular interventions being tenfold higher than other endovascular procedures [2]. This indicates that the operator is more exposed to a unit dose of radiation for these types of procedures than others, even if the overall radiation doses are lower than those of other endovascular procedures.

14.2.4 Diagnostic Reference Levels

Diagnostic reference levels (DRLs) were introduced in 1990 by the International Commission on Radiation Protection (ICRP) to provide an advisory reference for common procedures and to increase operator awareness of radiation safety [37]. They represent the 75% percentile radiation dose per procedure, calculated from multiple representational samples: the higher the number of samples, the more accurate the reference level [37]. We refer the reader to Hertault et al.'s comprehensive paper tabulating DRLs for a large number of previously published endovascular procedures [37].

14.3 Radiation Protection and Safety

14.3.1 Introduction

Three basic principles govern radiation safety: justification of the examination, optimisation of protection and application of dose limits [38]. This section will concentrate on optimisation of radiation protection, which in turn is shaped by knowledge, attitudes, behaviours and technical skills [39]. Despite the myriad of techniques discussed herein, they can all be reduced to three key concepts: limit fluoroscopy time, stay as far away from the source of radiation as possible and use all available methods of shielding available [38]. These all correspond to the ALARA principles [40].

Although some methods of radiation safety are not modifiable by the interventionalist, such as architectural shielding, the majority are entirely operator dependent and can easily be implemented in everyday practice [8, 38]. In addition, because the majority of radiation received by the interventionalist is scatter, any methods used to reduce patient exposure will reduce staff exposure too—a win-win situation [16, 38].

14.3.2 Team Behaviour

14.3.2.1 ALARA

ALARA (as low as reasonably achievable) encompasses a ubiquitous philosophy of radiation safety and is the responsibility of all operators [12]. It dictates that exposure to radiation should produce sufficient benefit to the patient to offset any risks [41]. When performing an examination, the radiation doses should be minimised, but not to the detriment of imaging quality, where studies become undiagnostic or procedures unsafe [8, 9, 39].

14.3.2.2 Team Dynamics

Crew resource management (CRM) is a collection of practices originating in the aviation industry in order to optimise outcomes by reducing human error. CRM focuses on communication, decision making, situational awareness, threat management and horizontal leadership. Because ALARA behaviours are the responsibility of the whole team, CRM can be applied to complex endovascular procedures to the same end, with team-based pre-procedural briefings, run-throughs and practice of high-value interactions or steps. More specifically, it can identify potential problems and their solutions, define roles, confirm planning and sizing and predict C-arm angulations [42]. Applying this to EVAR resulted in a reduction in fluoroscopy time and radiation dose [42]. In daily practice, the whole team should contribute to a 'radiation-conscious facility' [41]. For example, the role of the radiographer is key in monitoring radiation doses and prompting ALARA principles [9], particularly if the operator is focused on the technical aspects of the procedure.

14.3.2.3 Institutional Culture

There are specific cultural factors that may impede widespread adoption of radiation safety within the medical sector, as opposed to other sectors such as the nuclear industry, where radiation safety is firmly embedded within the culture [43]. These factors include:

1. A primary focus on diagnosis and treatment, with other more acute safety issues taking precedence
2. Radiation safety being considered as secondary importance to other issues
3. Poor understanding of radiation dose and risks
4. Highly variable education, training and supervision
5. Over-justification of medical exposures
6. Poor patient awareness of radiation safety
7. A large number of independent professional, commercial and government bodies contributing to inadequate inter-body communication [43]

The working group that identified these issues proposed a top-down and bottom-up approach to engage managers, regulators and staff utilising an easy-to-follow 10-point assessment framework constituting good radiation safety culture [43]. Key features of safety culture include the belief that everybody is personally responsible, with strong leaders providing a fundamental driving force by actively demonstrating commitment to safety. These leaders in turn need to be supported by management structures that provide adequate resources, facilities, equipment, policies and procedures through a formal radiation protection programme [44].

14.3.2.4 Leadership

It can be challenging to adopt a strong radiation safety culture within the apparent competing interests of a modern healthcare system. However, they are inextricably linked; good safety culture exemplified by priorities and patterns of behaviour inevitably leads to high quality care, safe and satisfied patients and cost-effective performance [17]. Key to this is leadership from senior clinicians and managers. By championing the cause, they can instil active support from their staff, permeating safety culture throughout the department [7, 17]. Trainees who observe their supervisors consistently practice ALARA principles are more likely to follow suit [40]. In a study highlighting inconsistent radiation safety practices across South Africa, a fundamental finding was an absence of senior leadership roles. The attitude of the head of unit was key to developing a culture of radiation safety, and units with inconsistent and ineffective leaders suffered [7]. Vascular surgeons are well placed to lead the charge in radiation safety [15], and the key to achieving essential 'buy-in' is to supplement strong leadership with adequate education and training [7].

14.3.2.5 Education and Training

Traditionally, little time has been dedicated to radiation safety education and training for interventionalists [13, 31, 40]. The training that does exist is often heterogeneous or incomplete, with large discrepancies in the curriculum [7, 37]. A survey of vascular surgeons in the USA revealed that 45% had not had any formal radiation training, 74% were unaware of their hospital's radiation safety work policy for pregnancy, 48% did not know how to contact their hospital's radiation safety officer and 43% were unaware of the yearly recommended dose limits [45]. Cardiology fellows appeared better trained; 82% having undergone radiation safety training, with those trained displaying more knowledge of basic radiation safety, adherence to ALARA and awareness of their personal radiation exposure from the previous year [46]. Issues that impede successful radiation safety training delivery include a lack of definition, extensive guidelines containing many aspects irrelevant to everyday practice, and a reliance on theoretical physics [39].

It is universally accepted that radiation safety education should be a mandatory and integral part of the training of a vascular interventionalist [4, 7–9, 20, 40]. The best way to ensure this is as part of the curriculum within a formal training programme [44, 47], with the requirement to obtain certification necessary for graduation [20]. For example, 15% of the interventional cardiology board examination includes questions relating to radiation safety and physics [41]. In addition to initial training, regular updates and retraining with refresher courses are imperative throughout one's career to address skills decay [37, 44, 48].

The IRCP recommends radiation safety training commensurate with the individual's use of radiation [49], with European legislation recommending expanded education for those using X-rays routinely, such as vascular surgeons [37]. The quality of education and training needs to be externally assessed in several ways:

1. Accreditation by a recognised body
2. Periodic review to ensure it remains current
3. Certification based on exams requiring revalidation every 3–5 years [37]

In order to determine what the most important competencies are for a radiation safety programme, an expert consensus was obtained from a wide range of European interventionalists [39]. They identified the following key components:

1. Knowledge skills (scatter, risks for healthcare workers and management of pregnant staff)
2. Technical skills (reducing exposure time, increasing distance from source, avoiding primary beam, use of shielding
3. Attitudes (personal and team protection) [39]

Interestingly, it was felt little was required in the way of theory and basic physics. It was felt that embracing modern and interactive training methods may improve the assimilation and practice of these skills. Alongside traditional lectures, these include e-learning, simulation and game-based learning to achieve skill acquisition in a safe environment without the use of X-rays [39].

Despite these recommendations, the delivery and content of such training still vary considerably from country to country [37], but there is evidence that education changes behaviour and reduces dose to patients and surgeons [4]. Vascular fellows who underwent radiation safety training were more knowledgeable regarding safety principles and adherence to ALARA principles [45]. Over a 3-year period, the introduction of a comprehensive radiation safety programme led to a 40% reduction in mean cumulative skin dose [50]. A 2-day training programme consisting of 15 hours education led to a 50% reduction in DAP over 3285 coronary procedures during a 2-year period [51]. An even shorter 90-minute 'mini-course' for 154 cardiologists led to a 48% reduction in DAP [52] and a 16% reduction in PSD was noted 8 months after an unspecified 'education event' taught by medical physicists [31].

14.3.3 Individual Behaviour

14.3.3.1 Distance from Source

If there is no requirement to be in close proximity to the X-ray source or patient, particularly during high-dose acquisitions (DSA runs), then staff should position themselves as far away as is practical, as the level of radiation decreases exponentially with distance according to the inverse square law [9]. For most endovascular procedures, the working distance from the arterial access site (usually the femoral artery) to the area of interest is fixed [19]. However, this distance can be extended using power injectors for DSA runs, and extension tubing attached to catheters or sheaths for manual injections [19, 53]. For operators who routinely hand-inject, 75% of their radiation exposure arises from DSA runs [54]. In cardiology, the influence of different arterial access sites on operator doses has been extensively investigated [55]. The simple but highly effective act of 'stepping away' from the patient during DSA can considerably reduce personal radiation dose [3, 9, 44]. A distance of 2 m is considered relatively 'safe' in terms of excess exposure [3], and taken to the extreme, operator dose can be effectively eliminated at 5 m [54]. If it is not practical to move 1–2 m back, even small changes can have a substantial effect, for example standing closer to the feet than the abdomen during pelvic interventions [38]. It has been suggested that 'stepping away' should be mandatory behaviour if it does not compromise the safety of the patient; however, it was only observed in 6% of complex aortic cases [9]. These manoeuvres are of even more importance to operators of short stature whose proximity to the radiation source and patient may result in their upper body being exposed to more scatter [16]. It is also important to convey this message to anaesthetic colleagues who are often at the head of the table and close to the source. Studies have demonstrated anaesthetists' doses are far greater than necessary, with one recording a dose at the anaesthetist's position significantly higher than the primary operator and 15-times that of the scrub nurse [3].

14.3.3.2 Position Around the Table

Due to the uneven distribution of scatter radiation, the position at the angiography table significantly dictates the amount of radiation exposure one receives. The highest intensity of scatter is located on the X-ray beam entrance side of the patient [44], usually under the table, with cranial left anterior oblique (LAO) projections resulting in high levels of operator scatter [44]. Generally, doses are significantly higher for primary operators compared to assistants and scrub nurses [9, 29]. In a study reporting personal exposure during complex aortic repairs according to position around the table, it was found that the principal operator received twice the dose of the first assistant standing next to them, with the third assistant/scrub nurse position enjoying undetectable levels for almost all cases [2]. The second highest dose after the primary operator was the position required for left brachial access.

As previously discussed, the inverse square law is fundamental to understanding the importance of reducing radiation dose by 'stepping away' from the source. However, it pertains to the behaviour of X-rays in a vacuum, and variation in room configurations, imaging techniques and patient characteristics create multiple variables that deviate scatter radiation from easily predictable patterns [10]. In an elegant cadaveric study, which mapped the scatter around the angiographic table, it was found that, although radiation exposure decreased with distance from the source, this decay in dose was asymmetrical, and rather than conforming to concentric circles as predicted by the inverse square law, they resembled a 'scatter cloud' [10]. With antero-posterior (AP) imaging, the radiation fields had a bimodal symmetric dumbbell shape, with maximum exposure adjacent to the table at positions typical for the operator and assistant. Lateral projections led to peaks on the emitter side, with a full left lateral projection creating almost seven times the radiation as a right anterior oblique (RAO) 45° projection. All of these radiation plots demonstrated nonconformity when compared to the inverse square law, and therefore, the authors suggested that simply taking a step back from the table may not be enough to provide the level of safety that has traditionally been ascribed to it. In concordance with other investigators, they suggest emphasis should be made to move personnel away from the patient when standing on the emitter side of the table during DSA runs, as this is where the highest radiation doses were observed.

14.3.3.3 Pregnancy

Exposure to radiation in vascular training occurs in peak childbearing years, but less than 50% of women in vascular surgery surveyed had any counselling regarding radiation protection during their pregnancy [56]. With more women training in vascular surgery, specific guidelines regarding radiation safety during pregnancy are lacking [56]. The risks of intrauterine radiation on the developing foetus include miscarriage, intrauterine growth retardation, small head size with associated mental retardation, and subsequent development of childhood cancers [37]. The most sensitive phases of pregnancy are those in which the interventionalist may not be aware that they are pregnant [56]. These include the pre-natal phase (0–8 days before implantation), with organogenesis occurring mostly in the first trimester [56] and weeks 8–15 where mental abnormalities are more prevalent [57]. Studies suggest that doses under 100 mGy do not represent an increased risk to the embryo or foetus [58]; a dose far in excess of the 20 mSv annual occupational exposure limit set by ICRP. Nevertheless, the dose limits for pregnant workers are even lower; in the USA, the foetal dose recommended by the NCRP is 5 mSv/pregnancy, with a 0.5 mSv/month limit once pregnancy is declared [37, 58]. In Europe, the foetal dose limit is lower than that recommended by the ICRP, at 1 mSv/pregnancy, the same dose limit for a member of the public [37, 58].

These limits are easily achievable if the operator is already in the habit of conforming to ALARA behaviours, with the vast majority of pregnant interventionalists able to continue performing endovascular procedures safely throughout their pregnancy without increased risk of foetal death or malformations [44, 56, 58].

Although foetal doses are negligible utilising standard radiation safety principles [58], there are some additional procedures that pregnant interventionalists may wish to employ to ensure their foetal dose remains as low as possible. Although standard 0.5 mmPb LE lead aprons in combination with ancillary shielding are extremely likely to provide sufficient protection [58], there is the option of wearing additional lead. Ideally, this is in the form of specially designed maternity gowns with a 1.0 mmPb LE insert around the abdomen and pelvis, providing an additional protection of almost 100-fold [56]. If unavailable, the option exists to wear an additional wrap-around apron across the abdomen or wear two standard wrap-around aprons [58]. The drawback of this additional protection is the added weight, and this needs to be balanced alongside the additional musculoskeletal strain that pregnancy already places on the operator. Foetal dose can be estimated by wearing an additional foetal dosimeter on the abdomen under lead, but it is essential that the wearer receives monthly feedback of results [44, 56]. Some flexibility in rostering has been suggested to reduce the radiation dose to trainees, at least during the most crucial gestational weeks, whilst continuing to fully participate in their training [56]. For more details, we refer the reader to 'suggested program guidelines for vascular surgery trainees' in Shaw et al. [56].

14.3.3.4 Dosimeters

Personal radiation monitoring in the form of an individual dosimeter is an essential line of defence against occupational radiation exposure [59]. The majority are thermoluminescent (TLD) [22] or optically stimulated luminescence (OSLD) dosimeters worn for weeks or months at a time. After this set period, they are evaluated, and a personal dose equivalent is calculated as the dose received in soft tissue at a certain depth under the dosimeter [37]. Because they provide an estimate of radiation dose well after actual exposure they are termed 'passive' dosimeters.

Although decades of monitoring thousands of interventionalists has demonstrated that only a minority receive concerning doses [59], dosimeters are the only real feedback available regarding personal Effective Dose and how efficacious one's radiation safety behaviour is. To quote Lord Kelvin 'If you cannot measure it, you cannot improve it' and optimising radiation protection is impossible without the data provided by personal dosimeters [59]. Analysis of personal data over a few months will provide information regarding the attenuation of lead garments and efficacy of additional safety practices [58]. Individuals and institutions should maintain lifelong exposure records, and staff working at multiple sites should collate their collective exposures [41].

Location of Dosimeters Dosimeters can be worn in specific locations to measure doses at those sites (e.g. eye, hand and gonads) [44], or in one location for an overall estimate of effective dose (e.g. trunk at waist or chest) [19]. Dosimeters placed on the abdomen may give a more accurate representation of whole-body dose rather than those worn on the chest [29]. Combining doses from multiple sites, usually the collar and trunk, will give more accurate information regarding occupational exposure and radiation safety behaviour [22]. A collar badge provides a direct measure of head and neck irradiation and ambient radiation fields [59]. Badges should be worn facing the radiation source, if working on the right of the patient this means wearing it on the left [19]. Dosimeters worn under lead in addition to over it will give additional information when working in heterogenous radiation fields [22].

Number of Dosimeters The wearing of two dosimeters is strongly recommended by the ICRP and American College of Surgeons to provide a more accurate estimate of personal occupational dose; one on the torso (chest or abdomen) under lead garments in order to estimate the dose to protected organs, and one outside lead, usually attached to the collar or left shoulder, to estimate the dose to unshielded areas, especially the head, eyes and skin [1, 37, 41, 44]. Effective Dose is estimated using the following formula:

$$ED = 0.5Hw + 0.025Hn$$

(ED = Effective Dose, Hw = under lead, Hn = over lead) [37].

Due to the potential issues associated with multiple dosimeters (loss, location swapping, or compliance) it has been argued that one worn correctly, on the front of the torso under lead between the shoulder and waist gives a good estimate of effective dose and is better than two worn incorrectly [44]. However, without an outside dosimeter, it is impossible to monitor eye doses, and to accurately estimate Effective Dose from personal dosimeter data; the most accurate algorithms require two dosimeter readings from inside and outside lead [44]. Other causes of inaccuracy include wearing dosimeters in the wrong location, back-to-front, leaving the dosimeter in an area of radiation exposure when not physically present, and not wearing it all times whilst in the hospital [44]. They may also underestimate exposure when angulated away from the radiation source [12].

Replacement Interval Endovascular surgeons should monitor their radiation use with the same rigour that they audit their morbidity and mortality [16]. In the same way that one could not use published, or even institutional data, to predict one's own complication rates, the same is true of personal occupational dose. In one study, there was a 60-fold whole body dose variation between interventionalists in the same institution, with equivalent lens doses varying 100-fold [38]. Therefore, periodic review of one's own personal dosimeter readings is essential. Dosimeters should therefore be changed monthly to facilitate quick identification of poor practices to allow implementation of better radiation safety practices [44]. High doses may indicate poor ALARA behaviours, and very low doses should raise the question of non-compliance of dosimeter use.

Dosimeter Compliance & Radiation Safety Culture In a survey of 615 European interventional cardiology healthcare professionals, only 64% wore their dosimeter at all times, 18% wore it most of the time, 6.5% some of the time and 4% occasionally [60]. Two-thirds of individuals viewed their radiation data regularly [60], with knowledge of personal doses reflecting good radiation safety practice [44]. Data pertaining to an institution's dosimeter practices, such as collective annual dose and number of late or non-returned dosimeters, reflect radiation safety culture as a whole within the organisation [17]. In a study of five UK hospital's global dosimeter data, there were 30% late returns and 10% non-returns, figures unheard of in other radiation industries such as nuclear sites, reflecting very different radiation safety cultures [17].

Real-time Dosimeters It could be argued that the role of passive dosimeters is more regulatory than educational. Even if operators analyse their data regularly and accurately, the time lag between recording and changing a behaviour is months at best. In addition, individual case dose data are not available, and operators must therefore infer their case exposure from the indirect metrics provided by the fluoroscopy machine (i.e. CAK, DAP and fluoroscopy time (FT)) [2, 16]. Therefore, behaviour that results in high doses during the case cannot be highlighted at the time, and remedial behaviours such as stepping back or more effective shielding use to reduce the dose cannot be instigated when it matters [2, 3]. In an attempt to provide some real-time feedback during a case, FDA regulations dictate that CAK and DAP are easily visible on the operator monitor, and an audible signal is activated after each 5-minute block of cumulative fluoroscopy time, which has to be acknowledged by manually silencing the alarm [61]. The use of 'active' dosimeters which sit over the top of lead aprons take these concepts a step further. They provide immediate feedback on occupational radiation exposure, either in the form of an auditory tone or a visual display, as well as recording data for case-by-case evaluation [37, 62]. The deficiency of passive dosimeters to change radiation safety lies in the protracted step of data feedback which is often in the order of several months. By bringing this step into real-time, active dosimeters highlight radiation safety behaviours to the interventionalist throughout the procedure. This can be especially useful when they are focused on the technical aspects of a case, often to the detriment of radiation safety [63]. In this manner, real-time dosimetry immediately alerts operators to harmful practices and allows them to change their behaviour instantaneously [3].

The use of dose-sensitive auditory dosimeters resulted in augmented safety behaviours such as utilising the inverse square law and minimising fluoroscopy, resulting in a significant reduction in staff exposure [62], with a randomised control trial demonstrating a 30% reduction in operator dose during coronary interventions [64]. A trial of real-time dosimeters during paediatric interventions resulted in significantly reduced primary operator doses, despite no change in procedure time, fluoroscopy time or patient dose, suggesting a positive influence on operator radiation safety practices [65]. However, in keeping with introducing any new technology into an established workflow, there can be issues. Miller et al. found no improvement in radiation dose during a range of endovascular procedures, despite the introduction of real-time dosimeters [63]. They cited a number of reasons including the inability to divide attention between the dosimeter feedback screen and that of the angiographic image, and the small screen not being visible from all angles of the room. In addition, prior to the introduction of the dosimeters, staff had already undergone radiation safety training and authors felt that dose-reduction behaviours may already have been optimised. Although Baumann at al highlighted a learning curve associated with the use of active dosimeters, this was only in the order of a few weeks and reported a 45% reduction in total staff dose associated with the introduction of these devices in their practice [66].

14.3.4 Machine Controls

14.3.4.1 Fluoroscopy Time & Last Image Hold

The time the interventionalist has their foot on the pedal is the single most important determinant of radiation exposure to both patient and staff [33], and behaviours aimed at limiting time of exposure are essential to master [67]. These include removal of wires and catheters using short taps of 'spot' fluoroscopy rather than continuous use [19, 33, 44], disengaging as soon as data acquisition is completed [37], and only using fluoroscopy when information is required such as observing objects in motion [44]. Fluoroscopic loop recordings can also be used to review dynamic processes rather than additional time on the pedal [44]. 'Last-image hold' capabilities is an FDA requirement of fluoroscopy units [33, 61] and should be relied on liberally for study, consultation and discussion during a case without the need for ongoing irradiation [16, 30, 68]. Perhaps most important is considering getting help if the fluoroscopy time is protracted or even aborting the case to continue on another day if truncation of the procedure is clinically feasible and there is a significant risk of deterministic radiation injury [67].

14.3.4.2 Automatic Dose Settings

Modern fluoroscopy machines have an Automatic Brightness Control (ABC)—also known as automatic exposure control—that optimises image quality by automatically increasing radiation dose if feedback from a photodiode within the image intensifier detects low light output [19, 23, 37]. Whilst this increases X-ray penetration to produce a good image quality, ABC can significantly increase radiation exposure silently without the operator being aware. The amount of radiation produced depends on the energy required to produce the X-ray beam [19], which in turn is determined by two factors used to generate the X-ray beam: milliamperage (mA) and peak kilovolts (kVp) [16, 19]. The mA setting controls the amount of current passing through the tube, and hence the number of X-ray photons (but not their energy) produced [69]. This influences beam intensity, referred to as 'Beam Quantity'. Because beam quantity is also influenced by pedal time, metrics of Beam Quantity can also be expressed as mAs in addition to mA. Low mA produces a mottled image, and the image quality is improved by increasing mA which increases the signal-to-noise ratio, but at the cost of increased radiation due to more electrons being produced [19]. kVp on the other hand controls the energy of the range of X-rays being produced [69]. This influences beam penetrance, and what is referred to as 'Beam Quality'. Image contrast (the differentiation of structures of differing densities) is inversely related to penetrance. A high kVp (known as a 'hard beam') is required for more penetration, such as in the obese. It must be remembered however that the radiation dose doubles for every 15% increase in kVp (if there is no reciprocal reduction in mA), because the kVp indicates the maximum kV in a non-linear spectrum of X-rays emitted. Conversely a 'soft beam', characterised by a lower kVp, contains a higher fraction of low energy X-rays producing better contrast between tissues and/or contrast agents [19, 69]. It can be seen that the interplay of kVp and mA is complex, and ABC juggles these factors to ensure kVp is adequate for sufficient exposure but not at the expense of loss of contrast, whilst mA is optimised for signal-to-noise ratio whilst maintaining adequate contrast [69].

Typical scenarios to be aware of in which ABC will significantly increase dose are when treating obese patients, a field containing extraneous radiodense material (such parts of the body outside of the area of interest), and steep gantry angulation angles. Although default settings on most modern machines are automatic and usually 'low dose' [11], if a combination of lower mA and increased kVp settings can be achieved these can further reduce exposure whilst not necessarily impacting greatly on image quality [16, 19, 32]. For example, increasing the kVp from 75 to 96 kVp can decrease entrance dose by 50% [19], and the routine use of half dose settings has been shown to reduce skin dose significantly with no reduction in image quality [70].

Whilst thoughtless use of ABC will significantly increase radiation dose, it must be appreciated that modern imaging equipment also offers many low-dose technological advances to reduce radiation dose [8]. Image processing can often compensate considerably for reduced image quality due to the interventionalist intentionally reducing dose as a result of reducing pulse and frame rates [44]. Terminology may differ between different machine manufacturers, and it is useful to consult with your manufacture representative, radiographer or medical physicist to become familiar with the features of your angiography equipment [44].

14.3.4.3 Fluoroscopy & Pulse Rate

Fluoroscopy can be produced in either a continuous manner, or pulsed, with X-rays generated in short bursts [1, 20, 36]. Continuous fluoroscopy is associated with blurred images due to patient and instrument movement [16]. Pulsed fluoroscopy counteracts these movements and reduces blurring whilst reducing radiation exposure and is therefore the default mode in modern X-ray systems [20, 33, 41]. Pulse rates are typically available at 30, 15, 7.5, 4 and 2 pulses per second. Due to initial analogue fluoroscopy being recorded at 30 frames per second, continuous fluoroscopy was produced at 30 pulses per second. However, the human eye and the brain's visual reception system can only analyse up to 12 images per second, any more than this are interpreted as an illusion of visual continuity [71]. Reducing fluoroscopy pulse rates from 30 to 15 or 7.5 pulses/second decreases radiation dose by 47% and 72% respectively [16, 36]. The lowest pulse rate possible should be chosen to produce an adequate image [16, 20, 30, 32, 36, 37], and at even three pulses a second it is possible to perform complex FEVAR [72].

14.3.4.4 Digital Subtraction Angiography & Frame Rate

Digital Subtraction Angiography (DSA) entails acquiring several images in succession in one field of view and then digitally subtracting the non-vascular structures, leaving contrast-enhanced images of the vessels. These high-quality images are often used for diagnosis and documentation purposes but at the cost of significant radiation dose compared to fluoroscopy [37].

There appears to be a general lack of awareness of the relatively high radiation associated with DSA compared to fluoroscopy [9]. Previous reports have documented the percentage of total dose during peripheral and cardiac interventions due to DSA to range between 70% and 90% [30, 54], and 50–80% of the radiation dose during TEVAR and EVAR, even with low frame rates (2/s) being employed [9, 34]. Compared to fluoroscopy, DSA is associated with a 6–10 times higher dose rate per frame [18], which contributes to 66% of the total radiation dose, whilst only accounting for 23% of total exposure time [12]. DSA also results in an eightfold higher staff radiation dose [30]. Therefore, documentation of the procedure by DSA results in significantly more radiation than the fluoroscopy-guided intervention itself [30].

One of the most effective techniques for reducing radiation dose during endovascular surgery is to reserve DSA for key scenes and critical steps [30]. DSA can often be replaced with fluoroscopy loops if high-quality imaging is not required [9, 10, 20, 30, 38, 41, 68], and in fact can replace most DSA runs [37]. The operating surgeon needs to balance how much suboptimal imaging is permissible to effectively diagnose, treat and assess the condition, as per ALARA principals [16].

The total number of images acquired during a procedure significantly affects radiation dose [44]. This in turn depends on number of pictures acquired per second (frame rate), time per run, and number of runs. The operator should reduce all of these factors to the minimum required to meet clinical need [44]. When DSA is required, reducing the frame rate will reduce dose in the same way as reducing pulse rate during fluoroscopy [9, 30, 32, 44], with number of frames correlating highly with total radiation dose [30]. Reducing frame rates from a continuous to 7.5 frames per second (fps) results in a 90% reduction in image numbers with an equivalent reduction in radiation dose [37]. Reducing frame rates to 2 fps for pelvic and upper leg interventions and 1 fps for lower leg and foot interventions appears adequate [30]. Other features of modern machines such as the ability to return the table to the exact position and overlay a fade of a previous DSA will reduce unnecessary repeated DSA examinations [30].

14.3.4.5 Collimation

Collimation uses filters within the X-ray source to reduce the radiation field size to the minimal required area of interest, thereby shielding the patient's body from radiation outside of the area of interest [38]. By shaping the beam and absorbing low-energy photons not useful in image generation, collimation not only produces a sharper image, but also reduces radiation exposure to the patient in proportion to the reduced image size, and consequently scatter is reduced [1, 16, 30, 32, 33, 37, 73]. During cardiac procedures the use of collimation reduced patient and staff radiation by 40% [74] and meticulously collimating on a modern machine reduced DAP by a factor of more than ten compared to wide-open shutters [59]. In a cadaveric study, investigators found that horizontal and vertical collimation significantly reduced scatter and were independent of each other [75]. By increasing horizontal and vertical collimation independently from 0 to 10 cm (5 cm each side) they reduced scatter to the operator, assistant and anaesthetist by 86%, 80% and 96% for horizontal collimation and 88%, 89% and 92% for vertical collimation respectively [75]. Collimation reduces scatter by focusing the radiation field to a smaller area on the patient, resulting on a larger volume of the patient's tissues available to attenuate scatter before exiting the patient and reaching the staff [75]. However, the cost of this is increased patient skin entrance dose [75], and care must be taken not to perform prolonged and highly collimated studies in one gantry position. Virtual collimation (where the collimation blades are projected on the monitor) eliminates the need for fluoroscopy to adjust collimation leaf position [37, 44]. Even when a full field is required the collimator blade edges should be just visible on the monitor thereby reducing radiation extending outside of the image receptor [38].

14.3.4.6 Magnification

The input Field of View (FOV) of modern Image intensifiers (II) is adjustable to a range of sizes. Using the largest FOV without magnification the output spatial resolution is lower, image distortion higher and in general radiation dose lowest. By using magnification, a smaller area of the II input phosphor is irradiated, giving the effect of enlarging the image, enabling improved visibility [76]. If the FOV is halved the spatial resolution is doubled. However, only a quarter of the input II is being irradiated as the area is proportional to the square of the FOV. If all other parameters were kept constant, halving the FOV would reduce the image brightness to a quarter of the original FOV, rending it unusable [76]. Therefore, the machine's automatic brightness controls quadruple the radiation to compensate and deliver a bright image [77]. As a result, the smaller the FOV the larger the magnification and the higher the patient dose [76]. Because collimation is automatically applied during magnification, in the same way that increased collimation increases entrance skin dose but reduces scatter, increasing magnification (a smaller FOV) increases CAK, but decreases DAP, thereby increasing the risk of deterministic effects to the patient, but reducing stochastic effects and scatter experienced by the staff [3]. However, the general advice is to use the highest FOV as possible with judicious use of magnification [19, 67, 68]. One method to provide improved detail whilst avoiding the additional radiation associated with magnification is to use the 'digital zoom' function on a large monitor [68]. This simply increases the size of the image on the screen without actually reducing the FOV of the input beam, thereby leaving the radiation dose unchanged.

14.3.4.7 Imaging Chain Geometry

Imaging Chain Geometry refers to the distances between the linear arrangement of the X-ray source-to-patient-to-detector (image intensifier) [44]. Both X-ray source-to-patient and patient-to-detector have a significant independent combined influence on scatter.

The X-ray source is located under the patient to ensure that maximum scatter is dispersed under the table with a drop-off in scatter as one moves towards the operator's head [44]. The distance between the X-ray source and the patient is set by the table height. As with collimation and magnification, a balance needs to be met between radiation dose delivered to the patient and that to the operator. Ensuring maximal table height from the X-ray source will reduce patient dose [41, 44, 68], but at the cost of significantly increased scatter, with maximal dose at around 5 feet (1.5 m) from the floor, exposing the operator's head, eyes and neck [68, 75]. Therefore, the table needs to be as low as feasible to ensure the distance from the primary X-rays (source), and more importantly scatter (patient), is as far away from the operator's chest and head as possible [37]. This is of particular importance for shorter interventionalists.

The next component of imaging chain geometry is the distance from the patient to the detector. The detector should be as close to the patient as possible [41, 44]. Unnecessary distance causes increased dispersion of the X-ray beam, with a subsequent reduction in signal reaching the II, and a resultant increase in dose initiated by the machine's ABC in order to compensate [33, 37]. Minimising the patient-to-detector distance has multiple benefits:

1. Reduces the amount of energy required to produce the image and thereby reduces scatter
2. Increases scatter absorption by the detector itself
3. Results in a sharper image [19, 75]

14.3.4.8 C-Arm Angulation

Appreciating the influence of the C-arm, or gantry, angulation on radiation dose complements optimised imaging chain geometry. It is important to keep steep C-arm angulation to an absolute minimum for four reasons [8, 10, 16, 20]:

1. It requires more radiation to produce images through the lateral torso than in an anterior-posterior (AP) projection as patient thickness is increased; this increases both scatter and skin dose.
2. More of this scatter hits the operator.
3. More of this scatter occurs above the table in the region of the operator's torso and head.
4. It places the X-ray source closer to the patient's skin, increasing skin dose and risk of deterministic injuries.

Frequent changes in gantry angulation have been recommended in prolonged exposures to reduce skin dose by changing the pattern of radiation [31, 32, 67]. This should be achieved by moving back towards the AP position, but steep cranial and lateral angulation should never be used for this purpose [31], as it has the same effect as obesity in creating more tissue for X-rays to penetrate [33]. The machine's ABC then detects a thicker tissue path and increases dose to achieve adequate penetration [33]. The use of steep angulation in the obese compounds the risks [78] and should be used sparingly [33]. Due to the increased proximity of the X-ray source to skin that occurs with steep beam angulation, one review reported steep beam angulation as the cause of 83% of radiation skin injuries [78]. Exposure to the operator increases exponentially with lateral angulation over 30° and cranial angulation exceeding 15° [37], reaching a maximum at full lateral projection [9]. On a phantom model, AP projections resulted in 5 mSv/hour operator exposure rising to 11 mSv/hour at a 45° projection, and 69 mSv/hour at 90° [10]. Steep angulation such as that required during complex aortic repairs lead to significantly higher scatter exposure to the operator, particularly at the head level [79]. Cranial left anterior oblique projections cause the most exposure [9, 41, 44, 79–81], because the radiation source is usually on the same side as the operator in this configuration, leading to maximum backscatter towards the operator [9, 75]. The source being on the same side as the operator can lead to six times more radiation exposure [1]. When steep angulation is essential for the case, it should be for the shortest period of time with application of adequate collimation [37].

14.3.5 Imaging Equipment & Workflow

14.3.5.1 Flat Panel Detectors

Flat panel detectors reduce radiation dose [52]. They have a high sensitivity to X-rays, high signal to noise ratio, wide dynamic range, limited geometric distortion and high uniformity across the field of view. This results in 30–50% less dose than traditional image intensifiers [82, 83]. Due to this sensitivity, 'low dose' or 'extra-low dose' modes should be chosen over the 'normal' modes, as these are associated with adequate imaging quality with much lower radiation requirements [83].

14.3.5.2 Fixed Systems Versus Mobile C-Arms

Endovascular surgery has evolved from procedures performed using a fluoroscopy machine with a mobile C-arm in a traditional operating room, into dedicated hybrid suites with fixed angiographic machines. Compared to fixed systems, C-arms have been associated with inferior imaging quality, overheating, higher operator doses due to a lack of table and ceiling-mounted shields, worse chain-geometry and less ability for the operator to move away from the source. Despite these limitations, they have been associated with a reduced overall radiation dose of about 3.5 times lower than fixed systems [21, 26, 84–87]. It has been suggested that, for standard EVAR, mobile C-arms are of sufficient quality to perform the task with less radiation than that in hybrid suites [84], with fluoroscopy times and outcomes being similar for EVAR performed with C-arm versus a fixed system [88, 89]. However, it must be considered whether it is safe to perform complex procedures with inferior imaging capabilities, particularly in an ever-growing obese population [87], and also foregoing the additional efficiencies and safety features that hybrid suites afford [88]. Modern fixed systems have more powerful X-ray systems operating at higher energies with larger beam sizes and detectors which contribute to a three to tenfold higher radiation dose compared to mobile C-arms [87, 90]. However improved imaging allows replacement of DSA and magnification with other methods. Combined with dose-reducing software capabilities, this enables a reduction in radiation use despite the higher quality imaging [91]. It has been shown that by strictly adhering to ALARA principles and utilising modern radiation reducing technologies, such as image fusion and fluoroscopy loops replacing DSA, moving from a C-arm to a hybrid suite can actually be associated with a halving of the median radiation dose associated with EVAR from 30 to 12 Gycm^2. Similarly, another group found radiation exposure associated with TEVAR was significantly reduced from 14.9 to 8.6 mSv with the move from mobile C-arm to a fixed system [92]. Other groups have described significant increases in operator radiation exposure during a range of endovascular procedures with the move from mobile to fixed systems [89, 90], noting that surgeons will use the best imaging available to them. Indeed, the fact that the surgeon no longer has to worry about an overheating mobile unit may result in more liberal use with fixed systems [86]. This underscores the importance of utilising all the radiation-reducing capabilities that a hybrid suite offers to offset the increased exposure that accompanies superior imaging. These include dose-reducing software, low-dose settings, ceiling-mounted shielding, operator-controlled imaging and of course always adhering to ALARA and utilising the inverse square law.

14.3.5.3 Operator-Controlled Imaging

One of the advantages of moving from mobile systems into a hybrid suite is the ability to control imaging by the surgical team [85] using tableside operator-controlled imaging (OCI). OCI removes potential misunderstanding between the operator's instructions and the radiographer's actions, thereby reducing unnecessary exposure [85]. Discrepancies in language, ambiguous words (e.g. 'up', 'rotate' and 'turn') and confusion about how best to describe certain C-arm movements can all lead to unnecessary radiation exposure [93]. In a retrospective study of OCI during EVAR, investigators reported a significant reduction in fluoroscopy time (16.2 versus 20 minutes) and radiation exposure (DAP 4.9 vs 6.9 mGym^2) [94]. Interestingly, the range of DAP was significantly reduced (1.9–95 mGym^2 vs 1.25–13.3 mGym^2), perhaps reflecting more accurate patient positioning prior to high-dose acquisition runs. If OCI is unavailable, then improving communication between the surgeon and the radiographer can significantly reduce the time taken to move the C-arm and unnecessary radiation exposure [95].

14.3.5.4 Advanced Dose-Reduction Software

Modern imaging equipment produces excellent quality images, but at the cost of increased radiation dose. This has prompted imaging equipment vendors to focus now on radiation safety strategies, particularly hardware and software modifications to reduce radiation dose whilst maintaining imaging quality [96]. Whilst all vendors have their own proprietary approach, two studies reported on upgrading to the

Philips AlluraClarity system ClarityIQ (Philips Healthcare) system [87, 97]. This system combines:

1. Machine controls (smaller focal spots, shorter pulses, lower tube current and additional beam filtration)
2. Image-processing algorithms (automatic pixel shifting, temporal averaging of consecutive imaging, spatial noise reduction, motion compensation and image enhancement)
3. Hardware configurations to reduce entrance dose (optimising acquisition chain for different anatomical regions) [87, 97]

Studies utilising the upgraded system software have reported an approximate halving of radiation associated with EVAR, 39% reduction with visceral embolisation and up to 70% reduction in lower extremity interventions [63, 87, 97–99].

14.3.5.5 Pre-operative Planning Software

Meticulous case planning based on pre-operative CT imaging post-processing software prior to complex interventions can negate unnecessary diagnostic runs, thereby reducing radiation dose [37, 42]. Iliac bifurcation profiling during EVAR often requires 20–30° of lateral angulation and the neck 5–15° of cranial angulation [100]. DSA runs in this position contribute to some of the highest radiation doses and operator scatter exposure during EVAR [101]. One study using SyngoVia® (Siemens) post-processing software to remove unnecessary diagnostic runs demonstrated a threefold reduction in mean DAP during EVAR [101]. Several other studies have demonstrated similar utility with the open-source software Osirix® (Pixmeo Labs, Switzerland); whilst not measuring radiation doses, they have demonstrated a reduction in operating time by one third by predicting C-arm angles pre-operatively [102, 103].

14.3.5.6 3D-Image Fusion Software

3D-image fusion (3D-IF) amalgamates pre-operative CT-A images with live fluoroscopy, resulting in a three-dimensional volume-rendered angiogram that can be used as a virtual roadmap during interventions, particularly useful during complex aortic repairs [104]. By co-registering bony landmarks on both pre-op and live images, the fused 3D model automatically follows the table and gantry movements [37], negating the need for repeated DSA and fluoroscopy during stent deployment and target vessel cannulation, thereby reducing procedure time, contrast use and radiation exposure [9, 105, 106]. Investigative and real-world studies using 3D-IF report a significant reduction in radiation during a full range of standard and complex fenestrated and branched aortic interventions by up to 70% [26, 107, 108].

One limitation of 3D-IF is the additional radiation required to co-register the images at the beginning of the case. Initial systems required a full or partial spin, such as cone-beam CT (CBCT), which could add approximately 5% of the total radiation dose [104]. This radiation dose can be reduced up to tenfold by replacing CBCT with two orthogonal AP and lateral fluoroscopic shots [72, 109]. More sophisticated systems have since been developed, such as the Cydar 3D-imaging system, which have simplified this process by developing auto-registration of overlays from pre-operative imaging [110].

The remaining limitation is inaccuracy of overlay, particularly vessel deformation following the passage of stiff wires, which can render the overlaid pre-op images inaccurate [9]. Recent advances in 3D-IF technology using a cloud-based artificial intelligence system correct in real-time for deformation throughout the case, significantly improved accuracy and functionality of the overlay system, with a consequential reduction in radiation exposure [111].

14.3.6 Shielding

Along with ALARA principles, shielding is one of the main pillars of protection against scatter for the operator. Shielding comes in many forms including architectural (built into the walls and viewing windows of angiography suites), equipment-mounted lead (e.g. table drapes), ceiling-mounted leaded acrylic, large floor-supported mobile shields and leaded personal protection equipment (e.g. gown, glasses, thyroid shield). As the patient is the main source of scatter, most shielding is designed to act as a barrier between the patient and operator, and as such, shielding should be arranged to leave minimal gaps between the patient and shielding [59]. A combination of all available modalities should be routinely used as it dramatically reduces operator exposure [44]. For example, just combining ceiling- and table-mounted shields in a phantom model has been shown to reduce radiation dose to the upper body by at least 80% [112]. However, in clinical practice, the maximum potential attenuation is not always achieved due to incorrect shield positioning, patient position, change in tube angles, operator position, misunderstanding of optimal position or perhaps most importantly not using available shielding. Large transparent floor-mounted mobile shields of 1–1.5 mmPb LE are useful for circulating staff during high-dose DSA [113].

14.3.6.1 Personal Lead Garments

Personal lead garments ('gowns' or 'aprons') come in a plethora of designs, thicknesses, materials and configurations. If the garments are sourced from shared collections around the hospital, then physical condition adds further variability; shared garments are often maltreated with rough handling and improper storage, such as hanging over the back of a chair, leading to damaged lead lining and diminished protection that is not apparent by external appearances [19, 56].

For angiography use, most national standards require a minimum of 0.35 mm of lead equivalence (mmPb LE) protection at the front and 0.25 mmPb LE at the back. Recognising that testing and reporting of garments is highly variable, garments of 0.35 mmPb LE have been reported to attenuate 93% of radiation [9], with 0.5 mmPb LE associated with protection between 95% and 99% of scatter and protecting 80% of active bone marrow [19, 41].

Although lead provides the best protection against radiation, its disadvantage is its weight, and long-term use can lead to career-shortening chronic musculoskeletal conditions [114, 115]. A vest and kilt design allows some of the weight to be carried by the hips rather than solely on the shoulders [113]. Although backless aprons are much lighter, they should only ever be worn if always facing the patient and radiation source [114], which can seldom be guaranteed. In response, manufacturers have developed lighter-weight garments made from materials other than lead, such as antimony and bismuth. These 'lead-free', 'low-lead' and 'lite-lead' composite garments are associated with a 25–40% reduction in weight [113]. However, significant concern exists regarding their ability to provide adequate protection against the wide range of radiation energies typically encountered in endovascular practice, with little evidence that they are even equivalent to the gold-standard attenuation material of lead [114, 116]. Current product testing and reporting methods leave users uncertain as to the level of protection they are receiving [117], with large variations in performance compared to the manufacturer's stated lead equivalence [116, 118]. Some studies have reported composites transmitting as much as double the radiation equivalent of lead-only aprons [119], and a comparison of real-world hospital garments reported a 38-fold difference in scatter protection in garments labelled as having the same protection [116].

The current recommendation for vascular interventionalists is to choose your own personal garment and look after it. It needs to fit properly, without large gaps at the arm holes, which can lead to high axilla exposures [120] and, if it is of an overlapping design, it needs to overlap adequately as the overlap design usually ensures the minimum protective thickness [44, 113]. It should predominantly be made from lead that provides 0.5 mmPb LE or greater anteriorly from each posterior axillary line, being careful to check for undisclosed labelling of double-panel thickness [56, 114]. When not in use, it should be stored on hangers and periodically checked for cracks with fluoroscopy [44, 113].

14.3.6.2 Leaded Eye Glasses

Although scatter levels diminish as one moves from the feet to the head, the eyes are one of the most radiosensitive tissues in the body and susceptible to cataract formation (see Chap. 13, Sects. 13.3 and 13.3.2.3). Without eye protection, deterministic thresholds may be exceeded in a matter of years [121], especially with unfavourable conditions commonly encountered such as a steep gantry angle and patient obesity, which significantly increase eye exposure [44]. The importance of the routine use of leaded eye glasses cannot be overstated, as they dramatically reduce the eye dose by a factor of 5–10 [122, 123], or to 2–3% of baseline dose [67], thereby reducing lens exposure far below occupational limits [2].

However, as with lead garments, the situation is somewhat more complicated. There has been a wide variation of radiation attenuation in glasses reported with the same lead equivalence (35–95%) and lens thickness. Radiation incident angle and frame fitting also play a role in proportion of radiation which is attenuated [68]. Eye doses differ between right and left depending on the proximity of the X-ray source [29]. However, the most important 'invisible' factor is that of absent lateral protection. Leaded glasses provide excellent protection front on, but the protective effect markedly diminishes when the head is turned to the side [4, 68, 113, 123, 124]. Up to 21% of ocular exposure is due to scatter from the operator's head, suggesting that side shields or a wrap-around frame with added lead protection is necessary to provide adequate protection [19, 44].

It is therefore recommended that eye protection is always worn, made from 0.75 mmPb LE leaded glass in a well-fitted frame with no gaps at the nose and cheek, with incorporated lateral leaded shield in the design [68, 113], combined with ceiling-mounted shields to achieve full protection [4, 29, 113]. This combination can result in an undetectable lens dose [122]. In clinical practice, the addition of ceiling-mounted shields to leaded glasses reduced radiation dose from 2.1- to 5.7-fold [123]. In a separate experiment, leaded glasses combined with a host of addition shielding including ceiling shields and table skirts reduced eye doses in excess of 25-fold [122].

Despite the overwhelming evidence that the eye is highly vulnerable to radiation-induced injury, and that a combination of leaded glasses and adjunctive shielding dramatically reduces lens exposure, such protection remains grossly underutilised [68]. In one study, the use of eye protection during cases among vascular surgeons varied considerably from 0%, 9%, 10.6% and 100% of the time [6]. In another study, only 25% of interventionalists and 36% of cardiologists utilised eye protection [125]. Such behaviour has been most kindly described as illogical [68].

14.3.6.3 Thyroid Shield

In order to prevent radiation-induced thyroid cancer, it is recommended that all staff under 40 years old who regularly receive a monthly collar radiation dose of >4 mSv wear a lead thyroid shield [126]. However, due to their small size and convenience, their use is often extended outside of these recommendations [113], resulting in almost ubiquitous use. A 0.5 mmPb LE thyroid shield substantially reduces thyroid radiation dose [22] but also has the added benefit of protecting all inferior neck structures. This includes the carotid arteries which receive 50% of the radiation detected at a left collar dosimeter [124].

14.3.6.4 Hats

Traditionally, the head has not received much attention regarding radiation shielding because scatter doses are lowest at head height, the brain is of low radiosensitivity, and the skull attenuates about 40% of scatter [127]. However, this topic has been gaining more interest recently (see Chap. 13, Sects. 13.3 and 13.3.4.4).

Interventionalists' head exposure has been found to be almost 10-times higher than whole body exposure [127], with the left side of the head receiving higher doses than the right and centre of the skull [128]. Several radiopaque surgical caps are commercially available, with claims that they substantially reduce brain dose, but their efficiency in reducing brain radiation remains inconclusive. Studies based on skull surface doses in humans report significant reductions in radiation of up to 16-fold [128], but these may not reflect deeper brain doses, as the majority of brain radiation comes from scatter arising at angles not covered by caps. One study using an anthropomorphic phantom head and brain found that whilst the cap attenuated direct tangential radiation by 65–70%, it only provided 4.9% protection to the left brain, 1.8% to the right brain and 3.3% to the whole brain [124]. A similar study using a sophisticated anthropomorphic head phantom with 15 separate detectors found the caps attenuated radiation at the temporal region outer skull in interventionalists by 60% and 71% in the phantoms, but only by 7% in the upper brain with no significant attenuation in midbrain [127]. It was suggested that if the cap truly decreased brain doses, the brain levels should mirror the attenuation achieved in the temporal surface region which was ten times higher. The conclusions of both studies were that these caps provided negligible protection to the brain and are ineffective, due to most scatter reaching the brain from a location below the physician's head, at angles outside of the cap's attenuation shadow [124, 127].

Radio-opaque surgical caps may therefore be of inadequate size and shape to provide a sufficient X-ray shadow, particularly from inferior scatter, and perhaps a different configuration may be required. A helmet design has previously demonstrated significant attenuation at the skull level [129]. A hood design made out of commercially available attenuating caps, fashioned to hang alongside the face and back of neck to the level of the chin, appears to provide much better protection than the cap [124]. In the anthropomorphic head phantom, this hood offered 70% protection to the left brain, 49% protection to the right brain and 55% protection to the whole brain compared to 4.9%, 1.8% and 3.3%, respectively, with the theatre cap design [124]. Current evidence does not support routine use, although there may be a role for shorter interventionalists who are more susceptible to higher radiation doses to the head [130].

14.3.6.5 Gloves

The hands are the most unprotected part of the operator's body in close proximity to the primary beam and scatter [4] and receive more radiation compared with other parts of the body [20], particularly the distal middle and ringer fingers [113]. Interestingly, there is a significant correlation between DAP and eye and finger doses, with eye and finger doses correlating with each other [4]. It is important for the operator to keep their hands and fingers out of the field at all times [113]. Even when kept out of the field, extensive instrument manipulation during screening can lead to high hand doses [29] and the exposure over a career can be substantial [67]. Chronic low dose may cause microvascular damage leading to radiodermatitis [4]. In addition to behaviour, some equipment can be used to increase the distance of the hands from the radiation field, such as utilising needle holders during fluoroscopic guided punctures [131, 132], and the use of longer sheaths [37]. The use of a leaded ceiling-mounted shield reduces finger exposure twofold [38]. The use of leaded gloves should be avoided as they can paradoxically lead to higher hand doses [113]. Although they can attenuate radiation by 15–30%, if they are misused and placed within the primary beam, they will not only increase forward and backscatter indefinitely within the glove but will lead to increased radiation dose via the machine's ABC to compensate for the increased attenuation within the field, further increasing hand doses [37, 41, 44, 113].

14.3.6.6 Ceiling-Mounted Shielding

The importance of the combined use of ceiling-mounted shields with leaded glasses has previously been discussed [122], providing better protection than leaded glasses alone [68]. In addition, ceiling-mounted shields provide full protection to the head and neck [113], potentially reducing brain, carotid and thyroid exposure. Studies have reported a 5.7–19-fold reduction in eye dose associated with their use [8, 113]. Their lack of availability during mobile C-arm procedures was cited as contributing to an 18-fold increase in operator dose [133]. As a consequence, ceiling-mounted shields should be available in any room where fluoroscopy is performed [68], but they are often underutilised. Even in studies designed to investigate radiation protection during complex aneurysm repairs, their use was inconsistent [3] or non-existent [9].

Another important factor is their correct positioning; if they are not precisely positioned, their ability to provide adequate protection is substantially compromised [68, 112, 134]. They need to be tightly applied between the patient's skin entrance of the X-ray beam and the operator, abutting the patient adjacent to the access site, rather than above the patient or pointed towards the X-ray source or receiver [2, 68]. For femoral access, this means positioning the cut-out contour tight on the leg just cephalad to the access, with the use of soft lead extension flaps helping to maintain contact between the patient and the shield [112]. Rather than having the shield as close to the scatter source as possible, it should be closer to the operator, with due attention paid to minimising the gap [112]. Moving the shield away from the patient surface or further cephalad will accentuate this gap, decreasing the efficacy of the shield [112]. In order to maintain correct positioning, the shield requires continual repositioning throughout the case, whenever there is a change to gantry angle, table position or table height [112, 134]. Therefore, to reap the significant benefit of ceiling-mounted shields, they need to be consistently used, precisely positioned, and frequently repositioned.

14.3.6.7 Leg and Foot Shielding

By design, the highest amount of scatter occurs under the table where the beam enters the patient [37]. The majority of forward scatter is absorbed by the patient, thereby exponentially attenuating any that reaches the operator's upper body [2]. Backward scatter however exposes the legs [37] with the highest operator dose occurring at the waist and knee level [135]. Doses to the unprotected legs are similar to those received by the hands [136]. A table-mounted side skirt, which hangs at the side of the bed and preferably extends upward several inches, significantly minimises this dose by a factor of 5–50 [2, 135, 136].

Leg exposure has received additional attention with the finding that circulating markers of DNA damage in endovascular interventionalists were elevated following complex aortic repairs, despite the presence of under-table lead shielding, but were completely absent in those wearing additional personal lower leg lead shielding [81]. This suggested that the majority of this DNA damage occurred in the long bones of the legs and that additional lower leg protection was essential to reduce scatter radiation-induced DNA damage [81].

Other investigators have demonstrated unequal leg and foot doses, with the highest closest to the source, postulating that the gap between the skirt and the floor, which is variable due to table height, may be responsible [137]. Even when table-mounted side skirts reduced mean procedural foot doses from 0.19–2.61 to 0.02–0.5 mSv, these investigators suggested that lower extremity annual doses could reach 110 mSv, approaching dose limits [137]. They suggested that further protective measures are taken to reduce foot and leg dose, such as stepping back or the use of a lead-lined protective clogs [137].

14.3.6.8 Drapes

Disposable sterile lead-free bismuth-barium drapes are commercially available to drape around the area of interest with the purpose of reducing scatter to the operator. Their attenuation is in the order of 0.4–0.8 mmPb LE, depending on beam energies encountered [138]. By redirecting scatter, the aim is to reduce operator-received radiation [4, 37, 68, 139], but in doing so, they may increase patient dose [37, 68]. They must never enter the field of view as they will activate the machines' ABC [37, 114] and may need to be repositioned during the procedure to avoid this [113].

Their use is more common in cardiac procedures, perhaps due to the relatively focused and static set-up, and in this setting has been associated with a significant reduction in operator exposure in the order of 20% [138, 139]. They have also been shown to reduce hand, eye and head doses by up to 50% [113, 114] and reduce eye dose by a factor of 1.2–24.6 [68].

In a small RCT during EVAR, two drapes were positioned around the site of femoral access and were associated with a reduction in scatter to the hands and chest of about 50% [138]. However, it must be noted that the procedures were performed using a mobile C-arm in a non-dedicated theatre with no additional shielding such as table-mounted skirts or ceiling-mounted shields.

14.3.7 Innovations

The inherent limitations of personal shielding, principally the musculoskeletal issues, associated with the weight of lead, and the incomplete protection afforded by the combination of even the best products, have led to the development of a number of novel solutions. The holy grail of personal radiation protection is total elimination of radiation exposure to the whole body and removal of the burden of lead on the musculoskeletal system, all within a user-friendly framework that does not impede workflow.

14.3.7.1 Zero Gravity Suspended System

Zero gravity (Biotronik Inc., Lake Oswego, OR) is a full-body lead personal protection device which is suspended from a complex overhead motion system that eliminates any weight on the operator. As a consequence, a thicker 1 mm lead can be used to provide protection from the top of the head to the calves, leaving only the right arm and left forearm uncovered [140]. It provides 5.9–46 times more attenuation over a wide range of beam energies [114], with an overall 78-fold decrease in radiation exposure compared to a 0.5 mmPb LE apron [140].

14.3.7.2 Trinity System

The Trinity Radiation Protection System (ECLS, Salt Lake City, UT) consists of fixed shields and skirts creating a complete radiation protection 'cocoon' around the patient to protect the operator, whilst allowing femoral access to the patient for cardiac interventions [141, 142]. A small study comparing ten cases performed with Trinity to nine with standard shielding reported undetectable radiation associated with Trinity with complete elimination of any exposure to operators [141]. Unfortunately, due to its configuration, it does not offer utility outside of interventions confined to the torso.

14.3.7.3 Cathpax Cabin

Cathpax® (Lemer Pax, Carquefou, France) is a single-operator mobile radiation protection cabin, designed principally for high-dose electrophysiology interventions. In a comparison to standard protection garments, its use was associated with full-body protection and negligible radiation exposure, whilst providing unimpeded access to perform complex interventions from a femoral access site [143]. Once again, it has a limited application for general vascular interventions.

14.3.7.4 EggNest Table

The EggNest (Egg Medical, Mapel Grove, MN) is a redesigned catheterisation table with more complete integrated shielding with the manufacture reporting a greater than 90% reduction in scatter [132] and has applicability for general interventions.

14.3.7.5 Endovascular Robotics

Robotic endovascular interventions eliminate operator exposure by freeing them entirely from the vicinity of scattered radiation. The use of endovascular robotics, principally steerable catheters, has been reported in many pre-clinical and small clinical reports of EVAR, BEVAR, FEVAR, arterial embolisations, iliac and SFA cannulations, IVC filter retrieval, pulmonary artery interventions, and the management of endoleak [107, 144–146]. Larger clinical studies are still required to determine the global applicability of this technology. The coupling of endovascular robotics with innovative navigation tracking systems such as electromagnetic tracking and fusion imaging may 1 day eliminate the need for fluoroscopy [146].

14.3.7.6 Non-radiation Imaging

There are currently a number of exciting innovations that use low or no-radiation technology to guide endovascular interventions. These include augmented reality, movement tracking, electromagnetic location tracking, optical coherence tomography and magnetic particle imaging. In addition, the expanded utility of already established technologies such as intravascular ultrasound should be encouraged.

14.4 Conclusion

Endovascular surgery will continue to evolve, perhaps utilising some of the novel technologies described above to eventually unshackle itself from its current reliance on ionising radiation. Until that time, a basic understanding of radiation biology and physics and a respect for radiation safety, coupled with a strict adherence to ALARA technique, using all and every shielding available, and reducing the time spent with 'foot on the pedal', will keep exposure to a minimum.

Multiple Choice Questions

1. Which of the following ALARA techniques is the single most effective way to reduce radiation exposure to the patient and staff?

   (a) Replace DSA with fluoro runs
   (b) Collimation
   (c) Reduce time on the pedal
   (d) Reduce fluoro and frame rate
   (e) Utilise all lead shielding available

   Answer: (c) Reduce time on the pedal

2. Which of the following C-Arm configurations (imaging chain geometry) is the best way to reduce the operator's head and torso exposure?

   (a) High bed and lowered receiver (image intensifier)
   (b) Waist-height bed and lowered receiver (image intensifier)
   (c) High bed and raised receiver (image intensifier)
   (d) Waist-height bed and raised receiver (image intensifier)
   (e) Low bed and raised receiver (image intensifier)

   Answer: (b) Waist-height bed and lowered receiver (image intensifier)

References

1. Walsh SR, Cousins C, Tang TY, Gaunt ME, Boyle JR. Ionizing radiation in endovascular interventions. J Endovasc Ther. 2008;15:680–7. https://doi.org/10.1583/08-2495.1.
2. Kirkwood ML, Guild JB, Arbique GM, Anderson JA, Valentine RJ, Timaran C. Surgeon radiation dose during complex endovascular procedures. J Vasc Surg. 2015;62:457–63. https://doi.org/10.1016/j.jvs.2015.02.050.
3. Mohapatra A, Greenberg RK, Mastracci TM, Eagleton MJ, Thornsberry B. Radiation exposure to operating room personnel and patients during endovascular procedures. J Vasc Surg. 2013;58:702–9. https://doi.org/10.1016/j.jvs.2013.02.032.
4. Attigah N, Oikonomou K, Hinz U, Knoch T, Demirel S, Verhoeven E, et al. Radiation exposure to eye lens and operator hands during endovascular procedures in hybrid operating rooms. J Vasc Surg. 2016;63:198–203. https://doi.org/10.1016/j.jvs.2015.08.051.
5. Kim JB, Lee J, Park K. Radiation hazards to vascular surgeon and scrub nurse in mobile fluoroscopy equipped hybrid vascular room. Ann Surg Treat Res. 2017;92:156–63. https://doi.org/10.4174/astr.2017.92.3.156.
6. Ho P, Cheng SW, Wu PM, Ting AC, Poon JT, Cheng CK, et al. Ionizing radiation absorption of vascular surgeons during endovascular procedures. J Vasc Surg. 2007;46:455–9. https://doi.org/10.1016/j.jvs.2007.04.034.
7. Rose A, Rae WI. Perceptions of radiation safety training among interventionalists in South Africa. Cardiovasc J Afr. 2017;28:196–200. https://doi.org/10.5830/cvja-2017-028.
8. Resch TA, Törnqvist P, Sonesson B, Dias NV. Techniques to reduce radiation for patients and operators during aortic endografting. J Cardiovasc Surg (Torino). 2016;57:178–84.

9. Patel AP, Gallacher D, Dourado R, Lyons O, Smith A, Zayed H, et al. Occupational radiation exposure during endovascular aortic procedures. Eur J Vasc Endovasc Surg. 2013;46:424–30. https://doi.org/10.1016/j.ejvs.2013.05.023.
10. Haqqani OP, Agarwal PK, Halin NM, Iafrati MD. Defining the radiation "scatter cloud" in the interventional suite. J Vasc Surg. 2013;58:1339–45. https://doi.org/10.1016/j.jvs.2013.01.025.
11. Bicknell CD. Occupational radiation exposure and the vascular interventionalist. Eur J Vasc Endovasc Surg. 2013;46:431. https://doi.org/10.1016/j.ejvs.2013.06.012.
12. Zhou W. Radiation exposure of vascular surgery patients beyond endovascular procedures. J Vasc Surg. 2011;53:39s–43s. https://doi.org/10.1016/j.jvs.2010.06.176.
13. Machado R, Ferreira VM, Loureiro L, Gonçalves J, Oliveira P, Almeida R. Radiation exposure in endovascular infra-renal aortic aneurysm repair and factors that influence it. Braz J Cardiovasc Surg. 2016;31:415–21. https://doi.org/10.5935/1678-9741.20160084.
14. Bannazadeh M, Altinel O, Kashyap VS, Sun Z, Clair D, Sarac TP. Patterns of procedure-specific radiation exposure in the endovascular era: impetus for further innovation. J Vasc Surg. 2009;49:1520–4. https://doi.org/10.1016/j.jvs.2009.02.015.
15. Mastracci TM. Radiation safety: a call to arms. Eur J Vasc Endovasc Surg. 2015;50:1–2. https://doi.org/10.1016/j.ejvs.2015.02.001.
16. Ketteler ER, Brown KR. Radiation exposure in endovascular procedures. J Vasc Surg. 2011;53:35s–8s. https://doi.org/10.1016/j.jvs.2010.05.141.
17. Cole P, Hallard R, Broughton J, Coates R, Croft J, Davies K, et al. Developing the radiation protection safety culture in the UK. J Radiol Prot. 2014;34:469–84. https://doi.org/10.1088/0952-4746/34/2/469.
18. Hirshfeld JW Jr, Ferrari VA, Bengel FM, Bergersen L, Chambers CE, Einstein AJ, et al. 2018 ACC/HRS/NASCI/SCAI/SCCT expert consensus document on optimal use of ionizing radiation in cardiovascular imaging: best practices for safety and effectiveness: a report of the American College of Cardiology Task Force on Expert Consensus Decision Pathways. J Am Coll Cardiol. 2018;71:e283–351. https://doi.org/10.1016/j.jacc.2018.02.016.
19. Lipsitz EC, Veith FJ, Ohki T, Heller S, Wain RA, Suggs WD, et al. Does the endovascular repair of aortoiliac aneurysms pose a radiation safety hazard to vascular surgeons? J Vasc Surg. 2000;32:704–10. https://doi.org/10.1067/mva.2000.110053.
20. Monastiriotis S, Comito M, Labropoulos N. Radiation exposure in endovascular repair of abdominal and thoracic aortic aneurysms. J Vasc Surg. 2015;62:753–61. https://doi.org/10.1016/j.jvs.2015.05.033.
21. Beathard GA, Urbanes A, Litchfield T. Radiation dose associated with dialysis vascular access interventional procedures in the interventional nephrology facility. Semin Dial. 2013;26:503–10. https://doi.org/10.1111/sdi.12071.
22. Kim KP, Miller DL, Berrington de Gonzalez A, Balter S, Kleinerman RA, Ostroumova E, et al. Occupational radiation doses to operators performing fluoroscopically-guided procedures. Health Phys. 2012;103:80–99. https://doi.org/10.1097/HP.0b013e31824dae76.
23. Kim KP, Miller DL, Balter S, Kleinerman RA, Linet MS, Kwon D, et al. Occupational radiation doses to operators performing cardiac catheterization procedures. Health Phys. 2008;94:211–27. https://doi.org/10.1097/01.Hp.0000290614.76386.35.
24. Geijer H, Larzon T, Popek R, Beckman KW. Radiation exposure in stent-grafting of abdominal aortic aneurysms. Br J Radiol. 2005;78:906–12. https://doi.org/10.1259/bjr/72629938.
25. de Ruiter QMB, Jansen MM, Moll FL, Hazenberg C, Kahya NN, van Herwaarden JA. Procedure and step-based analysis of the occupational radiation dose during endovascular aneurysm repair in the hybrid operating room. J Vasc Surg. 2018;67:1881–90. https://doi.org/10.1016/j.jvs.2017.09.043.
26. Hertault A, Rhee R, Antoniou GA, Adam D, Tonda H, Rousseau H, et al. Radiation dose reduction during EVAR: results from a prospective multicentre study (the REVAR study). Eur J Vasc Endovasc Surg. 2018;56:426–33. https://doi.org/10.1016/j.ejvs.2018.05.001.

27. Weerakkody RA, Walsh SR, Cousins C, Goldstone KE, Tang TY, Gaunt ME. Radiation exposure during endovascular aneurysm repair. Br J Surg. 2008;95:699–702. https://doi.org/10.1002/bjs.6229.
28. Howells P, Eaton R, Patel AS, Taylor P, Modarai B. Risk of radiation exposure during endovascular aortic repair. Eur J Vasc Endovasc Surg. 2012;43:393–7. https://doi.org/10.1016/j.ejvs.2011.12.031.
29. Bacchim Neto FA, Alves AF, Mascarenhas YM, Nicolucci P, Pina DR. Occupational radiation exposure in vascular interventional radiology: a complete evaluation of different body regions. Phys Med. 2016;32:1019–24. https://doi.org/10.1016/j.ejmp.2016.06.014.
30. Pitton MB, Kloeckner R, Schneider J, Ruckes C, Bersch A, Düber C. Radiation exposure in vascular angiographic procedures. J Vasc Interv Radiol. 2012;23:1487–95. https://doi.org/10.1016/j.jvir.2012.05.048.
31. Kirkwood ML, Arbique GM, Guild JB, Timaran C, Chung J, Anderson JA, et al. Surgeon education decreases radiation dose in complex endovascular procedures and improves patient safety. J Vasc Surg. 2013;58:715–21. https://doi.org/10.1016/j.jvs.2013.04.004.
32. Panuccio G, Greenberg RK, Wunderle K, Mastracci TM, Eagleton MG, Davros W. Comparison of indirect radiation dose estimates with directly measured radiation dose for patients and operators during complex endovascular procedures. J Vasc Surg. 2011;53:885–94.e1; discussion 94. https://doi.org/10.1016/j.jvs.2010.10.106.
33. Killewich LA, Falls G, Mastracci TM, Brown KR. Factors affecting radiation injury. J Vasc Surg. 2011;53:9s–14s. https://doi.org/10.1016/j.jvs.2010.07.025.
34. Usai MV, Schäfers J, Wunderle K, Torsello GF, Panuccio G. Radiation dose distribution in endovascular aneurysm repair in the hybrid operating room according to the specific phases of the procedure. Eur J Vasc Endovasc Surg. 2018;56:e17–e8.
35. Kiang SC, Ahmed KA, Cha VJ, Farley DV, Oyoyo UE, Abou-Zamzam AM, et al. Analysis of intraoperative radiation use in vascular surgery: catalyst for quality improvement in patient and personnel safety. Vascular. 2019;27:144–52. https://doi.org/10.1177/1708538118806749.
36. Miller DL, Balter S, Noonan PT, Georgia JD. Minimizing radiation-induced skin injury in interventional radiology procedures. Radiology. 2002;225:329–36. https://doi.org/10.1148/radiol.2252011414.
37. Hertault A, Maurel B, Midulla M, Bordier C, Desponds L, Saeed Kilani M, et al. Editor's choice – Minimizing radiation exposure during endovascular procedures: basic knowledge, literature review, and reporting standards. Eur J Vasc Endovasc Surg. 2015;50:21–36. https://doi.org/10.1016/j.ejvs.2015.01.014.
38. Miller DL. Make radiation protection a habit. Tech Vasc Interv Radiol. 2018;21:37–42. https://doi.org/10.1053/j.tvir.2017.12.008.
39. Doyen B, Maurel B, Cole J, Maertens H, Mastracci T, Van Herzeele I. Defining the key competencies in radiation protection for endovascular procedures: a multispecialty Delphi consensus study. Eur J Vasc Endovasc Surg. 2018;55:281–7. https://doi.org/10.1016/j.ejvs.2017.11.020.
40. Bordoli SJ, Carsten CG 3rd, Cull DL, Johnson BL, Taylor SM. Radiation safety education in vascular surgery training. J Vasc Surg. 2014;59:860–4. https://doi.org/10.1016/j.jvs.2013.10.085.
41. Ahmed TAN, Taha S. Radiation exposure, the forgotten enemy: toward implementation of national safety program. Egypt Heart J. 2017;69:55–62. https://doi.org/10.1016/j.ehj.2016.10.001.
42. Stansfield T, Parker R, Masson N, Lewis D. The endovascular preprocedural run through and brief: a simple intervention to reduce radiation dose and contrast load in endovascular aneurysm repair. Vasc Endovasc Surg. 2016;50:241–6. https://doi.org/10.1177/1538574416644527.
43. Chapple CL, Bradley A, Murray M, Orr P, Reay J, Riley P, et al. Radiation safety culture in the UK medical sector: a top to bottom strategy. Radiat Prot Dosim. 2017;173:80–6. https://doi.org/10.1093/rpd/ncw344.

44. Durán A, Hian SK, Miller DL, Le Heron J, Padovani R, Vano E. A summary of recommendations for occupational radiation protection in interventional cardiology. Catheter Cardiovasc Interv. 2013;81:562–7. https://doi.org/10.1002/ccd.24520.
45. Bordoli SJ, Carsten CG III, Cull DL, Johnson BL, Taylor SM. Radiation safety education in vascular surgery training: an unmet requirement. J Vasc Surg. 2013;27:297.
46. Kim C, Vasaiwala S, Haque F, Pratap K, Vidovich MI. Radiation safety among cardiology fellows. Am J Cardiol. 2010;106:125–8. https://doi.org/10.1016/j.amjcard.2010.02.026.
47. Limacher MC, Douglas PS, Germano G, Laskey WK, Lindsay BD, McKetty MH, et al. ACC expert consensus document. Radiation safety in the practice of cardiology. American College of Cardiology. J Am Coll Cardiol. 1998;31:892–913. https://doi.org/10.1016/s0735-1097(98)00047-3.
48. Gendelberg D, Hennrikus WL, Sawyer C, Armstrong D, King S. Decreased radiation exposure among orthopedic residents is maintained when using the mini C-arm after undergoing radiation safety training. Orthopedics. 2017;40:e788–e92. https://doi.org/10.3928/01477447-20170531-04.
49. European Commission D-GfE. Guidelines on radiation protection education and training of medical professionals in the European Union [Internet]. 2014 [cited 2019 Apr 28]. Available from: http://dx.publications.europa.eu/10.2833/19786.
50. Fetterly KA, Mathew V, Lennon R, Bell MR, Holmes DR Jr, Rihal CS. Radiation dose reduction in the invasive cardiovascular laboratory: implementing a culture and philosophy of radiation safety. JACC Cardiovasc Interv. 2012;5:866–73. https://doi.org/10.1016/j.jcin.2012.05.003.
51. Georges JL, Livarek B, Gibault-Genty G, Aziza JP, Hautecoeur JL, Soleille H, et al. Reduction of radiation delivered to patients undergoing invasive coronary procedures. Effect of a programme for dose reduction based on radiation-protection training. Arch Cardiovasc Dis. 2009;102:821–7. https://doi.org/10.1016/j.acvd.2009.09.007.
52. Kuon E, Weitmann K, Hoffmann W, Dörr M, Reffelmann T, Hummel A, et al. Efficacy of a minicourse in radiation-reducing techniques in invasive cardiology: a multicenter field study. JACC Cardiovasc Interv. 2014;7:382–90. https://doi.org/10.1016/j.jcin.2013.11.016.
53. Marque N, Jégou A, Varenne O, Salengro E, Allouch P, Margot O, et al. Impact of an extension tube on operator radiation exposure during coronary procedures performed through the radial approach. Arch Cardiovasc Dis. 2009;102:749–54. https://doi.org/10.1016/j.acvd.2009.09.006.
54. Layton KF, Kallmes DF, Cloft HJ, Schueler BA, Sturchio GM. Radiation exposure to the primary operator during endovascular surgical neuroradiology procedures. AJNR Am J Neuroradiol. 2006;27:742–3.
55. Pancholy SB, Joshi P, Shah S, Rao SV, Bertrand OF, Patel TM. Effect of vascular access site choice on radiation exposure during coronary angiography: the REVERE trial (randomized evaluation of vascular entry site and radiation exposure). JACC Cardiovasc Interv. 2015;8:1189–96. https://doi.org/10.1016/j.jcin.2015.03.026.
56. Shaw PM, Vouyouka A, Reed A. Time for radiation safety program guidelines for pregnant trainees and vascular surgeons. J Vasc Surg. 2012;55:862–8.e2. https://doi.org/10.1016/j.jvs.2011.11.045.
57. Shaw P, Duncan A, Vouyouka A, Ozsvath K. Radiation exposure and pregnancy. J Vasc Surg. 2011;53:28s–34s. https://doi.org/10.1016/j.jvs.2010.05.140.
58. Marx MV. Baby on board: managing occupational radiation exposure during pregnancy. Tech Vasc Interv Radiol. 2018;21:32–6. https://doi.org/10.1053/j.tvir.2017.12.007.
59. Balter S. Always on my mind. Tech Vasc Interv Radiol. 2018;21:26–31. https://doi.org/10.1053/j.tvir.2017.12.006.
60. Buchanan GL, Chieffo A, Mehilli J, Mikhail GW, Mauri F, Presbitero P, et al. The occupational effects of interventional cardiology: results from the WIN for safety survey. EuroIntervention. 2012;8:658–63. https://doi.org/10.4244/eijv8i6a103.

61. Killewich LA, Singleton TA. Governmental regulations and radiation exposure. J Vasc Surg. 2011;53:44s–6s. https://doi.org/10.1016/j.jvs.2010.06.177.
62. Hough DM, Brady A, Stevenson GW. Audible radiation monitors: the value in reducing radiation exposure to fluoroscopy personnel. AJR Am J Roentgenol. 1993;160:407–8. https://doi.org/10.2214/ajr.160.2.8424362.
63. Miller C, Kendrick D, Shevitz A, Kim A, Baele H, Jordan D, et al. Evaluating strategies for reducing scattered radiation in fixed-imaging hybrid operating suites. J Vasc Surg. 2018;67:1227–33. https://doi.org/10.1016/j.jvs.2017.08.083.
64. Christopoulos G, Papayannis AC, Alomar M, Kotsia A, Michael TT, Rangan BV, et al. Effect of a real-time radiation monitoring device on operator radiation exposure during cardiac catheterization: the radiation reduction during cardiac catheterization using real-time monitoring study. Circ Cardiovasc Interv. 2014;7:744–50. https://doi.org/10.1161/circinterventions.114.001974.
65. Racadio J, Nachabe R, Carelsen B, Racadio J, Hilvert N, Johnson N, et al. Effect of real-time radiation dose feedback on pediatric interventional radiology staff radiation exposure. J Vasc Interv Radiol. 2014;25:119–26. https://doi.org/10.1016/j.jvir.2013.08.015.
66. Baumann F, Katzen BT, Carelsen B, Diehm N, Benenati JF, Peña CS. The effect of realtime monitoring on dose exposure to staff within an interventional radiology setting. Cardiovasc Intervent Radiol. 2015;38:1105–11. https://doi.org/10.1007/s00270-015-1075-6.
67. Brown KR, Rzucidlo E. Acute and chronic radiation injury. J Vasc Surg. 2011;53:15s–21s. https://doi.org/10.1016/j.jvs.2010.06.175.
68. Machan L. The eyes have it. Tech Vasc Interv Radiol. 2018;21:21–5. https://doi.org/10.1053/j.tvir.2017.12.005.
69. Sy E, Samboju V, Mukhdomi T. X-ray image production procedures. StatPearls Publishing; 2022. Updated 2022 Oct 17.
70. Lederman HM, Khademian ZP, Felice M, Hurh PJ. Dose reduction fluoroscopy in pediatrics. Pediatr Radiol. 2002;32:844–8. https://doi.org/10.1007/s00247-002-0696-5.
71. Read P, Meyer MP. Light, sound and audiovisual perception. In: Restoration of motion picture film. Butterworth Heinemann; 2000.
72. Rolls AE, Rosen S, Constantinou J, Davis M, Cole J, Desai M, et al. Introduction of a team based approach to radiation dose reduction in the enhancement of the overall radiation safety profile of FEVAR. Eur J Vasc Endovasc Surg. 2016;52:451–7. https://doi.org/10.1016/j.ejvs.2016.05.010.
73. Tonnessen BH, Pounds L. Radiation physics. J Vasc Surg. 2011;53:6s–8s. https://doi.org/10.1016/j.jvs.2010.05.138.
74. Lindsay BD, Eichling JO, Ambos HD, Cain ME. Radiation exposure to patients and medical personnel during radiofrequency catheter ablation for supraventricular tachycardia. Am J Cardiol. 1992;70:218–23. https://doi.org/10.1016/0002-9149(92)91278-c.
75. Haqqani OP, Agarwal PK, Halin NM, Iafrati MD. Minimizing radiation exposure to the vascular surgeon. J Vasc Surg. 2012;55:799–805. https://doi.org/10.1016/j.jvs.2011.08.055.
76. Wang J, Blackburn T. Imaging and therapeutic technology – the AAPM/RSNA physics tutorial for residents: X-ray image intensifiers for fluoroscopy. Radiographics. 2000;20:1471–7.
77. SUNY Upstate Medical University [Internet]. 2019 [cited 2019 Jun 16]. Available from: http://www.upstate.edu/radiology/education/rsna/fluoro/iisize.php.
78. Koenig TR, Mettler FA, Wagner LK. Skin injuries from fluoroscopically guided procedures: part 2, review of 73 cases and recommendations for minimizing dose delivered to patient. AJR Am J Roentgenol. 2001;177:13–20. https://doi.org/10.2214/ajr.177.1.1770013.
79. Albayati MA, Kelly S, Gallagher D, Dourado R, Patel AS, Saha P, et al. Editor's choice–Angulation of the C-arm during complex endovascular aortic procedures increases radiation exposure to the head. Eur J Vasc Endovasc Surg. 2015;49:396–402. https://doi.org/10.1016/j.ejvs.2014.12.032.

80. Agarwal S, Parashar A, Bajaj NS, Khan I, Ahmad I, Heupler FA Jr, et al. Relationship of beam angulation and radiation exposure in the cardiac catheterization laboratory. JACC Cardiovasc Interv. 2014;7:558–66. https://doi.org/10.1016/j.jcin.2013.12.203.
81. El-Sayed T, Patel AS, Cho JS, Kelly JA, Ludwinski FE, Saha P, et al. Radiation-induced DNA damage in operators performing endovascular aortic repair. Circulation. 2017;136:2406–16. https://doi.org/10.1161/circulationaha.117.029550.
82. Axelsson B. Optimisation in fluoroscopy. Biomed Imaging Interv J. 2007;3:e47. https://doi.org/10.2349/biij.3.2.e47.
83. Tsapaki V, Kottou S, Kollaros N, Dafnomili P, Koutelou M, Vano E, et al. Comparison of a conventional and a flat-panel digital system in interventional cardiology procedures. Br J Radiol. 2004;77:562–7. https://doi.org/10.1259/bjr/83257582.
84. de Ruiter QM, Reitsma JB, Moll FL, van Herwaarden JA. Meta-analysis of cumulative radiation duration and dose during EVAR using mobile, fixed, or fixed/3D fusion C-arms. J Endovasc Ther. 2016;23:944–56. https://doi.org/10.1177/1526602816668305.
85. Fidalgo Domingos L, San Norberto García EM, Gutiérrez Castillo D, Flota Ruiz C, Estévez Fernández I, Vaquero Puerta C. Radioprotection measures during the learning curve with hybrid operating rooms. Ann Vasc Surg. 2018;50:253–8. https://doi.org/10.1016/j.avsg.2017.12.010.
86. Maurel B, Sobocinski J, Perini P, Guillou M, Midulla M, Azzaoui R, et al. Evaluation of radiation during EVAR performed on a mobile C-arm. Eur J Vasc Endovasc Surg. 2012;43:16–21. https://doi.org/10.1016/j.ejvs.2011.09.017.
87. Stangenberg L, Shuja F, van der Bom IMJ, van Alfen MHG, Hamdan AD, Wyers MC, et al. Modern fixed imaging systems reduce radiation exposure to patients and providers. Vasc Endovasc Surg. 2018;52:52–8. https://doi.org/10.1177/1538574417742211.
88. Varu VN, Greenberg JI, Lee JT. Improved efficiency and safety for EVAR with utilization of a hybrid room. Eur J Vasc Endovasc Surg. 2013;46:675–9. https://doi.org/10.1016/j.ejvs.2013.09.023.
89. Fossaceca R, Brambilla M, Guzzardi G, Cerini P, Renghi A, Valzano S, et al. The impact of radiological equipment on patient radiation exposure during endovascular aortic aneurysm repair. Eur Radiol. 2012;22:2424–31. https://doi.org/10.1007/s00330-012-2492-4.
90. Kendrick DE, Miller CP, Moorehead PA, Kim AH, Baele HR, Wong VL, et al. Comparative occupational radiation exposure between fixed and mobile imaging systems. J Vasc Surg. 2016;63:190–7. https://doi.org/10.1016/j.jvs.2015.08.062.
91. McAnelly AS, Kelleher D, Ibrahim R, Antoniou GA. Does the use of a hybrid theatre in vascular surgery result in improved clinical outcomes and radiation protection? Int Angiol. 2017;36:289–92. https://doi.org/10.23736/s0392-9590.16.03738-x.
92. Zoli S, Trabattoni P, Dainese L, Annoni A, Saccu C, Fumagalli M, et al. Cumulative radiation exposure during thoracic endovascular aneurysm repair and subsequent follow-up. Eur J Cardiothorac Surg. 2012;42:254–9; discussion 9–60. https://doi.org/10.1093/ejcts/ezr301.
93. Kaplan DJ, Patel JN, Liporace FA, Yoon RS. Intraoperative radiation safety in orthopaedics: a review of the ALARA (as low as reasonably achievable) principle. Patient Saf Surg. 2016;10:27. https://doi.org/10.1186/s13037-016-0115-8.
94. Peach G, Sinha S, Black SA, Morgan RA, Loftus IM, Thompson MM, et al. Operator-controlled imaging significantly reduces radiation exposure during EVAR. Eur J Vasc Endovasc Surg. 2012;44:395–8. https://doi.org/10.1016/j.ejvs.2012.08.001.
95. Yeo CH, Gordon R, Nusem I. Improving operating theatre communication between the orthopaedics surgeon and radiographer. ANZ J Surg. 2014;84:316–9. https://doi.org/10.1111/ans.12482.
96. Bang VV, Levy MS. Radiation safety with dose reduction technology: the buck stops at zero dose. Catheter Cardiovasc Interv. 2018;91:1200–1. https://doi.org/10.1002/ccd.27670.

97. Baumann F, Peña C, Kloeckner R, Katzen BT, Gandhi R, Benenati JB. The effect of a new angiographic imaging technology on radiation dose in visceral embolization procedures. Vasc Endovasc Surg. 2017;51:183–7. https://doi.org/10.1177/1538574417698903.
98. Kirkwood ML, Guild JB, Arbique GM, Tsai S, Modrall JG, Anderson JA, et al. New image-processing and noise-reduction software reduces radiation dose during complex endovascular procedures. J Vasc Surg. 2016;64:1357–65. https://doi.org/10.1016/j.jvs.2016.04.062.
99. van Strijen MJ, Grünhagen T, Mauti M, Zähringer M, Gaines PA, Robinson GJ, et al. Evaluation of a noise reduction imaging technology in iliac digital subtraction angiography: noninferior clinical image quality with lower patient and scatter dose. J Vasc Interv Radiol. 2015;26:642–50.e1. https://doi.org/10.1016/j.jvir.2015.01.007.
100. Kakkos SK, Tsolakis IA. Commentary on "pre-operative simulation of the appropriate C-arm position using computed tomography post-processing software reduces radiation and contrast medium exposure during EVAR procedures". Eur J Vasc Endovasc Surg. 2017;53:275. https://doi.org/10.1016/j.ejvs.2016.11.010.
101. Stahlberg E, Planert M, Panagiotopoulos N, Horn M, Wiedner M, Kleemann M, et al. Pre-operative simulation of the appropriate C-arm position using computed tomography post-processing software reduces radiation and contrast medium exposure during EVAR procedures. Eur J Vasc Endovasc Surg. 2017;53:269–74. https://doi.org/10.1016/j.ejvs.2016.10.016.
102. Molinari GJ, Guillaumon AT, Dalbem AM. Efficacy analysis of a script-based guide for EVAR execution: is it possible to reduce patient exposure to contrast, operative time and blood loss even when advanced technologies are not available? Braz J Cardiovasc Surg. 2015;30:650–6. https://doi.org/10.5935/1678-9741.20150079.
103. Molinari GP. About image manipulation of the CTA on software to simulate the appropriate intra-operative C-arm position. Eur J Vasc Endovasc Surg. 2018;55:902–3. https://doi.org/10.1016/j.ejvs.2018.02.036.
104. Hua L, Doan K, Bajic N, Fitridge R, Dawson J. Procedural benefits of three-dimensional image fusion angiography during EVAR are associated with improved postoperative outcomes. J Vasc Surg. 2015;62:536–7.
105. Sailer AM, de Haan MW, Peppelenbosch AG, Jacobs MJ, Wildberger JE, Schurink GW. CTA with fluoroscopy image fusion guidance in endovascular complex aortic aneurysm repair. Eur J Vasc Endovasc Surg. 2014;47:349–56. https://doi.org/10.1016/j.ejvs.2013.12.022.
106. Bastos Gonçalves F. Alas, ALARA! why the (con)fusion? Eur J Vasc Endovasc Surg. 2018;56:434. https://doi.org/10.1016/j.ejvs.2018.05.029.
107. Rolls A, Riga C. Endovascular robotics. Ann R Coll Surg Engl. 2018;100:14–7. https://doi.org/10.1308/rcsann.supp2.14.
108. Hertault A, Maurel B, Sobocinski J, Martin Gonzalez T, Le Roux M, Azzaoui R, et al. Impact of hybrid rooms with image fusion on radiation exposure during endovascular aortic repair. Eur J Vasc Endovasc Surg. 2014;48:382–90. https://doi.org/10.1016/j.ejvs.2014.05.026.
109. Goudeketting SR, Heinen SGH, Ünlü Ç, van den Heuvel DAF, de Vries JPM, van Strijen MJ, et al. Pros and cons of 3D image fusion in endovascular aortic repair: a systematic review and meta-analysis. J Endovasc Ther. 2017;24:595–603. https://doi.org/10.1177/1526602817708196.
110. Malkoc A, Gnanadev R, Shoemaker HB, Alach A, Vo TD, Behseresht J, et al. The use of advanced three-dimensional computed tomography during simple and complex endovascular aortic aneurysm repairs. Ann Vasc Surg. 2024;106:90–8. https://doi.org/10.1016/j.avsg.2024.03.004.
111. Sorondo SM, Fereydooni A, Ho VT, Dossabhoy SS, Lee JT, Stern JR. Significant radiation reduction using cloud-based AI imaging in manually matched cohort of complex aneurysm repair. Ann Vasc Surg. 2025;114:24–9. https://doi.org/10.1016/j.avsg.2024.12.081.
112. Fetterly KA, Magnuson DJ, Tannahill GM, Hindal MD, Mathew V. Effective use of radiation shields to minimize operator dose during invasive cardiology procedures. JACC Cardiovasc Interv. 2011;4:1133–9. https://doi.org/10.1016/j.jcin.2011.05.027.

113. Schueler BA. Operator shielding: how and why. Tech Vasc Interv Radiol. 2010;13:167–71. https://doi.org/10.1053/j.tvir.2010.03.005.
114. Rees CR, Duncan BWC. Get the lead off our backs! Tech Vasc Interv Radiol. 2018;21:7–15. https://doi.org/10.1053/j.tvir.2017.12.003.
115. Benjamin JL, Meisinger QC. Ergonomics in the development and prevention of musculoskeletal injury in interventional radiologists. Tech Vasc Interv Radiol. 2018;21:16–20. https://doi.org/10.1053/j.tvir.2017.12.004.
116. Lu H, Boyd C, Dawson J. Lightweight lead aprons: the emperor's new clothes in the angiography suite? Eur J Vasc Endovasc Surg. 2019;57:730–9. https://doi.org/10.1016/j.ejvs.2019.01.031.
117. Bartal G, Sailer AM, Vano E. Should we keep the lead in the aprons? Tech Vasc Interv Radiol. 2018;21:2–6. https://doi.org/10.1053/j.tvir.2017.12.002.
118. Fakhoury E, Provencher JA, Subramaniam R, Finlay DJ. Not all lightweight lead aprons and thyroid shields are alike. J Vasc Surg. 2019;70:246–50. https://doi.org/10.1016/j.jvs.2018.07.055.
119. Murphy PH, Wu Y, Glaze SA. Attenuation properties of lead composite aprons. Radiology. 1993;186:269–72. https://doi.org/10.1148/radiology.186.1.8416577.
120. Guersen J, Cassagnes L, Mechin G, Ravel A, Dumousset E, Boyer L, et al. Interventional radiologists: a necessary evolution of leaded protective aprons design. J Vasc Interv Radiol. 2013;24:443. https://doi.org/10.1016/j.jvir.2012.11.004.
121. Vano E, Gonzalez L, Fernández JM, Haskal ZJ. Eye lens exposure to radiation in interventional suites: caution is warranted. Radiology. 2008;248:945–53. https://doi.org/10.1148/radiol.2482071800.
122. Thornton RH, Dauer LT, Altamirano JP, Alvarado KJ, St Germain J, Solomon SB. Comparing strategies for operator eye protection in the interventional radiology suite. J Vasc Interv Radiol. 2010;21:1703–7. https://doi.org/10.1016/j.jvir.2010.07.019.
123. van Rooijen BD, de Haan MW, Das M, Arnoldussen CW, de Graaf R, van Zwam WH, et al. Efficacy of radiation safety glasses in interventional radiology. Cardiovasc Intervent Radiol. 2014;37:1149–55. https://doi.org/10.1007/s00270-013-0766-0.
124. Fetterly K, Schueler B, Grams M, Sturchio G, Bell M, Gulati R. Head and neck radiation dose and radiation safety for interventional physicians. JACC Cardiovasc Interv. 2017;10:520–8. https://doi.org/10.1016/j.jcin.2016.11.026.
125. Vanhavere F, Carinou E, Domienik J, Donadille L, Ginjaume M, Gualdrini G, et al. Measurements of eye lens doses in interventional radiology and cardiology: final results of the ORAMED project. Radiat Meas. 2011;46:1243–7. https://doi.org/10.1016/j.radmeas.2011.08.013.
126. Durán A, Hian SK, Miller DL, Le Heron J, Padovani R, Vano E. Recommendations for occupational radiation protection in interventional cardiology. Catheter Cardiovasc Interv. 2013;82:29–42. https://doi.org/10.1002/ccd.24694.
127. Kirkwood ML, Arbique GM, Guild JB, Zeng K, Xi Y, Rectenwald J, et al. Radiation brain dose to vascular surgeons during fluoroscopically guided interventions is not effectively reduced by wearing lead equivalent surgical caps. J Vasc Surg. 2018;68:567–71. https://doi.org/10.1016/j.jvs.2017.12.054.
128. Reeves RR, Ang L, Bahadorani J, Naghi J, Dominguez A, Palakodeti V, et al. Invasive cardiologists are exposed to greater left sided cranial radiation: the BRAIN study (brain radiation exposure and attenuation during invasive cardiology procedures). JACC Cardiovasc Interv. 2015;8:1197–206. https://doi.org/10.1016/j.jcin.2015.03.027.
129. Kuon E, Birkel J, Schmitt M, Dahm JB. Radiation exposure benefit of a lead cap in invasive cardiology. Heart. 2003;89:1205–10. https://doi.org/10.1136/heart.89.10.1205.
130. Modarai B, Haulon S, Ainsbury E, Böckler D, Vano-Carruana E, Dawson J, et al. Editor's choice – European Society for Vascular Surgery (ESVS) 2023 clinical practice guidelines on radiation safety. Eur J Vasc Endovasc Surg. 2023;65:171–222. https://doi.org/10.1016/j.ejvs.2022.09.005.

131. Christopoulos G, Makke L, Christakopoulos G, Kotsia A, Rangan BV, Roesle M, et al. Optimizing radiation safety in the cardiac catheterization laboratory: a practical approach. Catheter Cardiovasc Interv. 2016;87:291–301. https://doi.org/10.1002/ccd.25959.
132. Brilakis ES. Innovations in radiation safety during cardiovascular catheterization. Circulation. 2018;137:1317–9. https://doi.org/10.1161/circulationaha.117.032808.
133. Vano E, Fernandez JM, Resel LE, Moreno J, Sanchez RM. Staff lens doses in interventional urology. A comparison with interventional radiology, cardiology and vascular surgery values. J Radiol Prot. 2016;36:37–48. https://doi.org/10.1088/0952-4746/36/1/37.
134. Kirkwood ML, Guild J, Arbique G, Anderson JA, Valentine RJ, Timaran C. Surgeon radiation dose during complex endovascular procedures. J Vasc Surg. 2014;60:1721.
135. Gonzales JP, Moran C, Silberzweig JE. Reduction of operator radiation dose by an extended lower body shield. J Vasc Interv Radiol. 2014;25:462–8, 8.e1. https://doi.org/10.1016/j.jvir.2013.11.006.
136. Whitby M, Martin CJ. Radiation doses to the legs of radiologists performing interventional procedures: are they a cause for concern? Br J Radiol. 2003;76:321–7. https://doi.org/10.1259/bjr/65778215.
137. Artschan RE, Brettle DS, Chase K, Fender A, Howells PG, Buchan S. An investigation of the radiation doses to the lower legs and feet of staff undertaking interventional procedures. Br J Radiol. 2014;87:20130746. https://doi.org/10.1259/bjr.20130746.
138. Kloeze C, Klompenhouwer EG, Brands PJ, van Sambeek MR, Cuypers PW, Teijink JA. Editor's choice–Use of disposable radiation-absorbing surgical drapes results in significant dose reduction during EVAR procedures. Eur J Vasc Endovasc Surg. 2014;47:268–72. https://doi.org/10.1016/j.ejvs.2013.12.008.
139. Vlastra W, Delewi R, Sjauw KD, Beijk MA, Claessen BE, Streekstra GJ, et al. Efficacy of the RADPAD protection drape in reducing operators' radiation exposure in the catheterization laboratory: a sham-controlled randomized trial. Circ Cardiovasc Interv. 2017;10:e006058. https://doi.org/10.1161/circinterventions.117.006058.
140. Marichal DA, Anwar T, Kirsch D, Clements J, Carlson L, Savage C, et al. Comparison of a suspended radiation protection system versus standard lead apron for radiation exposure of a simulated interventionalist. J Vasc Interv Radiol. 2011;22:437–42. https://doi.org/10.1016/j.jvir.2010.12.016.
141. Fattal P, Goldstein JA. A novel complete radiation protection system eliminates physician radiation exposure and leaded aprons. Catheter Cardiovasc Interv. 2013;82:11–6. https://doi.org/10.1002/ccd.24625.
142. Khanal S. A novel complete radiation protection system eliminates physician radiation exposure and leaded aprons. Indian Heart J. 2013;65:633–5. https://doi.org/10.1016/j.ihj.2013.08.007.
143. Dragusin O, Weerasooriya R, Jaïs P, Hocini M, Ector J, Takahashi Y, et al. Evaluation of a radiation protection cabin for invasive electrophysiological procedures. Eur Heart J. 2007;28:183–9. https://doi.org/10.1093/eurheartj/ehl420.
144. Riga CV, Bicknell CD, Hamady MS, Cheshire NJ. Evaluation of robotic endovascular catheters for arch vessel cannulation. J Vasc Surg. 2011;54:799–809. https://doi.org/10.1016/j.jvs.2011.03.218.
145. Au S, Ko K, Tsang J, Chan YC. Robotic endovascular surgery. Asian Cardiovasc Thorac Ann. 2014;22:110–4. https://doi.org/10.1177/0218492313484736.
146. Carrell T, Dastur N, Salter R, Taylor P. Use of a remotely steerable "robotic" catheter in a branched endovascular aortic graft. J Vasc Surg. 2012;55:223–5. https://doi.org/10.1016/j.jvs.2011.07.032.

Key References

Durán A, Hian SK, Miller DL, Heron JL, Padovani R, Vano E. Recommendations for occupational radiation protection in interventional cardiology. Catheter Cardiovasc Interv. 2013;82:29–42. https://doi.org/10.1002/ccd.24694.

Hertault A, Maurel B, Midulla M, Bordier C, Desponds L, Saeed Kilani M, et al. Editor's choice – Minimizing radiation exposure during endovascular procedures: basic knowledge, literature review, and reporting standards. Eur J Vasc Endovasc Surg. 2015;50:21–36. https://doi.org/10.1016/j.ejvs.2015.01.014.

Hirshfeld JW, Ferrari VA, Bengel FM, Bergersen L, Chambers CE, Einstein AJ, et al. 2018 ACC/HRS/NASCI/SCAI/SCCT expert consensus document on optimal use of ionizing radiation in cardiovascular imaging: best practices for safety and effectiveness. J Am Coll Cardiol. 2018;71:e283–351. https://doi.org/10.1016/j.jacc.2018.02.016.

Modarai B, Haulon S, Ainsbury E, Böckler D, Vano-Carruana E, Dawson J, et al. European Society for Vascular Surgery (ESVS) 2023 clinical practice guidelines on radiation safety. Eur J Vasc Endovasc Surg. 2023;65:171–222. https://doi.org/10.1016/j.ejvs.2022.09.005.

Shaw PM, Vouyouka A, Reed A. Time for radiation safety program guidelines for pregnant trainees and vascular surgeons. J Vasc Surg. 2012;55:862–8.e2. https://doi.org/10.1016/j.jvs.2011.11.045.

Chapter 15
Multifaceted Applications of Artificial Intelligence in Vascular Surgery

Fabien Lareyre, Guilherme Pena, and Juliette Raffort

SN Flashcards
Test your learning and check your understanding of this book's contents: use the "Springer Nature Flashcards" app to access questions using ▶ https://sn.pub/wppvze. To use the app, please follow the instructions in Chap. 1.

Key Learning Points

- Artificial intelligence (AI) has brought new perspectives for applications in vascular surgery in three main fields: vision, machine learning-based prediction models, and natural language processing.

F. Lareyre (✉)
Department of Vascular Surgery, Hospital of Antibes Juan-les-Pins, Antibes, France

Université Côte d'Azur, CNRS, UMR7370, LP2M, Nice, France

Fédération Hospitalo-Universitaire (FHU) Plan & Go, Nice, France

G. Pena
Discipline of Surgery, Adelaide University, Adelaide, SA, Australia

Vascular Surgery Unit, Flinders Medical Centre, Adelaide, SA, Australia
e-mail: guilherme.pena@sa.gov.au

J. Raffort
Fédération Hospitalo-Universitaire (FHU) Plan & Go, Nice, France

Clinical Chemistry Laboratory, University Hospital of Nice, Nice, France

Institute 3IA Côte d'Azur, Université Côte d'Azur, Nice, France
e-mail: raffort-lareyre.j@chu-nice.fr

R. Fitridge et al. (eds.), *Pathophysiology of Vascular Disease*,
https://doi.org/10.1007/978-3-032-31459-8_15

- AI offers perspectives of applications in clinical practice, vascular research, and education in vascular surgery.
- Clinical applications of AI in vascular surgery include new tools for the diagnosis and detection of vascular diseases, for the evaluation of the prognosis, for pre-surgical planning, for endovascular navigation, and for the follow-up of patients.
- AI applications require careful validation and evaluation before implementation in clinical practice.
- Current challenges include medical, technical, economic, legal, regulatory, ethical, and human considerations.
- Future directions for implementing AI in clinical practice involve improving standardisation, building guidelines and regulation, and promoting interdisciplinary international collaboration.

15.1 Introduction

Healthcare systems are facing major challenges worldwide, with increased demand exceeding workforce and imposing economic pressure. Among them, cardiovascular diseases are one of the leading causes of mortality, with substantial financial impact on healthcare systems related to treatment, hospitalisation, and morbidities [1]. Improving prevention, early detection, and optimising care are thus a priority, and digital health technologies have offered new opportunities to overcome these challenges. Digital health, also called e-health, refers to the use of information technology to deliver care to patients. It includes a wide range of fields and tools including telemedicine, smart devices, wearable technology, web-based and mobile health applications, health information systems, and integrated networks [2, 3]. Artificial intelligence (AI) has accelerated the digital transformation, offering a wide range of potential applications [4–6].

The term 'AI' was introduced in the 1950s at the Dartmouth College Conference, and it encompasses a broad discipline that aims to understand and design systems that display properties of human intelligence, such as reasoning, learning, adaptation, interaction, decision-making or sensory interpretation [7, 8]. Machine learning (ML) and deep learning (DL) algorithms are techniques used to enable learning from large amounts of data, to identify hidden and complex patterns, and to make decisions or predictions [9]. AI regroups main domains including robotic, vision (applications to image or video analysis) and natural language processing (NLP, applications for language analysis). Given the diversity of AI, various applications are currently being developed and implemented in the field of vascular surgery.

The aim of this review is to provide an overview of clinical applications of AI in vascular surgery in the three main fields including vision, ML-prediction models, and NLP. After an introduction on the technical fundamentals in AI, we provide practical examples related to aortic aneurysm and peripheral artery disease (PAD), and based on the applications, technical issues as well as current challenges are discussed.

15.2 Introduction to AI

Artificial intelligence involves the creation of computer systems that can perform tasks typically requiring human intelligence. Within AI, machine learning focuses on training software models to make predictions or generate content from data. In the context of healthcare, ML algorithms are capable of analysing vast amounts of patient data, identifying patterns, and providing valuable insights that can aid in diagnosis, treatment, and prognosis. Deep learning is a specialised subset of ML that employs multi-layered neural networks inspired by human brain's structure. This enables DL models to excel at processing complex and unstructured data such as medical images and textual clinical notes [9, 10].

ML systems come in various types based on the learning styles. Supervised learning models learn from labelled examples, predicting outcomes like risk of death or risk of limb loss (regression) or classifying data (e.g. benign vs. malignant tumours). Unsupervised learning models, on the other hand, discover hidden patterns in unlabelled data, often employing clustering to group similar data points (e.g. identifying patient subgroups). Reinforcement learning models operate on a trial-and-error basis, receiving rewards or penalties for their actions, making them suitable for complex tasks like robot-assisted surgery. Finally, generative AI models create new content based on learned patterns, capable of producing synthetic medical images or text for training or research purposes [10–13].

In the healthcare domain, deploying AI models successfully involves three critical stages: training, validation, and deployment. During the training stage, models are developed using retrospective data, but challenges such as data sufficiency, type, and label quality need to be addressed. Deep learning models particularly excel when dealing with unstructured data like images and text. The validation stage rigorously tests the model's performance on unsee data and evaluates its effectiveness in real-world scenarios [14, 15]. Considerations such as population bias and seamless integration into clinical workflows are crucial at this point [16]. Finally, the deployment stage involves integrating the AI model into the clinical workflow, but it is important to remember that dataset shifts due to changes in healthcare environment can impact model performance. Hence, continuous monitoring and auditing are essential to ensure the model remains effective over time [15].

Evaluating the performance of AI models necessitates an understanding of various metrics available. Sensitivity and specificity are fundamental metrics that assess the model's ability to correctly identify positive and negative cases, respectively. The AUROC (area under the receiver operating characteristic curve), frequently referred to as AUC (area under the curve), is a powerful metric that provides a comprehensive picture of a model's discriminatory ability across various decision thresholds. It essentially captures the trade-off between sensitivity and specificity. A higher AUROC indicates a superior overall performance, meaning the model is better at distinguishing between positive and negative cases. An AUROC of 0.5 signifies a model no better than random guessing, while an AUROC of 1.0 represents perfect discrimination [17, 18].

Predictive values offer insight into the reliability of the model's predictions. Positive predictive values (PPV) quantify the probability that a positive result is actually true, while negative predictive value (NPV) represents the likelihood that a negative result is indeed accurate [18].

Calibration is another important metric that examines how well the model's predicted probabilities align with the observed probabilities in the real world. A well-calibrated model generates reliable risk estimates, which are invaluable for clinical decision-making [19].

Discrimination pertains to the model's ability to differentiate between patients with and without the condition of interest. This ability is often reflected in the AUROC value, where a higher AUROC indicates better discrimination [17].

Finally, generalisability is a critical aspect that evaluates the model's ability to perform well across diverse settings and populations. It ensures that the model's applicability extends beyond the specific training data it was exposed to. Factors such as variations in patient demographics, clinical practices, and data collection methods can all impact a model's generalisability [11, 20].

By grasping these key AI metrics and their clinical implications, vascular surgeons can actively participate in evaluating and adopting AI tools, ensuring their responsible and effective use to enhance patient care.

Below we discuss some specific examples of AI use in vascular surgery.

15.3 Vision

Imaging is a key step in the management of vascular diseases and several techniques are currently available including doppler ultrasound, computed tomography angiography (CTA), and magnetic resonance imaging (MRI). AI has brought new insights in cardiovascular imaging analysis, offering new opportunities to facilitate segmentation, automatic measurement, detection, quantification, classification of vascular lesions and identification of predictive radiomic patterns (see Glossary) [21].

15.3.1 Aortic Aneurysm

15.3.1.1 Vascular Segmentation and Characterisation

Vascular segmentation is challenging due to the size of the vessels, curvature, and pathophysiological variations among patients. Several investigators have explored the role of AI and ML algorithms to facilitate segmentation and automatic characterisation of abdominal aortic aneurysm (AAA) [22, 23].

Lareyre et al. developed a fully automatic method for segmentation of AAA based on a hybrid approach combining feature-based expert systems and supervised deep learning [24, 25]. The method demonstrated its accuracy as compared to manual segmentation performed by human experts, with a Dice score of 0.83 ± 0.04, sensitivity of 0.95 ± 0.04, specificity of 0.99 and volume similarity of 0.91 ± 0.06 for lumen segmentation [24, 25]. This approach demonstrated its potential application for clinical practice by enabling automatic measurements of AAA characteristics such as maximal diameter [26]. Another study showed the interest of active learning methods for segmentation of AAA using a dataset of 300 CTAs, with good efficiency and a significant reduction in the segmentation time compared to the manual approach [27].

Among pioneering AI tools, several start-ups were created and proposed innovative solutions to enable automated segmentation of AAA features. Among them, the software PRAEVAorta proposed by Nurea (https://www.nurea-soft.com/praevaorta-software/) showed good performances and accuracy for measurements of AAA volumes, surfaces and diameters as compared to human manual segmentation [28]. Interestingly, the software enabled measurements of AAA volumes on CTA on the arterial, venous, and non-contrast phases [29]. Augmented radiology for vascular aneurysm (ARVA) is another software developed by Predisurge to enable automatic characterisation of AAA based on DL algorithms (https://www.predisurge.com). The software was used to analyse pre- and post-operative CTA in patients managed with fenestrated endovascular repair (FEVAR) [30]. In a dataset of 100 CTA, diameter measurements by ARVA were comparable to clinician measurements, with a median absolute difference of 2.4 mm on the pre-operative CTAs and 1.6 mm on the post-operative CTAs. Of note, no significant difference was detected for the measurement of maximum outer-wall aortic diameters as compared to clinician measurements on pre-operative and post-operative scans (range 0.5–0.9 mm) [30]. A multi-centre validation study was then performed to confirm the accuracy of the fully automatic DL-based method for aortic segmentation and measurements of diameters and volumes [31]. Using a dataset of 350 CTAs from 216 patients, the study showed the reliability of the AI-based method, with a median volume similarity error ranging from 0.93 to 0.95 in the main trunk and of 0.88 in the iliac arteries [31]. Based on this technology, numerical simulation for standard and complex EVAR using digital twins is also proposed to facilitate and improve endograft design and planning. (https://www.predisurge.com). Finally, in addition to allowing automatic measurements to facilitate pre-surgical planning, AI-based methods cân help to better characterise associated lesions such as calcifications and intraluminal thrombus [27, 32–34].

15.3.1.2 Automatic Detection

Early screening and detection of AAA is a key point in the management of AAA as the disease may remain clinically asymptomatic until the patient develops complications and fatal rupture. Several studies have highlighted the potential interest of AI to enable AAA screening on CTA [35–37]. In a dataset of 187 CTAs, researchers trained a deep convolutional network to screen for AAA [35]. The model achieved an accuracy of 0.856 and an area under the curve (AUC) of 0.926. In another dataset of 106 scans, the model achieved an accuracy of 0.953 and an AUC of 0.971 [35]. Another study trained a CNN on a dataset composed of 200 CTAs from patients with infrarenal AAA and 200 matched control patients with non-aneurysmal aortas [37]. The accuracy of the model was 99.1%, with an AUC of 0.99 [37]. Finally, other investigators developed a DL-based segmentation pipeline using 73 CTAs from 48 AAA and 25 controls [36]. The pipeline consisted of three main steps: automatic lumen segmentation, automatic thrombus segmentation, and geometric analysis for AAA [36]. It correctly classified 47 AAA out of 48 and 24 control patients out of 25 with 97% accuracy, 98% sensitivity, and 96% specificity [36]. These studies showed a proof of concept of the potential of DL to enable automatic detection of AAA based on CTAs, and several start-ups propose AI-powered solutions for the detection of aortic diseases including AAA and dissection, with automatic measurements of aortic diameters (https://www.viz.ai/aortic, https://www.aidoc.com/eu/).

15.3.1.3 Prediction of Outcomes

Imaging provides valuable information on AAA morphological characteristics and ML was proposed to predict the outcomes of the disease such as the risk of growth and rupture. In a dataset of 195 patients with AAA, Wang et al. tested multiple ML models to predict rapid AAA growth, which was defined as growth >0.25 cm/year [38]. The best performing model used seven radiomic features of the intraluminal thrombus and wall and showed an AUC of 0.83 in the development cohort, and of 0.78 in the independent test cohort [38]. Other investigators showed the interest of CNN to predict AAA growth using different features including radius, intraluminal thrombus thickness, and time-average wall shear stress [39]. Another study built a prognosis classifier based on ML to predict the three following categories of outcomes based on imaging and clinical data: AAA will remain stable, AAA will require repair according to current indications based on maximal diameter, or AAA will rupture [40]. In a dataset composed of 352 stable aneurysms, 16 clinical interventions, and 13 rupture, the models achieved AUCs to classify the three categories (stable, repair, and rupture groups) of 0.82, 0.78, and 0.83, respectively, for the training dataset, and of 0.90, 0.80, and 0.91, respectively, for the test dataset [40]. Altogether, these results suggest that AI could help to identify predictive radiomic patterns of AAA outcomes and assist clinicians in therapeutic decision-making for patients with AAA.

15.3.1.4 Pre-surgical Planning and Endovascular Navigation

Elective EVAR relies on precise anatomic characterisation of the AAA and of the vessels to design endografts tailored to patients' anatomy. AI-driven imaging analysis has brought innovative solutions for endograft sizing and deployment simulation

[41–43]. Start-ups propose the use of digital twins to enhance custom-made aortic endograft design with the aim of improving safety and accuracy of the procedures (https://www.predisurge.com/planop™-aortic-fevar/), (https://www.piemedicalimaging.com/product/3mensio-vascular). Intra-operative guidance is also a key step, and AI image-guided surgery has been introduced to enhance real-time visualisation of 3D fusion images during endovascular procedures (https://cydarmedical.com/cydar-maps/). Such technology has the potential to improve the management of patients undergoing endovascular repair.

15.3.2 Peripheral Artery Disease (PAD)

Imaging takes a central role in the management of vascular diseases related to atherosclerosis including PAD [44]. Various imaging techniques are available, but most studies have focused on using AI to improve the detection and classification of PAD lesions based on Doppler ultrasound or CTA [45–47]. As an example, Luo et al. developed a DL model to classify aortoiliac, femoropopliteal, and trifurcation disease using a dataset of 5761 LEAD ultrasound studies [48]. The model achieved a 97.0% accuracy for predicting normal cases, 88.2% accuracy for aortoiliac disease, 90.1% accuracy for femoropopliteal disease, and 90.5% accuracy for trifurcation disease, suggesting the ability of AI models to differentiate normal from diseased arterial systems and to classify the extent of vascular diseases [48]. Other investigators used a dataset of 17,050 CTA axial images of iliac, femoropopliteal and infrapopliteal arteries from 265 patients to train a CNN [49]. The model exhibited 91.5% accuracy, 90.2% sensitivity and 97.7% specificity in classifying above-knee artery, 90.9% accuracy, 91.3% sensitivity and 95.2% specificity in classifying below-knee artery [49]. The current literature underlines the potential interest of AI to improve the detection, diagnosis and classification of vascular lesions based on imaging data.

15.4 Machine Learning Prediction Models

ML algorithms have provided new methods to enable risk prediction [7]. In supervised learning, the model is trained using label input and output data. This enables the identification of associations and the construction of a function that maps input to expected output values. The algorithm generalises from the training data to unseen and new situations, allowing it to predict or classify future events, or understand which input variables are relevant to the outcomes. In contrast, unsupervised learning does not require labelled data and allows the discovery of hidden patterns within complex data without any pre-defined assumptions.

15.4.1 Aortic Aneurysm

Risk stratification is crucial to improve the prognosis of patients with AAA. Clinical decision-making in patients with AAA is currently based on the balance between the risk of growth and rupture and the risk related to vascular intervention. ML-based prediction models were used to assess the risk of AAA expansion and rupture, and they have been mainly based on imaging and radiomic features [4, 23, 45]. Several AI models have been proposed to evaluate the risk of post-operative complications in patients with AAA, and they were based on clinical pre-operative data and/or AAA morphological characteristics [4, 50]. Various outcomes have been targeted including in-hospital stay, mortality, adverse cardiovascular events or complications related to endograft such as endoleaks [4, 23, 50]. Studies reporting the use of ML to predict outcomes of patients with AAA are diverse and heterogeneous in terms of targeted outcome, study design, number of patients included, and data used as input. The use of vascular registries and collaboratives may help to train and develop robust AI models on large datasets [51]. As an example, Li et al. used the vascular quality initiative (VQI) database to include 12,027 patients who underwent elective open AAA repair [52]. Using 52 pre-operative demographic and clinical variables as input features, they developed a ML model which achieved an AUROC of 0.93 (95% confidence interval, 0.92–0.94) to predict in-hospital major adverse cardiovascular events [52]. The authors also applied this methodology to predict 1-year mortality following EVAR [53]. Using the VQI database, 63,655 patients were included, and the best performing ML model achieved an AUROC of 0.96 (0.95–0.97), suggesting the ability of ML to assess the prognosis of patients undergoing AAA intervention [53].

15.4.2 Peripheral Artery Disease

Patients with PAD have an increased risk of morbidity and mortality related to cardiovascular events [44]. ML models have therefore been proposed to assess the cardiovascular risk, enabling personalised therapeutic approach and follow-up care [45–47]. Various outcomes were predicted including major adverse cardiac and cerebrovascular events, mortality, or the risk of developing chronic limb-threatening ischaemia [54–56]. As an example, Zhang et al. aimed to predict in-hospital mortality in patients hospitalised for PAD [55]. In a cohort of 150,921 inpatients diagnosed with PAD, the investigators developed 4 ML models based on a selection of variables, including patient characteristics, comorbidities, procedures, and hospital-related factors. The models showed an AUC ranging from 0.83 to 0.85, sensitivity of 77–82%, and specificity of 72–75%. The results suggested a moderate ability of such an approach to guide clinical decision-making.

In addition to predicting outcomes related to PAD and associated comorbidities, the evaluation of the risk of complications after revascularisation might help to determine the most appropriate therapeutic approach. Cox et al. aimed to develop ML models to stratify the risk of 30-day procedure-related mortality and 30-day unplanned readmission in patients undergoing lower extremity infra-inguinal endovascular interventions in a cohort of 14,444 cases [57]. The best performing model achieved an AUC of 0.75 (95% CI: 0.71–0.79) to predict mortality and an AUC of 0.68 (95% CI: 0.67–0.71) to predict unplanned readmission. In another study, investigators used ML algorithms to predict 30-day outcomes following lower extremity endovascular revascularisation [58]. Using 38 pre-operative demographic and clinical variables, 6 ML models were trained to predict major adverse limb events. The best performing model showed an AUC of 0.93 (95% CI, 0.92–0.94) and performed better than logistic regression [58].

The risk of amputation represents a serious burden that significantly impacts patients' quality of life. New tools to evaluate this risk might help to optimise care and follow-up strategies of patients with PAD. Using the American College of Surgeons National Surgical Quality Improvement Program database to collect preoperative clinical and laboratory information on 14,444 patients who underwent endovascular procedures for PAD, a random forest ML model was developed to predict 30-day amputation [59]. It achieved an AUC of 0.81 and identified the most important features as being elective surgery designation, claudication, open wound/wound infection, white blood cell count, and albumin [59]. Altogether, these results emphasise the role of ML to enable risk stratification in patients with vascular diseases and pave the way to develop precision medicine and personalised therapeutic approach.

15.5 Natural Language Processing (NLP)

NLP is a domain of AI that aims to process, analyse, and understand human language including oral and written language. It offers a wide range of potential applications in healthcare, and the field is very dynamic, as shown by a substantial increase in funded clinical NLP projects [60]. Technological advances have led to an exponential increase in health data generated, and NLP can provide innovative solutions to facilitate the identification and extraction of medical information [60].

15.5.1 Identification and Extraction of Health Data

15.5.1.1 Aortic Aneurysm

Several studies have shown the ability of NLP to identify patients with aortic diseases from health records [61–63]. As an example, a study tested the use of a program that uses an NLP algorithm applied to electronic medical records to identify patients with AAA from imaging reports [62]. In total, 6,340,505 imaging reports were processed by the NLP program, which allowed the identification of 6495 patients with AAA. The program allowed identification of those who did not require surveillance (2937 cases), and placed 1183 patients in ongoing surveillance [62]. This approach shows a proof of concept on how NLP can be leveraged to facilitate the detection, the orientation, and the follow-up of patients with AAA. It has the potential to improve screening and surveillance across a large health system [62]. Another study highlighted the capacity of NLP to identify patients with AAA, and to extract relevant information such as the maximal aortic diameter in a large dataset of imaging study reports [63]. It offers potential applications in public health, facilitating medical information retrieval at large scale. Such data can then be analysed to identify patterns and better understand the outcomes among patients [63].

15.5.1.2 Peripheral Artery Disease

Similar approaches were used to identify patients with PAD from health records [64]. As an example, clinical notes from a cohort of 6861 patients with PAD were used to train, test, and validate an NLP model [64]. Interestingly, the model achieved a median AUC of 0.888 and a median area under the precision curve of 0.909 to identify patients with PAD, suggesting its ability to improve a large-scale search from health records [64]. It paves the way to facilitate analysis of clinical data and can be leveraged to evaluate current practice in comparison to guideline-based care [65]. Another study aimed to investigate compliance with guideline recommendations for secondary prevention in patients with PAD [65]. The authors used an NLP model for automated identification of moderate to severe PAD cases from clinical notes in electronic health records, allowing them to investigate the proportion of patients treated with appropriate guideline-recommended strategies [65].

15.5.2 Virtual Assistants and Chatbots

15.5.2.1 Question Answering and Education

In parallel to the identification and extraction of information from health records, the development of large language models (LLM) has offered the opportunity to improve chatbots and develop virtual assistants. LLM chatbots have shown their ability to mimic human-like responses, and they have attracted increased attention in healthcare, with potential applications to use them as innovative support to interact with patients to provide medical information. Various LLMs are currently available, including ChatGPT (Generative Pre-trained Transformer developed by OpenAI), Med-PaLM (Med-Pathways Language Model, developed by Google) or Copilot (formerly Bing Chat, developed by Microsoft) [66]. The performances of LLM chatbots for answering questions specifically related to vascular surgery have been scarcely investigated [67, 68] so far. Melissano et al. investigated the accuracy of two LLM chatbots to answer questions that a patient with an aortic disease might ask [67]. Their results showed that 111/279 (39.8%) of the English questions were accurate, and the authors highlighted potential misleading and inaccurate content in some answers [67]. Another study queried two chatbots with 24 questions spanning seven vascular surgery disease domains [68]. Accuracy and completeness of responses were rated from 1 to 4 (1: completely inaccurate to 4: completely accurate), and the appropriateness was evaluated as a binary criterion. The average accuracies for the two chatbots were, respectively, 3.08 ± 0.33 and 2.82 ± 0.40; the completeness was 2.98 ± 0.34 and 2.62 ± 0.36. The responses were deemed appropriate in 75.0% and 45.8% of cases, respectively. Finally, a pioneering study suggested that LLMs could help to improve readability to create new materials for patient education, although the accuracy and quality of such an approach remain to be further investigated [69]. While LLMs have offered a new source of information, these results highlight that caution should be taken and patients should be warned about potential inaccurate, incomplete, or inappropriate information. An international open electronic survey investigated vascular surgeons' opinions and feedback regarding the use of LLM chatbots in vascular surgery [70]. Among the 318 participants, 95 (36.3%) found that LLM chatbots were very useful or somewhat useful in clinical practice at this very moment and 229 (87.4%) agreed that they should be systematically validated prior to being used. Eighty participants (30.5%) had tested it specifically for questions related to clinical practice, and among them, 59 (73.8%) experienced issues or limitations. The results of the survey highlighted potential pitfalls related to the use of LLMs and underlined the real need to improve the formation and training of health professionals in this technology.

15.5.2.2 Management of Health Data, Text Writing and Clinical Support

LLMs have offered new opportunities to facilitate the management of health data in clinical practice to alleviate repetitive tasks and administrative burden. They have shown potential in various tasks such as generating medical reports, discharge summaries, and writing medical prescriptions [71–73]. Although such applications have not been yet specifically investigated in the field of vascular surgery, it has the potential to assist clinicians to handle writing tasks under their supervision and responsibility. Multi-modal LLMs can process various types of data including text, sounds, and images [74]. They can potentially provide support for clinical decision-making by allowing the analysis and integration of various patients' health data. A study tested the performance of LLMs to process common consult requests encountered in vascular surgery [75]. In total, 25 fictional vascular surgery consultation queries were investigated, and for each consult, the LLM was asked whether the situation was an emergency or not, and what would be the next steps for clinical care (examination, additional imaging, or urgent operation). Interestingly, the 4 LLMs investigated showed an accuracy of 88%, 100%, 76%, and 88% to identify emergencies [75]. Although further validation is required, it suggests the potential of LLMs to provide support for clinical decision-making.

15.5.2.3 Scientific and Medical Knowledge

LLMs have brought new techniques to facilitate information retrieval, and such technology can be leveraged to improve access to medical and scientific knowledge. Commercially available applications are now proposed to enhance literature search and facilitate access to appropriate content. A pilot study tested the applicability of using an AI-based mobile application for literature searching on a topic related to research and vascular surgery [76]. Interestingly, the application enabled a focus and appropriate identification of the relevant articles related to the topic, although the selection was not completely exhaustive. LLMs could therefore be used to facilitate access and dissemination of relevant scientific content and could also help to perform systematic reviews [77]. Finally, LLMs offer various possibilities to assist academic and scientific writing from editing and translating to summarising and even generating scientific content [78]. We have thus entered a new era where AI may be used in various ways through the patients' course in vascular surgery including care, education, and vascular research.

15.6 Medical and Technical Challenges

While AI offers a wide range of applications in vascular surgery, it has to be tempered by current technical challenges that have to be overcome before implementing such innovation in daily clinical practice. ML algorithms need to be trained and learn from data, and their performance therefore depends on the volume and the quality of datasets. Hidden bias in the learning dataset can impact the generalisability of the model, and the performance can be limited in case of class imbalance. Health data are very heterogeneous in terms of content, format, sources, and quality. Building an international multi-centre standardised data repository is a critical and indispensable step to allow collaborative research and efficient development of AI applications. International, European networks and vascular research collaboratives are very dynamic toward that aim and will undoubtedly be part of the development, validation, and implementation of AI applications in vascular surgery [51, 79]. Another challenge raised by AI models, especially in healthcare, is the lack of explicability and accountability. As they function as a black box, it is difficult to know and understand how the model links the input with the input [80]. Caution should therefore be observed for the validation of AI models before their implementation in practice [81]. Studies performed so far have mainly used a retrospective study design, and prospective multi-centre studies as well as randomised clinical trials would help to enhance evidence generation. Given the complexity and challenges associated with AI, specific guidelines and recommendations are currently being built to help standardise methods used to develop, evaluate the performance, ensure safety, and assess the clinical risks and benefits of AI applications [81]. Finally, economic investment and adapted infrastructure are required to build AI models, and medico-economic impact and sustainability still need to be evaluated.

15.7 Legal and Ethical Considerations

The use of AI in vascular surgery and in healthcare in general raises major ethical concerns [82, 83]. A primary concern is the access, analysis, and utilisation of sensitive health data; confidentiality, privacy, and data protection must be ensured at every stage of the process. It also brings challenges related to data management including governance, definitions of data ownership, sharing, and valorisation. In addition to concerns related to health data, AI models bring concerns regarding transparency, accountability and explainability. Medicine relies on an evidence-based approach, and transparent information on how the AI reaches the output is needed for clinicians to gain trust and confidence, but also to clearly understand the limits and potential pitfalls of the applications. Patients' safety is at stake, and the definition of responsibilities still needs to be clearly defined, especially in case of adverse events. Additional concern related to risks associated with automation, with the fear that it might lead to an unanticipated decrease in human skills, know-how and training opportunities [84]. AI applications should also guarantee equity and fairness in healthcare. Finally, the impact of AI on human relationships is a major aspect raised by society, and patients might fear that it can impact the doctor/patient relationship. Physician-patient relationship is based on trust and empathy and is of importance to accompany and support patients and their relatives. Clearly, AI cannot provide this support, and it does not intend to replace health professionals. It aims to bring new tools for management of vascular diseases, while being kept under the supervision and expertise of health professionals who will explain and accompany patients during decision-making and care.

To ensure a fair and ethical use of AI in healthcare, ethical principles and commitments have been built by international societies and organisations including the EU's AI high-level expert group (https://digital-strategy.ec.europa.eu/en/library/ethics-guidelines-trustworthy-ai). While these commitments serve as general guidelines, AI innovations and medical devices must comply with current regulations and legislation. In Europe, the use of health data should be compliant with the General Data Protection Regulation (GDPR) (https://gdpr.eu), and medical devices are subject to the CE mark to meet conformity to the general safety and performance requirements to access the European market. The EU's AI Act has recently been voted and approved and should become the global standard in Europe regarding regulations of AI in healthcare.

15.8 Conclusion

AI has brought a wide range of applications in vascular surgery, including screening and diagnosis of vascular diseases, prediction and prognosis assessment, pre-surgical planning, endovascular navigation, and follow-up of patients. It has the potential to bring new tools for vascular surgeons but also to reshape the organisation of healthcare, education, and vascular research through various applications enhancing the management of medical information systems. While the field is very dynamic, with technical advances already in use, especially in the field of medical imaging, various challenges and concerns remain to be addressed to ensure patients' safety and clinical benefits. Interdisciplinary and collaborative efforts involving all stakeholders would help to move into a new era where AI and digital innovation will improve care provided to patients with vascular diseases.

Multiple Choice Questions

1. Within the context of machine learning, which specific type of learning model requires the use of labelled examples (input and output data) during its training phase to predict outcomes and classify data?

   (a) Unsupervised learning
   (b) Reinforcement learning
   (c) Deep learning (DL)
   (d) Generative AI
   (e) Supervised learning

   Answer: (e) Supervised learning

2. Which single metric provides a comprehensive picture of a machine learning model's discriminatory ability across various decision threshold and is better at distinguishing between positive and negative cases when its value is higher?

   (a) Sensitivity
   (b) Specificity
   (c) Positive predictive value (PPV)
   (d) Area under the receiver operating characteristic curve (AUC-ROC)
   (e) Calibration

   Answer: (d) Area under the receiver operating characteristic curve (AUC-ROC)

References

1. Pahigiannis K, Thompson-Paul AM, Barfield W, Ochiai E, Loustalot F, Shero S, et al. Progress toward improved cardiovascular health in the United States. Circulation. 2019;139:1957–73. https://doi.org/10.1161/circulationaha.118.035408.
2. Lareyre F, Behrendt CA, Raffort J. e-Health in vascular diseases: integrating digital innovation in everyday clinical practice. J Clin Med. 2022;11:4757. https://doi.org/10.3390/jcm11164757.

3. Lareyre F, Chaptoukaev H, Kiang SC, Chaudhuri A, Behrendt CA, Zuluaga MA, et al. Telemedicine and digital health applications in vascular surgery. J Clin Med. 2022;11:6047. https://doi.org/10.3390/jcm11206047.
4. Li B, Feridooni T, Cuen-Ojeda C, Kishibe T, de Mestral C, Mamdani M, et al. Machine learning in vascular surgery: a systematic review and critical appraisal. NPJ Digit Med. 2022;5:7. https://doi.org/10.1038/s41746-021-00552-y.
5. Thaxton C, Dardik A. Computer science meets vascular surgery: keeping a pulse on artificial intelligence. Semin Vasc Surg. 2023;36:419–25. https://doi.org/10.1053/j.semvascsurg.2023.05.003.
6. Raffort J, Adam C, Carrier M, Lareyre F. Fundamentals in artificial intelligence for vascular surgeons. Ann Vasc Surg. 2020;65:254–60. https://doi.org/10.1016/j.avsg.2019.11.037.
7. Dey D, Slomka PJ, Leeson P, Comaniciu D, Shrestha S, Sengupta PP, et al. Artificial intelligence in cardiovascular imaging: JACC state-of-the-art review. J Am Coll Cardiol. 2019;73:1317–35. https://doi.org/10.1016/j.jacc.2018.12.054.
8. Panch T, Szolovits P, Atun R. Artificial intelligence, machine learning and health systems. J Glob Health. 2018;8:020303. https://doi.org/10.7189/jogh.08.020303.
9. LeCun Y, Bengio Y, Hinton G. Deep learning. Nature. 2015;521:436–44. https://doi.org/10.1038/nature14539.
10. Rajkomar A, Dean J, Kohane I. Machine learning in medicine. New Engl J Med. 2019;380:1347–58. https://doi.org/10.1056/NEJMra1814259.
11. Deo RC. Machine learning in medicine. Circulation. 2015;132:1920–30. https://doi.org/10.1161/CIRCULATIONAHA.115.001593.
12. Koteluk O, Wartecki A, Mazurek S, Kołodziejczak I, Mackiewicz A. How do machines learn? Artificial intelligence as a new era in medicine. J Pers Med. 2021;11:32. 0.3390/jpm11010032
13. Zhang P, Kamel Boulos MN. Generative AI in medicine and healthcare: promises, opportunities and challenges. Future Internet. 2023;15:286.
14. Sidey-Gibbons JA, Sidey-Gibbons CJ. Machine learning in medicine: a practical introduction. BMC Med Res Methodol. 2019;19:1–18. https://doi.org/10.1186/s12874-019-0681-4.
15. de Hond AA, Leeuwenberg AM, Hooft L, Kant IM, Nijman SW, van Os HJ, et al. Guidelines and quality criteria for artificial intelligence-based prediction models in healthcare: a scoping review. NPJ Digit Med. 2022;5:2. https://doi.org/10.1038/s41746-021-00549-7.
16. Parikh RB, Teeple S, Navathe AS. Addressing bias in artificial intelligence in health care. JAMA. 2019;322:2377–8. https://doi.org/10.1001/jama.2019.18058.
17. Steyerberg EW, Vickers AJ, Cook NR, Gerds T, Gonen M, Obuchowski N, et al. Assessing the performance of prediction models: a framework for traditional and novel measures. Epidemiology. 2010;21:128–38. https://doi.org/10.1097/EDE.0b013e3181c30fb2.
18. Naidu G, Zuva T, Sibanda EM, editors. A review of evaluation metrics in machine learning algorithms. In: Computer science on-line conference. Springer; 2023. p. 15–25.
19. Van Calster B, McLernon DJ, Van Smeden M, Wynants L, Steyerberg EW, et al. Calibration: the Achilles heel of predictive analytics. BMC Med. 2019;17:230. https://doi.org/10.1186/s12916-019-1466-7.
20. Kelly CJ, Karthikesalingam A, Suleyman M, Corrado G, King D. Key challenges for delivering clinical impact with artificial intelligence. BMC Med. 2019;17:1–9. https://doi.org/10.1186/s12916-019-1426-2.
21. Sermesant M, Delingette H, Cochet H, Jaïs P, Ayache N. Applications of artificial intelligence in cardiovascular imaging. Nat Rev Cardiol. 2021;18:600–9. https://doi.org/10.1038/s41569-021-00527-2.
22. Huang L, Lu J, Xiao Y, Zhang X, Li C, Yang G, et al. Deep learning techniques for imaging diagnosis and treatment of aortic aneurysm. Front Cardiovasc Med. 2024;11:1354517. https://doi.org/10.3389/fcvm.2024.1354517.
23. Raffort J, Adam C, Carrier M, Ballaith A, Coscas R, Jean-Baptiste E, et al. Artificial intelligence in abdominal aortic aneurysm. J Vasc Surg. 2020;72:321–33.e1. https://doi.org/10.1016/j.jvs.2019.12.026.

24. Lareyre F, Adam C, Carrier M, Dommerc C, Mialhe C, Raffort J. A fully automated pipeline for mining abdominal aortic aneurysm using image segmentation. Sci Rep. 2019;9:13750. https://doi.org/10.1038/s41598-019-50251-8.
25. Lareyre F, Adam C, Carrier M, Raffort J. Automated segmentation of the human abdominal vascular system using a hybrid approach combining expert system and supervised deep learning. J Clin Med. 2021;10:3347. https://doi.org/10.3390/jcm10153347.
26. Lareyre F, Adam C, Raffort J. Automatic measurement of abdominal aortic aneurysm maximum diameter using artificial intelligence. Eur J Vasc Endovasc Surg. 2022;63:525. https://doi.org/10.1016/j.ejvs.2021.10.053.
27. Kim T, On S, Gwon JG, Kim N. Computed tomography-based automated measurement of abdominal aortic aneurysm using semantic segmentation with active learning. Sci Rep. 2024;14:8924. https://doi.org/10.1038/s41598-024-59735-8.
28. Caradu C, Spampinato B, Vrancianu AM, Bérard X, Ducasse E. Fully automatic volume segmentation of infrarenal abdominal aortic aneurysm computed tomography images with deep learning approaches versus physician controlled manual segmentation. J Vasc Surg. 2021;74:246–56.e6. https://doi.org/10.1016/j.jvs.2020.11.036.
29. Coastaliou Q, Webster C, Bicknell C, Pouncey A, Ducasse E, Caradu C. Artificial intelligence with deep learning enables assessment of aortic aneurysm diameter and volume through different computed tomography phases. Eur J Vasc Endovasc Surg. 2024;68:408–9. https://doi.org/10.1016/j.ejvs.2024.04.004.
30. Wegner M, Fontaine V, Nana P, Dieffenbach BV, Fabre D, Haulon S. Artificial intelligence-assisted sac diameter assessment for complex endovascular aortic repair. J Endovasc Ther. 2023:15266028231208159. https://doi.org/10.1177/15266028231208159.
31. Postiglione TJ, Guillo E, Heraud A, Rossillon A, Bartoli M, Herpe G, et al. Multicentric clinical evaluation of a computed tomography-based fully automated deep neural network for aortic maximum diameter and volumetric measurements. J Vasc Surg. 2024;79:1390–400.e8. https://doi.org/10.1016/j.jvs.2024.01.214.
32. Lyu Z, Mu N, Rezaeitaleshmahalleh M, Zhang X, McBane R, Jiang J. Automatic segmentation of intraluminal thrombosis of abdominal aortic aneurysms from CT angiography using a mixed-scale-driven multiview perception network (M^2Net) model. Comput Biol Med. 2024;179:108838. https://doi.org/10.1016/j.compbiomed.2024.108838.
33. Hwang B, Kim J, Lee S, Kim E, Kim J, Jung Y, et al. Automatic detection and segmentation of thrombi in abdominal aortic aneurysms using a mask region-based convolutional neural network with optimized loss functions. Sensors (Basel). 2022;22:3643. https://doi.org/10.3390/s22103643.
34. Wang Y, Zhou M, Ding Y, Li X, Zhou Z, Xie T, et al. Fully automatic segmentation of abdominal aortic thrombus in pre-operative CTA images using deep convolutional neural networks. Technol Health Care. 2022;30:1257–66. https://doi.org/10.3233/thc-thc213630.
35. Golla AK, Tönnes C, Russ T, Bauer DF, Froelich MF, Diehl SJ, et al. Automated screening for abdominal aortic aneurysm in CT scans under clinical conditions using deep learning. Diagnostics (Basel). 2021;11:2131. https://doi.org/10.3390/diagnostics11112131.
36. Spinella G, Fantazzini A, Finotello A, Vincenzi E, Boschetti GA, Brutti F, et al. Artificial intelligence application to screen abdominal aortic aneurysm using computed tomography angiography. J Digit Imaging. 2023;36:2125–37. https://doi.org/10.1007/s10278-023-00866-1.
37. Camara JR, Tomihama RT, Pop A, Shedd MP, Dobrowski BS, Knox CJ, et al. Development of a convolutional neural network to detect abdominal aortic aneurysms. J Vasc Surg Cases Innov Tech. 2022;8:305–11. https://doi.org/10.1016/j.jvscit.2022.04.003.
38. Wang Y, Xiong F, Leach J, Kao E, Tian B, Zhu C, et al. Contrast-enhanced CT radiomics improves the prediction of abdominal aortic aneurysm progression. Eur Radiol. 2023;33:3444–54. https://doi.org/10.1007/s00330-023-09490-7.
39. Kim S, Jiang Z, Zambrano BA, Jang Y, Baek S, Yoo S, et al. Deep learning on multiphysical features and hemodynamic modeling for abdominal aortic aneurysm growth prediction. IEEE Trans Med Imaging. 2023;42:196–208. https://doi.org/10.1109/tmi.2022.3206142.

40. Chung TK, Gueldner PH, Aloziem OU, Liang NL, Vorp DA. An artificial intelligence based abdominal aortic aneurysm prognosis classifier to predict patient outcomes. Sci Rep. 2024;14:3390. https://doi.org/10.1038/s41598-024-53459-5.
41. Saitta S, Sturla F, Caimi A, Riva A, Palumbo MC, Nano G, et al. A deep learning-based and fully automated pipeline for thoracic aorta geometric analysis and planning for endovascular repair from computed tomography. J Digit Imaging. 2022;35:226–39. https://doi.org/10.1007/s10278-021-00535-1.
42. Derycke L, Avril S, Vermunt J, Perrin D, El Batti S, Alsac JM, et al. Computational prediction of proximal sealing in endovascular abdominal aortic aneurysm repair with unfavorable necks. Comput Methods Prog Biomed. 2024;244:107993. https://doi.org/10.1016/j.cmpb.2023.107993.
43. Kliewer ME, Bordet M, Chavent B, Reijnen M, Frisch N, Midy D, et al. Assessment of fenestrated Anaconda stent graft design by numerical simulation: results of a European prospective multicenter study. J Vasc Surg. 2022;75:99–108.e2. https://doi.org/10.1016/j.jvs.2021.07.225.
44. Nordanstig J, Behrendt CA, Baumgartner I, Belch J, Bäck M, Fitridge R, et al. Editor's Choice European Society for Vascular Surgery (ESVS) 2024 clinical practice guidelines on the management of asymptomatic lower limb peripheral arterial disease and intermittent claudication. Eur J Vasc Endovasc Surg. 2024;67:9–96. https://doi.org/10.1016/j.ejvs.2023.08.067.
45. Lareyre F, Behrendt CA, Chaudhuri A, Lee R, Carrier M, Adam C, et al. Applications of artificial intelligence for patients with peripheral artery disease. J Vasc Surg. 2023;77:650–8.e1. https://doi.org/10.1016/j.jvs.2022.07.160.
46. Martelli E, Capoccia L, Di Francesco M, Cavallo E, Pezzulla MG, Giudice G, et al. Current applications and future perspectives of artificial and biomimetic intelligence in vascular surgery and peripheral artery disease. Biomimetics (Basel). 2024;9:465. https://doi.org/10.3390/biomimetics9080465.
47. Flores AM, Demsas F, Leeper NJ, Ross EG. Leveraging machine learning and artificial intelligence to improve peripheral artery disease detection, treatment, and outcomes. Circ Res. 2021;128:1833–50. https://doi.org/10.1161/circresaha.121.318224.
48. Luo X, Ara L, Ding H, Rollins D, Motaganahalli R, Sawchuk AP. Computational methods to automate the initial interpretation of lower extremity arterial Doppler and duplex carotid ultrasound studies. J Vasc Surg. 2021;74:988–96.e1. https://doi.org/10.1016/j.jvs.2021.02.050.
49. Dai L, Zhou Q, Zhou H, Zhang H, Cheng P, Ding M, et al. Deep learning-based classification of lower extremity arterial stenosis in computed tomography angiography. Eur J Radiol. 2021;136:109528. https://doi.org/10.1016/j.ejrad.2021.109528.
50. Lareyre F, Chaudhuri A, Behrendt CA, Pouhin A, Teraa M, Boyle JR, et al. Artificial intelligence-based predictive models in vascular diseases. Semin Vasc Surg. 2023;36:440–7. https://doi.org/10.1053/j.semvascsurg.2023.05.002.
51. Lareyre F, Behrendt CA, Chaudhuri A, Ayache N, Delingette H, Raffort J. Big data and artificial intelligence in vascular surgery: time for multidisciplinary cross-border collaboration. Angiology. 2022;73:697–700. https://doi.org/10.1177/00033197221113146.
52. Li B, Aljabri B, Verma R, Beaton D, Eisenberg N, Lee DS, et al. Using machine learning to predict outcomes following open abdominal aortic aneurysm repair. J Vasc Surg. 2023;78:1426–38.e6. https://doi.org/10.1016/j.jvs.2023.08.121.
53. Li B, Aljabri B, Verma R, Beaton D, Eisenberg N, Lee DS, et al. Machine learning to predict outcomes following endovascular abdominal aortic aneurysm repair. Br J Surg. 2023;110:1840–9. https://doi.org/10.1093/bjs/znad28.
54. Ross EG, Jung K, Dudley JT, Li L, Leeper NJ, Shah NH. Predicting future cardiovascular events in patients with peripheral artery disease using electronic health record data. Circ Cardiovasc Qual Outcomes. 2019;12:e004741. https://doi.org/10.1161/CIRCOUTCOMES.118.004741.
55. Zhang D, Li Y, Kalbaugh CA, Shi L, Divers J, Islam S, et al. Machine learning approach to predict in-hospital mortality in patients admitted for peripheral artery disease in the United States. J Am Heart Assoc. 2022;11:e026987. https://doi.org/10.1161/JAHA.122.026987.

56. Chung J, Freeman NLB, Kosorok MR, Marston WA, Conte MS, McGinigle KL. Analysis of a machine learning-based risk stratification scheme for chronic limb-threatening ischemia. JAMA Netw Open. 2022;5:e223424. https://doi.org/10.1001/jamanetworkopen.2022.3424.
57. Cox M, Panagides JC, Tabari A, Kalva S, Kalpathy-Cramer J, Daye D. Risk stratification with explainable machine learning for 30-day procedure-related mortality and 30-day unplanned readmission in patients with peripheral arterial disease. PLoS One. 2022;17:e0277507. https://doi.org/10.1371/journal.pone.0277507.
58. Li B, Aljabri B, Verma R, Beaton D, Hussain MA, Lee DS, et al. Predicting outcomes following lower extremity endovascular revascularization using machine learning. J Am Heart Assoc. 2024;13:e033194. https://doi.org/10.1161/JAHA.123.033194.
59. Cox M, Reid N, Panagides JC, Di Capua J, DeCarlo C, Dua A, et al. Interpretable machine learning for the prediction of amputation risk following lower extremity Infrainguinal endovascular interventions for peripheral arterial disease. Cardiovasc Intervent Radiol. 2022;45:633–40. https://doi.org/10.1007/s00270-022-03111-4.
60. Wu H, Wang M, Wu J, Francis F, Chang YH, Shavick A, et al. A survey on clinical natural language processing in the United Kingdom from 2007 to 2022. NPJ Digit Med. 2022;5:186. https://doi.org/10.1038/s41746-022-00730-6.
61. Lareyre F, Nasr B, Chaudhuri A, Di Lorenzo G, Carlier M, Raffort J. Comprehensive review of natural language processing (NLP) in vascular surgery. EJVES Vasc Forum. 2023;60:57–63. https://doi.org/10.1016/j.ejvsvf.2023.09.002.
62. Boitano LT, DeVivo G, Robichaud DI, Okuhn S, Steppacher RC, Simons JP, et al. Successful implementation of a nurse-navigator-run program using natural language processing identifying patients with an abdominal aortic aneurysm. J Vasc Surg. 2023;77:922–9. https://doi.org/10.1016/j.jvs.2022.10.034.
63. McLenon M, Okuhn S, Lancaster EM, Hull MM, Adams JL, McGlynn E, et al. Validation of natural language processing to determine the presence and size of abdominal aortic aneurysms in a large integrated health system. J Vasc Surg. 2021;74:459–66.e3. https://doi.org/10.1016/j.jvs.2020.12.090.
64. Weissler EH, Zhang J, Lippmann S, Rusincovitch S, Henao R, Jones WS. Use of natural language processing to improve identification of patients with peripheral artery disease. Circ Cardiovasc Interv. 2020;13:e009447. https://doi.org/10.1161/CIRCINTERVENTIONS.120.009447.
65. Chaudhry AP, Afzal N, Abidian MM, Mallipeddi VP, Elayavilli RK, Scott CG, et al. Innovative informatics approaches for peripheral artery disease: current state and provider survey of strategies for improving guideline-based care. Mayo Clin Proc Innov Qual Outcomes. 2018;2:129–36. https://doi.org/10.1016/j.mayocpiqo.2018.02.001.
66. Cascella M, Semeraro F, Montomoli J, Bellini V, Piazza O, Bignami E. The breakthrough of large language models release for medical applications: 1-year timeline and perspectives. J Med Syst. 2024;48:22. https://doi.org/10.1007/s10916-024-02045-3.
67. Melissano G, Tinelli G, Soderlund T. Current artificial intelligence based chatbots may produce inaccurate and potentially harmful information for patients with aortic disease. Eur J Vasc Endovasc Surg. 2024;67:683–4. https://doi.org/10.1016/j.ejvs.2023.10.042.
68. Chervonski E, Harish KB, Rockman CB, Sadek M, Teter KA, Jacobowitz GR, et al. Generative artificial intelligence chatbots may provide appropriate informational responses to common vascular surgery questions by patients. Vascular. 2024:17085381241240550. https://doi.org/10.1177/17085381241240550.
69. Rouhi AD, Ghanem YK, Yolchieva L, Saleh Z, Joshi H, Moccia MC, et al. Can artificial intelligence improve the readability of patient education materials on aortic stenosis? A pilot study. Cardiol Ther. 2024;13:137–47. https://doi.org/10.1007/s40119-023-00347-0.
70. Lareyre F, D'Oria M, Caradu C, Jongkind V, Di Lorenzo G, Smeds MR, et al. Open E-survey on the use and perception of chatbots in vascular surgery. EJVES Vasc Forum. 2024;62:57–63. https://doi.org/10.1016/j.ejvsvf.2024.07.037.

71. Patel SB, Lam K. ChatGPT: the future of discharge summaries? Lancet Digit Health. 2023;5:e107–8. https://doi.org/10.1016/s2589-7500(23)00021-3.
72. Ali SR, Dobbs TD, Hutchings HA, Whitaker IS. Using ChatGPT to write patient clinic letters. Lancet Digit Health. 2023;5:e179–81. https://doi.org/10.1016/s2589-7500(23)00048-1.
73. Decker H, Trang K, Ramirez J, Colley A, Pierce L, Coleman M, et al. Large language model-based chatbot vs surgeon-generated informed consent documentation for common procedures. JAMA Netw Open. 2023;6:e2336997. https://doi.org/10.1001/jamanetworkopen.2023.36997.
74. Qiu J, Yuan W, Lam K. The application of multimodal large language models in medicine. Lancet Reg Health West Pac. 2024;45:101048. https://doi.org/10.1016/j.lanwpc.2024.101048.
75. Le Q, Lavingia KS, Amendola M. The performance of large language models on fictional consult queries indicates favorable potential for AI-assisted vascular surgery consult handling. JVS Vasc Insights. 2024;2:1000522024. https://doi.org/10.1016/j.jvsvi.2023.100052.
76. Roumengas R, Di Lorenzo G, Salhi A, de Buyer P, Chaudhuri A, Lareyre F, et al. Natural language processing for literature search in vascular surgery: a pilot study testing an artificial intelligence based application. EJVES Vasc Forum. 2023;60:48–52. https://doi.org/10.1016/j.ejvsvf.2023.09.004.
77. Tian S, Jin Q, Yeganova L, Lai PT, Zhu Q, Chen X, et al. Opportunities and challenges for ChatGPT and large language models in biomedicine and health. Brief Bioinform. 2023;25:bbad493. https://doi.org/10.1093/bib/bbad493.
78. Janssen BV, Kazemier G, Besselink MG. The use of ChatGPT and other large language models in surgical science. BJS Open. 2023;7:zrad032. https://doi.org/10.1093/bjsopen/zrad032.
79. Lareyre F, Trenner M. Collaborative vascular research in Europe to improve care for patients with vascular diseases: what is out there, and how to participate? EJVES Vasc Forum. 2024;62:5–6. https://doi.org/10.1016/j.ejvsvf.2024.05.009.
80. Spanos K, Giannoukas AD, Kouvelos G, Tsougos I, Mavroforou A. Artificial intelligence application in vascular diseases. J Vasc Surg. 2022;76:615–9. https://doi.org/10.1016/j.jvs.2022.03.895.
81. Lareyre F, Wanhainen A, Raffort J. Artificial intelligence-powered technologies for the management of vascular diseases: building guidelines and moving forward evidence generation. J Endovasc Ther. 2023:15266028231187599. https://doi.org/10.1177/15266028231187599.
82. Lareyre F, Maresch M, Chaudhuri A, Raffort J. Ethics and legal framework for trustworthy artificial intelligence in vascular surgery. EJVES Vasc Forum. 2023;60:42–4. https://doi.org/10.1016/j.ejvsvf.2023.08.003.
83. Lareyre F, Raffort J. Ethical concerns regarding the use of large language models in healthcare. EJVES Vasc Forum. 2024;61:1. https://doi.org/10.1016/j.ejvsvf.2023.10.003.
84. Drabiak K, Kyzer S, Nemov V, El Naqa I. AI and machine learning ethics, law, diversity, and global impact. Br J Radiol. 2023;96:20220934. https://doi.org/10.1259/bjr.20220934.

Key References

Flores AM, Demsas F, Leeper NJ, Ross EG. Leveraging machine learning and artificial intelligence to improve peripheral artery disease detection, treatment, and outcomes. Circ Res. 2021;128:1833–50. https://doi.org/10.1161/circresaha.121.318224.

Lareyre F, Behrendt CA, Chaudhuri A, Lee R, Carrier M, Adam C, et al. Applications of artificial intelligence for patients with peripheral artery disease. J Vasc Surg. 2023;77:650–8. https://doi.org/10.1016/j.jvs.2022.07.160.

LeCun Y, Bengio Y, Hinton G. Deep learning. Nature. 2015;521:436–44. https://doi.org/10.1038/nature14539.

Li B, Feridooni T, Cuen-Ojeda C, Kishibe T, de Mestral C, Mamdani M, et al. Machine learning in vascular surgery: a systematic review and critical appraisal. NPJ Digit Med. 2022;5:7. https://doi.org/10.1038/s41746-021-00552-y.

Raffort J, Adam C, Carrier M, Ballaith A, Coscas R, Jean-Baptiste E, et al. Artificial intelligence in abdominal aortic aneurysm. J Vasc Surg. 2020;72:321–33 e1. https://doi.org/10.1016/j.jvs.2019.12.026.

Glossary

Anisotropic Having a physical property which has a different value when measured in different directions. For example, this occurs when the angle of the ultrasound beam is not perpendicular to the tissue being scanned.

Apoptosis Orderly programmed (gene-directed) cell death in which a programmed sequence of events leads to the elimination of cells without releasing harmful substances into the surrounding area. Apoptosis is marked by the fragmentation of nuclear DNA into apoptotic bodies.

Autophagy A self-degradative process that is important for balancing sources of energy at critical times in development and in response to nutrient stress. Autophagy also plays a housekeeping role in removing misfolded or aggregated proteins, clearing damaged organelles, such as mitochondria, endoplasmic reticulum, and peroxisomes, as well as eliminating intracellular pathogens.

Bioenergetic Mechanism of how cells transform energy, often by producing, storing, or consuming adenosine triphosphate (ATP); impaired oxidative phosphorylation and beta-oxidation.

Biofilm A complex, three-dimensional community of bacteria that are encased in a self-produced matrix of extracellular polymeric substances (EPS) and are attached to a surface or to each other.

Biotube A tissue-engineered, autologous vascular graft created by implanting a mould (the biotube maker) inside a patient's body to encourage the body to form its own tubular tissue around it.

CEAP Score Clinical (C), Etiological (E), Anatomical (A), and Pathophysiological (P) classification of venous disease

Cell Adhesion Molecules Proteins located on the cell surface which are involved in binding to other cells or with the extracellular matrix. This binding is crucial for processes including cell migration, tissue formation, and development. Key families of cell adhesion molecules include cadherins, integrins, selectins, and immunoglobulin superfamily members.

R. Fitridge et al. (eds.), *Pathophysiology of Vascular Disease*,
https://doi.org/10.1007/978-3-032-31459-8

Chemokines A family of small signalling proteins that guide immune cells and other cells to specific locations in the body through a process called chemotaxis. They are crucial for the immune system by recruiting immune cells to sites of infection and inflammation, but also play roles in development, wound healing, and cancer.

Cytokines Small secreted molecules that signal cell-to-cell communication in immune responses and stimulate the movement of cells towards sites of inflammation, infection, and trauma.

DAMPs Also known as danger-associated molecular patterns, these proteins are host biomolecules that can initiate and perpetuate a non-infectious inflammatory response. Protein DAMPs include intracellular proteins, such as heat-shock proteins and materials derived from the extracellular matrix that are generated following tissue injury, such as hyaluronan fragments. Non-protein DAMPs include ATP, uric acid, and DNA.

Densification An increase in density or compactness in a tissue, organ, or other body part. In radiology, densification is a term used to describe an area that appears brighter or whiter than the surrounding tissue on an X-ray or CT scan.

Diapedesis The passage of white blood cells through intact blood vessel walls into the tissues. This is a critical step in the immune response, allowing immune cells to reach sites of infection or inflammation to fight pathogens and promote tissue repair. It involves several steps, including rolling, adhesion to the vessel wall, and finally, migrating through the endothelial cells.

Dice score A metric for evaluating the performance of image segmentation models. It quantifies the spatial overlap between the predicted segmentation and the ground truth (the manually annotated or "correct" segmentation).

Digital twin A computer model that simulates an object or process in the physical world.

Electrospinning Fibre production method which uses electric force to draw charged threads of polymer solutions into fibres with diameters of approximately hundreds of nanometres.

Epigallocatechin gallate A polyphenol which has multiple interactions with cell surface receptors, intracellular signalling pathways, and nuclear transcription factors. Hence, it possesses a wide variety of anti-inflammatory, antioxidant, antifibrotic, and tissue-protective properties.

Filopodia Slender cytoplasmic projections in migrating cells. They contain actin filaments cross-linked into bundles by actin-binding proteins. Filopodia have roles in sensing, migration, and cell-cell interaction. To close a wound, growth factors stimulate the formation of filopodia in fibroblasts to direct fibroblast migration and wound closure.

Genipin A natural compound known for its ability to act as a cross-linking agent for proteins, collagen, gelatin, and chitosan, enhancing their properties.

Glutaraldehyde Organic compound with the formula $(CH_2)_3(CHO)_2$, used primarily for disinfection and sterilisation due to its potent biocidal properties.

Hyper-oncotic albumin Hyper-oncotic albumin (25%) stimulates the movement of endogenous extracellular fluids into the patients' blood vessels, as opposed to adding more volume which can increase the risk of volume overload.

Immune checkpoints Immune checkpoints are a normal part of the immune system. Their role is to prevent an immune response from being so strong that it destroys healthy cells in the body. Immune checkpoints engage when proteins on the surface of T lymphocytes recognise and bind to partner proteins on other cells. These proteins are called immune checkpoint proteins. When the checkpoint and partner proteins bind together, they send an "off" signal to the T cells and provide a physiological brake on T cell activation to curb inflammation-associated tissue destruction.

Integrins Transmembrane receptor proteins on cell surfaces that mediate cell-to-cell and cell-to-extracellular matrix (ECM) adhesion, playing crucial roles in cell signalling, cell growth, cell movement, wound healing, and the immune response.

Matricryptic Cryptic (hidden) sites within the extracellular matrix that are not exposed in the intact molecule but become exposed after structural changes, resulting in activation of cell surface receptors including integrins, scavenger receptors, and Toll-like receptors which activate downstream signalling pathways following tissue injury.

Matrix metalloproteinases Zinc-dependent enzymes that break down extracellular matrix components including collagen and elastin, thus playing crucial roles in wound healing, embryonic development, and tissue remodelling.

Mechanotransduction Cellular mechanisms by which load-bearing cells sense physical forces, transduce the forces into biochemical signals, and generate appropriate responses leading to alterations in cellular structure and function.

MicroRNA A small non-coding RNA molecule (containing about 22 nucleotides) that functions in RNA silencing and post-transcriptional regulation of gene expression.

Necroptosis A programmed form of necrosis, or inflammatory cell death.

Netosis Neutrophil-related cell death characterised by the secretion of large web-like structures described as NETs.

NETS Networks of extracellular fibres, primarily composed of DNA from neutrophils, which bind pathogens. NETs allow neutrophils to kill extracellular pathogens while minimising damage to the host cells.

PAMPs Pathogen-Associated Molecular Patterns are molecules that are found on microorganisms but not on host cells. These conserved molecular patterns, such as lipopolysaccharide (LPS) on Gram-negative bacteria and viral nucleic acids, are recognised by the immune system's pattern recognition receptors (PRRs). This recognition triggers an innate immune response to fight the pathogen.

Planktonic Free-living motile bacteria, usually growing in cultures in the microbiology laboratory. Planktonic bacteria have faster growth rates than biofilm bacteria because they are not limited by surface attachment, but they are generally more vulnerable to antibiotic therapies.

Polyethyleneimine A synthetic cationic polymer known for its ability to condense nucleic acids and is used in gene delivery, most notably as a nonviral gene delivery vector due to its ability to bind DNA and facilitate its entry into cells.

Polyhedral oligomeric silsesquioxane A type of nanomaterial with a well-defined cage-like structure composed of a silicon-oxygen core and organic groups on the corners.

Pyroptosis A highly inflammatory form of programmed cell death that occurs in response to cell damage. Triggered by inflammatory caspases, it leads to the formation of pores in the cell membrane, causing the cell to swell and lyse, releasing inflammatory molecules. While this can help eliminate pathogens and cancer cells, excessive pyroptosis can contribute to tissue damage and diseases including sepsis and neurodegenerative disorders.

Radiomic The process of extracting high-throughput quantitative features from medical images to turn them into mineable data that can provide deeper biological information than qualitative human interpretation alone. It involves using automated methods to extract a large number of features related to the shape, texture, and intensity of tissues or lesions, which can then be used to support diagnosis, predict treatment response, and guide clinical decision-making.

RASopathies RASopathies are a group of rare congenital disorders characterised by mutations in the RAS-MAPK pathway which affects cell growth, maturation, and death.

Roto-evaporation technique A technique used to quickly and efficiently concentrate a liquid sample by removing a volatile solvent. The process involves placing a solution in a rotating flask within a heated water bath, while a vacuum system reduces the solvent's boiling point. The evaporated solvent travels to a condenser, where it cools and turns back into a liquid, collecting in a separate flask.

Silsesquioxane Organic-inorganic hybrid compounds with a rigid silicon-oxygen backbone and organic groups attached to each silicon atom.

SMADs A family of structurally similar proteins that are the main signal transducers for receptors of the transforming growth factor beta (TGF-β) superfamily, which are critically important for regulating cell development and growth.

Substance P An 11-amino acid peptide that acts as a neuropeptide, neurotransmitter, and hormone, playing a role in pain transmission, inflammation, and immune responses. It influences a wide range of bodily functions, including mood, appetite, and wound healing.

Th1 Type 1 T helper cells which produce interferon-gamma, interleukin (IL)-2, and tumour necrosis factor (TNF)-beta, which activate macrophages and are responsible for cell-mediated immunity and phagocyte-dependent protective responses.

Th2 Type 2 T helper cells which produce Interleukins -4, -5, -10, and -13 and help regulate humoral immune responses to extracellular parasites and bacterial infections.

Valorisation The act of thinking or stating that something has value or is valuable.

Vascular dendritic cells Immune cells found in the blood vessel wall that act as sentinels for the immune system, especially in areas of inflammation like atherosclerotic lesions. They function as antigen-presenting cells, meaning they can activate T-cells to initiate and regulate immune responses. Vascular dendritic cells are involved in both the initiation and progression of vascular diseases, including atherosclerosis and vasculitis by contributing to the inflammatory processes.

GPSR Compliance

The European Union's (EU) General Product Safety Regulation (GPSR) is a set of rules that requires consumer products to be safe and our obligations to ensure this.

If you have any concerns about our products, you can contact us on ProductSafety@springernature.com

In case Publisher is established outside the EU, the EU authorized representative is:

Springer Nature Customer Service Center GmbH
Europaplatz 3
69115 Heidelberg, Germany

Batch number: 10852833

Printed by Printforce, the Netherlands